T0413911

Statistics Applied to Clinical Studies

Ton J. Cleophas • Aeilko H. Zwinderman

Statistics Applied to Clinical Studies

Fifth Edition

With the help from

Toine F. Cleophas, Eugene P. Cleophas, and Henny I. Cleophas-Allers

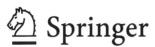 Springer

Ton J. Cleophas
Past-President American
College of Angiology
Co-Chair Module Statistics
Applied to Clinical Trials
European Interuniversity College
of Pharmaceutical Medicine, Lyon
France

Department of Medicine
Albert Schweitzer Hospital, Dordrecht
Netherlands

Aeilko H. Zwinderman
President-Elect International
Society of Biostatistics
Co-Chair Module Statistics
Applied to Clinical Trials
European Interuniversity College
of Pharmaceutical Medicine, Lyon
France

Department of Biostatistics
and Epidemiology, Academic Medical
Center, Amsterdam
Netherlands

ISBN 978-94-007-2862-2   e-ISBN 978-94-007-2863-9
DOI 10.1007/978-94-007-2863-9
Springer Dordrecht Heidelberg London New York

Library of Congress Control Number: 2012931360

Springer is part of Springer Science+Business Media (www.springer.com)

Foreword

In clinical medicine appropriate statistics has become indispensable to evaluate treatment effects. Randomized controlled trials are currently the only trials that truly provide evidence-based medicine. Evidence based medicine has become crucial to optimal treatment of patients. We can define randomized controlled trials by using Christopher J. Bulpitt's definition "a carefully and ethically designed experiment which includes the provision of adequate and appropriate controls by a process of randomization, so that precisely framed questions can be answered". The answers given by randomized controlled trials constitute at present the way how patients should be clinically managed. In the setup of such randomized trial one of the most important issues is the statistical basis. The randomized trial will never work when the statistical grounds and analyses have not been clearly defined before-hand. All endpoints should be clearly defined in order to perform appropriate power calculations. Based on these power calculations the exact number of available patients can be calculated in order to have a sufficient quantity of individuals to have the predefined questions answered. Therefore, every clinical physician should be capable to understand the statistical basis of well performed clinical trials. It is therefore a great pleasure that Drs. T. J. Cleophas, A. H. Zwinderman, and T. F. Cleophas have published a book on statistical analysis of clinical trials. The book entitled "Statistics Applied to Clinical Trials" is clearly written and makes complex issues in statistical analysis transparent. Apart from providing the classical issues in statistical analysis, the authors also address novel issues such as interim analyses, sequential analyses, and meta-analyses. The book is composed of 18 chapters, which are nicely structured. The authors have deepened our insight in the applications of statistical analysis of clinical trials. We would like to congratulate the editors on this achievement and hope that many readers will enjoy reading this intriguing book.

Professor of Cardiology, President Netherlands   E.E. van der Wall, M.D., Ph.D.
Association of Cardiology, Leiden, Netherlands

Preface to First Edition

The European Interuniversity Diploma of Pharmaceutical Medicine is a postacademic course of 2–3 years sponsored by the Socrates program of the European Community. The office of this interuniversity project is in Lyon and the lectures are given there. The European Community has provided a building and will remunerate lecturers. The institute which provides the teaching is called the European College of Pharmaceutical Medicine, and is affiliated with 15 universities throughout Europe, whose representatives constitute the academic committee. This committee supervises educational objectives. Start lectures February 2000.

There are about 20 modules for the first 2 years of training, most of which are concerned with typically pharmacological and clinical pharmacological matters including pharmacokinetics, pharmacodynamics, phase III clinical trials, reporting, communication, ethics and, any other aspects of drug development. Subsequent training consists of practice training within clinical research organisations, universities, regulatory bodies etc., and finally of a dissertation. The diploma, and degree are delivered by the Claude Bernard University in Lyon as well as the other participating universities.

The module "Statistics applied to clinical trials" will be taught in the form of a 3–6 day yearly course given in Lyon and starting February 2000. Lecturers have to submit a document of the course (this material will be made available to students). Three or four lecturers are requested to prepare detailed written material for students as well as to prepare examination of the students. The module is thus an important part of a postgraduate course for physicians and pharmacists for the purpose of obtaining the European diploma of pharmaceutical medicine. The diploma should make for leading positions in pharmaceutical industry, academic drug research, as well as regulatory bodies within the EC. This module is mainly involved in the statistics of randomized clinical trials.

The Chaps. 1–9, 11, 17, and 18 of this book are based on the module "Medical statistics applied to clinical trials" and contain material that should be mastered by the students before their exams. The remaining chapters are capita selecta intended for excellent students and are not included in the exams.

The authors believe that this book is innovative in the statistical literature because, unlike most introductory books in medical statistics, it provides an explanatory rather than mathematical approach to statistics, and, in addition, emphasizes non-classical but increasingly frequently used methods for the statistical analyses of clinical trials, e.g., equivalence testing, sequential analyses, multiple linear regression analyses for confounding, interaction, and synergism. The authors are not aware of any other work published so far that is comparable with the current work, and, therefore, believe that it does fill a need.

August 1999
Dordrecht, Leiden
Delft

Preface to Second Edition

In this second edition the authors have removed textual errors from the first edition. Also seven new chapters (Chaps. 8, 10, 13, 15–18) have been added. The principles of regression analysis and its resemblance to analysis of variance was missing in the first edition, and have been described in Chap. 8. Chapter 10 assesses curvilinear regression. Chapter 13 describes the statistical analyses of crossover data with binary response. The latest developments including statistical analyses of genetic data and quality-of-life data have been described in Chaps. 15 and 16. Emphasis is given in Chaps. 17 and 18 to the limitations of statistics to assess non-normal data, and to the similarities between commonly-used statistical tests. Finally, additional tables including the Mann-Whitney and Wilcoxon rank sum tables have been added in the Appendix.

December 2001
Dordrecht, Amsterdam
Delft

Preface to the Third Edition

The previous two editions of this book, rather than having been comprehensive, concentrated on the most relevant aspects of statistical analysis. Although well-received by students, clinicians, and researchers, these editions did not answer all of their questions. This called for a third, more comprehensive, rewrite. In this third edition the 18 chapters from the previous edition have been revised, updated, and provided with a conclusions section summarizing the main points. The formulas have been re-edited using the Formula-Editor from Windows XP 2004 for enhanced clarity. Thirteen new chapters (Chaps. 8–10, 14, 15, 17, 21, 25–29, 31) have been added. The Chaps. 8–10 give methods to assess the problems of multiple testing and data testing closer to expectation than compatible with random. The Chaps. 14 and 15 review regression models using an exponential rather than linear relationship including logistic, Cox, and Markow models. Chapter 17 reviews important interaction effects in clinical trials and provides methods for their analysis. In Chap. 21 study designs appropriate for medicines from one class are discussed. The Chaps. 25–29 review respectively (1) methods to evaluate the presence of randomness in the data, (2) methods to assess variabilities in the data, (3) methods to test reproducibility in the data, (4) methods to assess accuracy of diagnostic tests, and (5) methods to assess random rather than fixed treatment effects. Finally, Chap. 31 reviews methods to minimize the dilemma between sponsored research and scientific independence. This updated and extended edition has been written to serve as a more complete guide and reference-text to students, physicians, and investigators, and, at the same time, preserves the common sense approach to statistical problem-solving of the previous editions.

August 2005
Dordrecht, Amsterdam
Delft

Preface to Fourth Edition

In the past few years many important novel methods have been applied in published clinical research. This has made the book again rather incomplete after its previous edition. The current edition consists of 16 new chapters, and updates of the 31 chapters from the previous edition. Important methods like Laplace transformations, log likelihood ratio statistics, Monte Carlo methods, and trend testing have been included. Also novel methods like superiority testing, pseudo-R2 statistics, optimism corrected c-statistic, I-statistics, and diagnostic meta-analyses have been addressed.

The authors have given special efforts for all chapters to have their own introduction, discussion, and references section. They can, therefore, be studied separately and without need to read the previous chapters first.

September 2008
Dordrecht, Amsterdam, Gorinchem, and Delft

Preface to Fifth Edition

Thanks to the omnipresent computer, current statistics can include data files of many thousands of values, and can perform any exploratory analysis in less than seconds. This development, however fascinating, generally does not lead to simple results. We should not forget that clinical studies are, mostly, for confirming prior hypotheses based on sound arguments, and the simplest tests provide the best power and are adequate for such purposes. In the past few years the authors of this 5th edition, as teachers and research supervisors in academic and top-clinical facilities, have been able to closely observe the latest developments in the field of clinical data analysis, and they have been able to assess their performance. In this 5th edition the 47 chapters of the previous edition have been maintained and upgraded according to the current state of the art, and 20 novel chapters have been added after strict selection of the most valuable and promising novel methods. The novel methods are explained using practical examples and step-by-step analyses readily accessible not only to statisticians but also to non-mathematicians.

In order to keep up with the forefront of statistical analysis it was unavoidable to also include more complex data modeling and computationally intensive statistical methods. These methods include, e.g., multistage regression, neural networks, fuzzy modeling, mixed linear and non linear models, item response modeling, non linear regression methods, propensity score matching, Bhattacharya modeling and various regression models with multiple outcome variables. However, the authors have given every effort to review these methods in an explanatory rather than mathematical manner.

We should add that the authors are well-qualified in their field. Professor Zwinderman is president-elect of the International Society of Biostatistics, and Professor Cleophas is past-president of the American College of Angiology. From their expertise they should be able to make adequate selections of modern methods for clinical data analysis for the benefit of physicians, students, and investigators. The authors have been working and publishing together for over 10 years, and their research of statistical methodology can be characterized as a continued effort to demonstrate that statistics is not mathematics but rather a discipline at the interface of biology and mathematics.

September 2011
Dordrecht, Amsterdam, Lyon

Contents

1 Hypotheses, Data, Stratification 1
   1   General Considerations 1
   2   Two Main Hypotheses in Drug Trials: Efficacy and Safety 2
   3   Different Types of Data: Continuous Data 3
   4   Different Types of Data: Proportions,
        Percentages and Contingency Tables 8
   5   Different Types of Data: Correlation Coefficient 10
   6   Stratification Issues 12
   7   Randomized Versus Historical Controls 13
   8   Factorial Designs 13
   9   Conclusions 14
   References 14

2 The Analysis of Efficacy Data 15
   1   Overview 15
   2   The Principle of Testing Statistical Significance 16
   3   The t-Value = Standardized Mean Result of Study 18
   4   Unpaired t-Test 19
   5   Null-Hypothesis Testing of Three or More Unpaired Samples 21
   6   Three Methods to Test Statistically a Paired Sample 22
       6.1   First Method 22
       6.2   Second Method 23
       6.3   Third Method 24
   7   Null-Hypothesis Testing of Three or More Paired Samples 26
   8   Null-Hypothesis Testing with Complex Data 27
   9   Paired Data with a Negative Correlation 28
       9.1   Studies Testing Significance of Differences 28
       9.2   Studies Testing Equivalence 32
   10 Rank Testing 33
       10.1 Paired Test: Wilcoxon Signed Rank Test 34
       10.2 Unpaired Test: Mann-Whitney Test 35

11	Rank Testing for Three or More Samples	36
	11.1	The Friedman Test for Paired Observations	36
	11.2	The Kruskall-Wallis Test for Unpaired Observations	37
12	Conclusions	38
	References	38

3 The Analysis of Safety Data ... 41
1	Introduction, Summary Display	41
2	Four Methods to Analyze Two Unpaired Proportions	42
	2.1	Method 1	42
	2.2	Method 2	44
	2.3	Method 3	47
	2.4	Method 4	47
3	Chi-square to Analyze More Than Two Unpaired Proportions	48
4	McNemar's Test for Paired Proportions	51
5	Multiple Paired Binary Data (Cochran's Q Test)	52
6	Survival Analysis	54
	6.1	Survival Analysis	54
	6.2	Testing Significance of Difference Between Two Kaplan-Meier Curves	55
7	Odds Ratio Method for Analyzing Two Unpaired Proportions	56
8	Odds Ratios for One Group, Two Treatments	59
9	Conclusions	59

4 Log Likelihood Ratio Tests for Safety Data Analysis ... 61
1	Introduction	61
2	Numerical Problems with Calculating Exact Likelihoods	61
3	The Normal Approximation and the Analysis of Clinical Events	62
4	Log Likelihood Ratio Tests and the Quadratic Approximation	64
5	More Examples	66
6	Discussion	67
7	Conclusions	67
	References	68

5 Equivalence Testing ... 69
1	Introduction	69
2	Overview of Possibilities with Equivalence Testing	70
3	Calculations	72
4	Equivalence Testing, a New Gold Standard?	72
5	Validity of Equivalence Trials	73
6	Special Point: Level of Correlation in Paired Equivalence Studies	73
7	Conclusions	74

6 Statistical Power and Sample Size ... 77
| 1 | What Is Statistical Power | 77 |
| 2 | Emphasis on Statistical Power Rather Than Null-Hypothesis Testing | 78 |

3 Power Computations 80
  3.1 For t-Distributions of Continuous Data.................................. 80
  3.2 For Proportions.. 80
  3.3 For Equivalence Testing of Samples
       with t-Distributions and Continuous Data............................. 81
4 Examples of Power Computation Using the t-Table........................ 81
  4.1 First Example 81
  4.2 Second Example... 83
  4.3 Third Example.. 83
5 Calculation of Required Sample Size, Rationale............................. 86
6 Calculations of Required Sample Size, Methods............................. 87
  6.1 A Simple Method 87
  6.2 A More Accurate Method Is the Power Index Method............. 87
  6.3 Power Calculation for Parallel-Group Studies 89
  6.4 Required Sample Size Equation
       for Studies with Proportions.. 89
  6.5 Required Sample Size Formula for Equivalence Testing.......... 90
7 Testing Inferiority of a New Treatment (Type III Error).................... 91
8 Conclusions.. 93
Reference 93

7 Interim Analyses 95
1 Introduction.. 95
2 Monitoring 95
3 Interim Analysis.. 96
4 Group-Sequential Design of Interim Analysis................................ 99
5 Continuous Sequential Statistical Techniques 99
6 Conclusions.. 101
References... 101

8 Controlling the Risk of False Positive Clinical Trials 103
1 Introduction.. 103
2 Bonferroni Test 103
3 Least Significant Difference (LSD) Test.. 105
4 Other Tests for Adjusting the p-Values 105
5 Composite Endpoint Procedures... 106
6 No Adjustments at all, and Pragmatic Solutions 107
7 Conclusions.. 107
References... 107

9 Multiple Statistical Inferences 109
1 Introduction.. 109
2 Multiple Comparisons.. 109
3 Multiple Variables... 113
4 Conclusions.. 116
References... 117

10 The Interpretation of the p-Values 119
   1 Introduction 119
   2 Renewed Attention to the Interpretation
      of the Probability Levels, Otherwise Called the p-Values 119
   3 Standard Interpretation of p-Values 120
   4 Common Misunderstandings of the p-Values 122
   5 Renewed Interpretations of p-Values,
      Little Difference Between $p = 0.06$ and $p = 0.04$ 122
   6 The Real Meaning of Very Large p-Values Like $p > 0.95$ 123
   7 p-Values Larger than 0.95, Examples (Table 10.2) 124
   8 The Real Meaning of Very Small p-Values Like $p < 0.0001$ 124
   9 p-Values Smaller than 0.0001, Examples (Table 10.3) 126
  10 Discussion 127
  11 Recommendations 128
  12 Conclusions 129
   References 130

**11 Research Data Closer to Expectation
    than Compatible with Random Sampling** 133
   1 Introduction 133
   2 Methods and Results 134
   3 Discussion 135
   4 Conclusions 138
   References 138

**12 Statistical Tables for Testing Data Closer
    to Expectation than Compatible with Random Sampling** 139
   1 Introduction 139
   2 Statistical Tables of Unusually High p-Values 141
   3 How to Calculate the p-Values Yourself 141
      3.1 t-Test 141
      3.2 Chi-square Test 141
      3.3 F-Test 142
   4 Additional Examples Simulating Real Practice,
      Multiple Comparisons 144
   5 Discussion 146
   6 Conclusions 146
   References 147

13 Data Dispersion Issues 149
   1 Introduction 149
   2 Data Without Measure of Dispersion 150
      2.1 Numbers Needed to Treat in Clinical Trials 150
      2.2 Reproducibility of Quantitative Diagnostic Tests 151
      2.3 Sensitivity and Specificity 152
      2.4 Markov Predictors 153
      2.5 Risk Profiles from Multiple Logistic Models 154

3   Data with Over-Dispersion 155
4   Discussion 157
5   Conclusions 158
References 159

14 Linear Regression, Basic Approach 161
1   Introduction 161
2   More on Paired Observations 162
3   Using Statistical Software for Simple Linear Regression 164
4   Multiple Linear Regression 166
5   Multiple Linear Regression, Example 168
6   Purposes of Linear Regression Analysis 171
7   Another Real Data Example of Multiple
     Linear Regression (Exploratory Purpose) 173
8   It May Be Hard to Define What Is Determined
     by What, Multiple and Multivariate Regression 174
9   Limitations of Linear Regression 176
10   Conclusions 176

**15 Linear Regression for Assessing Precision,
     Confounding, Interaction, Basic Approach** 177
1   Introduction 177
2   Example 178
3   Model 178
4   (I.) Increased Precision of Efficacy 180
5   (II.) Confounding 181
6   (III.) Interaction and Synergism 182
7   Estimation, and Hypothesis Testing 183
8   Goodness-of-Fit 183
9   Selection Procedures 185
10   Main Conclusions 185
References 185

16 Curvilinear Regression 187
1   Introduction 187
2   Methods, Statistical Model 188
     2.1   Reproducibility of Means of the Population 189
     2.2   Reproducibility of Individual Data 189
3   Results 190
     3.1   Reproducibility of Means of Population 190
     3.2   Reproducibility of Individual Data 193
4   Discussion 194
5   Conclusions 196
References 196

17 Logistic and Cox Regression, Markov Models,
Laplace Transformations 199
  1   Introduction 199
  2   Linear Regression 199
  3   Logistic Regression 203
     3.1 Logistic Regression Analysis for Predicting
          the Probability of an Event 203
     3.2 Logistic Regression for Efficacy Data Analysis 207
  4   Cox Regression 209
  5   Markov Models 212
  6   Regression-Analysis with Laplace Transformations 213
  7   Discussion 216
  8   Conclusions 217
  References 218

18 Regression Modeling for Improved Precision 219
  1   Introduction 219
  2   Regression Modeling for Improved Precision
      of Clinical Trials, the Underlying Mechanism 220
  3   Regression Model for Parallel-Group Trials
      with Continuous Efficacy Data 220
  4   Regression Model for Parallel-Group Trials
      with Proportions or Odds as Efficacy Data 222
  5   Discussion 224
  6   Conclusions 225
  References 225

19 Post-hoc Analyses in Clinical Trials,
A Case for Logistic Regression Analysis 227
  1   Multiple Variables Methods 227
  2   Examples 228
  3   Logistic Regression Equation 230
  4   Conclusions 231
  References 231

20 Multistage Regression 233
  1   Introduction 233
  2   An Example, Usual Linear Regression Modeling 234
  3   Path Analysis 234
  4   Multistage Least Squares Method 237
  5   Bivariate Analysis Using Path Analysis 238
  6   Discussion 239
  7   Conclusions 240
  References 241

21 Categorical Data ... 243
    1 Introduction ... 243
    2 Races as a Categorical Variable ... 244
    3 Numbers of Co-medications as a Categorical Variable ... 248
    4 Discussion ... 250
        4.1 Multinomial Logistic Regression ... 251
    5 Conclusions ... 251
    References ... 252

22 Missing Data ... 253
    1 Introduction ... 253
    2 Current Methods for Missing Data Imputation ... 254
    3 A Proposed Novel Approach to Regression-Substitution ... 254
    4 Example ... 255
    5 Discussion ... 258
    6 Conclusions ... 262
    Appendix ... 262
    References ... 265

23 Poisson Regression ... 267
    1 Introduction ... 267
    2 Example 1 ... 267
    3 Example 2 ... 272
    4 Discussion ... 273
    5 Conclusions ... 274
    References ... 275

24 More on Non Linear Relationships, Splines ... 277
    1 Introduction ... 277
    2 Logit or Probit Transformation ... 278
    3 "Trial and Error" Method, Box Cox
      Transformation, ACE/AVAS Packages ... 280
    4 Curvilinear Data ... 281
    5 Spline Modeling ... 282
    6 Discussion ... 285
    7 Conclusions ... 286
    Appendix ... 287
    References ... 288

25 Multivariate Analysis ... 289
    1 Introduction ... 289
    2 Multivariate Regression Analysis Using Path Analysis ... 290
    3 Multiple Analysis of Variance, First Example ... 292
    4 Multiple Analysis of Variance, Second Example ... 294
    5 Multivariate Probit Regression ... 296
    6 Discussion ... 297
    7 Conclusions ... 298
    References ... 299

26 Bhattacharya Modeling 301
  1   Introduction.. 301
  2   Unmasking Normal Values 302
  3   Improving the p-Values of Data Testing 304
  4   Objectively Searching Subsets in the Data 307
  5   Discussion 309
  6   Conclusions.. 310
  References.. 311

27 Trend-Testing.. 313
  1   Introduction.. 313
  2   Binary Data, the Chi-Square-Test-for-Trends............................ 314
  3   Continuous Data, Linear-Regression-Test-for-Trends................ 315
  4   Discussion 316
  5   Conclusions.. 318
  References.. 318

28 Confounding 319
  1   Introduction.. 319
  2   First Method for Adjustment of Confounders:
      Subclassification on One Confounder..................................... 320
  3   Second Method for Adjustment of Confounders:
      Regression Modeling 321
  4   Third Method for Adjustment of Confounders:
      Propensity Scores... 323
  5   Discussion 325
  6   Conclusions.. 326
  References.. 327

29 Propensity Score Matching 329
  1   Introduction.. 329
  2   Calculation of Propensity-Scores.. 329
  3   Propensity-Scores for Adjusting Covariates 331
  4   Propensity-Scores for Matching 332
  5   Discussion 333
  6   Conclusions.. 334
  Appendix... 335
  References.. 336

30 Interaction 337
  1   Introduction.. 337
  2   What Exactly Is Interaction, a Hypothesized Example 337
  3   How to Test Interaction Statistically, a Real Data Example
      with a Concomitant Medication as Interacting Factor:
      Incorrect Method.. 339

4	Three Analysis Methods	340
	4.1 First Method, t-Test	341
	4.2 Second Method, Analysis of Variance (ANOVA)	341
	4.3 Third Method, Regression Analysis	342
5	Using a Regression Model for Testing Interaction, Another Real Data Example	343
6	Analysis of Variance for Testing Interaction, Other Real Data Examples	345
	6.1 Parallel-Group Study with Treatment × Health Center Interaction	345
	6.2 Crossover Study with Treatment × Subjects Interaction	347
7	Discussion	349
8	Conclusions	350
	References	351

31 Time-Dependent Factor Analysis 353
   1 Introduction 353
   2 Cox Regression Without Time-Dependent Predictors 354
   3 Cox Regression with a Time-Dependent Predictor 356
   4 Cox Regression with a Segmented Time-Dependent Predictor 359
   5 Multiple Cox Regression with a Time-Dependent Predictor 361
   6 Discussion 362
   7 Conclusions 363
      References 364

32 Meta-analysis, Basic Approach 365
   1 Introduction 365
   2 Examples 366
   3 Clearly Defined Hypotheses 367
   4 Thorough Search of Trials 368
   5 Strict Inclusion Criteria 368
   6 Uniform Data Analysis 368
      6.1 Individual Data 369
      6.2 Continuous Data, Means and Standard Errors of the Mean (SEMs) 369
      6.3 Proportions: Relative Risks (RRs), Odds Ratios (ORs), Differences Between Relative Risks (RDs) 369
      6.4 Publication Bias 371
      6.5 Heterogeneity 372
      6.6 Robustness 375
   7 Discussion, Where Are We Now? 376
   8 Conclusions 377
      References 377

33 Meta-analysis, Review and Update of Methodologies 379
    1   Introduction 379
    2   Four Scientific Rules 380
        2.1 Clearly Defined Hypothesis 380
        2.2 Thorough Search of Trials 380
        2.3 Strict Inclusion Criteria 380
        2.4 Uniform Data Analysis 381
    3   General Framework of Meta-analysis 381
    4   Pitfalls of Data Analysis 383
        4.1 Publication Bias 383
        4.2 Heterogeneity 384
        4.3 Investigating the Cause for Heterogeneity 385
        4.4 Lack of Robustness 386
    5   New Developments 386
    6   Conclusions 388
    References 388

34 Meta-regression 391
    1   Introduction 391
    2   An Example of a Heterogeneous Meta-analysis 391
    3   Discussion 394
    4   Conclusions 395
    References 396

35 Crossover Studies with Continuous Variables 397
    1   Introduction 397
    2   Mathematical Model 398
    3   Hypothesis Testing 399
    4   Statistical Power of Testing 400
    5   Discussion 403
        5.1 Analysis of Covariance (ANCOVA) 403
    6   Conclusion 404
    References 405

36 Crossover Studies with Binary Responses 407
    1   Introduction 407
    2   Assessment of Carryover and Treatment Effect 408
    3   Statistical Model for Testing Treatment and Carryover Effects 409
    4   Results 409
        4.1 Calculation of p_c Values Just Yielding
            a Significant Test for Carryover Effect 409
        4.2 Power of Paired Comparison for Treatment Effect 410
    5   Examples 410
    6   Discussion 412
    7   Conclusions 413
    References 413

**37 Cross-Over Trials Should Not Be Used
to Test Treatments with Different Chemical Class** 415
   1   Introduction.. 415
   2   Examples from the Literature in Which
       Cross-Over Trials Are Correctly Used... 417
   3   Examples from the Literature in Which
       Cross-Over Trials Should Not Have Been Used............................... 417
   4   Estimate of the Size of the Problem by Review
       of Hypertension Trials Published.. 419
   5   Discussion 421
   6   Conclusions 421
   References.. 422

38 Quality-Of-Life Assessments in Clinical Trials.................................. 423
   1   Introduction.. 423
   2   Some Terminology.. 423
   3   Defining QOL in a Subjective or Objective Way?............................ 425
   4   The Patients' Opinion Is an Important
       Independent-Contributor to QOL... 425
   5   Lack of Sensitivity of QOL-Assessments... 426
   6   Odds Ratio Analysis of Effects of Patient
       Characteristics on QOL Data Provides Increased Precision............... 427
   7   Discussion 429
   8   Conclusions 430
   References.. 430

39 Item Response Modeling 433
   1   Introduction.. 433
   2   Item Response Modeling, Principles 434
   3   Quality Of Life Assessment.. 435
   4   Clinical and Laboratory Diagnostic-Testing..................................... 438
   5   Discussion 439
   6   Conclusions 442
   References.. 442

40 Statistical Analysis of Genetic Data... 445
   1   Introduction.. 445
   2   Some Terminology.. 446
   3   Genetics, Genomics, Proteonomics, Data Mining............................ 447
   4   Genomics 448
   5   Conclusions 452
   References.. 453

41 Relationship Among Statistical Distributions 455
   1   Introduction.. 455
   2   Variances 456
   3   The Normal Distribution.. 456

4 Null-Hypothesis Testing with the Normal or t-Distribution 458
5 Relationship Between the Normal Distribution
and Chi-Square Distribution, Null-Hypothesis
Testing with Chi-Square Distribution 459
6 Examples of Data Where Variance
Is More Important Than Mean 462
7 Chi-Square Can Be Used for Multiple Samples of Data 462
7.1 Contingency Tables 462
7.2 Pooling Relative Risks or Odds Ratios
in a Meta-analysis of Multiple Trials 463
7.3 Analysis of Variance (ANOVA) 463
8 Discussion 465
9 Conclusions 466
Reference 467

42 **Testing Clinical Trials for Randomness** 469
1 Introduction 469
2 Individual Data Available 470
2.1 Method 1: The Chi-Square Goodness of Fit Test...................... 470
2.2 Method 2: The Kolmogorov-Smirnov
Goodness of Fit Test... 471
2.3 Randomness of Survival Data 472
3 Individual Data Not Available 473
3.1 Studies with Single Endpoints 473
3.2 Studies with Multiple Endpoints 475
4 Discussion 476
5 Conclusions 477
References 478

43 **Clinical Trials Do Not Use Random Samples Anymore** 479
1 Introduction 479
2 Non-normal Sampling Distributions,
Giving Rise to Non-normal Data 479
3 Testing the Assumption of Normality 481
4 What to Do in case of Non-normality 482
5 Discussion 483
6 Conclusions 484
References 485

44 **Clinical Data Where Variability
Is More Important Than Averages** 487
1 Introduction 487
2 Examples 488
2.1 Testing Drugs with Small Therapeutic Indices 488
2.2 Testing Variability in Drug Response 488
2.3 Assessing Pill Diameters or Pill Weights 488

2.4   Comparing Different Patient Groups
           for Variability in Patient Characteristics 488
    2.5   Assessing the Variability in Duration
           of Clinical Treatments 489
    2.6   Finding the Best Method for Patient Assessments 489
3   An Index for Variability in the Data 489
4   How to Analyze Variability, One Sample 490
    4.1 χ^2 Test 490
    4.2   Confidence Interval 491
    4.3   Equivalence Test 491
5   How to Analyze Variability, Two Samples 492
    5.1   F Test 492
    5.2   Confidence Interval 492
    5.3   Equivalence Test 493
6   How to Analyze Variability, Three or More Samples 493
    6.1   Bartlett's Test 493
    6.2   Levene's Test 494
7   Discussion 495
8   Conclusions 496
References 496

45   Testing Reproducibility 499
1   Introduction 499
2   Testing Reproducibility of Quantitative
    Data (Continuous Data) 500
    2.1   Method 1, Duplicate Standard
           Deviations (Duplicate SDs) 500
    2.2   Method 2, Repeatability Coefficients 500
    2.3   Method 3, Intraclass Correlation Coefficients (ICCS) 501
3   Testing Reproducibility of Qualitative
    Data (Proportions and Scores) 502
    3.1   Cohen's Kappas 502
4   Incorrect Methods to Assess Reproducibility 503
    4.1   Testing the Significance of Difference
           Between Two or More Sets of Repeated Measures 503
    4.2   Calculating the Level of Correlation Between
           Two Sets of Repeated Measures 504
5   Additional Real Data Examples 504
    5.1   Reproducibility of Ambulatory
           Blood Pressure Measurements (ABPM) 504
    5.2   Two Different Techniques to Measure
           the Presence of Hypertension 506
6   Discussion 507
7   Conclusions 508
References 508

46 Validating Qualitative Diagnostic Tests 509
  1   Introduction 509
  2   Overall Accuracy of a Qualitative Diagnostic Test 510
  3   Perfect and Imperfect Qualitative Diagnostic Tests 511
  4   Determining the Most Accurate Threshold
      for Positive Qualitative Tests 512
  5   Discussion 516
  6   Conclusions 517
  References 517

47 Uncertainty of Qualitative Diagnostic Tests 519
  1   Introduction 519
  2   Example 1 519
  3   Example 2 520
  4   Example 3 521
  5   Example 4 521
  6   Discussion 522
  7   Conclusion 523
  Appendix 1 523
  Appendix 2 524
  References 525

48 Meta-Analysis of Qualitative Diagnostic Tests 527
  1   Introduction 527
  2   Diagnostic Odds Ratios (DORS) 528
  3   Constructing Summary ROC Curves 531
  4   Discussion 531
  5   Conclusions 533
  References 534

**49 c-Statistic Versus Logistic Regression for Assessing
      the Performance of Qualitative Diagnostic Accuracy** 535
  1   Introduction 535
  2   The Performance of c-Statistics 538
  3   The Performance of Logistic Regression 541
  4   Discussion 541
      4.1   Conclusions 542
  5   Conclusions 543
  References 543

50 Validating Quantitative Diagnostic Tests 545
  1   Introduction 545
  2   Linear Regression Testing a Significant Correlation
      Between the New Test and the Control Test 545
  3   Linear Regression Testing the Hypotheses
      That the a-Value = 0.000 and the b-Value = 1.000 547

4 Linear Regression Using a Squared Correlation
Coefficient (r²-Value) of >0.95.. 548
5 Alternative Methods... 550
6 Discussion... 551
7 Conclusions... 552
References.. 552

51 Summary of Validation Procedures for Diagnostic Tests................... 555
1 Introduction... 555
2 Qualitative Diagnostic Tests... 556
  2.1 Accuracy.. 556
  2.2 Reproducibility.. 557
  2.3 Precision.. 558
3 Quantitative Diagnostic Tests... 558
  3.1 Accuracy.. 558
  3.2 Reproducibility.. 560
  3.3 Precision.. 562
4 Additional Methods... 564
5 Discussion... 566
6 Conclusions... 567
References.. 568

52 Validating Surrogate Endpoints of Clinical Trials.............................. 569
1 Introduction... 569
2 Some Terminology... 570
3 Surrogate Endpoints and the Calculation
of the Required Sample Size in a Trial.. 571
4 Validating Surrogate Markers Using 95% Confidence Intervals........ 572
5 Validating Surrogate Endpoints Using Regression Modeling............. 574
6 Discussion... 576
7 Conclusions... 578
References.. 578

53 Binary Partitioning.. 579
1 Introduction... 579
2 Example.. 579
3 ROC (Receiver Operating Characteristic)
Method for Finding the Best Cut-Off Level.. 580
4 Entropy Method for Finding the Best Cut-Off Level........................... 582
5 Discussion... 583
6 Conclusions... 584
References.. 585

54 Methods for Repeated Measures Analysis.. 587
1 Introduction... 587
2 Summary Measures... 588

3   Repeated Measures ANOVA Without
Between-Subjects Covariates.. 588
4   Repeated Measures ANOVA with
Between-Subjects Covariates.. 589
5   Conclusions... 592
References.. 592

55 Mixed Linear Models for Repeated Measures 593
1   Introduction... 593
2   A Placebo-Controlled Parallel Group
Study of Cholesterol Treatment 594
3   A Three Treatment Crossover Study
of the Effect of Sleeping Pills on Hours of Sleep 599
4   Discussion.. 603
5   Conclusion 604
References.. 605

**56 Advanced Analysis of Variance, Random
Effects and Mixed Effects Models** 607
1   Introduction... 607
2   Example 1, a Simple Example
of a Random Effects Model 608
3   Example 2, a Random Interaction Effect
Between Study and Treatment Efficacy.................................... 609
4   Example 3, a Random Interaction Effect
Between Health Center and Treatment Efficacy............................... 611
5   Example 4, a Random Effects Model
for Post-hoc Analysis of Negative Crossover Trials 614
6   Discussion.. 615
7   Conclusions... 616
References.. 617

57 Monte Carlo Methods for Data Analysis 619
1   Introduction... 619
2   Principles of the Monte Carlo Method
Explained from a Dartboard to Assess the Size of Π 620
3   The Monte Carlo Method for Analyzing Continuous Data 621
4   The Monte Carlo Method for Analyzing Proportional Data.............. 622
5   Discussion.. 623
6   Conclusions... 624
References.. 625

58 Artificial Intelligence 627
1   Introduction... 627
2   Historical Background 627
3   The Back Propagation (BP) Neural Network:
The Computer Teaches Itself to Make Predictions 628

4   A Real Data Example.. 630
5   Discussion... 633
6   Conclusions.. 634
References... 635

59 Fuzzy Logic.. 639
1   Introduction... 639
2   Some Fuzzy Terminology 640
3   First Example, Dose–Response Effects
     of Thiopental on Numbers of Responders 640
4   Second Example, Time-Response Effect
     of Propranolol on Peripheral Arterial Flow 644
5   Discussion... 647
6   Conclusions.. 648
References... 649

60 Physicians' Daily Life and the Scientific Method............................... 651
1   Introduction... 651
2   Example of Unanswered Questions
     of a Physician During a Single Busy Day.. 651
3   How the Scientific Method Can Be Implied
     in a Physician's Daily Life 652
     3.1 Falling Out of Bed.. 652
     3.2 Evaluation of Fundic Gland Polyps 653
     3.3 Physicians with a Burn-Out 653
     3.4 Patients' Letters of Complaints... 654
4   Discussion 655
5   Conclusions.. 656
References... 656

61 Incident Analysis and the Scientific Method 659
1   Introduction... 659
2   The Scientific Method in Incident-Analysis 660
3   Discussion 661
4   Conclusions.. 662
References... 663

62 Clinical Trials: Superiority-Testing... 665
1   Introduction... 665
2   Examples of Studies Not Meeting Their Expected Powers 666
3   How to Assess Clinical Superiority 667
4   Discussion 669
5   Conclusions.. 672
References... 672

63 Noninferiority Testing.. 675
  1   Introduction.. 675
  2   A Novel Approach 676
    2.1   Basing the Margins of Noninferiority
        on Counted Criteria... 676
    2.2   Testing the Presence of Both Noninferiority
        and a Significant Difference from Zero..................................... 677
    2.3   Testing the New Treatment Versus
        Historical Placebo Data.. 678
    2.4   Including Prior Sample Size
        Calculations and p-Values 678
  3   Examples.. 679
    3.1   Example 1... 680
    3.2   Example 2... 680
    3.3   Example 3... 681
    3.4   Example 4... 682
  4   Discussion 682
  5   Conclusions 685
  References... 686

64 Time Series... 687
  1   Introduction.. 687
  2   Autocorrelation 688
  3   Cross Correlation 688
  4   Change Points 689
  5   Discussion 690
  6   Conclusions 692
  References... 693

**65 Odds Ratios and Multiple Regression
Models, Why and How to Use Them**... 695
  1   Introduction.. 695
  2   Understanding Odds Ratios (ORS)... 695
    2.1   Odds Ratios (ORs) as an Alternative Method
        to χ^2-Tests for the Analysis of Binary Data 696
    2.2   How to Analyze Odds Ratios (ORs) 697
    2.3   Real Data Examples of Simple OR Analyses 701
    2.4   Real Data Examples of Advanced OR Analyses 702
  3   Multiple Regression Models to Reduce the Spread in the Data 704
    3.1   A Linear Regression Model for Increasing Precision............... 705
    3.2   A Logistic Regression Model for Increasing Precision 707
  4   Discussion 709
  5   Conclusions 710
  References... 711

66 Statistics Is No "Bloodless" Algebra 713
   1 Introduction... 713
   2 Statistics Is Fun Because It Proves
      Your Hypothesis Was Right.. 713
   3 Statistical Principles Can Help
      to Improve the Quality of the Trial 714
   4 Statistics Can Provide Worthwhile Extras to Your Research........... 714
   5 Statistics Is Not Like Algebra Bloodless 715
   6 Statistics Can Turn Art into Science... 716
   7 Statistics for Support Rather Than Illumination? 716
   8 Statistics Can Help the Clinician to Better Understand
      Limitations and Benefits of Current Research................................ 717
   9 Limitations of Statistics 717
  10 Conclusions... 718
   References.. 719

67 Bias Due to Conflicts of Interests, Some Guidelines 721
   1 Introduction... 721
   2 The Randomized Controlled Clinical
      Trial as the Gold Standard 721
   3 Need for Circumspection Recognized 722
   4 The Expanding Commend of the Pharmaceutical
      Industry Over Clinical Trials 722
   5 Flawed Procedures Jeopardizing Current Clinical Trials.................. 723
   6 The Good News 724
   7 Further Solutions to the Dilemma Between
      Sponsored Research and the Independence of Science 725
   8 Conclusions... 726
   References.. 726

Appendix.. 729

Index.. 735

Chapter 1
Hypotheses, Data, Stratification

1 General Considerations

Over the past decades the randomized clinical trial has entered an era of continuous improvement and has gradually become accepted as the most effective way of determining the relative efficacy and toxicity of new drug therapies. This book is mainly involved in the methods of prospective randomized clinical trials of new drugs. Other methods for assessment including open-evaluation-studies, cohort- and case-control studies, although sometimes used, e.g., for pilot studies and for the evaluation of long term drug-effects, are, however, not excluded in this course. Traditionally, clinical drug trials are divided into IV phases (from phase I for initial testing to phase IV after release for general use), but scientific rules governing different phases are very much the same, and can thus be discussed simultaneously.

A. Clearly Defined Hypotheses

Hypotheses must be tested prospectively with hard data, and against placebo or known forms of therapies that are in place and considered to be effective. Uncontrolled studies won't succeed to give a definitive answer if they are ever so clever. Uncontrolled studies while of value in the absence of scientific controlled studies, their conclusions represent merely suggestions and hypotheses. The scientific method requires to look at some controls to characterize the defined population.

B. Valid Designs

Any research but certainly industrially sponsored drug research where sponsors benefit from favorable results, benefits from valid designs. A valid study means a study unlikely to be biased, or unlikely to include systematic errors. The most dangerous errors in clinical trials are systematic errors otherwise called biases. Validity is the most important thing for doers of clinical trials to check. Trials should be made independent, objective, balanced, blinded, controlled, with objective measurements, with adequate sample sizes to test the expected treatment effects, with random assignment of patients.

T.J. Cleophas and A.H. Zwinderman, *Statistics Applied to Clinical Studies*,
DOI 10.1007/978-94-007-2863-9_1, © Springer Science+Business Media B.V. 2012

C. Explicit Description of Methods

Explicit description of the methods should include description of the recruitment procedures, method of randomization of the patients, prior statements about the methods of assessments of generating and analysis of the data and the statistical methods used, accurate ethics including written informed consent.

D. Uniform Data Analysis

Uniform and appropriate data analysis generally starts with plots or tables of actual data. Statistics then comes in to test primary hypotheses primarily. Data that do not answer prior hypotheses may be tested for robustness or sensitivity, otherwise called precision of point estimates e.g., dependent upon numbers of outliers. The results of studies with many outliers and thus little precision should be interpreted with caution. It is common practice for studies to test multiple measurements for the purpose of answering one single question. In clinical trials the benefit to health is estimated by variables, which can be defined as measurable factors or characteristics used to estimate morbidity/mortality/time to events etc. Variables are named exposure, indicator, or independent variables, if they predict morbidity/mortality, and outcome or dependent variables, if they estimate morbidity/mortality. Sometimes both mortality and morbidity variables are used in a single trial, and there is nothing wrong with that practice. We should not make any formal correction for multiple comparisons of this kind of data. Instead, we should informally integrate all the data before reaching conclusions, and look for the trends without judging one or two low P-values among otherwise high P-values as proof.

However, subgroup analyses involving post-hoc comparisons by dividing the data into groups with different ages, prior conditions, gender etc can easily generate hundreds of P-values. If investigators test many different hypotheses, they are apt to find significant differences at least 5% of the time. To make sense of these kinds of results, we need to consider the Bonferroni inequality, which will be emphasized in the Chaps. 7 and 8. It states that, if k statistical tests are performed with the cut-off level for a test statistic, for example t or F, at the α level, the likelihood for observing a value of the test statistic exceeding the cut-off level is no greater than k times α. For example, if we wish to do three comparisons with t-tests while keeping the probability of making a mistake less than 5%, we have to use instead of $\alpha = 5\%$ in this case $\alpha = 5/3\% = 1.6\%$. With many more tests, analyses soon lose any sensitivity and do hardly prove anything anymore. Nonetheless, a limited number of post-hoc analyses, particularly if a plausible theory is underlying, can be useful in generating hypotheses for future studies.

2   Two Main Hypotheses in Drug Trials: Efficacy and Safety

Drug trials are mainly for addressing the efficacy as well as the safety of the treatments to be tested in them. For analyzing efficacy data formal statistical techniques are normally used. Basically, the null hypothesis of no treatment effect is tested, and is rejected when difference from zero is significant. For such purpose a great variety of statistical significance tests has been developed, all of whom report P values, and compute confidence intervals to estimate the magnitude of the treatment effect. The appropriate test depends upon the type of data and will be discussed in the next chapter. Of safety data, such as adverse events, data are mostly collected with the hope of demonstrating that the test treatment is not different from control. This concept is based upon a different hypothesis from that proposed for efficacy data, where the very objective is generally to show that there actually is a difference between test and control. Because the objective of collecting safety data is thus different, the approach to analysis must be likewise different. In particular, it may be less appropriate to use statistical significance tests to analyze the latter data. A significance test is a tool that can help to establish whether a difference between treatments is likely to be real. It cannot be used to demonstrate that two treatments are similar in their effects. In addition, safety data, more frequently than efficacy data, consist of proportions and percentages rather than continuous data as will be discussed in the next section. Usually, the best approach to analysis of these kinds of data is to present suitable summary statistics, together with confidence intervals. In the case of adverse event data, the rate of occurrence of each distinct adverse event on each treatment group should be reported, together with confidence intervals for the difference between the rates of occurrence on the different treatments. An alternative would be to present risk ratios or relative risks of occurrence, with confidence intervals for the relative risk. Chapter 3 mainly addresses the analyses of these kinds of data.

Other aspects of assessing similarity rather than difference between treatments will be discussed separately in Chap. 6 where the theory, equations, and assessments are given for demonstrating statistical equivalence.

3 Different Types of Data: Continuous Data

The first step, before any analysis or plotting of data can be performed, is to decide what kind of data we have. Usually data are continuous, e.g., blood pressures, heart rates etc. But, regularly, proportions or percentages are used for the assessment of part of the data. The next few lines will address how we can summarize and characterize these two different approaches to the data.

Samples of **continuous data** are characterized by:

$$\textbf{Mean} = \frac{\Sigma \textbf{x}}{\textbf{n}} = \bar{x},$$

where Σ is the summation, x are the individual data, n is the total number of data.

$$\textbf{Variance} = \sum (x - \bar{x})^2$$

$$\textbf{Mean variance} = \frac{\sum (x - \bar{x})^2}{n - 1}$$

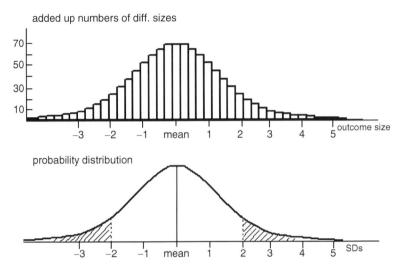

Fig. 1.1 Histogram and Gaussian curve representation of data

Mean variance is often briefly named variance. And, so, don't forget the term variance is commonly used to name mean variance. The famous term standard deviation is often abbreviated as, simply, s, and is equal to the square root of this mean variance.

$$\textbf{Standard deviation} \ (\textbf{SD}) = \sqrt{(\textbf{mean variance})}$$

Continuous data can be plotted in the form of a histogram (Fig. 1.1 upper graph). On the x-axis, frequently called z-axis in statistics, it has individual data. On the y-axis it has "how often". For example, the mean value is observed most frequently, while the bars on either side gradually grow shorter. This graph adequately represents the data. It is, however, not adequate for statistical analyses. Figure 1.1 lower graph pictures a Gaussian curve, otherwise called normal (distribution) curve. On the x-axis we have, again, the individual data, expressed either in absolute data or in SDs distant from the mean. On the y-axis the bars have been replaced with a continuous line. It is now impossible to determine from the graph how many patients had a particular outcome. Instead, important inferences can be made. For example, the total area under the curve (AUC) represents 100% of the data, AUC left from mean represents 50% of the data, left from −1 SDs it has 15.87% of the data, left from -2SDs it has 2.5% of the data. This graph is better for statistical purposes but not yet good enough.

Figure 1.2 gives two Gaussian curves, a narrow and a wide one. Both are based on the same data, but with different meaning. The wide one summarizes the data of our trial. The narrow one summarizes the mean of many trials similar to our trial. We will not try to make you understand why this is so. Still, it is easy to conceive

Fig. 1.2 Two examples of normal distributions

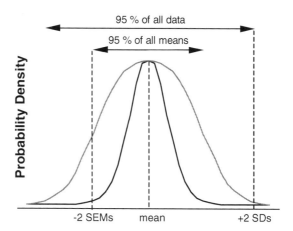

that the distribution of all means of many similar trials is narrower and has fewer outliers than the distribution of the actual data from our trial, and that it will center around the mean of our trial, because our trial is assumed to be representative for the entire population. You may find it hard to believe, but the narrow curve with standard errors of the mean (SEMs) or simply SEs on the x-axis can be effectively used for testing important statistical hypotheses, like (1) no difference between new and standard treatment, (2) a real difference, (3) the new treatment is better than the standard treatment, (4) the two treatments are equivalent. Thus, mean ± 2 SDs (or more precisely 1.96 SDs) represents 95% of the AUC of the wide distribution, otherwise called the 95% confidence interval of the data, which means that 95% of the data of the sample are within. The SEM-curve (narrow one) is narrower than the SD-curve (wide one) because SEM = SD/√n with n = sample size. Mean ± 2 SEMs (or more precisely 1.96 SEMs) represents 95% of the means of many trials similar to our trial.

$$\textbf{SEM} = \textbf{SD} / \sqrt{n}$$

As the size of SEM in the graph is about 1/3 times SD, the size of each sample is here about n = 10. The area under the narrow curve represents 100% of the sample means we would obtain, while the area under the curve of the wide graph represents 100% of all of the data of the samples.

Why is this SEM approach so important in statistics. Statistics makes use of mean values and their standard error to test the null hypotheses of finding no difference from zero in your sample. When we reject a null hypothesis at P < 0.05, it literally means that there is <5% chance that the mean value of our sample crosses the area of the null hypothesis where we say there is no difference. It does not mean that many individual data may not go beyond that boundary. Actually, it is just a matter of agreement. But it works well.

So remember:

Mean ± 2 SDs covers an area under the curve including 95% of the data of the given sample.
Mean ± 2 SEMs covers an area under curve including 95% of the means of many samples, and is sometimes called the 95% confidence interval (CI).

In statistical analysis we often compare different samples by taking their sums or differences. Again, this text is not intended to explain the procedures entirely. One more thing to accept unexplainedly is the following. The distributions of the sums as well as those of the difference of samples are again normal distributions and can be characterized by:

$$\text{Sum: mean}_1 + \text{mean}_2 \pm \sqrt{(SD_1^2 + SD_2^2)}$$

$$\text{Difference: mean}_1 - \text{mean}_2 \pm \sqrt{(SD_1^2 + SD_2^2)}$$

$$SEM_{sum} = \sqrt{(SD_1^2 / n_1 + SD_2^2 / n_2)}$$

$$SEM_{difference} = \quad \text{``}$$

Note: If the standard deviations are very different in size, then a more adequate calculation of the pooled SEM is given in the next chapter.

Sometimes we have paired data where two experiments are performed in one subject or in two members of one family. The variances with paired data are usually smaller than with unpaired because of the positive correlation between two observations in one subject (those who respond well the first time are more likely to do so the second). This phenomenon translates in a slightly modified calculation of variance parameters.

$$SD_{paired\ sum} = \sqrt{(SD_1^2 + SD_2^2 + 2\ r\ SD_1 \cdot SD_2)}$$

$$SD_{paired\ differrence} = \sqrt{(SD_1^2 + SD_2^2 - 2\ r\ SD_1 \cdot SD_2)}$$

Where r = correlation coefficient, a term that will be explained soon.
Likewise:

$$SEM_{paired\ sum} = \sqrt{SD_1^2 / n_1 + SD_2^2 / n_2 + (2\ r\ SD_2 \cdot SD_2)(1/2n_1 + 1/2n_2)}$$

$$SEM_{paired\ differrence} = \sqrt{SD_1^2 / n_1 + SD_2^2 / n_2 - (2\ r\ SD_1 \cdot SD_2)(1/2n_1 + 1/2n_2)}$$

Note that SEM does not directly quantify variability in a population. A small SEM can be mainly due to a large sample size rather than tight data.

With small samples the distribution of the means does not exactly follow a Gaussian distribution. But rather a t-distribution, 95% confidence intervals cannot

Fig. 1.3 Family of t-distributions: with n = 5 the distribution is wide, with n = 10 and n = 1,000 this is increasingly less so

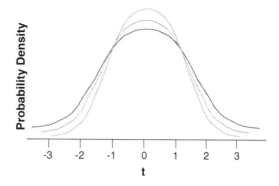

be characterized as the area under the curve between mean ± 2 SEMs but instead the area under curve is substantially wider and is characterized as mean ± t.SEMs where t is close to 2 with large samples but 2.5–3 with samples as small as 5–10. The appropriate t for any sample size is given in the t-table (Appendix).

Figure 1.3 shows that the t-distribution is wider than the Gaussian distribution with small samples. Mean ± t.SEMs presents the 95% confidence intervals of the means that many similar samples would produce.

Statistics is frequently used to compare more than two samples of data. To estimate whether differences between samples are true or just chance we first assess variances in the data between groups and within groups.

Group	n patients	Mean	SD
Group 1	n	$mean_1$	SD_1
Group 2	n	$mean_2$	SD_2
Group 3	n	$mean_3$	SD_3

This procedure may seem somewhat awkward in the beginning but in the next two chapters we will observe that variances, which are no less than estimates of noise in the data, are effectively used to test the probabilities of true differences between, e.g., different pharmaceutical compounds. The above data are summarized underneath.

Between-group variance:
Sum of $squares_{between} = SS_{between} = n$ $(mean_1 -$ overall $mean)^2 + n$ $(mean_2 - overall$ $mean)^2 + n$ $(mean_3 -$ overall $mean)^2$

Within-group variance:
Sum of $squares_{within} = SS_{within} = (n-1) SD_1^2 + (n-1) SD_2^2 + (n-1) SD_3^2$

The ratio of the sum of squares between-group/sum of squares within group (after proper adjustment for the sample sizes or degrees of freedom, a term which will be explained later on) is called the big F and determines whether variances between the sample means is larger than expected from the variability within the samples. If so, we reject the null hypothesis of no difference between the samples. With two samples the square root of big F, which actually is the test statistic of analysis of variance (ANOVA), is equal to the t of the famous t-test, which will further be explained in Chap. 2. These ten or so lines already brought us very close to what is currently considered the heart of statistics, namely ANOVA (analysis of variance).

4   Different Types of Data: Proportions, Percentages and Contingency Tables

Instead of continuous data, data may also be of a discrete character where two or more alternatives are possible, and, generally, the frequencies of occurrence of each of these possibilities are calculated. The simplest and commonest type of such data are the binary data (yes/no etc). Such data are frequently assessed as proportions or percentages, and follow a so-called binomial distribution. If $0.1 < $ proportion $(p) < 0.9$ the binomial distribution becomes very close to the normal distribution. If $p < 0.1$, the data will follow a skewed distribution, otherwise called Poisson distribution. Proportional data can be conveniently laid-out as contingency tables. The simplest contingency table looks like this:

	Numbers of subjects with side effect	Numbers of subjects without side effect
Test treatment (group$_1$)	a	b
Control treatment (group$_2$)	c	d

The proportion of subjects who had a side effect in group$_1$ (or the risk (**R**) or probability of having an effect):

$p = a/(a+b)$, in group$_2$ $p = c/(c+d)$,
The ratios $a/(a+b)$ and $c/(c+d)$ are called **risk ratios (RRs)**

Note that the terms proportion, risk and probability are frequently used in statistical procedures but that they basically mean the same.

Another approach is the **odds** approach where **a/b** and **c/d** are odds and their ratio is the **odds ratio (OR)**.

In clinical trials we use ORs as surrogate RRs, because here a/(a+b) is simply nonsense. For example:

	Treatment-group		Control-group		Entire-population
Sleepiness	32	a	4	b	4,000
No sleepiness	24	c	52	d	52,000

We assume that the control group is just a sample from the entire population but that the ratio b/d is that of the entire population. So, suppose $4 = 4{,}000$ and $52 = 52{,}000$, then we can approximate $\dfrac{a/(a \pm b)}{c/(c+d)} = \dfrac{a/b}{c/d} = RR$ of the entire population.

With observational cohort studies things are different. The entire population is used as control group. Therefore, RRs are better adequate. ORs and RRs are largely similar as long as they are close to 1.000. More information on ORs is given in the Chaps. 3, 17, 18, and 19.

Proportions can also be expressed as percentages:
p.100% = a/(a + b). (100%) etc

Just as with continuous data we can calculate SDs and SEMs and 95% confidence intervals of rates (or numbers, or scores) and of proportions or percentages.

SD of number $n = \sqrt{n}$
SD of difference between two numbers n_1 and $n_2 = (n_1 - n_2)/\sqrt{(n_1 + n_2)}$
SD proportion $= \sqrt{p(1-p)}$
SEM proportion $= \sqrt{p(1-p)/n}$

We assume that the distribution of proportions of many samples follows a normal distribution (in this case called the **z**-distribution) with 95% confidence intervals between:

$$p \pm 2\sqrt{p(1-p)/n}$$

a formula looking very similar to the 95% CI intervals formula for continuous data

$$\text{mean} \pm 2\sqrt{SD^2/n}$$

Differences and sums of the SDs and SEMs of proportions can be calculated similarly to those of continuous data:

$$SEM_{\text{of differences}} = \sqrt{\dfrac{p_1(1-p_1)}{n_1} + \dfrac{p_2(1-p_2)}{n_2}}$$

with 95% CI intervals: $p_1 - p_2 \pm 2$. SEMs

More often than with continuous data, proportions of different samples are assessed for their ratios rather than difference or sum. Calculating the 95% CI intervals of it is not simple. The problem is that the ratios of many samples do not follow a normal distribution, and are extremely skewed. It can never be less than 0 but can get very high. However, the logarithm of the relative risk is approximately symmetrical. Katz's method takes advantage of this symmetry:

$$95\% \text{ CI of } \log RR = \log RR \pm 2\sqrt{\dfrac{b/a}{a+b} + \dfrac{d/c}{c+d}}$$

Fig. 1.4 Ratios of proportions unlike continuous data usually do not follow a normal but a skewed distribution (values vary from 0 to ∞). Transformation into the logarithms provides approximately symmetric distributions (*thin curve*)

Probability distribution

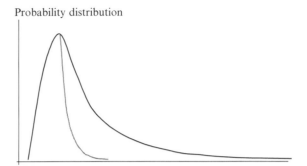

This equation calculates the CIs of the logarithm of the RR. Take the antilogarithm (shift and 10^x buttons of the pocket calculator) to determine the 95% CIs of the RR.

Figure 1.4 shows the distribution of RRs and the distribution of the logarithms of the RRs, and illustrates that the transformation from skewed data into their logarithms is a useful method to obtain an approximately symmetrical distribution, that can be analyzed according to the usual approach of SDs, SEMs and CIs.

5   Different Types of Data: Correlation Coefficient

The SD and SEM of paired data includes a term called r as described above. For the calculation of r, otherwise called R, we have to take into account that paired comparisons, e.g., those of two drugs tested in one subject generally have a different variance from those of comparison of two drugs in two different subjects. This is so, because between subjects variability of symptoms is eliminated and because the chance of a subject responding beneficially the first time is more likely to respond beneficially the second time as well. We say there is generally a positive correlation between the responses of one subject to two treatments.

Figure 1.5 gives an example of this phenomenon. X-variables, e.g., blood pressures after the administration of compound 1 or placebo, y-variables blood pressures after the administration of compound 2 or test-treatment.

The SDs and SEMs of the paired sums or differences of the x- and y-variables are relevant to estimate variances in the data and are just as those of continuous data needed before any statistical test can be performed. They can be calculated according to:

$$SD_{\text{paired sum}} = \sqrt{(SD_1^2 + SD_2^2 + 2 r \, SD_1 \cdot SD_2)}$$

Fig. 1.5 A positive correlation between the response of one subject to two treatments

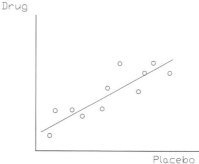

$$SD_{\text{paired differrence}} = \sqrt{(SD_1^2 + SD_2^2 - 2\,r\,SD_1 \cdot SD_2)}$$

where r = correlation coefficient, a term that will be explained soon.
  Likewise:

$$SEM_{\text{paired sum}} = \sqrt{(SD_1^2 + SD_2^2 + 2\,r\,SD_1 \cdot SD_2)/n}$$

$$SEM_{\text{paired differrence}} = \sqrt{(SD_1^2 + SD_2^2 - 2\,r\,SD_1 \cdot SD_2)/n}$$

where $n = n_1 = n_2$
  and that:

$$r = \frac{\sum(X - \bar{X})(Y - \bar{Y})}{\sqrt{\sum(X - \bar{X})^2 \sum(Y - \bar{Y})^2}}$$

r is between −1 and +1, and with unpaired data r = 0 and the SD and SEM formulas reduce accordingly (as described above). The figure also shows a line, called the regression line, which presents the best-fit summary of the data, and is the calculated method that minimizes the squares of the distances from the line.

  The 95% CIs of a regression line can be calculated and is drawn as area between the dotted lines in Fig. 1.6. It is remarkable that the borders of the straight regression line are curved although we do not allow for a non linear relationship between the x-axis and y-axis variables. More details on regression analysis will be given in Chaps. 2 and 3.

  In the above few lines we described continuous normally distributed or t-distributed data, and rates and their proportions or percentages. We did not yet address data ordered as ranks. This is a special method to transform skewed data into an approximately normal distribution, and is in that sense comparable with logarithmic transformation of relative risks (RRs). In Chap. 3 the tests involving this method will be explained.

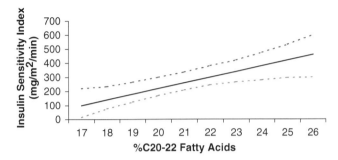

Fig. 1.6 Example of a linear regression line of two paired variables (x- and y-values), the regression line provides the best fit line. The dotted curves are 95% CIs that are curved, although we do not allow for a non linear relationship between x and y variables

6 Stratification Issues

When published, a randomized parallel-group drug trial essentially includes a table listing all of the factors, otherwise called baseline characteristics, known possibly to influence outcome. E.g., in case of heart disease these will probably include apart from age and gender, the prevalence in each group of diabetes, hypertension, cholesterol levels, smoking history. If such factors are similar in the two groups, then we can go on to attribute any difference in outcome to the effect of test-treatment over reference-treatment. If not, we have a problem. Attempts are made to retrieve the situation by multiple variables analysis allocating part of the differences in outcome to the differences in the groups, but there is always an air of uncertainty about the validity of the overall conclusions in such a trial. This issue is discussed and methods are explained in Chap. 8. Here we discuss ways to avoid this problem. Ways to do so, are stratification of the analysis and minimization of imbalance between treatment groups, which are both techniques not well-known. Stratification of the analysis means that relatively homogeneous subgroups are analyzed separately. The limitation of this approach is that it can not account for more than two, maybe three, variables, and that, thus, major covariates may be missed. Minimization can manage more factors. The investigators first classify patients according to the factors they would like to see equally presented in the two groups, then randomly assign treatment so that predetermined approximately fixed proportions of patients from each stratum receive each treatment. With this method the group assignment does not rely solely on chance but is designed to reduce any difference in the distribution of unsuspected contributing determinants of outcome so that any treatment difference can now be attributed to the treatment comparison itself. A good example of this method can be found in a study by Kallis et al. (1994). The authors stratified in a study of aspirin versus placebo before coronary artery surgery the groups according to age, gender, left ventricular function, and number of coronary arteries affected. Any other prognostic factors other than treatment can be chosen. If the treatments are given in a double-blind fashion, minimization influences the composition of the two groups but does not influence the chance of one group entering in a particular treatment arm rather than the other.

There is an additional argument in favor of stratification/minimization that counts even if the risk of significant asymmetries in the treatment groups is small. Some prognostic factors have a particularly large effect on the outcome of a trial. Even small and statistically insignificant imbalances in the treatment groups may then bias the results. E.g., in a study of two treatment modalities for pneumonia (Graham and Bradley 1978) including 54 patients, 10 patients took prior antibiotic in the treatment group and 5 did in the control group. Even though the difference between 5/27 and 10/27 is not statistically significant, the validity of this trial was being challenged, and the results were eventually not accepted.

7   Randomized Versus Historical Controls

A randomized clinical trial is frequently used in drug research. However, there is considerable opposition to the use of this design. One major concern is the ethical problem of allowing a random event to determine a patient's treatment. Freirich (1983) argued that a comparative trial, which shows major differences between two treatments, is a bad trial because half of the patients have received an inferior treatment. On the other hand, in a prospective trial randomly assigning treatments avoids many potential biases. Of more concern is the trial in which a new treatment is compared to an old treatment when there is information about the efficacy of the old treatment through historical data. In this situation the use of historical data for comparison with data from the new treatment will shorten the length of the study because all patients can be assigned to the new treatment. The current availability of multi-variable statistical procedures which can adjust the comparison of two treatments for differing presence of other prognostic factors in the two treatment arms, has made the use of historical controls more appealing. This has made randomization less necessary as a mechanism for ensuring comparability of the treatment arms. The weak point in this approach is the absolute faith one has to place in the multi-variable model. In addition, some confounding variables e.g., time effects, simply can not be adjusted, and remain unknown. Despite the ethical argument in favor of historical controls we must therefore emphasize the potentially misleading aspects of trials using historical controls.

8   Factorial Designs

The majority of drug trials are designed to answer a single question. However, in practice many diseases require a combination of more than one treatment modalities. E.g., beta-blockers are effective for stable angina pectoris but beta-blockers

Table 1.1 The factorial design for angina pectoris patients treated with calcium channel blockers with or without beta-blockers

	Calcium channel blocker	No calcium channel blocker
Beta-blocker	Regimen I	Regimen II
No beta-blocker	Regimen III	Regimen I

plus calcium channel blockers or beta-blockers plus calcium channel blockers plus nitrates are better (Table 1.1). Not addressing more than one treatment modality in a trial is an unnecessary restriction on the design of the trial because the assessment of two or more modalities in on a trial pose no major mathematical problems.

We will not describe the analytical details of such a design but researchers should not be reluctant to consider designs of such types. This is particularly so, when the recruitment of large samples causes difficulties.

9 Conclusions

What you should know after reading this chapter:

1. Scientific rules governing controlled clinical trials include prior hypotheses, valid designs, strict description of the methods, uniform data analysis.
2. Efficacy data and safety data often involve respectively continuous and proportional data.
3. How to calculate standard deviations and standard errors of the data.
4. You should have a notion of negative/positive correlation in paired comparisons, and of the meaning of the so-called correlation coefficient.
5. Mean ± standard deviation summarizes the data, mean ± standard error summarizes the means of many trials similar to our trial.
6. You should know the meaning of historical controls and factorial designs.

References

Freirich F (1983) Ethical problem of allowing a random event to determine a patient's treatment. In: Controversies in clinical trials. Philadelphia, Saunders, p 5

Graham WG, Bradley DA (1978) Efficacy of chest physiotherapy and intermittent positive-pressure breathing in the resolution of pneumonia. N Engl J Med 299:624–627

Kallis F et al (1994) Aspirin versus placebo before coronary artery surgery. Eur J Cardiovasc Surg 8:404–410

Chapter 2
The Analysis of Efficacy Data

1 Overview

Typical efficacy endpoints have their associated statistical techniques. For example, values of continuous measurements (e.g., blood pressures) require the following statistical techniques:

(a) if measurements are normally distributed: t-tests and associated confidence intervals to compare two mean values; analysis of variance (ANOVA) to compare three or more,
(b) if measurements have a non-normal distribution: Wilcoxon or Mann-Whitney tests with confidence intervals for medians.

Comparing proportions of responders or proportions of survivors or patients with no events involves binomial rather than normal distributions and requires a completely different approach. It requires a chi-square test, or a more complex technique otherwise closely related to the simple chi-square test, e.g., Mantel Haenszl summary chi-square test, logrank test, Cox proportional hazard test etc. Although in clinical trials, particularly phase III–IV trials, proportions of responders and proportion of survivors is increasingly an efficacy endpoint, in many other trials proportions are used mainly for the purpose of assessing safety endpoints, while continuous measurements are used for assessing the main endpoints, mostly efficacy endpoints. We will, therefore, focus on statistically testing continuous measurements in this chapter and will deal with different aspects of statistically testing proportions in the next chapter.

T.J. Cleophas and A.H. Zwinderman, *Statistics Applied to Clinical Studies*,
DOI 10.1007/978-94-007-2863-9_2, © Springer Science+Business Media B.V. 2012

Statistical tests all have in common that they try to estimate the probability that a difference in the data is true rather than due to chance. Usually statistical tests make use of a so-called **test statistic**:

Chi-square	For the chi-square test
t	For the t-test
Q	For nonparametric comparisons
Q^1	For nonparametric comparisons
q	For Newman-Keuls test
q^1	For Dunnett test
F	For analysis of variance
Rs	For Spearman rank correlation test.

These test statistics can adopt different sizes. In the Appendix of this book we present tables for t-, chi-square- and F-, Mann-Whitney-, and Wilcoxon-rank-sum-tests, but additional tables are published in most textbooks of statistics (see References). Such tables show us the larger the size of the test statistic, the more likely it is that the null-hypothesis of no difference from zero or no difference between two samples is untrue, and that there is thus a true difference or true effect in the data. Most tests also have in common that they are better sensitive or powerful to demonstrate such a true difference as the samples tested are large. So, the test statistic in most tables is adjusted for sample sizes. We say that the sample size determines the degrees of freedom, a term closely related to the sample size.

2   The Principle of Testing Statistical Significance

The human brain excels in making hypotheses but hypotheses may be untrue. When you were a child you thought that only girls could become a doctor because your family doctor was a female. Later on, this hypothesis proved to be untrue. Hypotheses must be assessed with hard data. Statistical analyses of hard data starts with assumptions:

1. our study is representative for the entire population (if we repeat the trial, difference will be negligible).
2. All similar trials will have the same standard deviation (SD) or standard error of the mean (SEM).

Because biological processes are *full* of variations, statistics will give no certainties only chances. What chances? Chances that hypotheses are true/untrue. What hypotheses?: e.g.:

1. our mean effect is not different from a 0 effect,
2. it is really different from a 0 effect,
3. it is worse than a 0 effect.

Statistics is about estimating such chances/testing such hypotheses. Please note that trials often calculate differences between a test treatment and a control treatment and, subsequently, test whether this difference is larger than 0. A simple way to

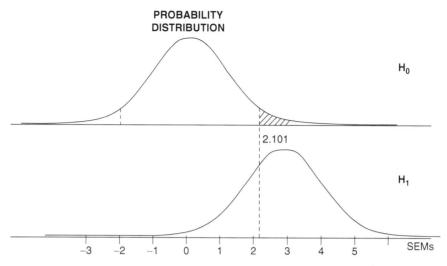

Fig. 2.1 Null-hypothesis (H_0) and alternative hypothesis H_1 of an example of experimental data with sample size (n) = 20 and mean = 2.9 SEMs, and a t-distributed frequency distribution

reduce a study of two groups of data and, thus, two means to a single mean and single distribution of data, is to take the difference between the two and compare it with 0.

In the past chapter we explained that the data of a trial can be described in the form of a normal distribution graph with SEMs on the x-axis, and that this method is adequate to test various statistical hypotheses. We will now focus on a very important hypothesis, the null-hypothesis. What it literally means is: no difference from a 0 effect: the mean value of our sample is not different from the value 0. We will try and make a graph of this null hypothesis.

What does it look like in graph? H1 in Fig. 2.1 is a graph based on the data of our trial with SEMs distant from mean on the x-axis (z-axis). H0 is the same graph with a mean value of 0 (mean ± SEM = 0 ± 1). Now, we will make a giant leap from our data to the entire population, and we can do so, because our data are representative for the entire population. H1 is also the summary of the means of many trials similar to ours (if we repeat, differences will be small, and summary will look alike). H0 is also the summary of the means of many trials similar to ours but with an overall effect of 0. Now our mean effect is not 0 but 2.9. Yet it could be an outlier of many studies with an overall effect of 0. So, we should think from now on of H0 as the distribution of the means of many trials with overall effect of 0. If H0 is true, then the mean of our study is part of H0. We can not prove anything, but we can calculate the chance/probability of this possibility.

A mean value of 2.9 is far distant from 0. Suppose it belongs to H0. Only 5% of the H0 trials have their means >2.1 SEMs distant from 0, because the area under the curve (AUC) >2.1 distant from 0 is only 5% of total AUC. Thus, the chance that our mean belongs to H0 is <5%. This is a small chance, and we reject this chance and conclude there is <5% chance to find this result. We, thus, reject the H0 of no difference from 0 at P<0.05. The AUC right from 2.101 (and left from −2.101 as will be soon explained) is called alpha=area of rejection of H0. Our result of 2.9 is far from 2.101. The probability of finding such a result may be a lot smaller than 5%. Table 2.1 shows the t-table that can tell us exactly how small this chance truly is.

The four right-hand columns are trial results expressed in SEM-units distant from 0 (=**also t-values**). The upper row gives the AUC-values right from trial results. The left-hand column presents adjustment for numbers of patients (degrees of freedom (dfs), in our example two samples of 10 gives $(20-2)=18$ dfs).

AUC right from 2.9 means → right from 2.878 means → this AUC<0.01. And so we conclude that our probability not<0.05 but even<0.01. Note: the t-distribution is just an adjustment of the normal distribution, but a bit wider for small samples. With large samples it is identical to the normal distribution. For proportional data always the normal distribution is applied.

Note: Unlike the t-table in the Appendix, the above t-table gives two-tailed=two-sided AUC-values. This means that the left and right end of the frequency distribution are tested simultaneously. A result >2.101 here means both >2.101 and < −2.101. If a result of + 2.101 was tested one sided, the p-value would be 0.025 instead of 0.05 (see t-table "Appendix").

3   The t-Value = Standardized Mean Result of Study

The t-table expresses the mean result of a study in SEM-units. Why does it make sense to express mean results in SEM-units? Consider a cholesterol reducing compound, which reduces plasma cholesterol by $1.7 \, mmol/l \pm 0.4 \, mmol/l$ (mean ± SEM). Is this reduction statistically significant? Unfortunately, there are no statistical tables for plasma cholesterol values. Neither are there tables for blood pressures, body weights, hemoglobin levels etc. The trick is to standardize your result.

$$\text{Mean} \pm \text{SEM} = \frac{\text{Mean}}{\text{SEM}} \pm \frac{\text{SEM}}{\text{SEM}} = t - \text{value} \pm$$

This gives us our test result in SEM-units with an SEM of 1. Suddenly, it becomes possible to analyze every study by using one and the same table, the famous t-table. How do we know that our data follow a normal or t frequency distribution? We have goodness of fit tests (Chap. 42).

How was the t-table made? It was made in an era without pocket calculators, and it was hard work. Try and calculate in three digits the square root of the number 5. The result is between 2 and 3. The final digits are found by a technique called "tightening the data". The result is larger than 2.1, smaller than 2.9. Also larger than 2.2, smaller than 2.8, etc. It will take more than a few minutes to find out the closest estimate of $\sqrt{5}$ in three digits. This example highlights the hard work done by the U.S. Government's Work Project Administration by hundreds of women during the economic depression in the 1930s.

Table 2.1 t-table

df	\multicolumn{4}{c}{Two-tailed P-value (df = degree of freedom)}
	0.1	**0.05**	**0.01**	**0.002**
1	6.314	12.706	63.657	318.31
2	2.920	4.303	9.925	22.326
3	2.353	3.182	5.841	10.213
4	2.132	2.776	4.604	7.173
5	2.015	2.571	4.032	5.893
6	1.943	2.447	3.707	5.208
7	1.895	2.365	3.499	4.785
8	1.860	2.306	3.355	4.501
9	1.833	2.262	3.250	4.297
10	1.812	2.228	3.169	4.144
11	1.796	2.201	3.106	4.025
12	1.782	2.179	3.055	3.930
13	1.771	2.160	3.012	3.852
14	1.761	2.145	2.977	3.787
15	1.753	2.131	2.947	3.733
16	1.746	2.120	2.921	3.686
17	1.740	2.110	2.898	3.646
18	1.734	2.101	2.878	3.610
19	1.729	2.093	2.861	3.579
20	1.725	2.086	2.845	3.552
21	1.721	2.080	2.831	3.527
22	1.717	2.074	2.819	3.505
23	1.714	2.069	2.807	3.485
24	1.711	2.064	2.797	3.467
25	1.708	2.060	2.787	3.450
26	1.706	2.056	2.779	3.435
27	1.701	2.052	2.771	3.421
28	1.701	2.048	2.763	3.408
29	1.699	2.045	2.756	3.396
30	1.697	2.042	2.750	3.385
40	1.684	2.021	2.704	3.307
60	1.671	2.000	2.660	3.232
120	1.658	1.950	2.617	3.160
∞	1.645	1.960	2.576	3.090

4   Unpaired t-Test

So far, we assessed a single mean versus 0, now we will assess two means versus each other. For example, a parallel-group study of two groups tests the effect of two beta-blockers on cardiac output.

	Mean ± SD	$SEM^2 = SD^2/n$
Group 1 (n =10)	5.9 ± 2.4 L/min	5.76/10
Group 2 (n =10)	4.5 ± 1.7 L/min	2.89/10

Calculate: $mean_1 - mean_2 = $ mean difference $= 1.4$

Then calculate pooled $SEM = \sqrt{SEM_1^2 + SEM_2^2} = 0.930$

Note: for SEM of difference: take the square root of the sums of squares of separate SEMs and so reduce analysis of two means and two SEMS to one mean and one SEM. The significance of difference between two unpaired samples of continuous data is assessed by the formula:

$$mean_1 - mean_2 \pm \sqrt{SEM_1^2 + SEM_2^2} = \text{mean difference} \pm \text{pooled SEM}$$

This formula presents again a t-distribution with a new mean and a new SEM, i.e., the mean difference and the pooled SEM. The wider this new mean is distant from zero and the smaller its SEM is, the more likely we are able to demonstrate a true effect or true difference from no effect. The size of the test statistic is calculated as follows.

$$\text{The size of t} = \frac{\text{mean difference}}{\text{pooled SEM}} = 1.4 / 0.930 = 1.505$$

With $n = 20$, and two groups we have $20 - 2 = 18$ degrees of freedom. The t-table shows that a t-value of 1.505 provides a chance of $>5\%$ that the null hypothesis of no effect can be rejected. The null-hypothesis cannot be rejected.

Note: If the standard deviations are very different in size, e.g., if one is twice the other, then a more adequate calculation of the pooled standard error is as follows.

$$\text{Pooled SEM} = \sqrt{\frac{(n_1 - 1)SD_1^2 + (n_2 - 1)SD_2^2}{n_1 + n_2 - 2} \times (\frac{1}{n_1} + \frac{1}{n_2})}$$

The lower graph of Fig. 2.2 is the probability distribution of this t-distribution. H0 (the upper graph) is an identical distribution with mean $= 0$ instead of mean $= mean_1$-$mean_2$ and with SEM identical to the SEM of H1, and is taken as the null- hypothesis in this particular approach. With $n = 20$ (18 dfs) we can accept that 95% of all t-distributions with no significant treatment difference from zero must have their means between -2.101 and $+2.101$ SEMs distant from zero. The chance of finding a mean value of 2.101 SEMs or more distant from 0 is 5% or less (we say $\alpha = 0.05$, where α is the chance of erroneously rejecting the null hypothesis of no effect). This means that we can reject the null-hypothesis of no difference at a probability (P) $= 0.05$. We have 5% chance of coming to this result, if there were no difference between the two samples. We, therefore, conclude that there is a true difference between the effects on cardiac output of the two compounds.

Also the F- and chi-square test reject, similarly to the t-test, reject the null-hypothesis of no treatment effect if the value of the test statistic is larger than would occur in 95% of the cases if the treatment had no effect. At this point we should emphasize that when the test statistic is not big enough to reject the null-hypothesis of no treatment effect, investigators often report no statistically

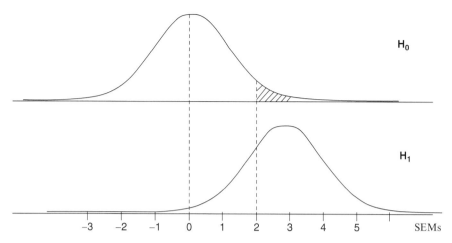

Fig. 2.2 Two t- distributions with n = 20: lower curve *H1* or actual SEM-distribution of the data, upper curve *H0* or null hypothesis of the study

significant difference and discuss their results in terms of documented proof that the treatment had no effect. All they really did, was, fail to demonstrate that it did have an effect. The distinction between positively demonstrating that a treatment had no effect and failing to demonstrate that it does have an effect, is subtle but very important, especially with respect to the small numbers of subjects usually enrolled in a trial. A study of treatments that involves only a few subjects and then fails to reject the null-hypothesis of no treatment effect, may arrive at that conclusion because the statistical procedure lacked power to detect the effect because of a too small sample size, even though the treatment did have an effect. We will address this problem in more detail in Chap. 6.

5   Null-Hypothesis Testing of Three or More Unpaired Samples

If more than two samples are compared, things soon get really complicated, and the unpaired t-test can no longer be applied. Usually, statistical software, e.g., SAS or SPSS Statistical Software, will be used to produce F- or P-values, but the Table 2.2 gives a brief summary of the principles of multiple groups analysis of variance (ANOVA) applied for this purpose. With ANOVA the outcome variable (Hb, hemoglobin-level in the example) is often called the dependent variable, while the groups-variable is called the independent factor (SPSS: Compare means; one-way ANOVA). If additional groups-variables are in the data (gender, age classes, comorbidities), then SPSS requires using the General Linear Model (univariate).

Table 2.2 Multiple groups ANOVA

Unpaired ANOVA 3 groups

Total variation

|

Between group variation   within group variation

In ANOVA:

Variations are expressed as sums of squares (SS) and can be added up to obtain total variation.
Assess whether between-group variation is large compared to within-group variation

Group	n patients	Mean	SD
1	–	–	–
2	–	–	–
3	–	–	–

Grand mean $= (\text{mean } 1+2+3)/3$

$SS_{\text{between groups}} = n\left(\text{mean}_1 - \text{grand mean}\right)^2 + n\left(\text{mean}_2 - \text{grand mean}\right)^2 + \dots$

$SS_{\text{within groups}} = (n-1)SD_1^2 + (n-1)SD_2^2 + \dots\dots$

$$F = \frac{SS \text{ between groups } /dfs}{SS \text{ within groups } / dfs} = MS_{\text{between}} / MS_{\text{within}}$$

F-table gives P-value

Effect of three compounds on Hb

Group	n patients	Mean	SD
1	16	8.7125	0.8445
2	16	10.6300	1.2841
3	16	12.3000	0.9419

Grand mean $= (\text{mean } 1+2+3)/3 = 10.4926$

$SS_{\text{between groups}} = 16(8.7125 - 10.4926)^2 + 16(10.6300 - 10.4926)^2 + \dots$

$SS_{\text{within groups}} = 15 \times 0.8445^2 + 15 \times 1.2841^2 + \dots\dots$

F=49.9 and so P<0.001

Note: In case two groups: ANOVA= unpaired T-test $(F=T^2)$. dfs means degrees of freedom, and
equals $3n-3$ for SS_{within}, and $(3-1)=2$ for SS_{between}

6   Three Methods to Test Statistically a Paired Sample

Table 2.3 gives an example of a placebo-controlled clinical trial to test efficacy of a
sleeping drug.

6.1   First Method

First method is simply calculating the SD of the mean difference d by looking at
the column of differences (d-values) and using the standard formula for variance
between data

Table 2.3 Example of a placebo-controlled clinical trial to test efficacy of a sleeping drug

| Patient | Hours of sleep | | | | |
	Drug	Placebo	Difference	Mean	SS
1	6.1	5.2	0.9	5.7	0.41
2	7.0	7.9	−0.9	7.5	
3	8.2	3.9	4.3		
4	7.6	4.7	2.9		
5	6.5	5.3	1.2		
6	7.8	5.4	3.0		
7	6.9	4.2	2.7		
8	6.7	6.1	0.6		
9	7.4	3.8	3.6		
10	5.8	6.3	−0.5		
Mean	7.06	5.28	1.78		
SD	0.76	1.26	1.77		
Grand mean	6.17				

$$SD_{\text{paired differences}} = \sqrt{\frac{\sum (d - \bar{d})^2}{n-1}} = 1.79$$

Next we find SEM of the mean difference by taking $SD / \sqrt{n} = 0.56$

Mean difference $\pm$ SEM $= 1.78 \pm 0.56$

Similarly to the above unpaired t-test we now can test the null hypothesis of no difference by calculating

$$t = \frac{\text{Mean difference}}{\text{SEM}} = 1.78 / 0.56 = 3.18 \text{ with a sample of 10 (degrees of freedom } = 10 - 1)$$

The t-table shows that P<0.02. We have <2% chance to find this result if there were no difference, and accept that this is sufficient to assume that there is a true difference.

6.2   Second Method

Instead of taking the column of differences we can take the other two columns and use the formula as described in Chap. 1 for calculating the SD of the paired differences $= SD_{\text{paired differrence}}$

$$= \sqrt{(SD_1^2 + SD_2^2 - 2r \cdot SD_1 \cdot SD_2)}$$

$$= \sqrt{(0.76^2 + 1.26^2 - 2r \cdot 0.76_1 \cdot 1.26)}$$

As r can be calculated to be +0.26, we can now conclude that

$$SD_{\text{paired differrence}} = 1.79$$

The remainder of the calculations is as above.

Table 2.4 ANOVA table of these data

Source of variation	Sum of squares (SS)	Degrees of freedom (dfs)	Mean square (MS = SS/dfs)	$F = \dfrac{\text{MS treatment}}{\text{MS residual}}$
Between subjects		2 (m)		F = 10.11, p < 0.02
Within subjects		10 (n × (m − 1))		
Treatments		1 (m − 1)		
Residual		9 (n − 1)		
Total		22		

Fig. 2.3 Paired data laid out in the form of linear regression

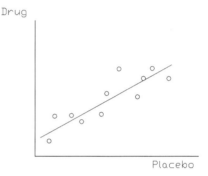

6.3   Third Method

The third method is the F test using analysis of variance (ANOVA). We have to calculate SS (sum of squares) e.g., for subject 1:

$SS_{\text{within subject 1}} = (6.1-5.7)^2 + (5.2-5.7)^2 = 0.41$ (Table 2.3)
grand mean $(7.06 + 5.28)/2 = 6.17$ (Table 2.3)
$SS_{\text{within subject}} = SS_{\text{within subject 1}} + SS_{\text{within subject 2}} + SS_{\text{within subject 3}} + \ldots$
$SS_{\text{treatment}} = (7.06-6.17)^2 + (5.28-6.17)^2$ (Table 2.3)
$SS_{\text{residual}} = SS_{\text{within subject}} - SS_{\text{treatment}}$

The ANOVA table (Table 2.4) shows the procedure. Note m is number of treatments, n is number of patients. The ANOVA is valid not only for two repeated measures but also for multiple repeated measures. For two repeated measures it is actually equal to the paired t-test (= first method). The results of the analysis of the two tests are similar, with F being equal to t^2.

Similarly, for unpaired samples, with two samples the one way ANOVA already briefly mentioned in Chap. 1 is equal to the unpaired t-test, but one-way ANOVA can also be used for multiple unpaired samples.

The above data can also be presented in the form of a linear regression graph.

Paired data can also be laid out in the form of linear regression (Fig. 2.3)

$$y = a + bx \ (\text{effect drug}) = a + b \,(\text{effect placebo})$$

Table 2.5 ANOVA table for the linear regression between paired samples

Source of variation	Sum of squares (SS)	Degrees of freedom (dfs)	Mean square (MS = SS/dfs)	$F = \dfrac{regression}{MS\ residual}$
Regression between samples	1.017	1	1.017	0.61, P > 0.05
Residual	14.027	8	1.753	
Total	15.044	9	1.672	

which can be assessed in the form of ANOVA:

$$F = r^2 = \frac{\text{regression sum of squares}}{\text{total sum of squares}} = \frac{(\sum(x-\bar{x})\,(y-\bar{y}))^2}{\sum(x-\bar{x})^2 \sum(y-\bar{y})^2} = \frac{SP^2 x \cdot y - \text{values}}{SS\ x-\text{values} \cdot SS\ y-\text{values}}$$

SS regression = SP^2 x·y -values / SS x -values
SS total = SS y
SS regression/SS total = r^2
SP indicates sum of products.

The ANOVA table (Table 2.5) gives an alternative interpretation of the correlation coefficient; the square of the correlation coefficient, r, equals the regression sum of squares divided by the total sum of squares ($0.26^2 = 0.0676 = 1.017/15.044$) and, thus, is the proportion of the total variation that has been explained by the regression. We can say that the variances in the drug data are only for 6.76% determined by the variances in the placebo data, and that they are for 93.24% independent of the placebo data. With strong positive correlations, e.g., close to +1 the formula for SD and thus SEM reduces to a very small size (because $[SD_1^2 + SD_2^2 - 2\ r\ SD_1 \cdot SD_2]$ will be close to zero), and the paired t-test produces huge sizes of t and thus huge sensitivity of testing. The above approach cannot be used for estimating significance of differences between two paired samples. And the method in the presented form is not very relevant. It starts, however, to be relevant, if we are interested in the dependency of a particular outcome variable upon several factors. For example, the effect of a drug is better than placebo but this effect still gets better with increased age. This concept can be represented by a multiple regression equation

$$y = a + b_1 x_1 + b_2 x_2$$

which in this example is

$$\text{drug response} = a + b_1 \cdot (\text{placebo response}) + b_2 \cdot (\text{age})$$

Although it is no longer easy to visualize the regression, the principles involved are the same as with linear regression. In the Chaps. 14 and 15 this subject will be dealt with more explicitly.

7 Null-Hypothesis Testing of Three or More Paired Samples

If more than two paired samples are compared, things soon get really complicated, and the paired t-test can no longer be applied. Usually, statistical software (SAS, SPSS) will be used to produce F- and P-values, but the Table 2.6 gives a brief summary of the principles of ANOVA for multiple paired observations, used for this purpose. A more in-depth treatment of repeated measures methods will be given in the Chaps. 54 and 55.

Table 2.6 Repeated measurements ANOVA

Paired ANOVA 3 treatments in single group

```
                              Total variation
                      |                    |
        Between subject variation    Within-subject variation
                      |                              |
            Between treatment variation         Residual variation
```

Variations expressed as sums of squares (SS) and can be added up

Assess whether between treatment variation is large compared to residual variation

Subject	Treatment 1	Treatment 2	Treatment 3	SD^2
1	–	–	–	–
2	–	–	–	–
3	–	–	–	–
4	–	–	–	–
Treatment mean	–	–	–	

Grand mean = (treatment mean $1 + 2 + 3$)$/ 3$ = …..

$$SS_{within\ subject} = SD_1^2 + SD_2^2 + SD_3^2 + \ldots$$

$$SS_{treatment} = \left(treatment\ mean\ 1 - grand\ mean\right)^2 + \left(treatment\ mean\ 2 - grand\ mean\right)^2 + \ldots..$$

$$SS_{residual} = SS_{within\ subject} - SS_{treatment}$$

$$F = \frac{SS_{treatment}\ /dfs}{SS_{residual}\ /\ dfs}$$

F table gives P-value.

Effect of three treatments on vascular resistance (blood pressure/cardiac output)

Person	Treatment 1	Treatment 2	Treatment 3	SD^2
1	22.2	5.4	10.6	147.95
2	17.0	6.3	6.2	77.05
3	14.1	8.5	9.3	18.35
4	17.0	10.7	12.3	21.4
Treatment mean	17.58	7.73	9.60	

Grand mean = 11.63   (continued)

Table 2.6   (continued)

$$SS_{within\ subj} = 147.95 + 77.05 + ...$$

$$SS_{treatment} = (17.58 - 11.63)^2 + (7.73 - 11.63)^2 + ...$$

$$SS_{residual} = SS_{within\ subject} - SS_{treatment}$$

F = 18.2 and so P < 0.025

Note: in case of two treatments: repeated measurements-ANOVA produces the same result as the paired t-test (F=t^2), dfs=degrees of freedom equals $(3-1)=2$ for $SS_{treatment}$, and $(4-1)=3$ for $SS_{residual}$

Table 2.7   ANOVA compares multiple cells with means, and can be classified in several ways

(1) One-way		Two-way			
Mean blood pressure		Mean results of treatments 1–3			
Group 1	......(SD...)		1	2	3
Group 2	......	Males	...	...	...
Group 3	......	Females	...	...	...
(2) Unpaired data		Unpaired data/paired data			
(3) With replication		With replication/without replication			
(4) Balanced/unbalanced		Balanced/unbalanced			

8   Null-Hypothesis Testing with Complex Data

ANOVA is briefly addressed in the above Sects. 6 and 7. It is a powerful method for the analysis of complex data, and will be addressed again in many of the following chapters of this book. ANOVA compares mean values of multiple cells, and can be classified in several manners: (1) one-way or two-way (Table 2.7, left example gives one-way ANOVA with three cells, right example two-way ANOVA with six cells), (2) unpaired or paired data, if the cells contain either non-repeated or repeated data (otherwise called repeated measures ANOVA), (3) data with or without replication, if the cells contain either multiple data or a single datum, (4) balanced or unbalanced, if the cells contains equal or differing numbers of data.

Sometimes samples consist of data that are partly repeated and partly non-repeated. For example, ten patients measured ten times produces a sample of n = 100. It is not appropriate to include this sample in an ANOVA-model as either entirely repeated or non-repeated. It may be practical, then, to use the means per patient as a summary measure without accounting its standard deviation, and perform simple tests using the summary measures per patient only. Generally, the simpler the statistical test the more statistical power.

9   Paired Data with a Negative Correlation

Not only crossover but also parallel-group studies often include an element of self-controlling. For example, observations before, during, and after treatment are frequently used as the main control on experimental variation. Such repeated measures will generally have a positive correlation: those who respond well during the first observation are more likely to do so in the second. This is, however, not necessarily so. When drugs of completely different classes are compared, patients may fall apart into different populations: those who respond better to one and those who respond better to the other drug. For example, patients with angina pectoris, hypertension, arrhythmias, chronic obstructive pulmonary disease, unresponsive to one class of drugs, may respond very well to a different class of drugs. This situation gives rise to a negative correlation in a paired comparison. Other examples of negative correlations between paired observations include the following. A negative correlation between subsequent observations in one subject may occur, because fast-responders are more likely to stop responding earlier. A negative correlation may exist in the patient characteristics of a trial, e.g., between age and vital lung capacity, and in outcome variables of a trial, e.g., between severity of heart attack and ejection fraction. Negative correlations in a paired comparison reduce the sensitivity not only of studies testing differences but also of studies testing equivalences (Chap. 4).

9.1   Studies Testing Significance of Differences

Figure 2.4 gives a hypothesized example of three studies: the left graph shows a parallel-group study of ten patients, the middle and right graph show self-controlled studies of five patients each tested twice. T-statistics is employed according to the formula

$$t = \frac{\overline{d}}{SE}$$

Where $\overline{d}$ is the mean difference between the two sets of data $(6-3=3)$ and the standard error (SE) of this difference is calculated for the left graph data according to

$$\sqrt{\frac{SD_1^2}{n_1} + \frac{SD_2^2}{n_2}} = 0.99$$

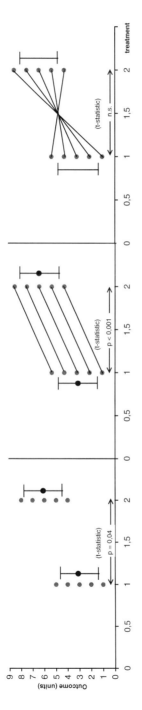

Fig. 2.4 Hypothesized examples of three studies: *left* graph parallel-group study of ten patients, *middle* and *right* graphs self-controlled studies of five patients each tested twice

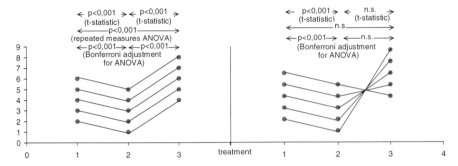

Fig. 2.5 Hypothesized example of two studies where five patients are tested three times. Due to negative correlation between treatment 2 and 3 in the right study, the statistical significance test is negative unlike the left graph study, despite the identical mean results

SD_1 and SD_2 are standard deviations and n_1 and n_2 are numbers of observations in each of the groups. We assume that $n_1 = n_2 = n$.

$$t = 3 / 0.99 = 3.0$$

With ten observations we can reject the null-hypothesis at $p = 0.04$.

With a positively paired comparison (middle graph) we have even more sensitivity. SE is calculated slightly different

$$SE = \frac{\sqrt{\sum (d - \bar{d})^2 / (n-1)}}{\sqrt{n}} = 0$$

where d is the observed change in each individual and $\bar{d}$ is its mean.

$$t = \bar{d} / SE = 3 / 0 = \infty$$

with $n = 5$ we can reject the null-hypothesis at $p < 0.001$.

The right graph gives the negative correlation situation. SE calculated similarly to the middle graph data is 1.58, which means that

$$t = 3 / 1.58 = 1.89$$

The null-hypothesis of no difference cannot be rejected. Differences are not significant (n.s.).

When more than two treatments are given to one sample of patients t-statistics is not appropriate and should be replaced by analysis of variance.

Figure 2.5 gives a hypothesized example of two studies where five patients are tested three times. In the left graph the correlation between treatment responses is positive, whereas in the right graph the correlation between treatment no.3 and no.2 is strong negative rather than positive. For the left graph data repeated measures ANOVA is performed.

Table 2.8 ANOVA table of the data

Source of variation	SS	dfs	MS
Within subjects	23.35	10	
Treatments	23.35	2	11.68
Residual	0	8	0

$$F = \frac{MS_{treatments}}{MS_{residual}} = \infty \qquad p < 0.001$$

The sum of squares (SS) of the different treatments is calculated according to

Patient	Treatment 1	Treatment 2	Treatment 3	Mean	SD^2
1	6	5	8	6.3	4.67
2	5	4	7	5.3	4.67
3	4	3	6	4.3	4.67
4	3	2	5	3.3	4.67
5	2	1	4	2.3	4.67
Treatment mean	4	3	6		

Grand mean 4.3

$SS_{within\ subjects} = 4.67 + 4.67 + \ldots = 23.3$

$SS_{treatments} = 5\ [(4-4.3)^2 + (3-4.3)^2 + (6-4.3)^2] = 23.35$

$SS_{residual} = SS_{within\ subjects} - SS_{treatments} = 0$

This analysis permits concluding that at least one of the treatments produces a change. To isolate which one, we need to use a multiple-comparisons procedure, e.g., the modified Bonferroni t-test for ANOVA where "$SE^2 = \Sigma(d-\bar{d})^2 / (n-1)$" is replaced with "$MS_{residual}$" (Table 2.8). So, to compare, e.g., treatment no. 2 with treatment no. 3

$$t = \frac{6-3}{\sqrt{(MS_{residual})/n}} = \infty \qquad p < 0.001$$

Of the right graph from Fig. 2.5 a similar analysis is performed.

Patients	Treatment 1	Treatment 2	Treatment 3	Mean	SD^2
1	6	5	4	5.0	1.0
2	5	4	5	4.7	0.67
3	4	3	6	4.3	4.67
4	3	2	7	4.0	14.0
5	2	1	8	3.7	28.49
Treatment mean	4	3	6		

Grand mean 4.3

$SS_{within\ subjects} = 1.0 + 0.67 + 4.67 + \ldots = 48.83$

$SS_{treatments} = 5\ [(4-4.3)^2 + (3-4.3)^2 + (6-4.3)^2] = 23.35$

$SS_{residual} = SS_{within\ subjects} - SS_{treatments} = 48.83 - 23.35 = 24.48$

Table 2.9 ANOVA table of
the data

Source of variation	SS	DF	MS
Within subjects	48.83	10	
Treatments	23.35	2	11.7
Residual	24.48	8	3.1

$$F = \frac{MS_{treatments}}{MS_{residual}} = 3.77 \qquad p = 0.20$$

This analysis does not permit concluding that one of the treatments produces a change (Table 2.9). The Bonferroni adjustment of treatments no. 2 and no. 3 of course, does not either (p=0.24 and p=0.34).

In conclusion, with negative correlations between treatment responses statistical methods including paired t-statistics, repeated measures ANOVA, and Bonferroni adjustments for ANOVA lack sensitivity to demonstrate significant treatment effects. The question why this is so, is not difficult to recognize. With t-statistics and a negative correlation between-patient-variation is almost doubled by taking paired differences. With ANOVA things are similar.

$SS_{within\ subjects}$ are twice the size of the positive correlation situation while $SS_{treatments}$ are not different. It follows that the positive correlation situation provides a lot more sensitivity to test than the negative correlation situation.

9.2   Studies Testing Equivalence

In an equivalence trial the conventional significance test has little relevance: failure to detect a difference does not imply equivalence, and a difference, which is detected may not have any clinical relevance and, thus, may not correspond to clinically relevant equivalence. In such trials the range of equivalence is usually predefined as an interval from −D to+D distant from a difference of 0. D is often set equal to a difference of undisputed clinical importance, and hence may be above the minimum of clinical interest by a factor two or three. The bioequivalence study design essentially tests both equivalence and superiority/inferiority. Let us assume that in an equivalence trial of vasodilators for Raynaud's phenomenon ten patients are treated with vasodilator 1 for one week and for a separate period of one week with vasodilator 2. The data below show the numbers of Raynaud attacks per week (Table 2.10).

Although samples have identical means and SEMs (25 ± 3.16 x-axis, 30 ± 3.16 y-axis) their correlation coefficients range from −1 to +1. The null hypothesis of no equivalence is rejected when the 95% CIs are entirely within the prespecified range of equivalence, in our case defined as between −10 and +10.

In the left trial 95% CIs are between −9.5 and +19.5, and thus the null hypothesis of no equivalence cannot be rejected. In the middle trial 95% CI are between −1.3 and 11.3, while in the right trial 95% CI are between −3.3 and 6.7. This means that the last trial has a positive outcome: equivalence is demonstrated, the null hypothesis of no equivalence can be rejected. The negative correlation trial and the zero

Table 2.10 Correlation levels and their influence on sensitivity of statistical tests

ρ=−1 Vasodilator			ρ=0 Vasodilator			ρ=+1 vasodilator		
One	Two	Paired differences	One	Two	Paired differences	One	Two	Paired differences
45	10	35	45	40	5	10	10	0
40	15	25	40	35	5	20	15	5
40	15	25	40	35	5	25	15	10
35	20	15	35	30	5	25	20	5
30	25	5	30	25	5	30	25	5
30	25	5	30	10	20	30	25	5
25	30	−5	25	15	10	35	30	5
25	35	−10	25	15	10	40	35	5
20	35	−15	20	20	0	40	35	5
10	40	−30	10	25	−15	40	40	5
Means								
30	25	5	30	25	5	30	25	5
SEMs								
3.16	3.16	6.46	3.16	3.16	2.78	3.16	3.16	0.76
t-values								
0.8			1.8			6.3		
95% CIs								
±14.5			±6.3			± 1.7		

SEM = standard error of the mean;

t means level of t according to t-test for paired differences;

CI means confidence interval calculated according to critical t value of t-distribution for 10−1 pairs = 9 degrees of freedom (critical t = 2.26, 95% CI = 2.26 x SEM);

ρ = correlation coefficient (the Greek letter is often used instead of r if we mean total population instead of our sample)

correlation trial despite a small mean difference between the two treatments, are not sensitive to reject the null-hypothesis, and this is obviously so because of the wide confidence intervals associated with negative and zero correlations.

10 Rank Testing

Non-parametric tests are an alternative for ANOVA or t-tests when the data do not have a normal distribution. In that case the former tests are more sensitive than the latter. They are quick and easy, and are based on ranking of data in their order of magnitude. With heavily skewed data this means that we make the distribution of the ranks look a little bit like a normal distribution. We have paired and unpaired non-parametric tests and with the paired test the same problem of loss of sensitivity with negative correlations is encountered as the one we observed with the paired normality tests as discussed in the preceding paragraph. Non-parametric tests are

Table 2.11 Paired comparison using Wilcoxon signed rank test: placebo-controlled clinical trial to test efficacy of sleeping drug

Hours of sleep				Rank
Patient	Drug	Placebo	Difference	(Ignoring sign)
1	6.1	5.2	0.9	3.5[a]
2	7.0	7.9	−0.9	3.5
3	8.2	3.9	4.3	10
4	7.6	4.7	2.9	7
5	6.5	5.3	1.2	5
6	8.4	5.4	3.0	8
7	6.9	4.2	2.7	6
8	6.7	6.1	0.6	2
9	7.4	3.8	3.6	9
10	5.8	6.3	−0.5	1

[a]number 3 and 4 in the rank are duplicate outcome values, otherwise called ties, so we use 3.5 for both of them

also used to test normal distributions, and provide hardly different results from their parametric counterparts when distributions are approximately normal. Most frequently used tests:

For paired comparisons:

Wilcoxon signed rank test = **paired Wilcoxon** test

For unpaired comparisons:

Mann – Whitney test = **Wilcoxon rank sum** test

10.1   Paired Test: Wilcoxon Signed Rank Test

The Wilcoxon signed rank test uses the signs and the relative magnitudes of the data instead of the actual data (Table 2.11). For example, the above table shows the number of hours sleep in ten patients tested twice: with sleeping pill and with placebo. We have three steps:

1. exclude the differences that are zero, put the remaining differences in ascending order of magnitude and ignore their sign and give them a rank number 1, 2, 3 etc (if differences are equal, average their rank numbers: 3 and 4 become 3.5 and 3.5);
2. add up the positive differences as well as the negative differences;
   + ranknumbers = 3.5 + 10 + 7 + 5 + 8 + 6 + 2 + 9 = 50.5
   − ranknumbers = 3.5 + 1 = 4.5
3. The null hypothesis is that there is no difference between + and − ranknumbers. We assess the smaller of the two ranknumbers. The test is significant if the value is smaller than could be expected by chance. We consult the Wilcoxon signed rank

Table 2.12 Two-samples of patients are treated with two different NSAIDs

Globulin concentration (g/l)	Rank number
26	1
27	**2**
28	**3**
29	4
30	5
31	6
32	7
33	8
34	**9**
35	10
36	11
38	12.5
38	**12.5**
39	**14.5**
39	**14.5**
40	**16**
41	17
42	**18**
45	**19.5**
45	**19.5**

Outcome variable is plasma globulin concentration (g/l). Sample one is printed in standard and sample two is printed in fat print

table showing us the upper values for 5%, and 1% significance, for the number of differences constituting our rank. In this example we have ten ranks: 5% and 1% points are respectively 8 and 3 (Wilcoxon table). The result is significant at P<0.05, indicating that the sleeping drug is more effective than the placebo.

10.2   Unpaired Test: Mann-Whitney Test

Table 2.12 shows two-samples of patients are treated with two different NSAID agents. Outcome variable is plasma globulin concentration (g/l). Sample one is printed in standard and sample two is printed in fat print.

We have two steps (Table 2.12):

1. The data from both samples are ranked together in ascending order of magnitude. Equal values are averaged.
2. Add up the rank numbers of each of the two samples. In sample-one we have 81.5, in sample-two we have 128.5. We now can consult the Table for Mann-Whitney tests and find with n = 10 and n = 10 (differences in sample sizes are no problem) that the smaller of the two sums of ranks should be smaller than 71 in order to conclude P<0.05 (Mann-Whitney table). We can therefore not reject the null hypothesis of no difference, and have to conclude that the two samples are not significantly different from each other.

11 Rank Testing for Three or More Samples

11.1 The Friedman Test for Paired Observations

The Friedman test is used for comparing three or more repeated measures that are not normally distributed, and is an extension of the Wilcoxon signed rank test. An example is given in Table 2.13. The data are ranked for each patient in ascending order of hours of sleep. If the hours are equal, then an average ranknumber is given. Then, for each treatment the squared ranksum is calculated: for dose 1 it equals $(2+1.5+2+2+2+3+2+2+2+1.5)^2 = 400$, for dose 2 it is 676, for placebo it is 196. The following equation is used:

$$\text{chi - square} = \frac{12}{nk(k+1)} \left(\text{ranksum}^2_{\text{dose1}} + \text{ranksum}^2_{\text{dose2}} + \text{ranksum}^2_{\text{placebo}} \right) - 3n(k+1)$$

where n = the number of patients and k = the number of treatments.

The chi-square value is calculated to be 7.2. The chi-square statistic will be addressed in Chap. 3. Briefly, it works very similar to the t-statistics. Chi-square values larger than the ones given in the chi-square table in the Appendix indicate that the null-hypothesis of no difference in the data can be rejected. In this example the calculated chi-square value is larger than the rejection chi-square for (3−1) degrees of freedom at p = 0.05, and, therefore, we conclude that there is a significant difference between the three treatments at p < 0.05. Post-hoc subgroups analyses (using Wilcoxon's tests) are required to find out exactly where the difference is situated, between group 1 and 2, between group 1 and 3, or between group 2 and 3 or between two or more groups. The subject of post-hoc testing will be further discussed in the Chaps. 8 and 19.

Table 2.13 Paired comparison to test efficacy of two dosages of a sleeping drug versus placebo on hours of sleep

| Patient | Hours of sleep | | | | | |
| | Dose 1 | Dose 2 | Placebo | Dose 1 | Dose 2 | Placebo |
	(hours)			(ranks)		
1	6.1	6.8	5.2	2	3	1
2	7.0	7.0	7.9	1.5	1.5	3
3	8.2	9.0	3.9	2	3	1
4	7.6	7.8	4.7	2	3	1
5	6.5	6.6	5.3	2	3	1
6	8.4	8.0	5.4	3	2	1
7	6.9	7.3	4.2	2	3	1
8	6.7	7.0	6.1	2	3	1
9	7.4	7.5	3.8	2	3	1
10	5.8	5.8	6.3	1.5	1.5	3

Table 2.14 Three-samples of patients are treated with placebo or two different NSAIDs

Globulin concentration (g/l)	Rank number
−17	*1*
−16	*2*
−5	*3*
−3	*4*
−2	5
16	*6*
18	*7*
26	8
27	**9**
28	*10.5*
28	**10.5**
29	12
30	14
30	*14*
30	*14*
31	16
32	17
33	18
34	**19**
35	20
36	21
38	22.5
38	**22.5**
39	**24.5**
39	**24.5**
40	**26**
41	27
42	**28**
45	**29.5**
45	**29.5**

The outcome variable is the fall in plasma globulin concentration (g/l). Group 1 patients are printed in italics, group 2 in normal standard and group 3 in fat standard print

11.2   The Kruskall-Wallis Test for Unpaired Observations

The Kruskall-Wallis test compares multiple groups that are unpaired and not normally distributed, and is an extension of the Mann-Whitney test. Three groups of patients with rheumatoid arthritis are treated with a placebo or one of two different NSAIDS (Table 2.14). The fall in plasma globulin (g/l) is used to estimate the effect of treatments. First, we give a ranknumber to every patient dependent on his/her magnitude of fall. If two or three patients have the dame fall, they are given an average ranknumber. Then, we calculate the sum of the ranks for the three groups.

For group 1 this amounts to $1+2+3+4+5+6+7+10.5+14+14=66.5$, for group 2–175.5, group 3–488.5. Then we use the equation:

$$\text{chi - square} = \frac{12}{30\,(30-1)} \left(\frac{\text{ranksum}^2_{\text{group1}}}{10} + \frac{\text{ranksum}^2_{\text{group2}}}{10} + \frac{\text{ranksum}^2_{\text{group3}}}{10} \right) - 3(30-1)$$

where the number 30 equals all values, 10 the patient number per group.

The chi-square equals 7744.3. The chi-square statistic will be further addressed in Chap. 3. It works very similar to the t-statistics. Briefly, chi-square values larger than the ones given in the chi-square table in the Appendix indicate that the null-hypothesis of no difference in the data can be rejected. In this example the calculated chi-square value is much larger than the rejection chi-square for $(3-1)$ degrees of freedom and, therefore, we conclude that there is a significant difference between the three treatments at $p < 0.001$. Post-hoc subgroups analyses (using Man-Whitney tests) are required to find out exactly where the difference is situated, between group 1 and 2, between group 1 and 3, or between group 2 and 3 or between two or more groups. The subject post-hoc testing will be further discussed in Chap. 8.

12   Conclusions

For the analysis of efficacy data we test null-hypotheses. The t-test is appropriate for two parallel-groups or two paired samples. Analysis of variance (ANOVA) is appropriate for analyzing more than two groups/treatments. For data that do not follow a normal frequency distribution non-parametric tests are available: for paired data the Wilcoxon signed rank or Friedman tests, for unpaired data the Mann-Whitney test or Kruskall-Wallis tests are adequate.

Note: In the references (1–20) an overview of relevant textbooks on the above subjects is given.

References

1. Bailar JC, Mosteller F (1986) Medical uses of statistics. N Engl J Med Books, Waltham
2. Campbell MJ (2006) Statistics at square two. BMJ Books/Blackwell Publishing, New Delhi
3. Cohen A, Posner J (1995) Clinical drug research. Kluwer Academic Publishers, Dordrecht
4. De Vocht A (1998) SPSS basic guide book. Bijleveld Press, Amsterdam
5. Field A (2005) Discovering statistics using SPSSD, 2nd edn. Sage Publications, Thousand Oaks
6. Glantz SA (1992) Primer of biostatistics. McGraw-Hill, Singapore
7. Glaser AN (2001) High yield statistics. Lippincott Williams & Wilkins, Baltimore
8. Hays WL (1988) Statistics. Holt, Rine and Winston, Toronto
9. Kirkwood BR (1990) Medical statistics. Blackwell Scientific Publications, Boston
10. Kuhlmann J, Mrozikiewicz A (1998) What should a clinical pharmacologist know to start a clinical trial? Zuckschwerdt Verlag, Munich

11. Lu Y, Fang JQ (2003) Advanced medical statistics. World Scientific, River Edge
12. Matthews DE, Farewell VT (1996) Using and understanding medical statistics. Karger, Melbourne
13. Motulsky H (1995) Intuitive statistics. Oxford University Press, New York
14. Peat J, Barton B (2005) Medical statistics, 5th edn. BMJ Books/Blackwell Publishing, New Delhi
15. Petrie A, Sabin C (2000a) Medical statistics at a glance. Blackwell Science, London
16. Petrie A, Sabin C (2000b) Medical statistics at a glance. Blackwell Science, Malden
17. Riegelman RK (2005) Studying a study and testing a test, 5th edn. Lippincott Williams & Wilkins, Philadelphia
18. Riffenburgh RH (1999) Statistics in medicine. Academic, New York
19. Swinscow TD (1996) Statistics at square one. BMJ Publishing Group, London
20. Utts JM (1999) Seeing through statistics. Brooks Cole Company, Pacific Grove

Chapter 3
The Analysis of Safety Data

1 Introduction, Summary Display

As discussed in Chap. 1 the primary object of clinical trials of new drugs is generally to demonstrate efficacy rather than safety. However, a trial in human beings not at the same time adequately addressing safety is unethical, and the assessment of safety variables is an important element of the trial.

An effective approach to the analysis of adverse effects is to present summaries of prevalences. We give an example (Table 3.1). Calculations of the 95% confidence intervals (CIs) of a proportion are demonstrated in Chap. 1. If $0.1 <$ proportion $(p) < 0.9$, then the binomial distribution is very close to the normal distribution, but if $p < 0.1$, the data follow a skewed, otherwise called Poisson distribution. 95% CIs are, then, more adequately calculated according to $\pm 1.96 \sqrt{p/n}$

$$\text{rather than} \pm 1.96 \sqrt{p(1-p)/n}$$

(confer page 9). Alternatively, tables (e.g., Wissenschaftliche Tabelle, Documenta Geigy, Basel, 1995) and numerous statistical software packages can readily provide you with the CIs.

Table 3.1 gives an example. The numbers in the table relate to the numbers of patients showing a particular side effect. Some questions were not answered by all patients. Particularly, sleepiness occurred differently in the two groups: 33% in the left, 60% in the right group. This difference may be true or due to chance. In order to estimate the size of probability that this difference occurred merely by chance we can perform a statistical test which in case of proportions such as here has to be a chi-square or given the small data a Fisher exact test. We should add at this point that although mortality/morbidity may be an adverse event in many trials, there are also trials that use them as primary variables. This is particularly so with mortality trials in oncology and cardiology research. For the analysis of these kinds of trials the underneath methods of assessments are also adequate.

T.J. Cleophas and A.H. Zwinderman, *Statistics Applied to Clinical Studies*, DOI 10.1007/978-94-007-2863-9_3, © Springer Science+Business Media B.V. 2012

Table 3.1 The prevalence of side-effects after 8 week treatment

| | Alpha blocker | | | Beta blocker | | |
| | n = 16 | | | n = 15 | | |
Side effect	Yes	No	95% CIs (%)	Yes	No	95% CIs (%)
Nasal congestion	10	6	35–85	10	5	38–88
Alcohol intolerance	2	12	2–43	2	13	4–71
Urine incontinence	5	11	11–59	5	10	12–62
Disturbed ejaculation	4	2	22–96	2	2	7–93
Disturbed potence	4	2	22–96	2	2	7–93
Dry mouth	8	8	25–75	11	4	45–92
Tiredness	9	7	30–80	11	4	45–92
Palpitations	5	11	11–59	2	13	2–40
Dizziness at rest	4	12	7–52	5	10	12–62
Dizziness with exercise	8	8	25–75	12	3	52–96
Orthostatic dizziness	8	8	25–75	10	5	38–88
Sleepiness	5	10	12–62	9	6	32–84

2   Four Methods to Analyze Two Unpaired Proportions

Many methods exists to analyze two unpaired proportions, like odds ratios analysis (this chapter) and logistic regression (Chap. 14), but here we will start by presenting the four most common methods for that purpose. Using the sleepiness data from above we construct a 2×2 contingency table:

	Sleepiness	No sleepiness
Left treatment (left group)	5 (a)	10 (b)
Right treatment (right group)	9 (c)	6 (d)

2.1   Method 1

We can test significance of difference similarly to the method used for testing continuous data (Chap. 2). In order to do so we first have to find the standard deviation (SD) of a proportion. The SD of a proportion is given by the formula $\sqrt{p(1-p)}$. Unlike the SD for continuous data (see formula Chap. 1), it is strictly independent of the sample size. It is not easy to prove why this formula is correct. However, it may be close to the truth considering an example (Fig. 3.1). Many samples of 15 patients are assessed for sleepiness. The proportion of sleepy people in the population is 10 out of every 15. Thus, in a representative sample from this population ten sleepy patients will be the number most frequently encountered. It also is the mean proportion, and left and right from this mean proportion proportions grow gradually smaller, according to a binomial distribution (which becomes normal distribution

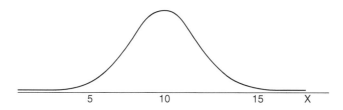

Fig. 3.1 Frequency distribution of numbers of sleepy people observed in multiple samples of 15 patients from the same population

with large samples). Figure 3.1 shows that the chance of eight or fewer sleepy patients is 15% (area under the curve, AUC, left from $8.3 = 15\%$). The chance of six or less sleepy patients is 2.5% (AUC left from $6.6 = 2.5\%$). The chance of five or less sleepy patients $= 1\%$. This is a so-called binomial frequency distribution with mean 10 and a standard deviation of $p(1-p) = 10/15(1-5/15) = 1.7$. -1SD means AUC of approximately 15%, -2SDs means AUC of approximately 2.5%. And, so, according to the curve below $SD = p(1-p)$ is close to the truth.

Note:For null-hypothesis-testing standard error (SE) rather than SD is required, and $SE = SD/\sqrt{n}$.

For testing we use the normal test (= z-test for binomial or binary data) which looks very much like the T-test for continuous data. $T = d/SE$, $z = d/SE$, where $d = $ mean difference between two groups or difference of proportions and SE is the pooled SE of this difference. What we test is, whether this ratio is larger than approximately 2 (1.96 for proportions, a little bit more, e.g., 2.1 or so, for continuous data).

Example of *continuous* data (testing two means).

	Mean ± SD	$SEM^2 = SD^2/n$
Group 1 (n=10)	5.9±2.4 l/min	5.76/10
Group 2 (n=10)	4.5±1.7 l/min	2.89/10

Calculate: $mean_1 - mean_2 = 1.4$.
Then calculate pooled $SEM = \sqrt{(SEM_1^2 + SEM_2^2)} = 0.930$.

Note:For SEM of difference: take square root of sums of squares of separate SEMs and, so, reduce the analysis of two means to one of a single mean.

$$T = \frac{mean_1 - mean_2}{Pooled\ SEM} = 1.4/0.930 = 1.505,\ \text{with degrees of freedom (dfs)}$$

18, [*]$p > 0.05$.

Example of *proportional* data (testing two proportions).

---

[*] We have two groups of n = 10 which means $2 \times 10 - 2 = 18$ dfs.

2×2 table	Sleepiness	No sleepiness
Left treatment (left group)	5	10
Right treatment (right group)	9	6

$$z = \frac{\text{difference between proportions of sleepers per group (d)}}{\text{pooled standard error difference}}$$

$$z = \frac{d}{\text{pooled SE}} = \frac{(9/15 - 5/15)}{\sqrt{(SE_1^2 + SE_2^2)}}$$

$$SE_1 \ (\text{or } SEM_1) = \sqrt{\frac{p_1(1-p_1)}{n_1}} \text{ where } p_1 = 5/15 \text{ etc.........,}$$

$z = 1.45$, not statistically significant from zero, because for a $p < 0.05$ a z-value of at least 1.96 is required.

Note: The z-test uses the bottom row of the t-table (see Appendix), because, unlike continuous data that follow a t-distribution, proportional data follow a normal distribution. The z-test is improved by inclusion of a continuity correction. For that purpose the term $-(1/2n_1 + 1/2n_2)$ is added to the denominator where n_1 and n_2 are the sample sizes. The reason is that a continuous distribution is used to approximate a proportional distribution which is discrete, in this case binomial.

2.2   Method 2

According to some a more easy way to analyze proportional data is the chi-square test. The chi-square test assumes that the data follow a chi-square frequency distribution which can be considered the square of a normal distribution (see also Chap. 41). First some philosophical considerations.

Repeated observations have both (1) a central tendency, and (2) a tendency to depart from an expected overall value, often the mean. In order to make predictions an index is needed to estimate the departures from the mean. Why not simply add up departures? However, this doesn't work, because, with normal frequency distributions, the add-up sum is equal to 0. A pragmatic solution chosen is taking the add-up sum of (departures)^2 = the variance of a data sample. Means/proportions follow normal frequency distributions, variances follow **(normal-distribution)^2**. The normal distribution is a biological rule used for making predictions from random samples.

With a normal frequency distribution in your data (Fig. 3.2 upper graph) you can test whether the mean of your study is significantly different from 0.

Fig. 3.2 Normal and
chi-square frequency
distributions

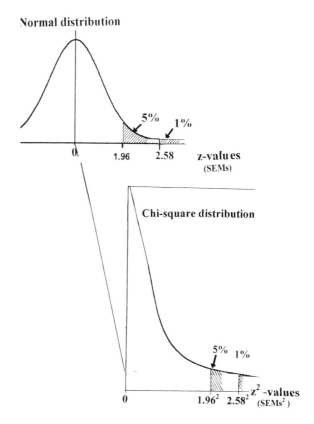

If the mean result of your study > approximately 2 SEMs distant from 0, then we have <5% chance of no difference from 0, and we are entitled to reject the 0 hypothesis of no difference.

With (normal frequency distributions)² (Fig. 3.2 lower graph) we can test whether the variance of our study is significantly different from 0. If the variance of our study is $>1.96^2$ distant from 0, then we have <5% chance of no difference from 0, and we are entitled to reject the 0-hypothesis of no difference.

The chi-square test, otherwise called χ^2 test can be used for the analysis of two unpaired proportions (2×2 table), but first we give a simpler example, a 1×2 table

Sleepy	Not-sleepy	Sleepy	Not-sleepy
Observed (O)		Expected from population (E)	
a (n=5)	b (n=10)	α (n=10)	β (n=5)

We wish to assess whether the observed proportion is significantly different from the established population data from this population, called the expected proportion?

$$O - E =$$
$$a - \alpha = 5 - 10 = -5$$
$$b - \beta = 10 - 5 = \frac{5+}{0} \quad \text{doesn't work}$$

The above method to assess a possible difference between the observed and expected data does not work. Instead, we take square values.

$$(a - \alpha)^2 = 25 \quad \text{divide by } \alpha \text{ to standardize} = 2.5$$
$$(b - \beta)^2 = 25 \quad \text{divide by } \beta \text{ to standardize} = \frac{5+}{7.5}$$

$$\chi^2 \text{ Value} = \text{the add-up variance in data} = 7.5$$

α is the standard error (SE) of $(a - \alpha)^2$ and is used to standardize the data, similarly to the standardization of mean results using the t-statistic (replacing the mean results with t-values, see Chap. 2).

This 1×2 table has 1 degree of freedom. The chi-square table (see Appendix) shows four columns of chi-square values (standardized variances of various studies), an upper row of areas under the curve (AUCs), and a left end column with the degrees of freedom. For finding the appropriate area under the curve (= p-value) of a 1×2 table we need the second row, because it has 1 degree of freedom. A chi-square value of 7.5 means an AUC=p-value of <0.01. The O-hypothesis can be rejected. Our observed proportion is significantly different from the expected proportion.

Slightly more complex is the chi-square test for the underneath table of observed numbers of patients in a random sample:

	Sleepiness(n)	No sleepiness(n)
Left treatment (left group)	5 (a)	10 (b)
Right treatment (right group)	9 (c)	6 (d)

n = numbers of patients in each cell

Commonly, no information is given about the numbers of patients to be expected, and, so, we have to use the best estimate based of the data given. The following procedure is applied:

$$\text{cell a}: (O - E)^2 / E = \left(5 - 14 / 30 \times 15\right)^2 / 14 / 30 \times 15 = ..$$
$$\text{cell b}: (O - E)^2 / E$$
$$\text{cell c}: (O - E)^2 / E$$
$$\text{cell d}: (O - E)^2 / E$$

$$\frac{\qquad\qquad\qquad +}{\text{chi - square} = 2.106}$$

(O = observed number; E = expected number = (proportion sleepers /total number) x number$_{\text{group}}$).

We can reject the 0-hypothesis if the squared distances from expectation > $(1.96)^2 = 3.841$ distant from 0, which is our critical chi-square value required to reject the 0-hypothesis. A chi-square value of only 2.106 means that the 0-hypothesis can not be rejected.

Note: A chi-square distribution = a squared normal distribution. When using the chi-square table, both the 1×2 and the 2×2 contingency tables have only 1 degree of freedom.

2.3   Method 3

Instead of the above calculations to find the chi-square value for a 2×2 contingency table, a simpler pocket calculator method producing exactly the same results is described underneath

	Sleepiness	No sleepiness	Total
Left treatment (left group)	5 (a)	10 (b)	a+b
Right treatment (right group)	9(c)	6 (d)	c+d
	a+c	b+d	

Calculating the chi-square (χ^2) – value is calculated according to:

$$\frac{(ad - bc)^2 (a+b+c+d)}{(a+b)(c+d)(b+d)(a+c)}$$

In our case the size of the chi-square is again 2.106 at 1 degree of freedom which means that the 0-hypothesis of no difference not be rejected. There is no significant difference between the two groups.

2.4   Method 4

Fisher-exact test is used as contrast test for the chi-square or normal test, and also for small samples, e.g., samples of $n < 100$. It, essentially, makes use of faculties expressed as the sign "!": e.g., 5! indicates $5 \times 4 \times 3 \times 2 \times 1$.

	Sleepiness	No sleepiness
Left treatment (left group)	5 (a)	10 (b)
Right treatment (right group)	9 (c)	6 (d)

$$P = \frac{(a+b)!(c+d)!(a+c)!(b+d)!}{(a+b+c+d)! \; a!b!c!d!} = 0.2 \, (\text{much larger than } 0.05)$$

Again, we can not reject the null-hypothesis of no difference between the two groups. This test is laborious but a computer can calculate wide faculties in seconds.

3   Chi-square to Analyze More Than Two Unpaired Proportions

As will be explained in Chap. 41, with chi-square statistics we enter the real world of statistics, because it is used for multiple tables, and it is also the basis of analysis of variance. Large tables of proportional data are more frequently used in business statistics than they are in biomedical research. After all, clinical investigators are, generally, more interested in the comparison between two treatment modalities than they are in multiple comparisons. Yet, e.g., in phase 1 trials multiple compounds are often tested simultaneously. The analysis of large tables is similar to that of the above method-2. For example:

	Sleepiness	No sleepiness
Group I	5 (a)	10 (b)
Group II	9 (c)	6 (d)
Group III	...(e)	...(f)
Group IV	...	
Group V		

cell a: $(O-E)^2 / E =$

b: $(O-E)^2 / E$

c: $(O-E)^2 / E$

d: $(O-E)^2 / E$

e: ..

f: ..

_____+

chi - square value = ..

For cell a $O = 5$

$$E = \frac{(5+9+...)}{(5+10+9+6+...)} x(5+10) \quad \text{etc}$$

Large tables have many degrees of freedom (dfs). For 2×2 cells, we have $(2-1) \times (2-1) = 1 \mathrm{df}$, 5% p-value at chi-square $= 3.841$. For 3×2 cells, we have

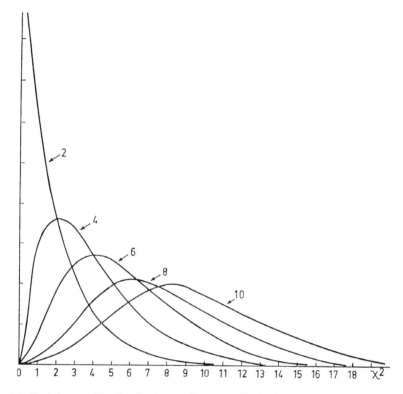

Fig. 3.3 Each degree of freedom has its own frequency distribution curve

$(3-1)\times(2-1)=2$dfs, 5% p-value at chi-square $= 5.991$. For 5×2 cells, we have $(5-1)(2-1)=4$ dfs, 5% p-value at chi-square $= 9.488$. Each degree of freedom has its own frequency distribution curve (Fig. 3.3):

$$dfs\ 2 \Rightarrow p = 0.05\ at\ \chi^2\quad 5.99$$
$$dfs\ 4\quad p = 0.05\ at\ \chi^2\quad 9.49$$
$$dfs\ 6\quad p = 0.05\ at\ \chi^2\quad 12.59$$
$$dfs\ 8\quad p = 0.05\ at\ \chi^2\quad 15.51$$
$$dfs\ 10\quad p = 0.05\ at\ \chi^2\quad 18.31.$$

As an example we give a χ^2 test for 3×2 table

Hypertension	Yes		No	
Group 1	a	n = 60	d	n = 40
Group 2	b	n = 100	e	n = 120
Group 3	c	n = 80	f	n = 60

Give the best estimate of the expected numbers in the cell according to the method described for the 2×2 contingency table above. Per cell: divide hypertensives in study by observations in study, multiply by observations in group. It gives you the best estimate. For cell a this is $\alpha=[(a+b+c)/(a+b+c+d+e+f)]\times(a+d)$. Do the same for each cell and add-up:

$$\alpha = \big[(a+b+c)/(a+b+c+d+e+f)\big]\times(a+d) \quad = \ 52.17$$
$$\beta \ldots \qquad\qquad\qquad\qquad\qquad\qquad\qquad\qquad = 114.78$$
$$\gamma \ldots \qquad\qquad\qquad\qquad\qquad\qquad\qquad\qquad = \ 73.04$$
$$\delta = [(d+e+f))/(a+b+c+d+e+f)]\times(a+d) \quad = \ 47.83$$
$$\varepsilon \ldots \qquad\qquad\qquad\qquad\qquad\qquad\qquad\qquad = \ 57.39$$
$$\xi \ldots \qquad\qquad\qquad\qquad\qquad\qquad\qquad\qquad = \ 66.96$$

$$a-\alpha)^2 / \alpha = 1.175$$
$$(b- \qquad = 1.903$$
$$(c- \qquad = 0.663$$
$$(d- \qquad = 1.282$$
$$(e- \qquad = 68.305$$
$$(f- \qquad = 0.723+$$
$$\chi^2 \text{value} \quad = 72.769$$

The p-value for $(3-1)\times(2-1)=3$ degrees of freedom is <0.001 according to the chi-square table (see Appendix).

Another example is given, a 2×3 table:

Hypertension	Hypertens-yes	Hypertens-no	Don't know
Group 1	(a) n=60	(c) n=40	(e) n=60
Group 2	(b) n=50	(d) n=60	(f) n=50

Give best estimate population. Per cell: divide hypertensives in population by all patients, multiply by hypertensives in group. For cell a this is:

$$\alpha = \big[(a+b)/(a+b+c+d+e+f)\big]\times(a+c+e)$$

Calculate every cell, add-up results.

$$\alpha = [(a+b)/(a+b+c+d+e+f)]\times(a+c+e) = 55.000$$
$$\beta\ldots \qquad\qquad\qquad\qquad\qquad\qquad\qquad = 55.000$$
$$\gamma = [(c+d)/(a+b+c+d+e+f)]\times(a+c+e) = 51.613$$
$$\delta = \ldots \qquad\qquad\qquad\qquad\qquad\qquad\qquad = 51.613$$
$$\varepsilon\ldots \qquad\qquad\qquad\qquad\qquad\qquad\qquad = 55$$
$$\xi\ldots \qquad\qquad\qquad\qquad\qquad\qquad\qquad = 55$$

$$(O-E)^2 / E =$$

$(a-\alpha)^2 / \alpha$	= 0.45
$(b-$	= 0.45
$(c-$	= 0.847
$(d-$	= 1.363
$(e-$	= 0.45
$(f-$	= 0.45 +
χ^2	= 4.01

For $(2-1)\times(3-1)=2$ degrees of freedom our p-value is <0.001 according to the chi-square table (see Appendix).

4   McNemar's Test for Paired Proportions

Paired proportions have to be assessed when e.g. different diagnostic tests are performed in one subject. For example, 315 subjects are tested for hypertension using both an automated device (test-1) and a sphygmomanometer (test-2), (Table 3.2).

184 subjects scored positive with both tests and 63 scored negative with both tests. These 247 subjects therefore give us no information about which of the tests is more likely to score positive. The information we require is entirely contained in the 68 subjects for whom the tests did not agree (the discordant pairs). Table 3.2 shows how the chi-square value is calculated. Here we have again 1 degree of freedom, and so, a chi-square value of 23.5 indicates that the two devised produce significantly different results at $p<0.001$.

To analyze samples of more than two pairs of data, e.g., 3, 4 pairs, etc., McNemar's test can not be applied. For that purpose Cochran's test or logistic regression analysis is adequate (next section).

Table 3.2 Finding discordant pairs

		Test 1		
		+	−	Total
Test 2	+	184	54	238
	−	14	63	77
	Total	198	117	315

$$\text{Chi - square McNemar} = \frac{(54-14)^2}{54+14} = 23.5$$

5   Multiple Paired Binary Data (Cochran's Q Test)

The scientific question of the underneath data is: is there a significant difference between the numbers of responders who have been treated differently three times (Table 3.3).

The above table shows three paired observations in one patient. The paired property of these observations has to be taken into account because of the, generally, positive correlation between paired observations. Cochran's Q test is appropriate for that purpose.

The following commands have to be given in SPSS (www.spss.com).

Command: Analyze – nonparametric tests – k related samples – mark: Cochran's Q – test variables: treatment 1, treatment 2, treatment 3 – ok

Test statistics	
N	139
Cochran's Q	10,133[a]
df	2
Asymp. Sig.	,006

[a] 0 is treated as a success

The test is highly significant with a p-value of 0.006. This means that there is a significant difference between the treatment responses. However, we do not know where: between treatments 1 and 2, 2 and 3, or between 1 and 3. For that purpose three separate McNemar's tests have to be carried out.

Test statistics[a]	
	Treat 1 and Treat 2
N	139
Chi-square[b]	4,379
Asymp. Sig.	,036

Test statistics[a]	
	Treat 1 and Treat 3
N	139
Chi-square[b]	8,681
Asymp. Sig.	,003

Test statistics[a]	
	Treat 2 and Treat 3
N	139
Chi-square[b]	,681
Asymp. Sig.	,409

[a] McNemar test
[b] Continuity corrected

Table 3.3 Responders (1) and non-responders (0) after treatment differently three times (variables 1, 2, and 3)

Variables											
1	2	3	1	2	3	1	2	3	1	2	3
0	0	0	0	1	0	0	1	0	1	0	0
0	0	1	0	0	1	0	0	0	1	0	0
0	0	0	0	1	1	0	0	0	1	0	1
0	0	1	0	1	0	0	1	1	1	0	1
0	0	1	0	0	0	0	0	1	1	1	0
0	0	1	0	1	0	0	1	1	1	1	1
0	0	1	0	0	1	0	0	1	1	1	0
0	0	0	0	1	1	0	0	0	1	1	1
0	1	0	0	0	1	0	0	0	1	0	0
0	1	1	0	1	0	0	1	0	1	0	1
0	1	1	0	1	0	0	1	0	1	0	0
0	0	1	0	0	0	0	1	1	1	0	1
0	1	1	0	0	1	0	0	0	1	1	1
0	0	1	0	0	1	0	0	1	1	0	1
0	1	0	0	1	0	0	0	0	1	1	0
0	0	0	0	1	1	0	1	1	1	0	1
0	1	0	0	1	0	0	0	0	1	1	0
0	0	1	0	0	1	0	1	1	1	1	1
0	0	1	0	0	0	0	0	0	1	0	0
0	0	1	0	1	1	0	0	1	1	0	1
0	0	1	0	1	0	0	1	0	1	1	0
0	1	0	0	0	0	0	0	0	1	1	1
0	0	0	0	1	1	0	1	0	1	0	0
0	1	0	0	0	1	0	0	1	1	0	0
0	0	0	0	1	0	0	1	1	1	1	0
0	0	1	0	0	0	1	0	1	1	1	0
0	0	1	0	0	0	1	0	1	1	0	1
0	0	1	0	0	1	1	1	0	1	0	0
0	1	1	0	1	1	1	1	0	1	1	1
0	1	1	0	1	1	1	1	1	1	1	0
0	1	0	0	0	0	1	0	1	1	0	1
0	1	0	0	0	0	1	1	0	1	0	0
0	0	1	0	1	1	1	0	0	1	1	1
0	0	1	0	1	1	1	1	1	1	1	1
0	0	0	0	1	1	1	1	1	1	0	0
									1	0	0

Var 1 = responder to treatment 1 (yes or no, 1 or 0) (Var = variable)
Var 2 = responder to treatment 2
Var 3 = responder to treatment 3

The above three separate McNemar's tests show that there is no difference between the treatments 2 and 3, but there are significant differences between 1 and 2, and 1 and 3. If we adjust the data for multiple testing, for example, by using p=0.01 instead of p=0.05 for rejecting the null-hypothesis, then the difference between 1 and 2 loses its significance, but the difference between treatment 1 and 3 remains statistically significant.

6   Survival Analysis

6.1   Survival Analysis

A survival curve plots percentage survival as a function of time. Figure 3.4 is an example. Fifteen patients are followed for 36 months. At time zero everybody is alive. At the end 40% (6/15) patients are still alive. Percentage decreased whenever a patient died. A problem with survival analysis generally is that of lost data: some patients may be still alive at the end of the study but were lost for follow-up for several reasons. We at least know that they lived at the time they were lost, and so they contribute useful information. The data from subjects leaving the study are called **censored** data and should be included in the analysis.

With the **Kaplan-Meier** method, survival is recalculated every time a patient dies (approaches to survival different from the Kaplan-Meier approach are (1) the actuarial method, where the x-axis is divided into regular intervals and (2) life-table analysis using tables instead of graphs). To calculate the fraction of patients who survive a particular day, simply divide the numbers still alive after the day by the number alive before the day. Also exclude those who are lost (= censored) on the very day and remove from both the numerator and denominator. To calculate the fraction of patients who survive from day 0 until a particular day, multiply the fraction who survive day-1, times the fraction of those who survive day-2, etc. This product of many survival fractions is called the **product-limit**. In order to calculate the 95% CIs, we can use the formula:

95% CI of the product of survival fractions (p) at time $k = p \pm 2 \cdot p \sqrt{\dfrac{(1-p)}{k}}$

The interpretation: we have measured survival in one sample, and the 95%CI shows we can be 95% sure that the true population survival is within the boundaries (see figure upper and lower boundaries). Instead of days, as time variable, weeks, months etc may be used.

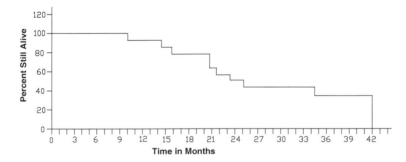

Fig. 3.4 Example of a survival curve plotting survival as a function of time

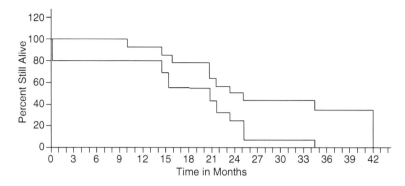

Fig. 3.5 Two Kaplan-Meier survival curves

6.2   Testing Significance of Difference Between Two Kaplan-Meier Curves

Survival is essentially expressed in the form of either proportions or odds, and statistical testing whether one treatment modality scores better than the other in terms of providing better survival can be effectively done by using tests similar to the above **chi-square tests** or chi-square-like tests in order to test whether any proportion of responders is different from another proportion, e.g., the proportion of responders in a control group. RRs or ORs are calculated for that purpose (review Chap. 1). For example, in the example in the i-th 2-month period we have left the following numbers: a_i and b_i in curve 1, c_i and d_i in curve 2,

Contingency table	Numbers of deaths	Numbers alive
Curve 1	a_i	b_i
Curve 2	c_i	d_i
$i = 1, 2, 3, \dots$		

$$\text{Odds ratio} = \frac{a_i / b_i}{c_i / d_i} = \frac{a_i d_i}{b_i c_i}$$

Significance of difference between the curves (Fig. 3.5) is calculated according to the added products "ad" divided by "bc". This can be readily carried out by the **Mantel-Haenszl summary chi-square test:**

$$\chi^2_{M-H} = \frac{(\sum a_i - \sum [(a_i + b_i)(a_i + c_i) / (a_i + b_i + c_i + d_i)])^2}{\sum [(a_i + b_i)(c_i + d_i)(a_i + c_i)(b_i + d_i) / (a_i + b_i + c_i + d_i)^3]}$$

where we thus have multiple 2×2 contingency tables e.g. one for every last day of a subsequent month of the study. With 18 months follow-up the procedure would yield eighteen 2×2-contingency-tables. This Mantel Haenszl summary chi square test is, when used for comparing survival curves, more routinely called **log rank test** (this name is rather confusing because there is no logarithm involved).

Note: An alternative more sophisticated approach to compare survival curves is the **Cox's proportional hazards model**, a method analogous to **multiple regression analysis** for multiple means of continuous data and to **logistic regression** for proportions (Chap. 17).

7   Odds Ratio Method for Analyzing Two Unpaired Proportions

Odds ratios increasingly replace chi/square tests for analyzing 2×2 contingency tables.

	Illness	No illness
Group 1	a	b
Group 2	c	d

The odds ratio $(OR) = a / b / \ c / d$

$\qquad\qquad\qquad$ = odds of illness group1 / odds illness group 2

$\qquad\qquad\qquad$ = chance illness......... / ....

We want to test whether the OR is significantly different from an OR of 1.0.

For that purpose we have to use the logarithmic transformation, and so we will start by recapitulating the principles of logarithmetic calculations.

Log = log to the base 10; Ln = natural log = log to the base e (e = 2.71...)

$\log 10 = {}^{10}\log 10 = 1$
$\log 100 = {}^{10}\log 100 = 2$
$\log 1 = {}^{10}\log 1 = {}^{10}\log 10^0 = 0$
antilog $1 = 10$
antilog $2 = 100$
antilog $0 = 1$

$\ln e = {}^{e}\log e = 1$
$\ln e^2 = {}^{e}\log e^2 = 2$
$\ln 1 = {}^{e}\log 1 = {}^{e}\log e^0 = 0$
antiln $1 = e$
antiln $2 = e^2$
antiln $0 = 1$

The frequency distributions of samples of continuous numbers or proportions are normal. Those of many odds ratios are not. The underneath example is an argument that odds ratios may follow an exponential pattern, while the normal distribution has been approximated by mathematicians by means of the underneath exponential formula

$$\frac{a/b}{c/d} = \frac{1/10}{1/100} = 10 \qquad \frac{a/b}{c/d} = \frac{1/10}{1/10} = 1 \qquad \frac{a/b}{c/d} = \frac{1/10}{1/10} = 1$$

$$y = (\frac{1}{\sqrt{2\pi}})e^{\frac{-1}{2}x^2}$$

x individual data, y how often, $e = 2.718$.

It was astonishing but not unexpected that mathematicians discovered that frequency distributions of log OR followed a normal distribution, and that results were even better if ln instead of log was used.

	Event	No event
Group 1	a	b
Group 2	c	d

If OR $= \dfrac{a/b}{c/d} = 1$, this means that no difference exists between group 1 and 2.

If OR $= 1$, then lnOR $= 0$. With a *normal distribution* if the result >2 standard errors (SEs) distant from 0, then the result is significantly different from 0 at $p < 0.05$. This would also mean that, if ln OR >2 SEs distant from 0, then this result would be significantly different from 0 at $p < 0.05$. There are three possible situations:

Study 1	< --.-- >	lnOR >2 SEs dist 0 $p < 0.05$
Study 2	< -.-- >	lnOR <2 SEs dist 0 ns
Study 3	< --.-- >	lnOR >2 SEs dist 0 $p < 0.05$

ln OR $= 0$
(OR $= 1.0$)

Using this method we can test the OR. However, we need to know how to find the SE of our OR. SE of lnOR is given by the formula $\sqrt{(\frac{1}{a} + \frac{1}{b} + \frac{1}{c} + \frac{1}{d})}$.

This relatively simple formula is not a big surprise, considering that the SE of a number $g = \sqrt{g}$, and the SE of $1/g = \sqrt{\frac{1}{g}}$. We can now assess our data by the OR method as follows:

	Hypertension yes		Hypertension no	
Group 1	a	n $= 5$	b	n $= 10$
Group 2	c	n $= 10$	d	n $= 5$

OR $= \dfrac{a/b}{c/d} = 0.25$

$$\text{lnOR} = -1.3863$$

$$\text{SEM lnOR} = \sqrt{(\frac{1}{a}+\frac{1}{b}+\frac{1}{c}+\frac{1}{d})} = 0.7746$$

$$\text{ln OR} \pm 2 \text{ SEMs} = -1.3863 \pm 1.5182$$
$$= \text{between} - 2.905 \text{ and } 0.132,$$

Now turn the ln numbers into real numbers by the antiln button of your pocket calculator.

$$= \text{between} \, 0.055 \text{ en } 1.14.$$

The result "crosses" 1.0, and, so, it is not significantly different from 1.0.

A second example answers the question: is the difference between the underneath group 1 and 2 significant?

	Orthostatic hypotension	
	Yes	No
Group 1	77	62
Group 2	103	46

$$OR = \frac{103/46}{77/62} = \frac{2.239}{1.242} = 1.803$$

$$\text{lnOR} = 0.589$$

$$\text{SEM lnOR} = \sqrt{\left(\frac{1}{103}+\frac{1}{46}+\frac{1}{77}+\frac{1}{62}\right)} = 0.245$$

$$\text{lnOR} \pm 2 \text{ SEMs} = 0.589 \pm 2(0.245)$$
$$= 0.589 \pm 0.482$$
$$= \text{between } 0.107 \text{ and } 1.071.$$

Turn the ln numbers into real numbers by use of antiln button of your pocket calculator.

$$= \text{between } 1.11 \text{ and } 2.92, \text{ and, so, significantly different from } 1.0.$$

What p-value do we have: $t = \text{lnOR/SEM} = 0.589/0.245 = 2.4082$. The bottom row of the t-table is used for proportional data (z-test), and give us a p-value < 0.02.

Note: A major problem with odds ratios is the ceiling problem. If the control group $n = 0$, then it is convenient to replace 0 with 0.5 in order to prevent this problem.

8   Odds Ratios for One Group, Two Treatments

So far we assessed two groups, one treatment. Now we will assess one group, two treatments and use for that purpose the **McNemar's OR**.

		Normotension with drug 1	
		Yes	No
Normotension with drug 2 Yes		(a) 65	(b) 28
	No	(c) 12	(d) 34

Here the OR$= b/c$, and the SE is not $\sqrt{(\frac{1}{a}+\frac{1}{b}+\frac{1}{c}+\frac{1}{d})}$,but rather $\sqrt{(\frac{1}{b}+\frac{1}{c})}$.

$$OR = 28/12 = 2.33$$

$$lnOR = ln2.33 = 0.847$$

$$SE = \sqrt{\left(\frac{1}{b}+\frac{1}{c}\right)} = 0.345$$

$$lnOR \pm 2\ SE = 0.847 \pm 0.690$$
$$= \text{between } 0.157 \text{ and } 1.537,$$

Turn the ln numbers into real numbers by the anti-ln button of your pocket calculator.

$$= \text{between } 1.16 \text{ and } 4.65$$
$$= \text{sig diff from } 1.0.$$

Calculation p-value: $t = lnOR/SEM = 0.847: 0.345 = 2.455$. The bottom row of the t-table produces a p-value of <0.02, and the two drugs produce, thus, significantly different results at $p < 0.02$.

9   Conclusions

1. For the analysis of efficacy data we test null-hypotheses, safety data consist of proportions, and require for statistical assessment different methods.
2. 2×2 tables are convenient to test differences between 2 proportions.
3. Use chi-square or t-test for normal distributions (z-test) for that purpose.
4. For paired proportions the McNemar's test is appropriate.
5. Kaplan Meier survival curves are also proportional data: include lost patients.
6. Two Kaplan-Meier Curves can be compared using the Mantel-Haenszl = Log rank test
7. Odds ratios with logarithmic transformation provide an alternative method for analyzing 2×2 tables.

In the past two chapters we discussed different statistical methods to test statistically experimental data from clinical trials. We did not emphasize correlation and regression analysis. The point is that correlation and regression analysis test correlations, rather than causal relationships. Two samples may be strongly correlated e.g., two different diagnostic tests for assessment of the same phenomenon. This does, however, not mean that one diagnostic test causes the other. In testing the data from clinical trials we are mainly interested in causal relationships. When such assessments were statistically analyzed through correlation analyses mainly, we would probably be less convinced of a causal relationship than we are while using prospective hypothesis testing. So, this is the main reason we so far did not address correlation testing extensively. With epidemiological observational research things are essentially different: data are obtained from the observation of populations or the retrospective observation of patients selected because of a particular condition or illness. Conclusions are limited to the establishment of relationships, causal or not. We, currently, believe that relationships in medical research between a factor and an outcome can only be proven to be causal when between the factor is introduced and subsequently gives rise to the outcome. We are more convinced when such is tested in the form of a controlled clinical trial. A problem with multiple regression and logistic regression analysis as method for analyzing of multiple samples in clinical trials is closely related to this point. There is always an air of uncertainty about such regression data. Many trials use null-hypothesis testing of two variables, and use multiple regression data only to support and enhance the impact of the report, and to make readership more willing to read the report, rather than to prove the endpoints. It is very unsettling to realize that clinicians and clinical investigators often make bold statements about causalities from multivariable analyses. We believe that this point deserves full emphasis, and will, therefore, address it again in the Chaps. 14, 15, 16, 17, 18, and 19.

Chapter 4
Log Likelihood Ratio Tests
for Safety Data Analysis

1 Introduction

For Gandhi non-violence was a primary invariance principle, while for his political successor Nehru justice was so. Invariance principles signify that while everything changes in life, some laws of life do not. Consequently, these laws of life do not include a measure of error. For example, Einstein's invariance principle is expressed in the famous equation $E = mc^2$. Most statistical tests, including t- (and z-) tests, F-tests, chi-square tests, odds ratio tests, do not meet the invariance principle, because they apply *estimated* likelihoods like averages and proportions that have their standard errors as a measure of uncertainty. However, a few statistical tests use likelihoods without standard error. These tests, called exact tests, should, by their very nature, provide the best precision and sensitivity of testing. They include, among others, the Fisher exact test and the log likelihood ratio test. Particularly, the log likelihood ratio test, avoiding some of the numerical problems of the other exact likelihood tests, is straightforward, and is available through most major software programs (BUGS y WinBUGS 2011; S plus 2011; Stata 2011; StatsDirect 2011; StatXact 2011; True Epistat 2011; SAS 2011; SPSS 2011), although infrequently used so far. This chapter reviews the advantages and problems of the log likelihood ratio test, and gives real and hypothesized data examples supporting its better sensitivity. We do hope that the chapter will stimulate researchers to more often apply this test.

2 Numerical Problems with Calculating Exact Likelihoods

Proportions of patients with events are an important endpoint in cardiovascular research. They are traditionally analyzed in the form of a contingency table of four cells, otherwise called 2×2 contingency table, using chi-square tests or odds ratio tests.

	Number patients with events	Number patients without
Group 1	a	b
Group 2	c	d

The problem with the traditional tests is that sensitivity is limited. As an alternative, the log likelihood ratio test, based on exact rather than estimated likelihoods, can be used. The general problem with exact likelihoods is, that they can be very complicated and may run into numerical problems that even modern computers can not handle. Let us assume that on average the proportion of patients with an event in a target population equals p. The likelihood of getting exactly y events in a sample of n individuals in this population can be calculated according to the underneath binomial equation:

$$\text{Likelihood p} = \frac{n!}{y!(n-y!)} \qquad p^y (1-p)^{(n-y)}$$

$$n! = n \text{ faculty} = n(n-1)(n-2)(n-3)\ldots\ldots$$

For example, a group of citizens was taking a pharmaceutical company to court for misrepresenting the danger of fatal rhabdomyolysis due to a statin treatment:

	Patients with rhabdomyolysis	Patients without
Company	1 (a)	309,999 (b)
Citizens	4 (c)	300,289 (d)

p_{co} = proportion given by the pharmaceutical company = $a/(a+b)$ = 1/310,000
p_{ci} = proportion given by the citizens = $c/(c+d)$ = 4/300,293

$$\text{likelihood } p_{co} = \frac{310000!}{1!(310000-1)!} \cdot (1/310000)^1 \cdot (1-1/310000)^{(310000-1)}$$

Likelihood p_{ci} can be calculated similarly.

The numerical problem of calculating likelihoods in the above way can be largely circumvented by taking the (log) ratios of two equations as will be demonstrated underneath. Log means natural logarithm, otherwise called naperian logarithm, otherwise called logarithm to the base e.

3   The Normal Approximation and the Analysis of Clinical Events

If we take many samples from a target population, the mean results of those samples usually follow a normal frequency distribution, meaning that the value in the middle will be observed most frequently and the more distant from the middle the less

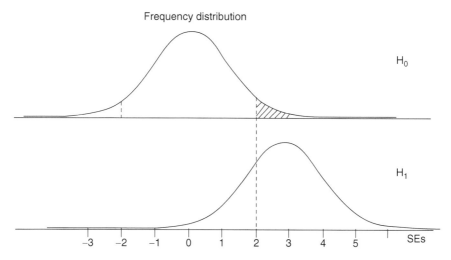

Fig. 4.1 H1 = graph based on the data of a sample with standard errors distant from zero (*SEs*) as unit on the x-axis, often called z-axis in statistics. H0 = same graph with a mean value of 0. We make a giant leap from the sample to the entire population, and we can do so because the sample is assumed to be representative for the entire population. H1 = also the summary of the means of many samples similar to our sample. H0 = also the summary of the means of many samples similar to our sample, but with an overall effect of 0. Our mean not 0 but 2.9. Still it could be an outlier of many samples with an overall effect of 0. If H0 is true, then our sample is an outlier. We can't prove, but calculate the chance/probability of this possibility. A mean result of 2.9 SEs is far distant from 0: suppose it belongs to H0. Only 5% of H0 trials >2.0 SEs distant 0. The chance that it belongs to H0 is thus <5%. We conclude that we have <5% chance to find this result, and, therefore, reject this small chance

frequently a value will be observed. For example, we will have only 5% chance to find a result more than 2 standard errors (SEs) (or more precisely 1.96 SEs) distant from the middle. The same is true with proportional data like events. Many statistical tests make use of the normal distribution to make predictions. Figure 4.1 shows, e.g., how the normal distribution theorem is used to reject the null-hypothesis of no difference from zero.

Assume on average that 10 of 15 patients in a population will have some kind of cardiovascular event within a certain period of time. Then, 10/15 will be the proportion most frequently encountered when randomly sampling from this population. The chance of finding <10 or >10 gets gradually smaller. Figure 4.2 gives on the x-axis (often called z-axis in statistics) the results from many samples, the y-axis shows "how often". The chance of 8 or less is only 15%, of 7 or less only 2.5%, and of 5 or less only 1%. With many samples the graph follows a normal frequency distribution with 95% of the sample results between ±2 SEs distant from the mean value, a proportion of 10/15. Most of the approaches to test the significance of difference between the events in a treatment and control group make use of this normal approximation. This includes the z-test, the chi-square test, and the odds ratio test. Also, the log likelihood ratio test does so.

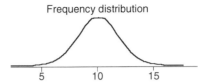

Frequency distribution

Fig. 4.2 Assume that, on average, 10 of 15 patients in a population will have some kind of cardiovascular event within a certain period of time. Then, 10/15 will be the proportion most frequently encountered when taking many random samples of 15 patients from this population. The chance of finding <10 or >10 gets gradually smaller. On the x-axis the numbers of events from many samples is given, the y-axis shows "how often". The chance of 8 or less is only 15%, of 7 or less only 2.5%, and of 5 or less only 1%. With many samples the graph follows a normal frequency distribution with 95% of the sample results between ±2standard errors distant from the mean value

4   Log Likelihood Ratio Tests and the Quadratic Approximation

Assume, like in the above example, that 10/15 has the maximum likelihood, while all other proportions have less than that. The likelihood ratio is defined as the measured proportion/maximum likelihood. The likelihood ratio for 10/15 thus equals 1. Instead of frequency distribution of many samples, Fig. 4.2 can also be interpreted as a likelihood ratio curve of many samples. If $p = 10/15$ is given place 0 on the z-axis, with standard error-units on the z-axis and the top of the curve $= 1$, then the underneath normal distribution equation and the corresponding curve (Fig. 4.3) are adequate.

$$\text{Likelihood ratio} = e^{-1/2\, z^2}$$

If we transform the likelihood ratio values of the y-axis from Fig. 4.3 to log likelihood ratio values, leaving the z-axis unchanged, then the next equations and their corresponding curve (Fig. 4.4) are adequate.

$$\log \text{likelihood ratio} = -1/2\, z^2$$

$$-2 \log \text{likelihood ratio} = z^2$$

With normal distributions, if $z > 2$ or < -2, we conclude a significant difference from zero in the data at $p < 0.05$. Here if -2 log likelihood ratio > 2 or < -2, then the difference between the proportions of events in a two-group comparison is significant at $p < 0.05$.

We now calculate the exact likelihoods for either of the two proportions using the underneath binomial equation.

$$\text{Likelihood p} = \frac{n!}{y!(n-y!)}\, p^y\, (1-p)^{(n-y)}$$

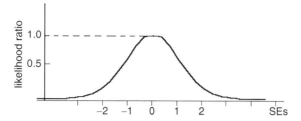

Fig. 4.3 Assume like in Fig. 4.2 that 10/15 has the maximum likelihood, while all other proportions have less likelihood. The likelihood ratio is defined as the measured proportion/maximum likelihood. The likelihood ratio for 10/15 thus equals 1. If p=10/15 is given place 0 on the z-axis with standard errors as unit, and the top of the curve=1, then Fig. 4.2 can also be interpreted as a likelihood ratio curve

Fig. 4.4 If we transform the likelihood ratio values of the y-axis from Fig. 4.3 to log likelihood ratio values, leaving the z-axis unchanged, then the above curve is observed

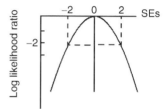

$$\text{log likelihood } p = \log \frac{n!}{y!(n-y)!} + y.\log p + (n-y)\log(1-p)$$

If the data produce two proportions, we can deduce from the above formula the exact (log) likelihood ratio of the two, where log is the natural logarithm. We take the previously used example.

	Patients with rhabdomyolysis	Patients without
Company	1 (a)	309,999 (b)
Citizens	4 (c)	300,289 (d)

p_{co} =proportion given by the pharmaceutical company=$a/(a+b)$=1/310000
p_{ci} =proportion given by the citizens=$c/(c+d)$=4/300293

$$\text{log likelihood ratio} = \log \frac{\text{likelihood } p_{co}}{\text{likelihood } p_{ci}}$$

$$= \log \text{likelihood } p_{co} - \log \text{likelihood } p_{ci}$$

$$= y \log p_{co}/p_{ci} + (n-y)\log(1-p_{co})/(1-p_{ci})$$

As -2 log likelihood ratio equals z^2, we can now test the significance of difference between the two proportions.

$$\text{Log likelihood ratio} = 4 \log \frac{1/310000}{4/300293} + 300289 \log \frac{1-1/310000}{1-4/300293}$$
$$= -2.641199$$

We should note that both the odds ratio test and chi-square test produced a non-significant result here ($p > 0.05$).

5   More Examples

Example 1

Two group of 15 patients at risk for arrhythmias were assessed for the development of torsade de points after calcium channel blockers treatment

	Patients with torsade de points	Patients without
Calcium channel blocker 1	5	10
Calcium channel blocker 2	9	6

The proportion of patients with event from calcium channel blocker 1 is 5/15, from blocker 2 it is 9/15.

$$\text{Log likelihood ratio} = 9 \log \frac{5/15}{9/15} + 6 \log \frac{1-5/15}{1-9/15}$$
$$= -2.25$$

-2 log likelihood ratio $= 4.50$ ($p < 0.05$, because $z > 2$).

Both odds ratio test and chi-square test were again non-significant ($p > 0.05$).

Example 2

Two groups of patients with stage IV New York Heart Association heart failure were assessed for hospitalizations after two beta-blockers.

	Patients with hospitalization	Patients without
Beta blocker 1	77	62
Beta blocker 2	103	46

The proportion of patients with event from beta blocker 1 is 77/139, from beta blocker 2 it is 103/149.

$$\text{Log likelihood ratio} = 103 \log \frac{77/139}{103/149} + 46 \log \frac{1-77/139}{1-103/149}$$
$$= -5.882$$

−2 log likelihood ratio = 11.766 (p < 0.002, because z > 3.090).

Both the odds ratio test and chi-square test were also significant. However, at lower levels of significance, both p-values $0.01 < p < 0.05$.

6 Discussion

The chi-square test for events uses the observed cells in a contingency table to approximate the expected cells, a rather imprecise method. The odds ratio test uses the log transformation of a skewed frequency distribution as a rather imprecise approximation of the normal distribution. Sensitivity of these tests is, obviously, limited, and tests with potentially better sensitivity like exact tests are welcome.

At first sight, we might doubt about the precision of the log likelihood ratio test for events, because it is based on no less than three approximations: (1) the binomial formula as an estimate for likelihood, (2) the binomial distribution as an estimate for the normal distribution, (3) the quadratic approximation as an estimate for the normal distribution. However, the approximations (1) and (3) provide exact rather than estimated likelihoods, and it turns out from the above examples that de log likelihood ratio test is, indeed, more sensitive than the standard tests. In addition, the log transformation of the exponential binomial data is convenient, because exponents become simple multiplification factors. Also, the quadratic approximation is convenient, because an exponential equation is turned into a simpler quadratic equation (parabola).

Likelihood ratio statistics has a relatively short history. It was begun independently by Barnard (1947) and Fisher (1956) in the past World War II era. In this paper the log likelihood ratio test was used for the analysis of events only. The test can be generalized to other types of data including continuous data and the data in regression models, whereby the advantage of better sensitivity remains equally true. The test is, therefore, increasingly important in modern statistics.

We conclude that the log likelihood ratio test is more sensitive than traditional statistical tests including the t-(and z)-test, chi-square test and odds ratio test. Other advantages are the following: exponents can be conveniently handled by the log transformation and an exponential equation is turned into a simpler quadratic equation. A potential disadvantage of numerical problems is avoided by taking ratios of likelihoods instead of separate likelihoods in the final analysis.

7 Conclusions

Traditional statistical tests for the analysis of clinical events have limited sensitivity, particularly with smaller samples. Exact tests, although infrequently used so far, should have better sensitivity, because they do not include standard errors as a measure of uncertainty. The log likelihood ratio test is one of them. The objective of the current chapter was to assess the above question using real and hypothesized data examples. In three studies of clinical events the log likelihood ratio test was consistently more sensitive than traditional tests, including the chi-square and the odds ratio test, producing p-values respectively between <0.05 and <0.002 and between not-significant and <0.05. This was true both with larger and smaller samples. Other advantages of the log likelihood ratio were: exponents can be conveniently handled by the log transformation and an exponential equation is turned into a simpler quadratic equation. A potential disadvantage of numerical problems is avoided by taking in the final analysis the ratios of likelihoods instead of separate likelihoods. Log likelihood ratio tests are consistently more sensitive than traditional statistical tests. We hope that this chapter will stimulate clinical researchers to more often apply them.

References

Barnard GA (1947) A review of sequential analysis. J Am Stat Ass 422:658–64
BUGS y WinBUGS. http://www.mrc-bsu.cam.ac.uk/bugs http://cran.r-project.org. Accessed 15 Dec 2011
Fisher RA (1956) Statistical methods and scientific inferences. Oliver & Boyd, Edinburgh
S-plus. http://www.mathsoft.com/splus. Accessed 15 Dec 2011
SAS. http://www.prw.le.ac.uk/epidemiol/personal/ajs22/meta/macros.sas. Accessed 15 Dec 2011
SPSS Statistical Software. http://www.spss.com. Accessed 15 Dec 2011
Stata. http://www.stata.com. Accessed 15 Dec 2011
StatsDirect. http://www.camcode.com. Accessed 15 Dec 2011
StatXact. http://www.cytel.com/products/statxact/statact1.html. Accessed 15 Dec 2011
True Epistat. http://ic.net/~biomware/biohp2te.htm. Accessed 15 Dec 2011

Chapter 5
Equivalence Testing

1 Introduction

A study unable to find a difference is not the same as an equivalent study. For example, a study of three subjects does not find a significant difference simply because the sample size is too small. Equivalence testing is particularly important for studying the treatment of diseases for which a placebo control would unethical. In the situation a new treatment must be compared with standard treatment. The latter comparison is at risk of finding little differences.

Figure 5.1 gives an example of a study where the mean result is little different from 0. Is the result equivalent then? H1 represent the distribution of our data and H0 is the null-hypothesis (this approach is more fully explained in Chap. 2). What we observe is that the mean of our trial is only 0.9 standard errors of the mean (SEMs) distant from 0, which is far too little to reject the null-hypothesis. Our result is not significantly different from 0. Whether our result is equivalent to 0, depends on our prior defined criterium of equivalence. In the figure D sets the defined interval of equivalence. If 95% CIs of our trial is completely within this interval, we conclude that equivalence is demonstrated. This mean that with D_1 boundaries we have no equivalence, with D_2 boundaries we do have equivalence. The striped area under curve (=the socalled 95% CIs) is the interval approximately between -2 SEMs and $+2$ SEMs (i.e., 1.96) SEMs with normal distributions, a little bit more than 2 SEMs with t-distributions. It is often hard to prior define the D boundaries, but they should be based not on mathematical but rather on clinical arguments, i.e., the boundaries where differences are undisputedly clinically irrelevant.

Figure 5.2 gives another example. The mean result of our trial is larger now: mean value is 2.9 SEMs distant from 0, and, so, we conclude that the difference from 0 is > approximately 2 SEMs and, that we can reject the null-hypothesis of no difference. Does this mean that our study is not equivalent? This again depends on our prior defined criterium of equivalence. With D_1 the trial is not completely within the boundaries and equivalence is thus not demonstrated. With D_2 the striped area of the trial is completely within the boundaries and we conclude that equivalence has been demonstrated. Note that with D_1 we have both significant difference and equivalence.

T.J. Cleophas and A.H. Zwinderman, *Statistics Applied to Clinical Studies*, DOI 10.1007/978-94-007-2863-9_5, © Springer Science+Business Media B.V. 2012

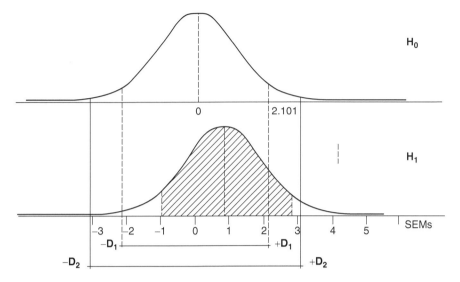

Fig. 5.1 Null-hypothesis testing and equivalence testing of a sample of t-distributed data

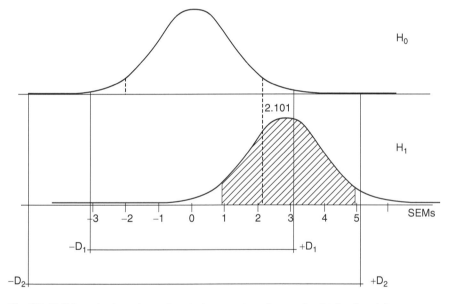

Fig. 5.2 Null-hypothesis testing and equivalence testing of a sample of t-distributed data

2   Overview of Possibilities with Equivalence Testing

Table 5.1 shows that any confidence interval (95% CIs intervals between the brackets in each of the examples) that does not overlap zero is statistically different from zero. Only intervals between the prespecified range of equivalence $-D$ to $+D$

Table 5.1 Any confidence interval (95% CIs intervals between the brackets in each of the examples) that does not overlap zero is statistically different from zero. Only intervals between the prespecified range of equivalence −D to +D present equivalence

Study (1-8)	Statistical significance demonstrated	equivalence demonstrated

```
1.  Yes--------------------------------------------------------------------< not equivalent >
2.  Yes-----------------------------------------------------------------<    uncertain    >-------------
3.  Yes --------------------------------------------------------<    equivalent  >------------------------
4.  No ------------------------------------------<     equivalent        >----------------------------------
5.  Yes----------------------------< equivalent    >--------------------------------------------------
6.  Yes------------<    uncertain       >--------------------------------------------------------------
7.  Yes-< not equivalent   >-------------------------------------------------------------------------
8.  No--------<_____     uncertain           _____>--------
```

```
                        !                                        !
_____
                       -D                    O                   +D
                                     true difference
```

present equivalence. Thus, situations 3, 4 and 5 demonstrate equivalence, while 1 and 2, just like 6 and 7 do not. Situations 3 and 5 present equivalence and at the same time significant difference. Situation 8 presents nor significant difference, nor equivalence.

Testing equivalence of two treatments is different from testing their difference. We will in this chapter use the term comparative studies to name the latter kind of studies. In a comparative study we use statistical significance tests to determine whether the null hypothesis of no treatment difference can be rejected, frequently together with 95% CIs to better visualize the size of the difference. In an equivalence study this significance test has little relevance: failure to detect a difference does not imply equivalence; the study may have been too small with corresponding wide standard errors to allow for such a conclusion. Also, not only difference but also equivalence are terms that should be interpreted within the context of clinical relevance. For that purpose we have to predefine a range of equivalence as an interval from −D to +D. We can then simply check whether our 95% CIs as centered on the observed difference lies entirely between −D and +D. If it does equivalence is demonstrated if not, there is room for uncertainty. The above table shows the discrepancies between significance and equivalence testing. The procedure of checking whether the 95% CIs are within a range of equivalence does look somewhat similar to a significance testing procedure, but one in which the role of the usual null and alternative hypothesis are reversed. In equivalence testing the relevant null hypothesis is that a difference of at least D exists, and the analysis is targeted at rejecting this "null-hypothesis". The choice of D is difficult, is often chosen on clinical arguments: the new agent should be sufficiently similar to the standard agent to be clinically indistinguishable.

3   Calculations

95% CIs intervals are calculated according to the standard formulas

Continuous data paired or unpaired and normal distributions (with t-distribution **2**, which is actually 1.96, should be replaced by the appropriate t-value dependent upon sample size).

$$\text{Mean}_1 - \text{mean}_2 \pm \mathbf{2} \text{ SEMs where}$$

$$\text{SEM}_{\text{unpaired differences}} = \sqrt{SD_1^2 / n_1 + SD_2^2 / n_2}$$

$$\text{SEM}_{\text{paired differences}} = \sqrt{\frac{(SD_1^2 + SD_2^2 - 2r \cdot SD_1 \cdot SD_2)}{n}} \quad \text{if } n_1 = n_2 = n$$

Binary data

$$\text{SEM}_{\text{of differences}} = \sqrt{\frac{p_1(1-p_1)}{n_1} + \frac{p_2(1-p_2)}{n_2}}$$

$$\text{With 95\% CIs}: p_1 - p_2 \pm 2. \text{ SEM}$$

More details about the calculation of SEMS of samples are given in Chap. 1.

The calculation of required samples size of the trial based on expected treatment effects in order to test our hypothesis reliably, will be explained in the next chapter together with sample size calculations for comparative studies.

It is helpful to present the results of an equivalence study in the form of a graph (Table 5.1). The result may be:

1. The confidence interval for the difference between the two treatments lies entirely between the equivalence range so that we conclude that equivalence is demonstrated.
2. The confidence interval covers at least several points outside the equivalence range so that we conclude that a clinically important difference remains a possibility, and equivalence cannot be safely concluded.
3. The confidence interval is entirely outside the equivalence range.

4   Equivalence Testing, a New Gold Standard?

The classic gold standard in drug research is the randomized placebo controlled clinical trial. This design is favored for confirmatory trials as part of the phase III development of new medicines. Because of the large numbers and classes of medicines already available, however, new medicines are increasingly being developed for indications for which a placebo control group would be unethical. In such situations an obvious solution is to use as comparator an existing drug already licensed and regularly used for the indications in question. When an active comparator is used, the expectation may sometimes be that the new treatment will be better than the standard, the objective of the study may be to demonstrate this. This situation would be similar to a placebo control and requires no special methodology. More probably, however, the new treatment is expected to simply largely match the efficacy of the standard treatment but to have some advantages in terms of safety, adverse effects, costs, pharmacokinetic properties. Under these circumstances the objective of the trial is to show equivalent efficacy.

5   Validity of Equivalence Trials

A comparative trial is valid when it is blinded, randomized, explicit, accurate statistically and ethically. The same is true for equivalence trial. However, a problem arises with the intention to treat analysis. Intention to treat patients are analyzed according to their randomized treatment irrespective of whether they actually received the treatment. The argument is that it mirrors what will happen when a treatment is used in practice. In a comparative parallel group study the inclusion of protocol violators in the analysis tend to make the results of the two treatments more similar. In an equivalence study this effect may bias the study towards a positive result, being the demonstration of equivalence. A possibility is to carry out both intention-to-treat-analysis and completed-protocol-analysis. If no difference is demonstrated, we conclude that the study's data are robust (otherwise called sensitive, otherwise called precise), and that the protocol-analysis did not introduce major sloppiness into the data. Sometimes, efficacy and safety endpoints are analyzed differently: the former according to the protocol analysis simply because important endpoint variables are missing in the population that leaves the study early, and intention to treat analysis for the latter, because safety variables frequently include items such as side effects, drop-offs, morbidity and mortality during trial. Either endpoint can of course be assessed in an equivalence assessment trial, but we must consider that an intention to treat analysis may bias the equivalence principle towards overestimation of the chance of equivalence.
Note: Statistical power of equivalence testing is explained in the next chapter.

6   Special Point: Level of Correlation in Paired Equivalence Studies

Figure 5.3 shows the results of three crossover trials with two drugs in patients with Raynaud's phenomenon. In the left trial a negative correlation exists between the treatments, in the middle trial the correlation level is zero, while in the right trial a

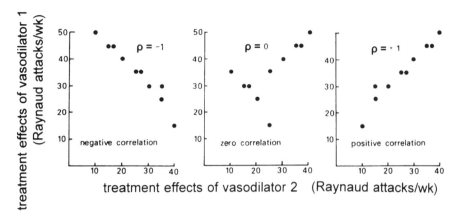

Fig. 5.3 Example of three crossover studies of two treatments in patients with Raynaud's phenomenon. The Pearson's correlation coefficient ρ varies from −1 to 1

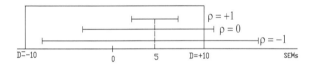

Fig. 5.4 The mean difference between the two treatments of each of the treatment comparison of Fig. 5.3 is 5 Raynaud attacks/week. However, standard errors, and, thus, 95% confidence intervals are largely different. With a D-boundary of ±10 Raynaud attacks/week only the positive correlation study (ρ=+1) can demonstrate equivalence

strong postive correlation is observed. It is calculated that the mean difference between the treatments in each trial equals 5 Raynaud attacks/week but that the standard errors of the differences are different, left trial 6.46, middle trial 2.78, right trial 0.76 Raynaud attacks/week. Figure 5.4 shows that with a D-boundary of ±10 Raynaud attacks/week only the positive correlation study is able to demonstrate equivalence. Fortunately, most crossover studies have a positive correlation between the treatments, and, so, the crossover design is generally quite sensitive to assess equivalence.

7   Conclusions

1. The use of placebos is unethical if an effective active comparator is available.
2. With an active comparator the new treatment may simply match the standard treatment.

3. Predefined areas of equivalence have to be based on clinical arguments.
4. Equivalence testing is indispensable in drug development (for comparison versus an active comparator).
5. Equivalence trials have to be larger than comparative trials. You will understand this after reviewing the next chapter.

Chapter 6
Statistical Power and Sample Size

1 What Is Statistical Power

Figure 6.1 shows two graphs of t-distributions. The lower graph (H1) could be a probability distribution of a sample of data or of a sample of paired differences between two observations. N=20 and so 95% of the observations is within 2.901 ± 2.101 standard errors of the mean (SEMs) on the x-axis (usually called z-axis in statistics). The upper graph is identical, but centers around 0 instead of 2.901. It is called the null-hypothesis H0, and represents the data of our sample if the mean results were not different from zero. However, our mean result is 2.901 SEMs distant from zero. If we had many samples obtained by similar trials under the same null-hypothesis, the chance of finding a mean value of more than 2.101 is <5%, because the area under the curve (AUC) of H0 right from 2.101 <5% of total AUC. We, therefore, reject the assumption that our results indicate a difference just by chance and decide that we have demonstrated a true difference. What is the power of this test. The power has as prior assumption that there is a difference from zero in our data. What is the chance of demonstrating a difference if there is one. If our experiment would be performed many times, the distribution of obtained mean values of those many experiments would center around 2.901, and about 70% of the AUC of H1 would be larger than 2.101. When smaller than 2.101, our statistical analysis would not be able to reject the null-hypothesis of no difference, when larger, it would rightly be able to reject the null-hypothesis of no difference. So, in fact $100\% - 70\% = 30\%$ of the many trials would erroneously be unable to reject the null-hypothesis of no difference, even when a true difference is in the data. We say the power of this experiment $= 1 - 0.3 = 0.7$ (70%), otherwise called the chance of finding a difference when there is one (area under curve $(1-\beta) \times 100\%$). β is also called the chance of making a type II error=chance of finding no difference when there is one. Another chance is the chance of finding a difference where there is none, otherwise called the type I error (area under the curve ($2x \; \alpha/2) \times 100\%$). This type of error is usually set to be 0.05 (5%).

T.J. Cleophas and A.H. Zwinderman, *Statistics Applied to Clinical Studies*,
DOI 10.1007/978-94-007-2863-9_6, © Springer Science+Business Media B.V. 2012

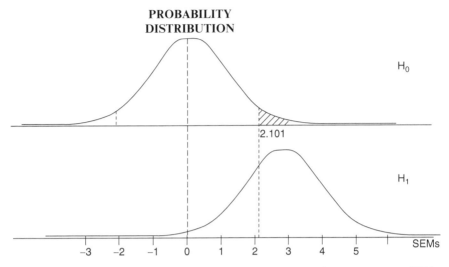

Fig. 6.1 H1 is the given distribution of our data with mean value of 2.901 (= t=mean/SEM). β=area under curve (*AUC*) of H1 *left* from the *dotted vertical line*=±0.3 (±30% of the total AUC). 1−β=±0.7=± 70% of total AUC of H1. Statistical power=± 0.7=chance of finding a difference when there is one

2 Emphasis on Statistical Power Rather Than Null-Hypothesis Testing

Generally, statistical tests reach their conclusions by seeing how compatible the observations were with the null-hypothesis of no treatment effect or treatment difference between test-treatment and reference-treatment. In any test we reject the null-hypothesis of no treatment effect if the value of the test statistic (F, t, q, or chi-square) was bigger than 95% of the values that would occur if the treatment had no effect. When this is so, it is common for medical investigators to report a statistically significant effect at P (probability) <0.05 which means that the chance of finding no difference if there is one, is less than 5%. On the other hand, when the test statistic is not big enough to reject this null-hypothesis of no treatment effect, the investigators often report no statistically significant difference and discuss their results in terms of documented proof that the treatment had no effect. All they really did, was fail to demonstrate that it did have an effect. The distinction between positively demonstrating that a treatment had no effect and failing to demonstrate that it does have an effect, is subtle but very important, especially with respect to the small numbers of subjects usually enrolled in a trial. A study of treatments that involves only a few subjects and then fails to reject the null hypothesis of no treatment effect, may arrive at this result because the statistical procedure lacked

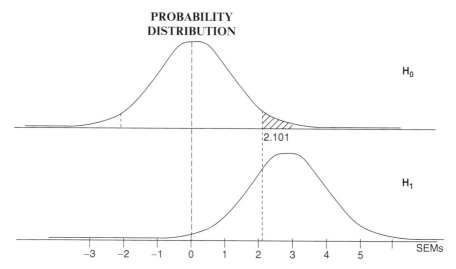

Fig. 6.2 Example of t-distribution with n=20 and its null- hypothesis of no effect. *Lower curve H1* or actual SEM distribution of the data, *upper curve H0* or null-hypothesis of the study

power to detect the effect because of a too small sample size, even though the treatment did have an effect.

Figure 6.2 gives an example of a t-distribution with n=20 (H1) and its null-hypothesis of no effect (H0). 95% of all similar trials with no significant treatment difference from zero must have their means between −2.101 and +2.101 SEMs from zero. The chance of finding a mean value of 2.101 SEMs or more is 5% or less ($\alpha=0.05$ or α. 100%=5%, where α is the chance of finding a difference when there is none−erroneously rejecting the null-hypothesis of no effect, also called type I error). The figure shows that in this particular situation the chance of β is 0.5 or β times 100%=50% (β is the chance of finding no difference where there is one=the chance of erroneously accepting the null-hypothesis of no treatment difference, also called type II error).

Statistical power, defined as $1-\beta$, can be best described as the chance of finding a difference where there is one=the chance of rightly rejecting the null-hypothesis of no effect. The figure shows that this chance of detecting a true-positive effect, i.e., reporting a statistically significant difference when the treatment really produces an effect is only 50%, and likewise that the chance of no statistically significant difference is no less than 50% either ($\beta=0.5$). It means that if we reject the null-hypothesis of no effect at P=0.05, we still have a chance of 50% that a real effect in our data is not detected. As a real effect in the data rather than no effect is the main underlying hypothesis of comparative drug trials, a 50% chance to detect it, is hardly acceptable for reliable testing. A more adequate cut-off level of rejecting would be, e.g., a

90–95% power level, with corresponding α level of 0.005–0.001. Many physicians and even some investigators never confront these problems because they never heard of power. An additional advantage of power analysis is the possibility to use power computations on hypothesized results a priori in order to decide in advance on sample size for a study.

3   Power Computations

Calculating power can be best left over to a computer, because other approaches are rather imprecise. For example, with normal distributions or t-distributions power $=1-\beta$ can be readily visualized from a graph as estimated percentage of the $(1-\beta) \times 100\%$ area under the curve. However, errors as large as 10–20% are unavoidable with this approach. We may alternatively use tables for t- and z-distributions, but as tables give discrete values this procedure is rather inaccurate either.

A computer will make use of the following equations.

3.1   For t-Distributions of Continuous Data

$$\text{Power} = 1-\beta = 1 - \text{probability}\left[z_{power} \leq (t-t')\right] = \text{probability}\left[z_{power} > (t-t')\right]$$

where z_{power} represents a position on the x-axis of the z-distribution (or in this particular situation more correctly t-distribution), and t' represents the level of t that for the given degrees of freedom ($\approx$ sample size) yields an α of 0.05. Finally, t in the equation is the actual t as calculated from the data.

Let's assume we have a parallel-group data comparison with test statistic of $t=3.99$ and $n=20$ ($P<0.001$). What is the power of this test? $Z_{power}=(t'-t)=3.99-2.101=1.89$. This is so, because $t'=$ the t that with 18 degrees of freedom (dfs) ($n=20$, $20-2$) yields an α of 0.05. To convert z_{power} into power we look up in the t-table with dfs $=18$ the closest level of probability and find approximately 0.9 for 1.729. The power of this test thus is approximately 90%.

3.2   For Proportions

$$z_{power} = 2.\left(\text{arcsine }\sqrt{p_1} - \text{arcsine }\sqrt{p_2}\right)\sqrt{\frac{n}{2}} - z'$$

where z_{power} is a position on the x-axis of the z-distribution and z^1 is 2 if $\alpha = 0.05$ (actually 1.96). It is surprising that arcsine (= 1/sine) expressed in radians shows up but it turns out that power is a function of the square roots of the proportions, which has a 1/sine like function.

A computer turns z_{power} into power. Actually, power graphs as presented in many current texts on statistics can give acceptable estimates for proportions as well.

3.3 For Equivalence Testing of Samples with t-Distributions and Continuous Data

$$\text{Power} = 1 - \beta = 1 - \text{probability}\left[z < (D/SEM - z_{1-\alpha})\right]$$

where z is again a position on the x-axis of the z- or t-distribution, D is half the interval of equivalence (see previous chapter), and $z_{1-\alpha}$ is 2 (actually 1.96) if α is set at 5%.

4 Examples of Power Computation Using the t-Table

4.1 First Example

Although a table gives discrete values, and is somewhat inaccurate to precisely calculate the power size, it is useful to master the method, because it is helpful to understand what statistical power really is. The example of Fig. 6.3 is given. Our trial mean is 2.878 SEMs distant from 0 (= the t-value of our trial). We will try to find beta by subtracting $t - t^1$ where is the t-value that yields an area under the curve (AUC) of 5% = 2.101. $t - t^1 = 2.878 - 2.101 = 0.668$. Now we can use the t-table to find 1-beta = power.

The t-table (Table 6.1) gives eight columns of t-values and one column (left one) of degrees of freedom. The upper rows give an overview of AUCs corresponding to various t-values and degrees of freedom. In our case we have two groups of ten subjects and thus $(20 - 2) = 18$ degrees of freedom (dfs). The AUC right from $2.101 = 0.05$ (tested 2-sided = tested for both > +2.101 and < −2.101 distant from 0). Now for the power analysis. The t-value of our trial = 2.878. The t^1 − value = approximately 2.101; $t - t^1$ = approximately 0.777. The AUC right from 0.777 is right from 0.688 corresponding with an area under the curve (AUC) <0.25 (25%). Beta, always tested one-sided, is, thus, < 25%; 1−beta = power => 75%.

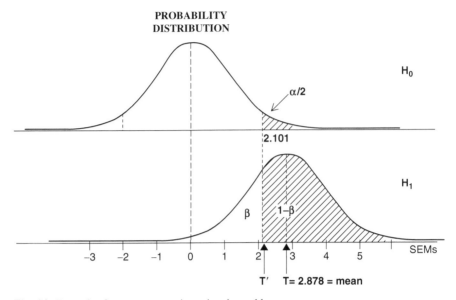

Fig. 6.3 Example of power computation using the t-table

Table 6.1 t-Table: ν=degrees of freedom for t-variable, Q=proportion of cases cut off on the upper tail of the t-distribution

	Q=0.4	0.25	0.1	0.05	0.025	0.01	0.005	0.001
	2Q=0.8	0.5	0.2	0.1	0.05	0.02	0.01	0.002
1	0.325	1.000	3.078	6.314	12.706	31.821	63.657	318.31
2	.289	0.816	1.886	2.920	4.303	6.965	9.925	22.326
3	.277	.765	1.638	2.353	3.182	4.547	5.841	10.213
4	.171	.741	1.533	2.132	2.776	3.747	4.604	7.173
5	0.267	0.727	1.476	2.015	2.571	3.365	4.032	5.893
6	.265	.718	1.440	1.943	2.447	3.143	3.707	5.208
7	.263	.711	1.415	1.895	2.365	2.998	3.499	4.785
8	.262	.706	1.397	1.860	2.306	2.896	3.355	4.501
9	.261	.703	1.383	1.833	2.262	2.821	3.250	4.297
10	0.261	0.700	1.372	1.812	2.228	2.764	3.169	4.144
11	.269	.697	1.363	1.796	2.201	2.718	3.106	4.025
12	.269	.695	1.356	1.782	2.179	2.681	3.055	3.930
13	.259	.694	1.350	1.771	2.160	2.650	3.012	3.852
14	.258	.692	1.345	1.761	2.145	2.624	2.977	3.787
15	0.258	0.691	1.341	1.753	2.131	2.602	2.947	3.733
16	.258	.690	1.337	1.746	2.120	2.583	2.921	3.686
17	.257	.689	1.333	1.740	2.110	2.567	2.898	3.646
18	.257	688	1.330	1.734	2.101	2.552	2.878	3.610
19	.257	.688	1.328	1.729	2.093	2.539	2.861	3.579

(continued)

Table 6.1 (continued)

	$Q=0.4$	0.25	0.1	0.05	0.025	0.01	0.005	0.001
	$2Q=0.8$	0.5	0.2	0.1	0.05	0.02	0.01	0.002
20	0.257	0.687	1.325	1.725	2.086	2.528	2.845	3.552
21	.257	.686	1.323	1.721	2.080	2.518	2.831	3.527
22	.256	.686	1.321	1.717	2.074	2.508	2.819	3.505
23	.256	.685	1.319	1.714	2.069	2.600	2.807	3.485
24	.256	.685	1.318	1.711	2.064	2.492	2.797	3.467
25	0.256	0.684	1,316	1.708	2.060	2.485	2.787	3.450
26	.256	.654	1,315	1.706	2.056	2.479	2.779	3.435
27	.256	.684	1,314	1.701	2.052	2.473	2.771	3.421
28	.256	.683	1,313	1.701	2.048	2.467	2.763	3.408
29	.256	.683	1.311	1.699	2.045	2.462	2.756	3.396
30	0.256	0.683	1.310	1.697	2.042	2.457	2.750	3.385
40	.255	.681	1.303	1.684	2.021	2.423	2.704	3.307
60	.254	.679	1.296	1.671	2.000	2.390	2.660	3.232
120	.254	.677	1.289	1.658	1.950	2.358	2.617	3.160
∞	.253	.674	1.282	1.645	1.960	2.326	2.576	3.090

4.2 Second Example

The mean result from the example in Fig. 6.4 is 2.1 SEMs distant from zero, which is equal to the t-value in the underneath t-table. We find beta by subtracting $t-t^1$ where t^1 is the t yielding AUC of 5% = 2.101. $t-t^1 = 0.0$. Now we use t-table to find $1-$beta. The t- value = 2.1, $t^1 = 2.1$, $t-t^1 = 0.0$, close to 0.257.

The AUC is, thus, close to 0.4 and will be approximately 0.50. Beta (1-sided) = approximately 50%, $1-$beta = power = $1-0.50$ = approximately 0.50 = approximately 50%, power is 50%. This little power is not acceptable for accurate testing (Table 6.2).

4.3 Third Example

Things may get worse. The mean result of the study from Fig. 6.5 is 0.9 SEMs distant from zero. The t-value = 0.9. We find beta by subtracting $t-t^1$ where t^1 is the t yielding an AUC of 0.05 = 2.101; $t-t^1 = -1.20$.

Our t–value is, thus, 0.9, t^1 is 2.1, $t-t^1 = -1.2$, 1.2 is between 0.68 and 1.33, and close to 1.33, and corresponds with an AUC a bit more than 10%: 15% or so, -1.2 corresponds with an AUC 100% $-$ 15% = 85%, beta = 85%, $1-$beta = 15% = STATISTICAL POWER. Notice that this procedure is getting rather imprecise with extreme values (Table 6.3).

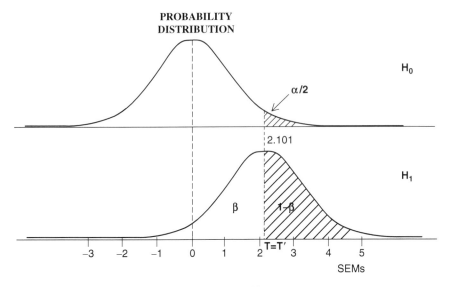

Fig. 6.4 Example of power computation using the t-table

Table 6.2 t-Table: ν=degrees of freedom for t-variable, Q=proportion of cases cut off on the upper tail of the t-distribution

	Q=0.4	0.25	0.1	0.05	0.025	0.01	0.005	0.001
Q=0.5	2Q=0.8	0.5	0.2	0.1	0.05	0.02	0.01	0.002
1	0.325	1.000	3.078	6.314	12.706	11.821	63.657	318.31
2	.289	0.816	1.886	2.920	4.303	6.965	9.925	22.326
3	.277	.765	1.638	2.353	3.182	4.547	5.841	10.213
4	.171	.741	1.533	2.132	2.776	3.747	4.604	7.173
5	0.267	0.727	1.476	2.015	2.571	3.365	4.032	5.893
6	.265	.718	1.440	1.943	2.447	3.143	3.707	5.208
7	.263	.711	1.415	1.895	2.365	2.998	3.499	4.785
8	.262	.706	1.397	1.860	2.306	2.896	3.355	4.501
9	.261	.703	1.383	1.833	2.262	2.821	3.250	4.297
10	0.261	0. 700	1.372	1.812	2.228	2.764	3.169	4.144
11	.269	.697	1.363	1.796	2.201	2.718	3.106	4.025
12	.269	.695	1.356	1.782	2.179	2.681	3.055	3.930
13	.259	.694	1.350	1.771	2.160	2.650	3.012	3.852
14	.258	.692	1.345	1.761	2.145	2.624	2.977	3.787
15	0.258	0.691	1.341	1.753	2.131	2.602	2.947	3.733
16	.258	.690	1.337	1.746	2.120	2.583	2.921	3.686
17	0.0 .257	.689	1.333	1.740	2.110	2.567	2.898	3.646
18	.257	688	1.330	1.734	2.101	2.552	2.878	3.610
19	.257	.688	1.328	1.729	2.093	2.539	2.861	3.579

(continued)

Table 6.2 (continued)

	Q = 0.4	0.25	0.1	0.05	0.025	0.01	0.005	0.001
Q = 0.5	2Q = 0.8	0.5	0.2	0.1	0.05	0.02	0.01	0.002
20	0.257	0.687	1.325	1.725	2.086	2.528	2.845	3.552
21	.257	.686	1.323	1.721	2.080	2.518	2.831	3.527
22	.256	.686	1.321	1.717	2.074	2.508	2.819	3.505
23	.256	.685	1.319	1.714	2.069	2.600	2.807	3.485
24	.256	.685	1.318	1.711	2.064	2.492	2.797	3.467
25	0.256	0.684	1,316	1.708	2.060	2.485	2.787	3.450
26	.256	.654	1,315	1.706	2.056	2.479	2.779	3.435
27	.256	.684	1,314	1.701	2.052	2.473	2.771	3.421
28	.256	.683	1,313	1.701	2.048	2.467	2.763	3.408
29	.256	.683	1.311	1.699	2.045	2.462	2.756	3.396
30	0.256	0.683	1.310	1.697	2.042	2.457	2.750	3.385
40	.255	.681	1.303	1.684	2.021	2.423	2.704	3.307
60	.254	.679	1.296	1.671	2.000	2.390	2.660	3.232
120	.254	.677	1.289	1.658	1.950	2.358	2.617	3.160
∞	.253	.674	1.282	1.645	1.960	2.326	2.576	3.090

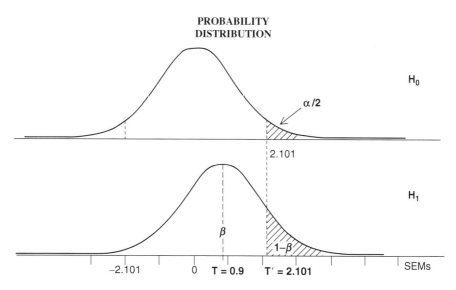

Fig. 6.5 Example of power computation using the t-table

Table 6.3 t-Table: v=degrees of freedom for t-variable, Q=proportion of cases cut off on the upper tail of the t-distribution

v	Q=0.4	0.25	0.1	0.05	0.025	0.01	0.005	0.001
	2Q=0.8	0.5	0.2	0.1	0.05	0.02	0.01	0.002
1	0.325	1.000	3.078	6.314	12.706	31.821	63.657	318.31
2	.289	0.816	1.886	2.920	4.303	6.965	9.925	22.326
3	.277	.765	1.638	2.353	3.182	4.547	5.841	10.213
4	.171	.741	1.533	2.132	2.776	3.747	4.604	7.173
5	0.267	0.727	1.476	2.015	2.571	3.365	4.032	5.893
6	.265	.718	1.440	1.943	2.447	3.143	3.707	5.208
7	.263	.711	1.415	1.895	2.365	2.998	3.499	4.785
8	.262	.706	1.397	1.860	2.306	2.896	3.355	4.501
9	.261	.703	1.383	1.833	2.262	2.821	3.250	4.297
10	0.261	0.700	1.372	1.812	2.228	2.764	3.169	4.144
11	.269	.697	1.363	1.796	2.201	2.718	3.106	4.025
12	.269	.695	1.356	1.782	2.179	2.681	3.055	3.930
13	.259	.694	1.350	1.771	2.160	2.650	3.012	3.852
14	.258	.692	1.345	1.761	2.145	2.624	2.977	3.787
15	0.258	0.691	1.341	1.753	2.131	2.602	2.947	3.733
16	.258	.690	1.337	1.746	2.120	2.583	2.921	3.686
17	.257	.689	1.333	1.740	2.110	2.567	2.898	3.646
18	.257	688	1.330	1.734	2.101	2.552	2.878	3.610
19	.257	.688	1.328	1.729	2.093	2.539	2.861	3.579
20	0.257	0.687	1.325	1.725	2.086	2.528	2.845	3.552
21	.257	.686	1.323	1.721	2.080	2.518	2.831	3.527
22	.256	.686	1.321	1.717	2.074	2.508	2.819	3.505
23	.256	.685	1.319	1.714	2.069	2.600	2.807	3.485
24	.256	.685	1.318	1.711	2.064	2.492	2.797	3.467
25	0.256	0.684	1,316	1.708	2.060	2.485	2.787	3.450
26	.256	.654	1,315	1.706	2.056	2.479	2.779	3.435
27	.256	.684	1,314	1.701	2.052	2.473	2.771	3.421
28	.256	.683	1,313	1.701	2.048	2.467	2.763	3.408
29	.256	.683	1.311	1.699	2.045	2.462	2.756	3.396
30	0.256	0.683	1.310	1.697	2.042	2.457	2.750	3.385
40	.255	.681	1.303	1.684	2.021	2.423	2.704	3.307
60	.254	.679	1.296	1.671	2.000	2.390	2.660	3.232
120	.254	.677	1.289	1.658	1.950	2.358	2.617	3.160
∞	.253	.674	1.282	1.645	1.960	2.326	2.576	3.090

5 Calculation of Required Sample Size, Rationale

An essential part of planning a clinical trial is to decide how many people need to be studied in order to answer the study objectives. Just pulling the sample sizes out of a hat gives rise to:

1. Ethical problems, because if too many patients are given a potentially inferior treatment, this is not ethical to do.

2. Scientific problems, because negative studies require the repetition of the research.
3. Financial problems, because extra costs are involved in too small and too large studies.

If we have no prior arguments to predict the outcome of a trial, we at least will have an idea of the kind of result that would be clinically relevant. This is also a very good basis to place prior sample size requirement on. For example, a smaller study, for example, will be needed to detect a fourfold increase than a twofold one. So the sample size also depends on the size of result we want to demonstrate reliably.

6 Calculations of Required Sample Size, Methods

An essential part of planning a clinical trial is to decide: how many people need to be studied in order to answer the study objectives.

6.1 A Simple Method

Mean should be at least 1.96 or approximately 2 SEMs distant from 0 to obtain statistical significance.

Assume: mean $= 2$ SEM
Then   mean $/$ SEM $= 2$
Then   mean $/$ SD $/ \sqrt{n} = 2$
Then $\sqrt{n} = 2.\text{SD} / \text{mean}$
Then $n = 4 . (\text{SD} / \text{mean})^2$

For example, with mean $= 10$ and SD $= 20$ we will need a sample size of at least $n = 4$ $(20/10)^2 = 4 \times 4 = 16$. P-value is then 0.05 but power is only 50%.

6.2 A More Accurate Method Is the Power Index Method

The statistical power (1) of a trial assessing a new treatment versus control is determined by three major variables:

(2) D (mean difference or mean result),
(3) Variance in the data estimated as SD or SEM,
(4) Sample size.

It follows that we can calculate (4) if we know the other three variables.

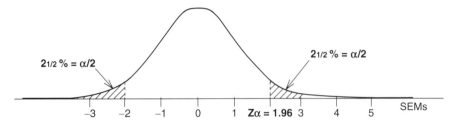

Fig. 6.6 Calculating power indexes

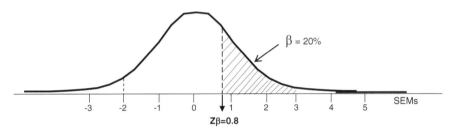

Fig. 6.7 Calculating power indexes

The relationship between (4) and the three other variables can be expressed in fancy formulas with $(z_\alpha + z_\beta)^2 = $ **power index** as an important element in all of them. Here is the formula for continuous variables

$$n = (SD \, / \, mean)^2 \, (z_\alpha + z_\beta)^2$$

If the power index for null-hypothesis is $(z_\alpha + z_\beta)^2$, what is the size of this $(z_\alpha + z_\beta)^2$?

What does for example $Z_{(alpha)}$ exactly mean? $Z_{(alpha)}$ **means "a place" on the Z-line. What place?** If **alpha** is defined 5%, or rather $2 \times 2\ 1/2\%$, then right from this place on the Z-line AUC=5%, or rather $2 \times 2\ 1/2\%$. So this place must be 1.96 SEMs distant from 0, or a bit more with t-distribution. **So $Z_{alpha} = 1.96 = $ approximately 2.0** (Fig. 6.6).

What does $Z_{(beta)}$ exactly mean? If **beta** is defined 20%, what is the place on Z-line of $Z_{(beta)}$? Right from this place the AUC=20% of the total AUC. This means that this place must be approximately 0.6 SEMs distant from 0. **So $Z_{beta} = $ approximately 0.8** (Fig. 6.7).

Now we can calculate the power index $(z_\alpha + z_\beta)^2$.

$Z_{(alpha)} = $ approximately 2.0
$Z_{(beta)} = $ approximately 0.8
power index $= (z_\alpha + z_\beta)^2 = 2.8^2 = 7.8$

As the formula for continuous variables is $n = (SD/mean)^2 (z_\alpha + z_\beta)^2$, we can now conclude that with $\alpha = 5\%$ and power $= 1 - \beta = 80\%$ the required sample size is $n = 7.8$ $(SD/mean)^2$. For example, with $SD = 20$ and mean $= 10$, we will need a sample size of $n = 7.8 \, (20/10)^2 = \mathbf{32.}$

So, accounting a power of 80% requires 32, rather than the 16 patients, required according to the simple method.

6.3 Power Calculation for Parallel-Group Studies

For parallel-group studies including two groups larger sample sizes are required. Each group produces its own mean and standard deviation (SD).

The pooled $SD = \sqrt{(SD_{group1}^2 + SD_{group2}^2)}$

The equation for sample size is given by:

$$n = 2 \, (z_\alpha + z_\beta)^2 \, (\text{pooled SD} / \text{mean difference})^2$$

If the mean difference $= 10$, and the pooled $SD = \sqrt{(20^2 + 20^2)} = 28.3$, then the required sample size is given by

$$n = 2 \times 7.8 \times (28.3/10)^2 = 2 \times 7.8 \times 8.01 = 126$$

Thus, 63 subjects per group are required for the purpose of 80% power with alpha $= 0.05$.

6.4 Required Sample Size Equation for Studies with Proportions

If we have arguments to expect events in 10% of the subjects included, then $p = $ proportion $= 0.1$. The SD of this proportion $= \sqrt{[p(1-p)]}$.

The equations for continuous data and proportions are very similar.

$$\text{Continuous data}: n = \text{powerindex} \times (SD/mean)^2$$
$$\text{Proportions} \quad : n = \text{powerindex} \times (SD/proportion)^2$$

So, if $p = 0.10$, then the required sample size is given by

$$n = 7.8 \times [(0.1 \times 0.9)/0.1]^2$$

For parallel-group studies with two proportions we again have to pool the SDs.

$$\text{pooled SDs} = \sqrt{(SD_{group1}^2 + SD_{group2}^2)}$$

For example

	Number of subjects with an event		
	Yes	No	
Group 1	a	b	proportion $p_1 = a/(a+b)$ $SD_1 = \sqrt{[p_1(1-p_2)]}$
Group 2	c	d	proportion $p_2 = c/(c+d)$ $SD_2 = \ldots\ldots$
			pooled $SD = \sqrt{(SD_1^2 + SD_2^2)}$

It is hard to recognize the equation from the equation of continuous data, but it is actually very similar:

$$n = 2(z_\alpha + z_\beta)^2 \cdot \frac{p_1(1-p_1)+p_2(1-p_2)}{(p_1-p_2)^2}$$

(where p_1 and p_2 are the proportions to be compared).

As an example a standard and new treatment are compared.

The standard treatment produces a proportion of responders of $p_1 = 0.1$, the new treatment of $p_2 = 0.2$. The required sample size is calculated according to

$$n = 2 \times 7.8 \times \frac{0.1(1-0.1)+0.2(1-0.2)}{(0.1-0.2)^2} = 390$$

The required sample per group is, thus, 195.

Note that a requested power of 90% means a power index of 10.5. In this study 526 subjects would have to be included.

6.5   Required Sample Size Formula for Equivalence Testing

$$N = 2(\text{between subject variance})(z_{1-1/2\alpha} + z_{1-1/2\beta})^2 / D^2$$

(where D is minimal difference we wish to detect).

What size is the **power index of equivalence test** $(z_{1-1/2\alpha}+z_{1-1/2\beta})^2$?
If the power index of equivalence testing $= (z_{1-1/2\alpha}+z_{1-1/2\beta})^2$
What is the size of this power index?

If alpha is defined 5%, then ½ alpha = 2 ½%. What is the place on the Z-line of $Z_{(1-1/2\alpha)}$? **Left from this place the AUC = $1-$½ alpha = $100-2$ ½% = 97 ½% of total AUC.** So this place is, just like Z_{alpha}, 1.96 SEMs distant from 0, or bit more with t-distribution. So, $Z_{(1-½\,alpha)} = 1.96$ **or approximately 2.0** (Fig. 6.8).

Now, if beta is defined 20%, then ½ beta = 10% What is the place on the Z-line of $Z_{(1-1/2\,beta)}$? **Left from the place the AUC = 100% $-$ 10% = 90% of total AUC.**

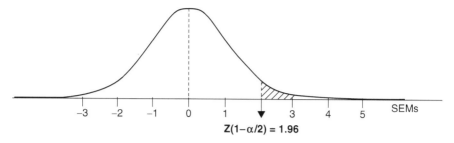

Fig. 6.8 Calculating power indexes

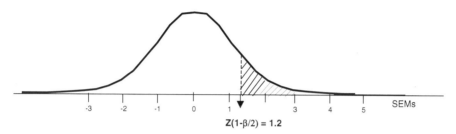

Fig. 6.9 Calculating power indexes

This means that this place must be approximately 1.2 SEMs distant from 0, or a bit more, and, thus, $\mathbf{Z}_{(1-\frac{1}{2}\,\mathbf{beta})}=\mathbf{approximately\ 1.2}$ (Fig. 6.9).

Now we can calculate this power index. $Z_{(1-\frac{1}{2}\alpha)}=$approximately 2.0. $Z_{(1-\frac{1}{2}\beta)}=$app 1.2. The power index for equivalence testing$=(2.0+1.2)^2=$approximately 10.9.

Note: power index null hypothesis testing =   7.8
         power index equivalence testing = 10.9

Obviously, for equivalence testing larger sample sizes are required !

Equivalence trials often include too few patients. The conclusion of equivalence becomes meaningless if, due to this, the design lacks power. Testing equivalence usually requires a sample larger than that of comparative null hypothesis testing studies. Required numbers of patients to be included should be estimated at the design stage of such studies.

7   Testing Inferiority of a New Treatment (Type III Error)

An inferior treatment may sometimes mistakenly be believed to be superior. "Negative" studies, defined as studies that do not confirm their prior hypotheses, may be "nega-tive" because an inferior treatment is mistakenly believed to be superior. However, from a statistical point of view this possibility is unlikely, because the possibility of a

PROBABILITY
DISTRIBUTION

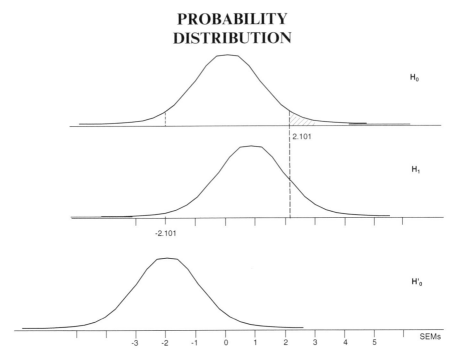

Fig. 6.10 Study with n = 20 and mean results + 1 SEM distant from the mean of the null-hypothesis of no treatment effect (H₀). For testing the chance that our treatment is significantly inferior, a new null hypothesis at approximately – 2SEMs left from zero is required

type III error can not be rejected. Suppose in a study the mean results is+1 SEM distant from the mean of the null hypothesis of no treatment effect (Fig. 6.10).

This means that we are unable to reject this null hypothesis, because a null hypothesis is rejected when the mean result of a study is more than about 2 SEMs distant from zero (P<0.05), and the study is thus "negative". For testing the chance that our treatment is significantly inferior, a new null-hypothesis at approximately – 2SEMs distant from zero is required (Fig. 6.10). This null-hypothesis is about 3 SEMs distant from our mean result, which means that this chance is <0.001. So, it seems that even statistically "negative" trials give strong evidence that the favored treatment is, indeed, not inferior. This issue can be illustrated by an example. The treatment of hypertension is believed to follow a J-shape curve, where overtreatment produces increased rather than reduced mortality/morbidity. A different theory would tell you that the more intensive the therapy the better the result. This latter theory was recently tested in the HOT trial (HOT investigators 1998), but could not be confirmed: high dosage antihypertensive therapy was not significantly better than medium-dosage therapy. Probably it was not worse either, however, unfortunately, this was not tested in the report. The study would definitely have been powerful to test this question, and, moreover, it would have solved a major so far unsolved discussion.

An additional advantage of testing type III errors is, that it helps preventing well-designed studies from going down in history as just "negative" studies that did not prove anything and are more likely not to be published, leading to unnecessary and costly repetition of research. If such "negative" studies are capable of rejecting the chance of a type III error, they may be reconsidered as a study that is not completely negative and may be rightly given better priority for being published.

The issue of non-inferiority has developed tremendously in the past years, and this subject will be re-addressed in a broader perspective in Chapter 63.

8 Conclusions

1. If underlying hypothesis is that one treatment is really different from control, power analysis is a more reliable to evaluate the data than null hypothesis testing; Power level of at least 80% is recommended. Power=chance of finding a difference where there actually is one.
2. Despite speculative character of prior estimates, it is inappropriate not to calculate required sample size based on expected results.
3. Type III error demonstrates in negative trial whether the new treatment is worse than control.
4. Important formulas:

$$\text{Power} = 1 - \text{prob}\left(z < (t - t^1)\right) \quad \text{where prob} = \text{probability}$$

Power index needed for calculating sample size $(z_\alpha + z_\beta)^2$ is generally 7.8.

$$\text{Required sample size} = 2.(SD / \text{mean})^2 (z_\alpha + z_\beta)^2$$

5. Required knowledge after studying this chapter: to calculate power from simple example of (continuous) trial data using t-table, to calculate required sample size for continuous data trial with alpha=0.05 and beta=0.20 using power index.

Reference

HOT investigators (1998) The HOT trial. Lancet 87:133–142

Chapter 7
Interim Analyses

1 Introduction

Clinical trials tend to have a long duration, because mostly patients are enrolled one by one, and their responses to treatment are observed sequentially. For the organizers this part of the trial is an exciting phase because after all the hard work involved in planning and getting the trial started, finally concrete data will become available. Immediately, there is the possibility to look at the data in order to check that the trial protocol is pursued appropriately by the investigators and to look at any difficulties, e.g., those with patient and/or doctor compliance, and to see whether there is any need for protocol alterations (Pocock 1988a). "Looking at the data" for such purposes should, however, be done carefully. In this chapter we will discuss questions such as:

1. why should we monitor a trial;
2. who should monitor a trial;
3. what should be monitored;
4. why should we be careful.

2 Monitoring

Careful conduct of a clinical trial according to the protocol has a major impact on the credibility of the results (Department of Health and Human Services, Food and Drug Administration 1998); to ensure patient/doctor compliance with the protocol, careful monitoring of the trial is a prerequisite. In large-scale pharmaceutical phase III trials, mainly two types of monitoring are being used: one is concerned with quality assessment of trial, and the other with the assumptions that were made in the protocol concerning treatment differences, power, and adverse effects. The quality of the trial is greatly enhanced when checks are performed to ensure that:

1. the protocol requirements are appropriately met by investigators and patients;
2. inclusion and exclusion criteria are appropriately met;
3. the rate of inclusion of patients in the trial is in accordance with the trial plan;
4. the data are being accrued properly, and;
5. design assumptions are met.

This type of monitoring does not require access to the data in the trial, nor is unblinding necessary, and therefore has no impact on the Type I error of finding a difference where there is none (Department of Health and Human Services, Food and Drug Administration 1998) (see also Sects. 6.1 and 6.2 of the current book). Usually, this type of monitoring is carried out by a specialized monitoring team under the responsibility of the steering committee of the trial. The period for this type of monitoring starts with the selection of the trial centers and ends with the collection and cleaning of the last patient's data.

Inclusion and exclusion criteria should be kept constant, as specified in the protocol, throughout the period of patient recruitment. In very long-term trials accumulating medical knowledge either from outside the trial, or from interim analyses, may warrant a change in inclusion or exclusion criteria. Also, very low recruitment rates due to over-restrictive criteria, may sometimes favor some change in the criteria. These should be made without breaking the blinding of the trial and should always be described in a protocol amendment to be submitted to the ethic committee for their approval. This amendment should also cover any statistical consequences such as sample size, and alterations to the planned statistical analysis.

The rate of subject accrual should be monitored carefully, especially with long-term trials. If it falls below the expected level, the reasons why so should be identified, and action taken not to jeopardize the power of the trial. Naturally, the quality of the data should be assessed carefully. Attempts should be made to recover missing data and to check the consistency of the data.

3   Interim Analysis

The other type of monitoring requires the comparison of treatment results, and it, therefore, generally requires at least partly unblinded access to treatment group assignment. This type of monitoring is actually called interim analysis. It refers to any analysis intended to compare treatment arms with respect to efficacy or safety at any time prior to formal completion of the trial.

The primary goals for monitoring trial data through interim analysis include

1. ethical concerns to avoid any patient receiving a treatment the very moment it is recognized to be inferior;
2. (cost-)efficiency concerns of avoiding undue prolongation of a trial once the treatment differences are reasonably clear-cut, and;

3. checking whether prior assumptions concerning sample size, treatment efficacy and adverse effects are still valid.

As the sample-size of the trial is generally based on preliminary and/or uncertain information, an interim check on the unblinded data may also be useful to reveal whether or not overall response variances, event rates or survival experience are as anticipated. A revised sample size may then be required using suitable modified assumptions. As a matter of course, such modification should be documented in a protocol amendment and in the clinical study report. Steps taken to preserve blindness during the rest of the trial and consequences for the risk of type I errors and the width of the confidence intervals should be accounted for.

Particularly, severe toxic reactions, as well as other adverse effects, are important and need careful observation and reporting to the steering committee, so that prompt action can be taken. Investigators need to be warned to look out for such events and dose modifications may be necessary.

Every process of examining and analyzing data as accumulated in a clinical trial, either formally or informally, can introduce bias and/or increase of type I errors. Therefore, all interim analyses, formal or informal, preplanned or ad hoc, by any study participant, steering committee member, or data monitoring group should be described in full in the clinical study report, even if their results were disclosed to the investigators while on trial (Drug Administration 1996).

For the purpose of reducing the risk of biases there are a number of important points in the organisation of the analysis and the interpretation of its results to keep in mind.

I – In most trials there are many outcome variables, but in interim analyses it is best to limit the number to only the major variables in order to avoid the multiple comparison problem (referred to in Sect. 1.1). Pocock (1988a) recommends to use only one main treatment comparison for which a formal 'stopping rule' may be defined, and to use the other treatment comparisons only as an informal check on the consistency of any apparent difference in the main comparison.

II – It is important to perform the interim analysis on correct and up-to-date data. The data monitoring and data checks should be performed on all of the data generated at the time of the interim analysis in order to avoid any selection bias in the patients.

III – The interim analysis should be performed only when there is a sufficient number of patients. Any comparison is academic when the sample size is so small that even huge treatment differences will not be significant.

IV – The interim analysis should not be too elaborate, because there is a limited goal, namely to check whether differences in the main treatment comparison are not huge to the extent that further continuation of the trial would seem unethical.

V – The interim analysis should be planned only when a decision to stop the trial is a serious possibility. With very long-term treatment periods in a trial when the period between patient entry and observance of patient outcome is very long, the patient accrual may be completed before any interim analysis can be performed and the interim analysis results will have no impact on the trial anymore.

VI – The decision to stop the trial must be made according to a predefined stopping rule. The rule should be formulated in terms of magnitude and statistical significance of treatment differences and must be considered in the light of adverse effects, current knowledge, and practical aspects such as ease of administration, acceptability and cost. We must decide in advance what evidence of a treatment difference is sufficiently strong to merit stopping the trial. Statistical significance is a commonly used criterion, but the usual P-level is not appropriate. The problem with statistical significance testing of interim data is that the risk of a type I error may be considerably increased because we perform more than one analysis. Hence, for a sequence of interim analyses we must set a more stringent significance level than the usual P<0.05. We may use a Bonferroni adjustment (see also Chap. 1 introduction), i.e., use as significance level the value 0.05 divided by the number of planned interim analyses, but this leads in most cases to a somewhat overconservative significance level. Therefore, in most trials a so-called group-sequential design is employed. This subject will be discussed in the next section. A practical guideline is to use Pocock's criteria (Pocock 1988b): **if one anticipates no more than 10 interim analyses and there is one main response variable, one can adopt p < 0.01 as the criterion for stopping the trial.** An example of this approach is the following: "stop the trial if the treatment difference is 20% or larger and this difference is statistically significant with a p-value less than 0.01, and the proportion patients with adverse effects is less than 10%." The outcome of the interim analysis may also be such that the treatments differ far less than expected. In such case the trial might be stopped for lack of efficacy. Again, it is essential that a formal stopping rule is formulated in advance specifying the boundary for the treatment difference for the given confidence intervals (CIs). In this case statistical significance is not helpful as an additional criterion, but it is helpful to calculate the confidence interval of the observed treatment difference and to see whether the expected treatment difference, specified in the protocol, is far outside that interval.

VII – It is necessary to keep the results of the interim analysis as confidential as possible. Investigators may change their outlook and future participation to the trial, and might even change their attitudes towards treatment of patients in the trial if he/she is aware of any interim results. This may cause a serious bias to the overall trial results. The U.S. Food and Drug Administration (FDA) therefore recommends not only that the execution of the interim analysis be highly confidential (Department of Health and Human Services, Food and Drug Administration 1998), but also that the investigators not be informed about its results unless a decision to stop the trial has been made. An external independent group of investigators should ideally perform the interim analysis, for the benefit of the objectivity of the research (although complete independence may be an illusion, it is still better to have some other persons with their own ethical and scientific principles look at your data than do it yourself). The steering committee should be informed about the decisions to continue or discontinue or the implementation of protocol amendments only.

VIII – There is little advantage to be gained from carrying out a large number of interim analyses: the consequences of executing many interim analyses are that the sample sizes are small (at least in the first analyses), and that a smaller significance level must be used. Pocock (1988c) recommends never to plan more than five interim analyses, but at the same time to plan at least one interim analysis, in order to warrant scientific and ethical validity of the trial.

4 Group-Sequential Design of Interim Analysis

Group sequential design is the most widely used method to define the stopping rule precisely and it was introduced by Pocock (1977). The FDA (Department of Health and Human Services, Food and Drug Administration 1998) advocates the use of this design, though it is not the only acceptable type of design, and the FDA does so particularly for the purpose of safety assessment, one of its major concerns.

In a group-sequential trial we need to decide about the number (N) of interim analyses and the number (n) of patients per treatment that should be evaluated in between successive analyses: i.e. if the trial consists of two treatment arms 2n patients must be evaluated in each interim analysis. Pocock (1977) (and extensively explained in Pocock (Food and Drug Administration 1996)) provides tables for the exact nominal significance levels depending on the number of interim analyses N and the overall significance level,. For instance if a trial is evaluated using a normal distributed response variable with known variance and one wishes the overall significance level to be,$= 0.05$ and one plans $N = 2$ analyses, then the nominal significance level must be set at 0.0294. If $N = 3$ or 4 or 5, the nominal significance levels must be set at 0.0221, 0.0182, and 0.0158, respectively. For other types of response variables, Pocock (1977) provides similar tables. Pocock (1977) also provides tables of the optimal sample size numbers of patients to be included in successive interim analyses.

Several extensions of the practical rules of Pocock were developed, for instance rules for letting the nominal significance level vary between interim analyses. In practice a far more stringent p-value is suggested for earlier interim analyses and a less stringent one for later analyses. Pocock (1988a) claimed that such a variation might be sensible for studies with a low power, but that almost no efficiency is gained in studies with powers of 90% or higher. Other extensions concern one-sided testing (Demets and Ware 1980) and skewed designs where a less stringent rule might be adopted for stopping if the new treatment is worse than the standard and a more stringent rule if the new treatment appears to be better than the standard.

5 Continuous Sequential Statistical Techniques

Historically, the statistical theory for stopping rules in clinical trials has been largely concerned with sequential designs for continuous monitoring of treatment differences. The basic principle is that after every additional patient on each treatment has been evaluated, some formal statistical rule is applied to the whole data so far to determine whether the trial should stop. The theory of sequential techniques is

Treatment difference (z)

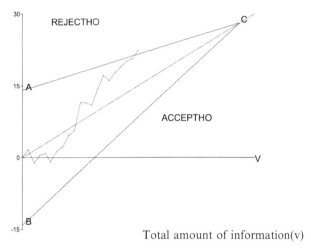

Fig. 7.1 Typical example of a sequential trial with a so-called triangular test. The *undulating line* illustrates a possible realisation of a clinical trial: after each time a new patient could be evaluated, Z and V are calculated and the line is extended a little further. The line-sections AC and BC are the stopping boundaries, and the triangular region ABC is the continuation region. If the sample path crosses AC, the null hypothesis is rejected at the 5% significance level, and if BC is crossed then H_0 is accepted. When Z is replaced by t or chi-square statistic, and V by degrees of freedom, the graph represents very much the same as the t- or chi-square tables (Appendix) respectively do

already quite old (developed in the early 1940s and even earlier than that (Wald 1947)), and many excellent textbooks have been published (Armitage 1975); here we adopt the arguments of Whitehead (1983).

The central idea is to calculate after each additional patient (or after I additional patients) (a function of) the treatment difference, called Z, and the total amount of information, called V, sampled thus far. These two statistics are plotted graphically against each other each time a new patient is evaluated. The stopping rule of the trial entails evaluating whether a boundary is crossed. In Fig. 7.1 a typical example of a sequential trial with a so-called triangular test is illustrated.

The undulating line illustrates a possible realisation of a clinical trial: after each time a new patient could be evaluated, Z and V are calculated and the line is extended a little further. The line-sections AC and BC are the stopping boundaries, and the triangular region ABC is the continuation region. If the sample path crosses AC, the null hypothesis is rejected at the 5% significance level, and if BC is crossed then H_0 is accepted. The triangular test is one of many possible sequential trial designs; but the triangular test has some very attractive characteristics. If the treatment difference is large, it will lead to a steeply increasing sample path, and consequently to a small trial because the AC boundary is reached quickly. If there is no difference between treatment, the sample path will move horizontally and will cross the BC boundary quickly which also leads to a small trial. If the treatment difference is negative, the BC boundary will be crossed even quicker.

The trick is to devise sensible boundaries. Whitehead (1983) gives an elaborate discussion on how to do this (as well as how to calculate Z and V). Whitehead (1983) also discussed many different sequential plans for many different types of clinical trials and data-types. Whitehead and his associates have also developed a user-friendly computer program to design and analyze sequential clinical trials (Whitehead 1998).

6   Conclusions

Interim analyses in clinical trials can be of great importance in maintaining quality standards of the entire investigation and such analyses may be of crucial importance if clinical trials are to be ethically acceptable. Drawbacks of interim analyses are the increased risk of the type I error and the potential introduction of several kinds of biases, such as loss of validity factors, including blinding and randomization. It is rarely sensible to perform more than five interim analyses and usual one interim analysis before the final assessment suffices. It is crucial to specify in advance in the study protocol, how many analyses are to be performed and on how many patients, and which decisions are to be made on the basis of the interim results. It is best to let an external independent group, often called Independent Data Monitoring Committee (IDMC), execute the job and to keep its results as confident as is ethically possible. To do so, will be difficult but rewarding, and contribute to the credibility and scientific value of the trial results.

References

Armitage P (1975) Sequential medical trials. Blackwell, Oxford

Demets DL, Ware JH (1980) Group sequential methods in clinical trials with a one-sided hypothesis. Biometrika 67:651–660

Department of Health and Human Services, Food and Drug Administration (1998) International conference on harmonisation; guidance on statistical principles for clinical trials availability. Fed Regist 63(179):49583–49598

Food and Drug Administration (1996) Guideline for industry. Structure and content of clinical study reports. FDA. At internet website WWW.DFA.GOV/CDER/REGGUIDE.HTM/GUIDANCEDOCUMENTS

Pocock SJ (1977) Group sequential methods in the design and analysis of clinical trials. Biometrika 64:191–199

Pocock SJ (1988a) Clinical trials. A practical approach. Wiley, New York, p 62

Pocock SJ (1988b) Clinical trials. A practical approach. Wiley, New York, p 147

Pocock SJ (1988c) Clinical trials. A practical approach. Wiley, New York, p 153

Pocock SJ (1988d) Clinical trials. A practical approach. Wiley, New York, p 149

Wald A (1947) Sequential analysis. Wiley, New York

Whitehead J (1983) The design and analysis of sequential clinical trials. Ellis Horwood publishers, Chichester

Whitehead J (1998) Planning and evaluating sequential trials (PEST, version 3). University of Reading, Reading. www.reading.ac.uk/mps/pest/pest.html

Chapter 8
Controlling the Risk of False Positive Clinical Trials

1 Introduction

Statistical hypothesis testing is much like gambling. If, with gambling once, your chance of a prize is 5%, then, with gambling 20 times, this chance will be close to 40%. The same is true with statistical testing of clinical trials. If, with one statistical test, your chance of a significant result is 5%, then after 20 tests, it will increase to 40%. This result is, however, not based on a true treatment effect, but, rather, on the play of chance. In current clinical trials, instead of a single efficacy-variable of one treatment, multiple efficacy-variables of more than one treatment are increasingly assessed. For example, in 16 randomized controlled trials with positive results, published in the British Medical Journal (BMJ) in 2004 (Table 8.1), the numbers of primary efficacy-variables varied from 4 to 13. This phenomenon introduces the statistical problem of multiple comparisons and multiple testing, which increases the risk of false positive results, otherwise called type I errors. There is no consensus within the statistical community on how to cope with this problem. Also, the issue has not been studied thoroughly for every type of variable. Clinical trials rarely adjust their data for multiple comparisons. For example, none of the underneath BMJ papers did. The current chapter briefly summarizes the main methods for control in order to further emphasize the importance of this issue, and it gives examples.

2 Bonferroni Test

If more than two samples are compared in a clinical trial, multiple groups analysis of variance (ANOVA) is often applied for the analysis. For example, three groups of patients were treated with different hemoglobin improving compounds with the following results:

T.J. Cleophas and A.H. Zwinderman, *Statistics Applied to Clinical Studies*,
DOI 10.1007/978-94-007-2863-9_8, © Springer Science+Business Media B.V. 2012

Table 8.1 Positive randomized controlled trials published in the BMJ in 2004

	Numbers of primary efficacy variables	Smallest p-values	Positive study after Bonferroni adjustment
Adjustment			
1. Schroter et al. 328: 742–3	5	0.001	Yes
2. Laurant et al. 328: 927–30	12	0.006	No
3. Yudkin et al. 328: 989–90	10	0.001	Yes
4. Craig et al. 328: 1067–70	6	0.030	No
5. Kalra et al. 328: 1099–101	7	0.001	Yes
6. Hilten et al. 328: 1281–1	5	0.05	No
7. James et al. 328: 1237–9	10	0.003	Yes
8. Logan et al. 328: 1372–4	6	0.01	No
9. Cairns S Smith et al. 328: 1459–63	13	0.002	Yes
10. Powell et al. 329: 89–91	10	0.001	Yes
11. Henderson et al. 329: 136–9	6	0.03	No
12. Collins et al. 329: 193–6	4	0.03	No
13. Svendsen et al. 329: 253–8	7	0.02	No
14. McKendry M 329: 258–61	9	0.001	Yes
15. Van Staaij et al. 329: 651–4	8	0.01	No
16. Norman et al. 329: 1259–62	10	0.02	Yes

	Sample size	Mean hemoglobin mmol/l	Standard deviation mmol/l
Group 1	16	8.725	0.8445
Group 2	10	10.6300	1.2841
Group 3	15	12.3000	0.9419

The F test produces a p-value <0.01, indicating that a highly significant difference is observed between the three groups. This leads to the not-too-informative information that not all group means were equal. A question encountered is, which group did and which one did not differ from the others. This question involves the problem of multiple comparisons. As there are three different treatments, three different pairs of treatments can be compared: groups 1 versus 2, groups 1 versus 3, and groups 2 versus 3. The easiest approach is to calculate the Student's t-test for each comparison. It produces a highly significant difference at $p<0.01$ between treatment 1 versus 3 with no significant differences between the other comparisons. This highly significant result is, however, unadjusted for multiple comparisons. If the chance of a falsely positive result is, e.g. α with one comparison, it should be 2α with two, and close to 3α with three comparisons. Bonferroni recommends to reject the null-hypothesis at a lower level of significance according to the formula

$$\text{rejection p - value} = \alpha \times 2/k\,(k-1)$$

k = number of comparisons, α = agreed chance of falsely positive result (mostly 0.05).

In case of three comparisons the rejection p-value will be $0.05 \times \dfrac{2}{3(3-1)} = 0.0166$.

A p-value of 0.0166 is still larger than 0.01, and, so, the difference observed remains significant, but using a cut-off p-value of 0.0166, instead of 0.05, the difference is not highly significant anymore.

3   Least Significant Difference (LSD) Test

As an alternative to the Bonferroni test a refined t-test, the least significant difference (LSD) test, can be applied. This refined t-statistic has n-k degrees of freedom, where n is the number of observations in the entire sample and k is the number of treatment groups. In the denominator of this refined t-test the pooled-within-group variance from the F-test mentioned in the previous section, is used (see also page 114, Eq. 1). For the application of the LSD procedure, it is essential to perform it sequentially to a significant F-test of the ANOVA procedure. So, if one chooses to perform the LSD procedure, one first calculates the ANOVA procedure and stops if it is not significant, and calculates the LSD test only if the F-test is statistically significant. Otherwise, the test is similar to the Bonferroni-test, and yields with the above example a p-value smaller than 0.05. Like with Bonferroni, the difference is still significant, but not highly significant anymore.

4   Other Tests for Adjusting the p-Values

None of the 16 BMJ trials discussed in the introduction were adjusted for multiple testing. When we performed a Bonferroni adjustment of them, only eight trials continued to be positive, while the remainder turned into negative studies. This does not necessarily indicate that all of these studies were truly negative. Several of them had more than five efficacy-variables, and, in this situation, the Bonferroni test is somewhat conservative, meaning that power is lost, and the risk of falsely negative results is raised. This is particularly so, if variables are highly correlated. A somewhat less conservative variation of the Bonferroni correction was suggested by Hochberg: if there are k primary values multiply the highest p-value with 1, the second-largest p-value with 2, the third largest with 3…, and the smallest p-value with k (Hochberg 1988).

Calculated p-values	Reject null-hypothesis at
(1) Largest p-value	$\alpha_1 = 0.05 \times 1 = 0.05$
(2) Second largest p-value	$\alpha_2 = 0.05 \times 2 = 0.10$
(3) Third largest p-value	$\alpha_3 = 0.05 \times 3 = 0.15$
(k) kth largest p-value	$\alpha_k = 0.05 \times k = \ldots.$

The mathematical arguments of this procedure goes beyond this paper. What happens is, that the lowest and highest p-values will be less different from one another. There are other less conservative methods, like Tukey's honestly significant difference (HSD) test, Dunnett's test, Student-Newman-Keuls test, and the Hotelling Q-square test. Most of them have in common that they produce their own test-statistics. Tables of significance levels are available in statistical software packages including SAS and SPSS.

5 Composite Endpoint Procedures

A different solution for the multiple testing problem is to construct a composite endpoint of all of the efficacy-variables, and, subsequently, to perform a statistical analysis on the composite only. For example, it is reasonable to believe that statin treatment has a beneficial effect on total cholesterol (Tc), high density cholesterol (HDL), low density cholesterol (LDL), and triglycerides (Tg). We can perform a composite analysis of the four variables according to

$$\text{Composite variable} = \left(T_c + HDL + LDL + Tg \right) / 4$$

$$T_c = \frac{\left(T_c - \text{mean}(T_c) \right)}{SDT_c} \text{ etc}$$

A simple t-test produces
Placebo: mean result composite variable $= -0.23$ (SD 0.59)
Statin: mean result composite variable $= 0.15$ (SD 0.56)
$p = 0.006$

This p-value is lower than that obtained by a Bonferroni or LSD procedure. This is probably so, because of the added power provided by the positive correlation between the repeated observations in one subject. If no strong correlation between the variables is to be expected, the composite endpoint procedure provides power similar to that of the Bonferroni or LSD procedure.

Largely similar to the composite endpoint procedure are the index methods. If the efficacy-variables are highly correlated, because they more or less measure the same patient characteristic, then they be best replaced with their add-up sum. In this way the number of primary variables is reduced, and an additional advantage is that the standardized add-up sum of the separate variables is more reliable than the separate variables. For example, the Disease Activity Score (DAS) for the assessment of patients with rheumatoid arthritis, including the Ritchie joint pain score, the number of swollen joints, and the erythrocyte sedimentation rate, is an example of this approach (Fuchs 1993).

6 No Adjustments at all, and Pragmatic Solutions

A more philosophical approach to the problem of multiple comparisons is to informally integrate the data, look for trends without judging one or two low p-values among otherwise high p-values as proof of a significant difference in the data. However, both the medical community and the investigators may be unhappy with this solution, because they want the hard data to provide unequivocal answers to their questions, rather than uncertainties. An alternative and more pragmatic solution could be the standard use of lower levels of significance to reject the null-hypothesis. For the statistical analysis of interim analyses, that suffer from the same risk of increased type I errors due to multiple testing, Pocock's recommendation to routinely use $p < 0.01$ instead of $p < 0.05$ has been widely adopted (Pocock 1988). A similar rule could, of course, be applied to any multiple testing situation. The advantage would be that it does not damage the data, because the data remain undamaged. Moreover, any adjustments may produce new type I errors, particularly, if they are post-hoc, and not previously described in the study protocol.

7 Conclusions

Approaches to reducing the problem of multiple testing include (1) the Bonferroni, test, (2) the LSD method, (3) other less conservative, more rarely used methods like Tukey's honestly significant (HSD) method, Dunnett's test, Student-Newman-Keuls test, Hochberg's adjustment, and the Hotelling Q-square test. Alternative approaches to the problems of multiple testing include (4) the construct of composite endpoints, (5) no adjustment at all, but a more philosophical approach to the interpretation of the p-values, and (6) the replacement of the traditional 5% rejection level with a 1% rejection level or less.

Evidence-based medicine is increasingly under pressure, because clinical trials do not adequately apply to their target populations (Furberg 2002; Julius 2003; Cleophas and Cleophas 2003). Many causes are mentioned. As long as the issue of multiple testing is rarely assessed in the analysis of randomized controlled trials, it can not be excluded as one of the mechanisms responsible. We recommend that the increased risk of false positive results should be taken into account in any future randomized clinical trial which assesses more than one efficacy-variable and/or treatment modality. The current chapter provides six possible methods for assessment.

References

Cleophas GM, Cleophas TJ (2003) Clinical trials in jeopardy. Int J Clin Pharmacol Ther 41:51–56

Fuchs HA (1993) The use of the disease activity score in the analysis of clinical trials in rheumatoid arthritis. J Rheumatol 20:1863–1866

Furberg C (2002) To whom do the research findings apply? Heart 87:570–574

Hochberg Y (1988) A sharper Bonferroni procedure for multiple tests of significance. Biometrika 75:800–802

Julius S (2003) The ALHATT study: if you believe in evidence-based medicine. Stick to it. J Hypertens 21:453–454

Pocock SJ (1988) Clinical trials. A practical approach. Wiley, New York

Chapter 9
Multiple Statistical Inferences

1 Introduction

Clinical trials often assess the efficacy of more than one new treatment and often use mquestions about subgroups differences or about what variables do or do not contribute to the efficacy results, remain. Assessment of such questions introduces the statistical problem of multiple comparison and multiple testing, which increases the risk of false positive statistical results, and thus increases the type-I error risk. In the previous chapter six commonly-used methods for controlling the risk of this problem have been addressed. This chapter gives a more mathematical approach of the problem, and gives examples in which different methods are compared with one another.

2 Multiple Comparisons

When in a trial three of more treatments are compared to each other, the typical first statistical analysis is to test the null hypothesis (H_0) of no difference between treatments versus the alternative hypothesis (H_a) that at least one treatment deviates from the others. Suppose that in the trial k different treatments are compared, then the null hypothesis is formulated as $H_0 : \vartheta_1 = \vartheta_2 = ... = \vartheta_j$, where ϑ_i is the expected treatment-effect of treatment i. When the efficacy variable is quantitative (and normally distributed), then ϑ is the mean value. When the efficacy variable is binary (e.g. healthy or ill), then ϑ is the proportion of positive (say healthy) patients. When the efficacy variable is of ordinal character, or is a survival time, ϑ can have different quantifications. For the remainder of this paragraph we assume that the efficacy is quantitative and normally distributed, because for this situation the multiple comparison procedure has been studied thoroughestly.

Consider the randomized clinical trial comparing five different treatments for ejaculation praecox (Waldinger et al. 1998): one group of patients received a placebo

T.J. Cleophas and A.H. Zwinderman, *Statistics Applied to Clinical Studies*, DOI 10.1007/978-94-007-2863-9_9, © Springer Science+Business Media B.V. 2012

Table 9.1 Randomized clinical trial comparing five different treatments for ejaculation praecox (Waldinger et al. 1998): one group of patients received a placebo treatment (group 1), and the four other groups received different serotonin reuptake inhibitors (*SSRI*)

Treatment	Sample size (n)	Mean (x)	Standard deviation (S)
Placebo	9	3.34	1.14
SSRI A	6	3.96	1.09
SSRI B	7	4.96	1.18
SSRI C	12	5.30	1.51
SSRI D	10	4.70	0.78

The primary variable for evaluating the efficacy was the logarithmically transformed intravaginal ejaculation latency time (*IELT*) measured after 6 weeks of treatment

treatment (group 1), and the four other groups received different serotonin reuptake inhibitors (SSRI). The primary variable for evaluating the efficacy was the logarithmically transformed intravaginal ejaculation latency time (IELT) measured after 6 weeks of treatment. The null hypothesis in this trial was that there was no difference between the five groups of patients with respect to the mean of the logarithmically transformed IELT: $H_0 : \vartheta_1 = \vartheta_2 = \vartheta_3 = \vartheta_4 = \vartheta$. The summarized data of this trial are listed in Table 9.1.

The first statistical analysis was done by calculating the analysis of variance (ANOVA) table. The F-test for the testing the null hypothesis had value 4.13 with 4 and 39 degrees of freedom and p-value 0.0070. The within group sums of squares was 55.16 with 39 degrees of freedom, thus the mean squared error was $S = 1.41$. Since the p-value was far below the nominal level of $\alpha = 0.05$, the null hypothesis could be rejected. This led to the not-too-informative conclusion that not all population averages were equal. A question immediately encountered is which one of the different population did and which one did not differ from each other. This question concerns the problem of multiple comparisons or post-hoc comparison of treatment groups.

The only way of finding out which one of the populations means differ from each other is to compare every treatment group with all of the other groups or with a specified subset receiving other treatments. When there are five different treatments, $5 \times 4/2 = 10$ different pairs of treatments can be compared. In general, when there are k treatments, $k(k-1)/2$ different comparisons can be made.

The easiest approach to this question is to calculate the Student's t-test for each comparison of the groups i and j. This procedure may be refined by using in the denominator of the t-test the pooled-within-group variance S_w^2, as already calculated in the above F-test according to:

$$t_{ij} = \frac{\overline{x}_i - \overline{x}_j}{\sqrt{S_w^2 \left(\dfrac{1}{n_i} + \dfrac{1}{n_j} \right)}}. \tag{9.1}$$

This t-statistic has n-k degrees of freedom, where n is the total number of observations in the entire sample and k is the number of treatment groups. This procedure is called the "least significant difference" procedure (LSD procedure). For the application of the LSD procedure, it is essential to perform it sequentially to a significant F-test of the ANOVA procedure. So if one chooses to perform the LSD procedure, one first calculates the ANOVA procedure and stops if the F-test is non-significant, and calculates the LSD tests only when the F-test is statistically significant.

When the different treatment groups are compared without performing ANOVA first, or when you do so without the F-test being significant, then the problem of multiple comparisons is, particularly, enhanced. This means that when you make enough comparisons, the chance of finding a significant difference will be substantially larger than the nominal level of $\alpha = 0.05$: thus the risk of a type-I error will be (far) too large. There may be situations where we want to further the analysis all the same.

There are several ways, then, of dealing with the problem of an increased risk of type-I-error. The easiest method is to use the Bonferroni-correction, sometimes known as the modified LSD procedure. The general principle is that the significance level for the experiment, α_E is less than or equal to the significance level for each comparison, α_C, times the number of comparisons that are made (remember α is the chance of a type-I-error or the chance of finding a difference where there is none):

$$\alpha_E \leq \frac{k(k-1)}{2} \alpha_C \qquad (9.2)$$

If $\alpha_E \leq 0.05$, then this level of α is maintained if, α_c is taken to be, divided by the number of comparisons:

$$\alpha_C = \alpha \frac{2}{k(k-1)}. \qquad (9.3)$$

When k is not too large, this method performs well. However, if k is large (k>5), then the Bonferroni correction is overconservative, meaning that the nominal significance level soon will be much lower than $\alpha = 0.05$ and loss of power occurs accordingly.

There are several alternative methods (Multiple comparisons boek 2008), but here we will discuss briefly three of them: Tukey's honestly significant difference (HSD) method, the Student-Newman-Keuls method, and the method of Dunnett. Tukey's HSD method calculates the test-statistic from the above Eq. 9.1, but determines the significance level slightly differently, by considering the distribution of the largest standardized difference $\left| x_i - x_j \right| / se\, (x_i - x_j)$. This distribution is somewhat more complex than that of the t-distribution or of the LSD procedure. A table of significance levels is available in all major statistical books as well as statistical software packages such as SAS (2011) and SPSS (2011). The HSD procedure controls the maximum experiment wise error rate, and performs well in simulation studies, especially when sample sizes are unequal.

The Student-Newman-Keuls (SNK) procedure is a so-called multiple-stage or multiple range test. The procedure first tests the homogeneity of all k means at the nominal level α_k. When the homogeneity is rejected, then each subset of (k−1) means is tested for homogeneity at the nominal level α_{k-1}, and so on. It does so by calculating the studentized statistic in the above Eq. 9.1 for all pairs. The distribution of this statistic is again rather complex, and it depends on the degrees of freedom n-k (from ANOVA), on the number of comparisons that are made, and on α_k. The table of significance levels is likewise available in most statistical packages. The conclusions of the SNK procedure critically depend on the order of the pair wise comparisons being made. The proper procedure is to compare first the largest mean with the smallest, then the largest with the second-smallest, and so on. An important rule is that if no significant difference exists between two means, it should be concluded that no difference exists between any means enclosed by the two, without further need of testing.

There are many multiple range tests (Multiple comparisons boek 2008), mainly differing in their use of the significance level α_k, and α_{k-1}. The Student-Newman-Keuls procedure uses $\alpha_k = \alpha = 0.05$, and therefore does not control the maximum experimentwise error rate.

Finally, there is a special multiple comparison procedure for comparing all active treatments to a control or placebo group. This is the Dunnett's procedure. For all treatments the studentized statistic of above Eq. 9.1 compared to the placebo group is calculated. In case of Dunnett's procedure, this statistic again has a complex distribution (many-one t-statistic) which depends on the number of active treatment groups, the degrees of freedom and a correlation term which depends on the sample sizes in each treatment group. Tables are likewise available in statistical packages. If sample sizes are not equal, it is important to use the harmonic mean of the sample sizes when calculating the significance of the Dunnett's test.

Most of the statistical packages compute common multiple range tests, and provide associated confidence intervals for the difference in means. In our trial comparing four SSRIs and placebo in patients with ejaculation praecox, we were interested in all of the possible comparisons between the five treatment groups. Since the ANOVA F-test was statistically significant, we applied the LSD procedure to find out which treatment differed significantly from each other. We found the following results. HSD procedure, the Bonferroni correction, and Dunnett's procedure of the same data were applied for control (Table 9.2).

The mean difference indicates the differences of the means of the groups as shown in Table 9.1. The standard error as calculated from the studentized statistic in the Eq. 9.1, and is required in order to construct confidence intervals. The critical values for the construction of such confidence intervals are supplied by appropriate tables for the HSD, and Dunnett's procedure, but are also calculated by most statistical software programs. In our case it is obvious that the LSD procedure provides the smallest p-values, and significant differences between SSRIs B, C and D and placebo results, as well as between A and C results. When using the Bonferroni test or the HSD procedure, only SSRI C is significantly different from placebo. Dunnett's test agrees with the LSD procedure with respect to the differences of the SSRIs compared to placebo, but has no information on the differences between the SSRIs.

There is no general consensus on what post-hoc test to use or when to use it; as the statistical community has not yet reached agreement on this issue. The US Food

Table 9.2 In the trial from Table 9.1 the investigators were interested in all of the possible comparisons between the five treatment groups

Private		Difference Mean (SE)	P value LSD	HSD	Bonferroni	Dunnett
Placebo vs	A	−0.62 (0.63)	0.33	0.86	0.99	0.73
	B	−1.62 (0.60)	0.01	0.07	0.10	0.035
	C	−1.96 (0.52)	0.001	0.005	0.006	0.002
	D	−1.36 (0.55)	0.017	0.12	0.17	0.058
A vs	B	−1.00 (0.66)	0.14	0.56	0.99	
	C	−1.34 (0.60)	0.03	0.18	0.30	
	D	−0.74 (0.61)	0.24	0.75	0.99	
B vs	C	−0.34 (0.57)	0.56	0.98	0.99	
	D	0.26 (0.59)	0.66	0.99	0.99	
C vs	D	0.60 (0.51)	0.25	0.76	0.99	

Since the ANOVA F-test was statistically significant, we applied the LSD procedure to find out which treatment differed significantly from each other. We found the following results. HSD procedure, the Bonferroni correction, and Dunnett's procedure of the same data were applied for control
SE = standard error

and Drug Agency suggests in its clinical trial handbook for in house usage to describe in the study protocol the arguments for using a specific method, but refrains from making any preference. We have a light preference for calculating an overall test first such as is done with ANOVA, and subsequently proceed with the LSD test.

Unfortunately, so far multiple comparisons methods have not been developed much for discrete, ordinal and censored data. When dealing with such data, it is best to perform first an overall test by chi-square, Kruskal-wallis or logrank methods, and afterwards perform pairwise comparisons with a Bonferroni correction.

Whatever method for multiple comparisons, its use or the lack of its use should be discussed in the statistical analysis, and preferably be specified in the analysis plan of the study protocol.

3 Multiple Variables

Most clinical trials use several, and sometimes many, endpoints to evaluate the treatment efficacy. The use of significance tests separately for each endpoint comparison increases the risk of a type-I error of finding a difference where there is none. The statistical analysis should reflect awareness of this very problem, and in the study protocol the use or non-use of statistical adjustments or their lack must be explained. There are several ways of handling this problem of multiple testing.

I. The most obvious way is to simply reduce the number of endpoint parameters otherwise called primary outcome variable. Preferably, we should include one primary parameter, usually being the variable that provides the most relevant and convincing evidence of the primary objective of the trial. The trial success is formulated in terms of results demonstrated by this very variable, and prior sample size determination is also based on this variable. Other endpoint variables are placed on a lower level of importance and are defined secondary variables. The secondary variable results may be used to support the evidence provided by the primary variable.

It may sometimes be desirable to use two or more primary variables, each of which sufficiently important for display in the primary analysis. The statistical analysis of such an approach should be carefully spelled in the protocol. In particular, it should be stated in advance what result of any of these variables is least required for the purpose of meeting the trial objectives. Of course, if the purpose of the trial is to demonstrate a significant effect in two or more variables, then there is no need for adjustment of the type-I error risk, but the consequence is that the trial fails in its objectives if one of these variables do not produce a significant result. Obviously, such a rule enhances the chance of erroneously negative trials, in a way similar to the risk of negative trials due to small sample sizes.

II. A different more philosophical approach to the problem of multiple outcome variables is to look for trends without judging one or two low P-values among otherwise high P-values as proof. This requires discipline and is particularly efficient when multiple measurements are performed for the purpose of answering one single question, e.g., the benefit to health of a new drug estimated in terms of effect on mortality in addition to a number of morbidity variables. There is nothing wrong with this practice. We should not make any formal correction for multiple comparisons of this kind (see also Chap. 1, Sect. 1). Instead, we should informally integrate all the data before reaching a conclusion.

III. An alternative way of dealing with the multiple comparison problem when there are many primary variables, is to apply a Bonferroni correction. This means that *the p-value of every variable is multiplied by the number of endpoints k.* This ensures that if treatments were truly equivalent, the trial as a whole will have less than a 5% chance of getting any p-value less than 0.05; thus the overall type-I error rate will be less than 5%.

IV. The Bonferroni correction, however, is not entirely correct when multiple comparisons are dependent of each other (multiple comparisons in one subject cannot be considered independent of each other, compare Chap. 2, Sect. 3, for additional discussion of this issue). Also the Bonferroni correction is an overcorrection in case of larger numbers of endpoints, particularly when different endpoints are (highly) correlated. A somewhat more adequate variation of the Bonferroni correction, was suggested by Hochberg (1988). *When there are k primary values, the idea is to multiply the largest p-value with 1, the second-largest p-value with 2, the third largest p-value with 3, ..., and the smallest p-value with k.* We do not attempt to explain the mathematical arguments of this procedure, but conclude that lowest and highest –values will be less different from each other. In practice, Hochberg's procedure is frequently hardly less conservative than is the Bonferroni correction.

V. A further alternative for analyzing two or more primary variables is to design a summary measure or composite variable. With such an approach endpoint and primary variables must, of course, be assessed in advance, and the algorithm to calculate the composite must also be specified a priori. Since in this case primary variables are reduced to one composite, there is no need to make adjustments to salvage the type-I error rate. For the purpose of appropriate composite variables there are a few sensible rules to bear in mind:

- Highly correlated variables, measuring more or less the same patient characteristic can best be replaced by their average. In this way the number of primary variables is reduced, and an additional advantage is that the mean is more reliable than both single measurements.
- When the variables have different scales (e.g. blood pressure is measured in mm Hg units, and cholesterol in mmol/L units), the composite variables are best calculated as standardized variables. This means that the overall mean is subtracted from each measurement and that the resulting difference is divided by the overall standard deviation. In this way all variables will have zero mean and unit standard deviation in the total sample.

Well-known examples of composite variables are rating scales routinely used for the assessment of health-related quality of life, as well as disease-activity-scales (e.g., the disease activity scale of Fuchs for patients with rheumatoid arthritis, DAS (Fuchs 1993)). The DAS is a composite based on the Ritchie joint pain score, the number of swollen joints, and, in addition, the erythrocyte sedimentation rate:

$$DAS = 0.53938\sqrt{ritchie\ index} + 0.06465(number\ of\ swollen\ joints)$$
$$+ 0.330\ \ln(erythocyte\ sedimentation\ rate) + 0.224.$$

For the statistical analysis of a composite variable, standard methods may be used without adjustments. Lauter (1996) showed that the statistical test for the composite has 5% type-I error rate. He also showed that such a statistical test is especially sensitive when each endpoint variable has more or less the same individual p-value, but that it has little sensitivity when one endpoint variable is much more significant than others.

We applied these methods to a clinical trial of patients with atherosclerosis comparing 2-year placebo versus pravastatin medication (Jukema et al. 1995). The efficacy of this medication was evaluated by assessing the change of total cholesterol, HDL cholesterol, LDL cholesterol, and triglycerides. The mean changes and standard deviations (mmol/L) are given in Table 9.3, while also the uncorrected p-values, and the corrected p-values according to Bonferroni and Hochberg are reported.

It is obvious that none of the changes are statistically significant using a standard t-test, but it is also clear that all four efficacy variables have a treatment difference that points in the same direction, namely of a positive pravastatin effect. When correcting for multiple testing, the p-values are

Table 9.3 Clinical trial of patients with atherosclerosis comparing 2-year placebo versus pravastatin medication (Jukema et al. 1995)

Change of:	Placebo (n = 31)	Pravastatin (n = 48)	P[a]	P[b]	P[c]
Total cholesterol decrease	−0.07 (0.72)	0.25 (0.73)	0.06	0.24	0.11
HDL cholesterol increase	−0.02 (0.18)	0.04 (0.12)	0.07	0.28	0.11
LDL cholesterol decrease	0.34 (0.60)	0.59 (0.65)	0.09	0.36	0.11
Triglycerides increase	0.03 (0.65)	0.28 (0.68)	0.11	0.44	0.11

The efficacy of this medication was evaluated by assessing the change of total cholesterol, HDL cholesterol, LDL cholesterol, and triglycerides. The mean changes and standard deviations (mmol/L) are given, while also the uncorrected p-values, and the corrected p-values according to Bonferroni and Hochberg are reported
[a]p-value of Student's t-test
[b]Bonferroni corrected p-value
[c]p-value corrected using Hochberg's methods

nowhere near statistical significance. A composite variable of the form $z = $ (total cholesterol + HDL + LDL + triglycerides)/4, where the four lipid measurements are standardized, however, did show statistically significant results: the mean of Z in the placebo group was −0.23 (SD 0.59), and the mean of Z in the pravastatin group was 0.15 (SD 0.56), different $p < 0.01$, and so, it is appropriate to conclude that pravastatin significantly reduced the composite variable.

VI. Finally, there are several multivariate methods to perform an overall statistical test for which the type-I error risk equals 5%. Equivalently to the situation comparing many different treatment groups, one might argue that the overall test controls the type-I error, and that subsequently to the overall test, one can perform t-tests and the like without adjustment to explore which variables show significant differences. For comparing two treatment groups on several (normally distributed) variables, one may use Hotelling's T-square, which is the multivariate generalization of the Student's t-test. Other methods to compare different groups of patients on several variables are discriminant analysis, variants of principal components analysis and multinominal logistic regression. The discussion of these methods falls outside the scope of this chapter, but will be addressed in more detail in the Chaps. 21 and 25. It suffices to remark that Hotelling's T-square and the other multivariate methods are readily available through most statistical packages.

4   Conclusions

Multiple group comparison and multiple variable testing is a very common problem when analyzing clinical trials. There is no consensus within the statistical community on how to cope with these problems. It is therefore essential that awareness of the existence of these problems is reflected in the study protocol and the statistical analysis.

References

Fuchs HA (1993) The use of the disease activity score in the analysis of clinical trials in rheumatoid arthritis. J Rheumatol 20(11):1863–1866

Hochberg Y (1988) A sharper Bonferroni procedure for multiple tests of significance. Biometrika 75:800–802

Jukema JW, Bruschke AV, Van Boven AJ, Zwinderman AH et al (1995) Effects of lipid lowering by pravastatin on the regression of coronary artery disease in symptomatic men. Circulation 91:2528–2540

Lauter J (1996) Exact t and F-tests for analyzing studies with multiple endpoints. Biometrics 52:964–970

Multiple comparisons boek (2008) Edition University of Leiden, Neth

SAS (2011) Statistical software

SPSS (2011) Statistical software. Chicago, IL

Waldinger MD, Hengeveld MW, Zwinderman AH, Olivier B (1998) Effect of SSRI antidepressants on ejaculation: a double-blind, randomized, placebo-controlled study with fluoxetine, fluvoxamine, paroxetine, and sertraline. J Clin Psychopharmacol 18(4):274–281

Chapter 10
The Interpretation of the p-Values

1 Introduction

In randomized controlled trials, prior to statistical analysis, the data are checked for outliers and erroneous data. Data-cleaning is defined as deleting-the-errors/ maintaining-the-outliers. Statistical tests are, traditionally, not very good at distinguishing between errors and outliers. However, they should be able to point out main endpoint results that are closer to expectation than compatible with random sampling. For example, a difference from control of 0.000 is hardly compatible with random sampling. As it comes to well-balanced random sampling of representative experimental data, nature will be helpful to provide researchers with results close to perfection.

However, because biological processes are full of variations, nature will never allow for 100% perfection. Statistical distributions can account for this lack of perfection in experimental data sampling, and provide exact probability levels of finding results close to expectation.

2 Renewed Attention to the Interpretation of the Probability Levels, Otherwise Called the p-Values

The p-values tell us the chance of making a type I error of finding a difference where there is none. Generally, a cut-off p-value of 0.05 is used to reject the null-hypothesis (H_0) of no difference. In the 1970s exact p-values were laborious to calculate, and they were, generally, approximated from statistical tables, in the form of $p < 0.01$ or $0.05 < p < 0.10$ etc. In the past decades with the advent of computers the job became easy (SAS 2011; SPSS 2011; S plus 2011; Stata 2011). Exact p-values such as 0.84 or 0.007 can now be calculated fast and accurately. This development lead to a renewed attention to the interpretation of p-values. In business statistics (Levin and Rubin 1998; Utts 1999), the 5% cut-off p-value has been largely abandoned and

T.J. Cleophas and A.H. Zwinderman, *Statistics Applied to Clinical Studies*,
DOI 10.1007/978-94-007-2863-9_10, © Springer Science+Business Media B.V. 2012

replaced with exact p-values used for making decisions on the risk business men are willing to take, mostly in terms of costs involved. In medicine, the cut-off p-values have not been completely abandoned, but broader attention is given to the interpretation of the exact p-values, and rightly so, because they can tell us a number of relevant things in addition to the chance of making type I errors. In the current chapter standard and renewed interpretations of p-values are reviewed as far as relevant to the interpretation of clinical trials and evidence-based medicine.

3   Standard Interpretation of p-Values

Statistics gives no certainties, only chances. What chances? Chances that hypotheses are true/untrue (we accept 95% truths). What hypotheses? For example, no difference from a 0 effect, a real difference from a 0 effect, worse than a 0 effect. Statistics is about estimating such chances/testing such hypotheses. Trials often calculate differences between test treatment and control (for example, standard treatment, placebo, baseline), and, subsequently, test whether the difference-between-the-two is different from 0.

Important hypotheses are Hypothesis 0 (H_0, i.e., no difference from a 0 effect), and Hypothesis 1 (H_1, the alternative hypothesis, i.e., a real difference from a 0 effect). What do these two hypotheses look like in graph? Figure 10.1 gives an example.

- H_1 = graph based on the data of our trial (mean ± standard error (SEM) = 2.1 ± 1).
- H_0 = same graph with mean 0 (mean ± SEM = 0 ± 1).

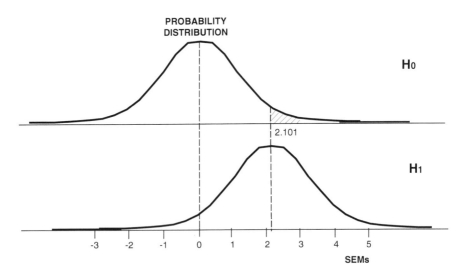

Fig. 10.1 Null-hypothesis and alternative hypothesis of a parallel group study of two groups $n = 10$ (18 degrees of freedom)

- Now we make a giant leap from our data to the population from which the sample was taken (we can do so, because our data are supposed to be representative of the population).
- H_1 = also summary of means of many trials similar to ours (if we repeated trial, difference would be small, and distribution of means of many such trials would look like H_1).
- H_0 = summary of means of many trials similar to ours, but with overall effect 0 (our mean not 0 but 2.1). Still, it could be an outlier of many studies with an overall effect of 0.
- So, we should think of H_0 and H_1 as summaries of means of many trials.
- If hypothesis 0 is true, then mean of our study is part of H_0.
- If hypothesis 1 is true, then mean of our study is part of H_1.
- We can't prove anything, but we can calculate the chance of either of these possibilities.
- A mean result of 2.1 is far distant from 0:

Suppose it belongs to H_0.
Only 5% of the H_0 trials >2.1 SEM distant from 0.
The chance that it belongs to H0 is <5%.
We reject this possibility if probability is <5%.

Suppose it belongs to H_1.
50% of the H_1 trials >2.1 SEM distant from 0. These 50% cannot reject null hypothesis, only the remainder, here also 50%, can do so.

Conclude here if H_0 is true, we have <5% chance to find it, if H1 is true, we have 50% chance to find it.
Or in statistical terms: we reject null hypothesis of no effect at $p < 0.05$ and with a statistical power of 50%.

Obviously, a p-value of <0.05 does not indicate a true effect, and allows for very limited conclusions (Cleophas et al. 2004a, b):

1. <5% chance to find this result if H_0 is true (H_0 is probably untrue, and so, this statement does not mean too much anyway);
2. only 50% chance to find this result if H_1 is true.
   The conclusions illustrate the uncertainties involved in H_0 – testing. With lower p-values, better certainty is provided, e.g., with $p < 0.01$ we have around 80% chance to find this result if H_1 were true, with $p < 0.001$ even 90%. However, even then, the chance of a type II error of finding no difference where there is one is still 10%. Also, we must realize that the above conclusions are appropriate only if
3. the data follow a normal distribution, and
4. they follow exactly the same distribution as that of the population from which the sample was taken.

4   Common Misunderstandings of the p-Values

The most common misunderstanding while interpreting the p-values is the concept that the p-value is actually the chance that the H_0 is true, and, consequently, that $p > 0.05$ means H_0 is true. Often, this result, expressed as "not significantly different from zero", is then reported as documented proof that the treatment had no effect. The distinction between demonstrating that a treatment had no effect and failing to demonstrate that it did have an effect, is subtle but very important, because the latter may be due to inadequate study methods or lack of power rather than lack of effect. Moreover, in order to assess whether the H_0 is true, null-hypothesis testing can never give the answer, because this is not the issue. The only issue here is: H_0 is rejected or not, no matter if it is true or untrue. To answer the question whether no-difference-in-the-data is true, we need to follow a different approach: similarity testing. With similarity (otherwise called equivalence)-testing the typical answer is: similarity is or is not demonstrated, which can be taken synonymous for no-difference-in-the-data being true or not (see also Chap. 5).

5   Renewed Interpretations of p-Values, Little Difference
Between p = 0.06 and p = 0.04

H_0 is currently less dogmatically rejected, because we believe that such practice mistakenly attempts to express certainty of statistical evidence in the data. If the H_0 is rejected, it is also no longer concluded that there is no difference in the data. Instead, we increasingly believe that there is actually little difference between $p = 0.06$ and $p = 0.04$. Like with business statistics clinicians now have the option to use p-values for an additional purpose, i.e., for making decisions about the risks they are willing to take.

Also an advantage of the exact p-value approach is the possibility of more refined conclusions from the research: instead of concluding significantly yes/no, we are able to consider levels of probabilities from very likely to be true, to very likely to be untrue (Michelson and Schofield 1996). The p-value which ranges from 0.0 to 1.0 summarizes the evidence in the data about H_0. A large p-value such as 0.55 or 0.78 indicates that the observed data would not be unusual if H_0 were true. A small p-value such as 0.001 denotes that these data would be very doubtful if H_0 were true. This provides strong support against H_0. In such instances results are said to be significant at the 0.001 level, indicating that getting a result of this size might occur only 1 out of 1,000 times.

Exact p-values are also increasingly used for comparing different levels of significance. The drawback of this approach is that sampled frequency distributions are approximations, and that it can be mathematically shown that exactly calculated p-values are rather inaccurate (Petrie and Sabin 2000). However, this drawback is outweighed by the advantages of knowing the p-values especially when it gets to extremes (Matthews and Farewel 1996).

6   The Real Meaning of Very Large p-Values Like p>0.95

Let us assume that in a Mendelian experiment the expected ratio of yellow-peas/green-peas = 1/1. A highly representative random sample of n = 100 might consist of 50 yellow and 50 green peas. However, the larger the sample the smaller the chance to find exactly fifty/fifty. The chance of exactly 5,000 yellow/5,000 green peas or even the chance of a result very close to this result is, due to large variability in biological processes, almost certainly zero.

Statistical distributions like the chi-square distribution can account for this lack of perfection in experimental data sampling, and provide exact probability levels of finding results close to "expected". Chi-squares curves are skewed curves with a lengthy right-end (Fig. 10.2).

We reject the null-hypothesis of no difference between "expected and observed", if the area under curve (AUC) on the right side of the calculated chi-square value is <5% of the total AUC. Chi-square curves do, however, also have a short left-end which ends with a chi-square value of zero. If the chi-square value calculated from our data is close to zero, the left AUC will get smaller and smaller, and as it becomes <5% of the total AUC, we are equally justified not to accept the null hypothesis as we are with large chi-square values. For example, in a sample of 10,000 peas, you might find 4,997 yellow and 5,003 green peas. Are these data representative for a population of 1/1 yellow/green peas? In this example a chi-square value of $<3.9 \cdot 10^{-3}$ indicates that the left AUC is <5% and, so, we have a probability <5% to find it (Table 10.1) (Riffenburgh 1999).

Chi-square value is calculated according to:

(Observed yellow − Expected yellow)^2 = $(4,997 − 5,000)^2$: 5,000 to standardize = $1.8 \cdot 10^{-3}$

(Observed green − Expected green)^2 = $(5,003 − 5,000)^2$: 5,000 to standardize = $1.8 \cdot 10^{-3}$

chi-square (1 degree of freedom) = $3.6 \cdot 10^{-3}$

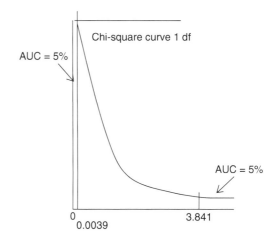

Fig. 10.2 Probability of finding χ^2 value >3.841 is <0.05, so is probability of finding a χ^2 value <0.0039 (*AUC* area under the curve, *df* degree of freedom)

Table 10.1 Left end χ^2 table: seven columns of χ^2 values, upper two rows areas under the curve (*AUCs*) of left and right end of χ^2 curves, left column: adjustments for degrees of freedom (*dfs*)

AUC left end	0.0005	0.001	0.005	0.01	0.025	0.05	0.10
AUC right end	0.9995	0.999	0.995	0.99	0.975	0.95	0.90
Degrees of freedom							
1	0.0000004	0.0000016	0.000039	0.00016	0.00091	0.0039	0.016
2	0.00099	0.0020	0.010	0.020	0.051	0.10	0.21
3	0.015	0.024	0.072	0.12	0.22	0.35	0.58
4	0.065	0.091	0.21	0.30	0.48	0.71	1.06
5	0.6	0.21	0.41	0.55	0.83	1.154	1.61

   This result is smaller than $3.9 \cdot 10^{-3}$ and, thus, it is so close to what was expected that we can only conclude that we have <5% probability to find it. We have to scrutinize these results, and must consider and examine the possibility of inadequate data improvement. The above example is actually based on some true historic facts (Mendel indeed improved his data) (Cleophas and Cleophas 2001).

7   p-Values Larger than 0.95, Examples (Table 10.2)

We searched for main endpoint p-values close to 0.95 in randomized controlled trials published in recent issues of the Lancet and the New England Journal of Medicine, and found four studies. Table 10.2 gives a summary. All of these studies aimed at demonstrating similarities rather than differences. Indeed, as can be observed, proportions of patients with events in the treatment and control groups were very similar. For example, the percentages in treatment and control groups of patients with sepsis were 1.3% and 1.3% (study 1, Table 10.2), and of patients with cardiovascular events 79.2% and 79.8% (study 5, Table 10.2). The investigators of the studies calculated p-values from p>0.94 to p>0.995, which, according to the chi-square table (Table 10.1), would provide left-end p-values between ≤0.06 and ≤0.005. This would mean, that, for whatever reason, these data were probably not completely random. Unwarranted exclusion of, otherwise, appropriate outliers is one of the possible explanations.

8   The Real Meaning of Very Small p-Values Like p<0.0001

Statistics gives no certainties, only chances. A generally accepted concept is "the smaller the p-value the better reliable the results". This is not entirely true with current randomized controlled trials. First, randomized controlled trials are designed to

Table 10.2 Study data with p-values close to 0.95, as published in recent Lancet and N Engl J Med issues

	Result (numbers)	Results (%)	Sample size requirement	Alpha-level	p-values
Hansson et al. (1998)	107/6,264 vs 107/6,262	1.7 vs 1.7	Yes	0.05	>0.995
Sandham et al. (2003)	88/965 vs 84/941	9.1 vs 8.9	Yes	0.05	>0.95
Sandham et al. (2003)	13/965 vs 12/941	1.3 vs 1.3	Yes	0.05	>0.95
LIPID Study Group (2002)	214/1,338 vs 319/2,319	15.9 vs 13.8	Yes	0.05	>0.99
Heart Protection Study Collaborative Group (2002)	285/360 vs 1,087/1,363	79.2 vs 79.8	Yes	0.05	>0.94

(1) Proportions of patients with heart infarction in patients with diastolic blood pressure $80 < <85$ vs <80 mmHg, (2) Proportion of patients with arrhythmias in patients with standard perioperative treatment vs Swann-Ganz catheter-guided perioperative treatment, (3) Proportion of patients with sepsis in patients with standard perioperative treatment vs Swann-Ganz catheter-guided perioperative treatment, (4) Proportions of patients with cardiovascular events in patients with LDL-cholesterol, <3.5 mmol/l vs $3.5 < <4.5$ mmol/l, and (5) Proportions of patients with cardiovascular events in patients with LDL-cholesterol <2.6 mmol/l vs >3.4 mmol/l

Alpha type I error, *vs* versus

test small differences. A randomized controlled trial with major differences between old and new treatment is unethical because half of the patients have been given an inferior treatment.

Second, they are designed to confirm prior evidence. For that purpose, their sample size is carefully calculated. Not only too small but also too large a sample size is considered unethical and unscientific, because negative studies have to be repeated and a potentially inferior treatment should not be given to too many patients. Often in the study protocol a statistical power of 80% is agreed, corresponding with a p-value of approximately 0.01.

The ultimate p-value may then be a bit larger or smaller. However a p-value of >0.05 will be rarely observed, because current clinical trials are confirmational and, therefore, rarely negative. Also a p-value much smaller than 0.01 will be rarely observed, because it would indicate that either the power assessment was inadequate (the study is overpowered) or the data have been artificially improved. With p = 0.0001 we have a peculiar situation. In this situation the actual data can not only reject the null-hypothesis, but also the hypothesis of significantly better Thus, a p-value <0.0001, if the power was set at 80%, does not completely confirm its prior expectations and must be scrutinized for data improvement. (This issue is explained more in detail in the next chapter).

9   p-Values Smaller than 0.0001, Examples (Table 10.3)

Table 10.3 gives an overview of five published studies with main endpoint p-values <0.0001. All of these studies were published in the first six issues of the 1992 volume of the New England Journal of Medicine. It is remarkable that so many overpowered studies were published within six subsequent months of a

Table 10.3 Study data with p-values as low as < 0.0001, published in the first six issues of the 1992 volume of the N Engl J Med. In the past 4 years p-values smaller than p < 0.001 were never published in this journal

	Result	Sample size requirement	Alpha-level	p-values
Parisi et al. (1992)	+0.5 vs +2.1%	Yes	0.05	<0.0001
Parisi et al. (1992)	−2.8 vs +1.8%	Yes	0.05	<0.0001
Seppälä et al. (1992)	11 vs 19%	No	0.05	<0.0001
Rafal et al. (1992)	r = −0.53	No	0.05	<0.0001
Barrett et al. (1992)	213 vs 69	No	0.05	<0.0001

(1) Duration exercise in patients after medical therapy vs percutaneous coronary angioplasty, (2) Maximal double product (systolic blood pressure times heart rate) during exercise in patients after medical treatment vs percutaneous coronary angioplasty, (3) Erythromycin resistance throat swabs vs pus samples, (4) Correlation between reduction of epidermal pigmentation during treatment and baseline amount of pigmentation, and (5) Adverse reactions of high vs non-high osmolality agents during cardiac catheterization
Alpha type I error, *vs* versus

single volume, while the same journal published not any study with p-values below 0.001 in the past 4 years' full volumes. We do not know why, but this may be due to the journal's policy not to accept studies with very low p-values anymore. In contrast, many other journals including the Lancet, Circulation, BMJ, abound with extremely low p-values. It is obvious that these journals still believe in the concept "the lower the p-value, the better reliable the research". The concept may still be true for observational studies. However, in confirmational randomized controlled trials, p-values as low as 0.0001 do not adequately confirm prior hypotheses anymore, and have to be checked for adequacy of data management.

10 Discussion

In 1948 the first randomized controlled trial was published by the BMJ (Medical Research Council 1948). Until then, observations had been mainly uncontrolled. Initially, trials were frequently negative due to little sensitivity as a consequence of too small samples, and inappropriate hypotheses based on biased prior data. Nowadays, clinical trials are rarely negative, and they are mainly confirmational rather than explorative. This has consequences for the p-values that can be expected from such trials. Very low p-values like $p < 0.0001$ will be rarely encountered in such trials, because it would mean that the study was overpowered and should have had a smaller sample size. Also very large p-values like $p > 0.95$ will be rare, because they would indicate similarities closer than compatible with a normal distribution of random data samples.

We should emphasize that the above-mentioned interpretation of very low/high p-values is only true within the context of randomized controlled trials. For example, unrandomized observational data can easily produce very low and very high p-values, and there is nothing wrong with that. Also the above interpretation is untrue in clinical trials that test multiple endpoints rather than a single main endpoint or a single composite endpoint. Clinical trials testing multiple rather than single endpoints, often do so for the purpose of answering a single question, e.g., the benefit of health of a new drug may be estimated by mortality in addition to various morbidity variables. If investigators test many times, they are apt to find differences, e.g., 5% of the time, but this may not be due to significant effects but rather to chance. In this situation, one should informally integrate all of the data before reaching conclusions, and look for the trends in the data without judging one or two low p-values, among otherwise high p-values, as proof (see also the Chaps. 7 and 8).

In the present chapter, for the assessment of high p-values, the chi-square test is used, while for the assessment of low p-values the t-test is used. Both tests are, however, closely related to one another, and like other statistical tests, including the F-test, regression analysis, and other tests based on normal distributions. The conclusions drawn from our assessments are, therefore, equally true for alternative statistical tests and data.

We should add that the nominal p-values have to be interpreted with caution in case of multiple testing, as already discussed in the previous two chapters. A not yet mentioned but straightforward way to correct this is to calculate an E-value, i.e. the product of the p-value and the number of tests.

11   Recommendations

p-values <0.0001 will be rarely encountered in randomized controlled clinical trials, because it would mean that the study is overpowered and should have had a smaller sample size. Also p-values >0.95 will be rare, because they would indicate similarities closer than compatible with a normal distribution of random samples. It would seem appropriate, therefore, to require investigators to explain such results, and to consider rejecting the research involved. So far, in randomized controlled trials the null-hypothesis is generally rejected at p <0.05. Maybe, we should consider rejecting the entire study if the main endpoint p-values are >0.95 or <0.0001.

The concept of the p-value is notoriously poorly understood. Some physicians even comfortably think that the p-value is a measure of effect (Motulsky 1995). When asked whether a drug treatment worked, their typical answer would be: "Well, p is less than 0.05, so I guess it did". The more knowledgeable among us know that p stands for chance (probability = p), and that there must be risks of errors. The current paper reviews the standard as well as renewed interpretations of the p-values, and was written for physicians accepting statistical reasoning as a required condition for an adequate assessment of the benefits and limitations of evidence-based medicine.

Additional points must be considered when interpreting the p-values. In the first place, the interpretation of low p-values is different in studies that test multiple endpoints rather than a single main endpoint or a single composite endpoint. Studies testing multiple rather than single endpoints, often do so for the purpose of answering a single question, e.g., the benefit of health of a new drug may be estimated by mortality in addition to various morbidity variables. If investigators test many times, they are apt to find differences, e.g., 5% of the time, but this may not be due to significant effects but rather to chance. In this situation, one should informally integrate all of the data before reaching conclusions, and look for the trends in the data without judging one or two low p-values, among otherwise high p-values, as proof.

Special attention in this respect deserves the issue of multiple low-powered studies. One might consider this situation to be similar to the above one, and conclude that such studies be similarly integrated. Actually, this is one of the concepts of the method of meta-analysis. Second, the point of one sided testing versus two-sided testing must be considered. Studies testing both ends of a normal frequency distribution have twice the chance of finding a significant difference compared to those testing only one end. If our research assesses whether there is any difference in the data, no matter in what direction, either the positive or the negative one, then we have a two-sided design and the p-values must doubled. It is then, consequently, harder to obtain a low p-value.

Recommendations regarding the interpretation of main-endpoint-study p-values either two-sided or not, include the following.

1. $p < 0.05$ gives a conditional probability: H0 can be rejected on the limitations/assumptions that (1) we have up to 5% chance of a type I error of finding a difference where there is none, (2) we have 50% chance of a type II error of finding no difference where there is one, (3) the data are normally distributed, (4) they follow exactly the same distribution as that of the population from which the sample was taken.
2. A common misunderstanding is the concept that the p-value is actually the chance that H_0 is true, and, consequently that a $p > 0.05$ indicates a significant similarity in the data. $p > 0.05$ may, indeed, indicate similarity. However, also a study-sample too small or study design inadequate to detect the difference must be considered.
3. An advantage of the exact p-values is the possibility of more refined conclusions from the research: instead of concluding significantly yes/no, we are able to consider levels of probabilities from very likely to be true, to very likely to be untrue.
4. $p > 0.95$ suggests that the observed data are closer to expectation than compatible with a Gaussian frequency distribution, and such results must, therefore, be scrutinized.
5. A $p < 0.0001$, if power was set at 80%, does not completely confirm the prior expectations of the power assessment. Therefore, such results must be scrutinized.

12 Conclusions

The p-values tell us the chance of making a type I error of finding a difference where there is none. In the 1970s exact p-values were laborious to calculate, and they were, generally, approximated from statistical tables, in the form of $p < 0.01$ or $0.05 < p < 0.10$ etc. In the past decades with the advent of computers it became easy to calculate exact p-values such as 0.84 or 0.007. The cut-off p-values have not been completely abandoned, but broader attention is given to the interpretation of the exact p-values. The objective of this chapter was to review standard and renewed interpretations of p-values:

1. Standard interpretation of cut-off p-values like $p < 0.05$.
   The null-hypothesis of no difference can be rejected on the limitations/assumptions that (1) we have up to 5% chance of a type I error of finding a difference where there is none, (2) we have 50% chance of a type II error of finding no difference where there is one, (3) the data are normally distributed, (4) they follow exactly the same distribution as that of the population from which the sample was taken.

2   A common misunderstanding of the p-value.

It is actually the chance that the null-hypothesis is true, and, consequently that a $p > 0.05$ indicates a significant similarity in the data. $p > 0.05$ may, indeed, indicate similarity. However, a study-sample too small or study design inadequate to detect the difference must be considered.

3.   Renewed interpretations of the p-values.

Exact p-values enable to more refined conclusions from the research than cut-off levels: instead of concluding significantly yes/no, we are able to consider levels of probabilities from very likely to be true, to very likely to be untrue. Very large p-values are not compatible with a normal Gaussian frequency distribution, very small p-values do not completely confirm prior expectations. They must be scrutinized, and may have been inadequately improved.

References

Barrett BJ, Parfrey PS, Vavasour HM, O'Dea F, Kent G, Stone E (1992) A comparison of nonionic, low-osmolality radiocontrast agents with ionic, high-osmolality agents during cardiac catheterization. N Engl J Med 326:431–436

Cleophas TJ, Cleophas GM (2001) Sponsored research and continuing medical education. JAMA 286:302–304

Cleophas TJ, Zwinderman AH, Cleophas AF (2004a) P-values. Review. Am J ther 11:317–322

Cleophas TJ, Zwinderman AH, Cleophas AF (2004b) P-values, beware of the extremes. Clin Chem Lab Med 42:300–305

Hansson L, Zanchetti A, Carruthers SG, Dahlof B, Elmfeldt D, Julius S, et al., for the HOT Study Group (1998) Effects of intensive blood pressure lowering and low-dose aspirin in patients with hypertension: principal results of the Hypertension Optimal Treatment (HOT) randomised trial. Lancet 351:1755–1762

Heart Protection Study Collaborative Group (2002) MRC/BHF Heart Protection Study of cholesterol lowering with simvastatin in 20536 high-risk individuals: a randomised placebo-controlled trial. Lancet 360:7–22

Levin RI, Rubin DS (1998) P-value. In: Levin RI, Rubin DS (eds) Statistics for management. Prentice-Hall, Englewood Cliffs, pp 485–496

LIPID Study Group (2002) Long-term effectiveness and safety of pravastatin in 9014 patients with coronary heart disease and average cholesterol concentrations: the LIPID trial follow-up. Lancet 359:1379–1387

Matthews DE, Farewel VT (1996) P-value. In: Matthews DE, Farewell VT (eds) Using and understanding medical statistics. Karger, New York, pp 15–18

Medical Research Council (1948) Streptomycin treatment of pulmonary tuberculosis. Br Med J 2:769–782

Michelson S, Schofield T (1996) p-values as conditional probabilities. In: Michelson S, Schofield T (eds) The biostatistics cookbook. Kluwer Academic Publishers, Boston, pp 46–58

Motulsky H (1995) P-values, definition and common misinterpretations. In: Motulsky H (ed) Intuitive biostatistics. Oxford University Press, New York, pp 96–97

Parisi AF, Folland ED, Hartigan P, on behalf of the Veterans Affairs ACME Investigators (1992) A comparison of angioplasty with medical therapy in the treatment of single-vessel coronary artery disease. N Engl J Med 326:10–16

Petrie A, Sabin C (2000) Explanation of p-values. In: Petrie A, Sabin C (eds) Medical statistics at glance. Blackwell Science, Oxford, pp 42–45

Rafal ES, Griffiths CE, Ditre CM, Finkel LJ, Hamilton TA, Ellis CN et al (1992) Topical retinoin treatment for liver spots associated with photodamage. N Engl J Med 326:368–374

Riffenburgh RH (1999) P-values. In: Riffenburgh RH (ed) Statistics in medicine. Academic, San Diego, pp 95–96, 105–106

S-plus. www.splus.com. Accessed 14 Dec 2011

Sandham JD, Hull RD, Brand RF, Knox L, Pineo GF, Doig CJ, et al., for the Canadian Critical Care Clinical Trials Group (2003) A randomized, controlled trial of the use of pulmonary-artery catheters in high-risk surgical patients. N Engl J Med 348:5–14

SAS. www.sas.com. Accessed 14 Dec 2011

Seppälä H, Nissinen A, Järvinen H, Huovinen S, Henrikson T, Herva E et al (1992) Resistance to erythromycin in group A streptococci. N Engl J Med 326:292–297

SPSS. www.spss.com. Accessed 14 Dec 2011

Stata. www.stata.com. Accessed 14 Dec 2011

Utts JM (1999) P-value. In: Utts JM (ed) Seeing through statistics. Duxbury Press, Detroit, pp 375–386

Chapter 11
Research Data Closer to Expectation than Compatible with Random Sampling

1 Introduction

Research data may be close to expectation. However, a difference from control of 0.000 is hardly compatible with random sampling. As it comes to well-balanced random sampling of representative experimental data, nature will be helpful to provide researchers with results close to perfection. However, because biological processes are full of variations, nature will never allow for 100% perfection. Statistical distributions can account for this lack of perfection in experimental data sampling, and provide exact probability levels of finding results close to expectation.

As an example, in a Mendelian experiment the expected ratio of yellow-peas/green-peas is 1/1. A highly representative random sample of $n = 100$ might consist of 50 yellow and 50 green peas. However, the larger the sample the smaller the chance of finding exactly fifty/fifty. The chance of exactly 5,000 yellow/5,000 green peas or even the chance of a result very close to this result is, due to large variability in biological processes, almost certainly zero. In a sample of 10,000 peas, you might find 4,997 yellow and 5,003 green peas. What is the chance of finding a result this close to expectation? A simple chi-square test produces here a $p > 0.95$ of finding a result less close, which means a chance of $< (1-0.95)$, i.e., < 0.05 of finding a result this close or closer. Using the traditional 5% decision level, this would mean, that we have a strong argument that these data are not completely random. The example is actually based on some true historic facts, Mendel improved his data (Cleophas and Cleophas 2001).

Mendel's data were unblinded and unrandomized. Currently interventional data are obtained through randomized controlled trials. The phenomenon of data closer to expectation than compatible with random sampling is not considered anymore. But it is unknown whether it has actually disappeared. In the previous chapter the subject of extreme p-values as a result of research data closer to expectation than compatible with random sampling has been briefly addressed. The current chapter provides additional methods and examples in order to further emphasize the importance of this issue.

T.J. Cleophas and A.H. Zwinderman, *Statistics Applied to Clinical Studies*,
DOI 10.1007/978-94-007-2863-9_11, © Springer Science+Business Media B.V. 2012

2   Methods and Results

In order to assess this issue we defined data closer than random according to:

1. *An observed p-value of >95%.*

This literally means that we have >95% chance of finding a result less close expectation, and, consequently, <5% chance of finding a result this close or closer.

2. *An observed p-value of <0.0001.*

Often in the study protocol a statistical power of 80% is agreed, corresponding with a p-value of approximately 0.01. The ultimate p-value may then be a bit larger or smaller. However a p-value of >0.05 will be rarely observed, because current clinical trials are conformational and, therefore, rarely negative. Also a p-value much smaller than 0.01 will be rarely observed, because it would indicate that the study is overpowered. If the p-values can be assumed to follow a normal distribution around $p = 0.01$, then we will have less than 5% chance of observing a p-value of <0.0001.

3 *An observed standard deviation (SD) <50% the SD expected from prior population data.*

From population data we can be pretty sure about SDs to be expected. For example, the SDs of blood pressures are close to 10% of their means, meaning that for a mean systolic blood pressures of 150 mmHg the expected SD is close to 15 mmHg, for a mean diastolic blood pressure of 100 mmHg the expected SD is close to 10 mmHg. If such SDs can be assumed to follow a normal distribution, we will have <5% chance of finding SDs <7.5 and <5 mmHg respectively.

4. *An observed standard deviation (SD) >150% the SD expected from prior population data.*

With SDs close to 10% of their means, we, likewise, will have <5% chance of finding SDs >150% the size of the SDs expected from population data.

We, then, searched randomized controlled trials of the 1999–2002 volumes of four journals accordingly. However, we decided to early terminate our search after observing respectively 7, 14, 8 and 2 primary endpoint results closer than random in a single random issue from the journals (Table 11.1). We have to conclude that the phenomenon of research data closer to expectation than compatible with random sampling has not at all disappeared. We assume that, like with the above Mendelian example, inappropriate data cleaning is a major factor responsible. We recommend that the statistical community develop guidelines for assessing appropriateness of data cleaning, and that journal editors require submitters of research papers to explain their results if they provide extremely high or low p-values or unexpectedly small or large SDs. Maybe, they should even consider, like the New England Journal of Medicine, not to publish p-values smaller than 0.001 anymore.

Evidence-based medicine is under pressure due to the conflicting results of recent trials producing different answers to similar questions (Julius 2003; Cleophas and Cleophas 2003). Many causes are mentioned. As long as the possibility of

Table 11.1 Numbers of primary endpoint results closer to expectation than compatible with random sampling observed in a single issue from four journals

	p>0.95	p<0.0001	SD<50% of expected SD	>150% of expected SD
Cardiovascular Research 1999; 43: issue 1	1 (1)[a]	5 (1)	3 (2)	1 (1)
Current Therapeutic Research 2000; 61: issue 1	0 (0)	3 (1)	3 (1)	0 (0)
International Journal of Clinical Pharmacology and Therapeutics 2001; 39: issue 12	3 (2)	1 (1)	0 (0)	0 (0)
Journal of Hypertension 2002; 20: issue 10	3 (2)	5 (1)	2 (1)	1 (1)
Total	7 (5)	14 (4)	8 (4)	2 (2)

[a]Between brackets numbers of studies

inappropriate data cleaning has not been addressed, this very possibility cannot be excluded as potential cause of the obvious lack of homogeneity in current research.

3   Discussion

In randomized controlled trials, prior to statistical analysis, the data are checked for outliers and erroneous data. Statistical tests are, traditionally, not very good at distinguishing between errors and outliers, but they should be able to point out main endpoint results closer to expectation than compatible with random sampling. In the current chapter we propose some criteria to assess main endpoint results for such purpose. One of the criteria proposed is a <5% probability to observe p-values of <0.0001 in studies planned at a power of 80% (Cleophas 2004). Kieser and Cleophas (2005) takes issue with this proposed criterion, and states that, based on the two-sample normally distributed model of Hung et al. (1997), this probability should be much larger than 5%. We used a different, and, in our view, more adequate model for assessment, based on the t-distribution and a usual two-sided type I error of 5%, rather than a one-sided type I error of 1%. We here take the opportunity to explain our assessment a little bit further and, particularly, to explain the arguments underlying it.

In statistics, a generally accepted concept is "the smaller the p-value, the better reliable the results". This is not entirely true with current randomized controlled trials. First, randomized controlled trials are designed to test small differences. A randomized controlled trial with major differences between old and new treatment is unethical because half of the patients have been given an inferior treatment. Second, they are designed to confirm prior evidence. For that purpose, their sample size is carefully calculated. Not only too small, but also too large a sample size is considered unethical and unscientific, because negative studies have to be repeated and a potentially inferior treatment should not be given to too many patients. Often in the study

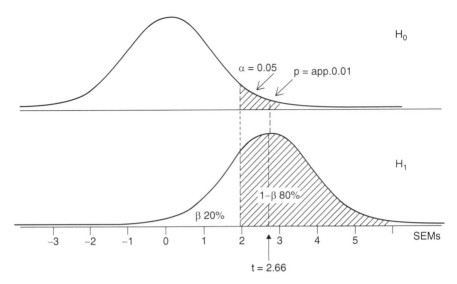

Fig. 11.1 Null-hypothesis (H0) and alternative hypothesis (H1) of an example of experimental data with sample size $n = 60$ and mean $= 2.66$, and a t-distributed frequency distribution. The null-hypothesis is rejected with a p-value of approximately 0.01 and a statistical power $(=1-\beta)$ of 80% ($\alpha =$ type I error $= 5\%$; $\beta =$ type II error $= 20\%$; *app.* approximately; *SEM* standard error of the mean)

protocol a statistical power of 80% is agreed, corresponding with a p-value of approximately 0.01 (Fig. 11.1). The ultimate p-value may then be a little bit larger or smaller. However, a p-value > 0.05 will be rarely observed, because most of the current clinical trials are conformational, and, therefore, rarely negative. Also, a p-value much smaller than 0.01 will be rarely observed, because it would indicate that either the power assessment was inadequate (the study is overpowered) or data management was not completely adequate. With $p = 0.0001$ we have a peculiar situation. In this situation the actual data can not only reject the null-hypothesis (H_0, Fig. 11.2) at $p = 0.0001$, but also the hypothesis of significantly better (H_1, Fig. 11.2) at $p = 0.05$. This would mean that not only H_0 but also H_1 is untrue.

Table 11.2 gives an overview of five published studies with main endpoint p-values <0.0001. All of these studies were published in the first six issues of the 1992 volume of the New England Journal of Medicine. It is remarkable that so many overpowered studies were published within six subsequent months of a single volume, while the same journal published not any study with p-values below 0.001 in the past 4 years' full volumes. We do not know why, but this may be due to the journal's policy not to accept studies with very low p-values anymore. In contrast, many other journals including the Lancet, Circulation, BMJ (British Medical Journal), abound with extremely low p-values. We should add that, while preparing this chapter, we noticed that, in the past 2 months, also JAMA (Journal of American Medical Association) did not publish p-values below 0.001 anymore. It is obvious,

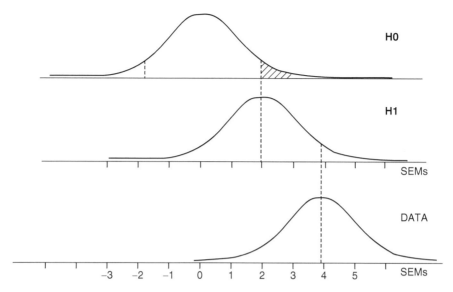

Fig. 11.2 Null-hypothesis (H0), hypothesis of significantly better (H1), and actual data distribution (*DATA*) of an example of experimental data with n = 120 and mean = 3.90 SEMs and a t-distributed frequency distribution. The actual data can not only reject H0 (t = 3.90, p = 0.0001), but also H1 (t = 1.95, p = 0.05). This would mean that not only H0 but also H1 is untrue (*SEM* standard error of the mean)

Table 11.2 Study data with p-values as low as <0.0001, published in the first six issues of the 1992 volume of the New England Journal of Medicine. In the past 4 years p-values smaller than p < 0.001 were never published in this journal

	Result	Sample size requirement	Alpha-level	p-values
1. Parisi et al. (1992)	+0.5 vs +2.1%	Yes	0.05	<0.0001
2. Parisi et al. (1992)	−2.8 vs +1.8%	Yes	0.05	<0.0001
3. Seppälä et al. (1992)	11 vs 19%	No	0.05	<0.0001
4. Rafal et al. (1992)	r = −0.53	No	0.05	<0.0001
5. Barrett et al. (1992)	213 vs 69	No	0.05	<0.0001

(1) Duration exercise in patients after medical therapy vs percutaneous coronary angioplasty, (2) Maximal double product (systolic blood pressure times heart rate) during exercise in patients after medical treatment vs percutaneous coronary angioplasty, (3) Erythromycin resistance throat swabs vs pus samples, (4) Correlation between reduction of epidermal pigmentation during treatment and baseline amount of pigmentation, and (5) Adverse reactions of high vs non-high osmolality agents during cardiac catheterization
Alpha type I error, *vs* versus

however, that most of the other journals still believe in the concept "the lower the p-value, the better reliable the research". The concept may still be true for observational studies. However, in conformational randomized controlled trials, p-values as low as 0.0001 do not adequately confirm prior hypotheses anymore, and have to be checked for adequacy of data management.

4   Conclusions

The following results may be closer to expectation than compatible with random.

1. An observed p-value of >0.95.
2. An observed p-value of <0.0001.
3. An observed standard deviation (SD) <50% the SD expected from prior population data.
4. An observed standard deviation (SD) >150% the SD expected from prior population data.

Additional assessments to identify data at risk of unrandomness will be reviewed in the Chaps. 42 and 43.

References

Barrett BJ, Parfrey PS, Vavasour HM, O'Dea F, Kent G, Stone E (1992) A comparison of nonionic, low-osmolality radiocontrast agents with ionic, high-osmolality agents during cardiac catheterization. N Engl J Med 326:431–436

Cleophas TJ (2004) Research data closer to expectation than compatible with random sampling I. Stat Med 23:1015–1017

Cleophas TJ, Cleophas GM (2001) Sponsored research and continuing medical education. JAMA 286:302–304

Cleophas GM, Cleophas TJ (2003) Clinical trials in jeopardy. Int J Clin Pharmacol Ther 41:51–56

Hung HMJ, O'Neill RT, Bauer P, Köhne K (1997) The behavior of the p-value when the alternative hypothesis is true. Biometrics 53:11–22

Julius S (2003) The ALLHAT study: if you believe in evidence-based medicine, stick to it. J Hypertens 21:453–454

Kieser M, Cleophas TJ (2005) Research data closer to expectation than compatible with random sampling II. Stat Med 24:321–323

Parisi AF, Folland ED, Hartigan P, on behalf of the Veterans Affairs ACME Investigators (1992) A comparison of angioplasty with medical therapy in the treatment of single-vessel coronary artery disease. N Engl J Med 326:10–16

Rafal ES, Griffiths CE, Ditre CM, Finkel LJ, Hamilton TA, Ellis CN et al (1992) Topical retinoin treatment for liver spots associated with photodamage. N Engl J Med 326:368–374

Seppälä H, Nissinen A, Järvinen H, Huovinen S, Henrikson T, Herva E et al (1992) Resistance to erythromycin in group A streptococci. N Engl J Med 326:292–297

Chapter 12
Statistical Tables for Testing Data Closer to Expectation than Compatible with Random Sampling

1 Introduction

A p-value <0.05 is generally used as a cut-off level to indicate a significant difference from what we expect. A p-value of >0.05, then, indicates no significant difference. The larger the p-value the smaller the chance of a difference. A p-value of 1.00 means 0% chance of a difference, while a p-value of 0.95 means a chance of difference close to 0. A p-value of >0.95 literally means that we have >95% chance of finding a result less close to expectation, which means a chance of <(1−0.95), i.e., <0.05 of finding a result this close or closer. Using the traditional 5% decision level, this would mean, that we have a strong argument that such data are not completely random. The example from the previous chapter is used once more. In a Mendelian experiment the expected ratio of yellow-peas/-green peas is 1/1. A highly representative random sample of n = 100 might consist of 50 yellow and 50 green peas. However, the larger the sample the smaller the chance of finding exactly fifty/fifty. The chance of exactly 5,000 yellow/5,000 green peas or even the chance of a result very close to this result is, due to large variability in biological processes, almost certainly zero. In a sample of 10,000 peas, you might find 4,997 yellow and 5,003 green peas. What is the chance of finding a result this close to expectation? A chi-square test produces here a p > 0.95 of finding a result less close, and consequently, <0.05 of finding a result this close or closer. Using the 5% decision level, this would mean, that we have a strong argument that these data are not completely random. The example is actually based on some true historic facts, Mendel improved his data (Cleophas and Cleophas 2001).

Some readers might be confused by the assertion that a p-value >0.95 implies that the data are closer to expectation than compatible with random sampling. A large p-value, indeed, generally, means that the data behave very similar to that which one would expect under the null hypothesis. Yet, a p-value >0.95 will be rarely observed, because not only data but also *mean outcomes of data-samples* follow (normal or chi-square) frequency distributions. Figure 12.1 displays a

T.J. Cleophas and A.H. Zwinderman, *Statistics Applied to Clinical Studies*,
DOI 10.1007/978-94-007-2863-9_12, © Springer Science+Business Media B.V. 2012

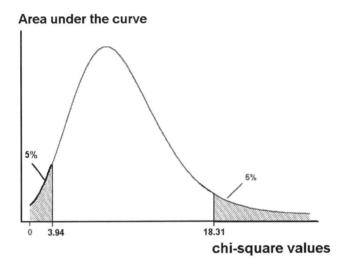

Fig. 12.1 Null hypothesis of chi-square distributed samples with 10 degrees of freedom. The area under the curve for chi-square values larger than 18.31 or smaller than 3.94 is <5%. This means we have <5% chance to find a variability thát large or thát small, and so, we are entitled to reject the null hypothesis in either case

chi-square-distributed null hypothesis curve (10 degrees of freedom). On the x-axis we have the so-called chi-square values which can be interpreted as estimates of variabilities of studies that have 10 degrees of freedom. On the y-axis we have p-values (= areas under the curve). The curve presents the collection of all of the variabilities one can expect. The area under the curve for chi-square values larger than 18.31 is <5%. This means we have <5% chance to find a variability thát large or thát small, and so, we are entitled to reject the null hypothesis in either case. The left end of the chi-square curve, although routinely used for testing appropriateness of data distributions, is little used for the above purpose so far.

In a recent search of randomized trials published in four journals we found main-endpoint results with p-values >95% in every single issue of the journals (Cleophas 2004). We assumed that inappropriate data cleaning was a major factor responsible. In clinical research the appropriateness of data cleaning is rarely assessed. The current paper was written to facilitate the assessment of this issue. We present tables of unusually large p-values to assess data closer to expectation than compatible with random sampling. We also give examples showing how to calculate such p-values from published data yourself, and examples to simulate real practice. The chapter tries to address a phenomenon, rather than accuse research groups. Therefore, only simulated examples are given.

2 Statistical Tables of Unusually High p-Values

Statistical tests estimate the probability that a difference in the data is true rather than due to chance, otherwise called random. For that purpose they make use of test-statistics:

Test-statistic	Test
t-value	For the t-test
Chi-square	For the chi-square test
F-value	For the F-test

The t-statistic (t-value) is used for the assessment of the means of continuous data, odds ratios and regression coefficients. The chi-square statistic (chi-square-value) is used for the analysis of proportional data, and survival data. The f-statistic (f-value) is used for comparing continuous data from more than two groups or more than two observations in one person, and for additional purposes such as testing correlation coefficients. The Tables 12.1, 12.2, and 12.3 give overviews of the unusual sizes these test-statistics and their corresponding p-values can adopt if data are closer to expectation than compatible with random sampling.

3 How to Calculate the p-Values Yourself

3.1 t-Test

In a parallel-group study two cholesterol reducing drugs are assessed.

Group1 (n=50), mean result 3.42 mmol/l, standard error of the mean (SEM) 0.06 mmol/l.

Group2 (n=50), mean result 3.38 mmol/l, SEM 0.06 mmol/l.

Difference between results 0.04 mmol/l, pooled SEM = $\sqrt{SEM_1^2 + SEM_2^2}$ = 0.848.

T-value = 0.04/0.848 = 0.0472 for (50 + 50) − 2 = 98 degrees of freedom. T-value is <0.0619, and according to the t-table (Table 12.1) the p-value is thus >0.95. These data are closer to expectation than compatible with random.

3.2 Chi-square Test

The underneath example is given in the form of a 2×2 contingency table which follows a chi-square distribution with 1 degree of freedom.

Pea phenotype		P	p
	R	PR 27 (a)	pR 271(b)
	r	Pr 9 (c)	pr 92 (d)

Table 12.1 t-values with unusually high p-values

p-value (two sided)			
0.999	0.99	0.95	0.90
Degrees freedom			
1 0.0015	0.154	0.0770	0.1580
2 0.0014	0.141	0.0707	0.1419
3 0.0014	0.136	0.0681	0.1366
4 0.0013	0.0133	0.0667	0.1338
5 0.0013	0.0132	0.0659	0.1322
6 0.0013	0.0132	0.0654	0.1311
7 0.0013	0.0130	0.0650	0.1303
8 0.0013	0.0129	0.0647	0.1297
9 0.0013	0.0129	0.0647	0.1293
10 0.0013	0.0129	0.0643	0.1289
15 0.0013	0.0127	0.0638	0.1278
20 0.0013	0.0127	0.0635	0.1273
30 0.0013	0.0126	0.0632	0.1267
40 0.0013	0.0126	0.0631	0.1265
50 0.0013	0.0126	0.0630	0.1263
60 0.0013	0.0126	0.0630	0.1262
70 0.0013	0.0126	0.0629	0.1261
80 0.0013	0.0126	0.0629	0.1261
100 0.0013	0.0126	0.0629	0.1261
∞ 0.0013	0.0126	0.0629	0.1261

The appropriate chi-square value according to:

$$\frac{(ad-bc)^2(a+b+c+d)}{(a+b)(c+d)(b+d)(a+c)} = 0.00205$$

The chi-square table (Table 12.2) gives in four columns various chi-square values corresponding to the p-values given in the upper row. The left hand column adjusts for degrees of freedom. The above result of 0.00205 is on the left side of the critical chi-square value of 0.0039, and, so, we can reject the possibility that our data are so close to each other by chance even if there were no difference in the data. We may worry that these data are not randomly sampled.

3.3 F-Test

The effect of three compounds improving Hemoglobin levels is assessed in three parallel groups.

Table 12.2 Chi-square values with unusually high p-values

p-value(two sided)

Degrees freedom	0.999	0.99	0.95	0.90
1	0.0000016	0.0016	0.0039	0.016
2	0.0020	0.020	0.10	0.21
3	0.024	0.12	0.35	0.58
4	0.091	0.30	0.71	1.06
5	0.21	0.55	1.15	1.61
6	0.38	0.87	1.64	2.20
7	0.60	1.24	2.17	2.83
8	0.86	1.65	2.73	3.49
9	1.15	2.09	3.33	4.17
10	1.48	2.56	3.94	4.87
15	3.48	5.23	7.26	8.55
20	5.92	8.26	10.85	12.44
25	8.66	11.52	14.61	16.47
30	11.58	14.95	18.49	20.60
35	14.68	18.51	22.46	24.80
40	17.93	22.16	26.51	29.05
50	24.68	29.71	34.76	37.69
60	31.73	37.49	43.19	46.46
70	39.02	45.44	45.74	55.33
80	46.49	53.54	60.39	64.28
100	61.92	70.07	77.93	82.36

Group	n patients	Mean (mmol/l)	SD (mmol/l)
1	16	10.6300	1.2840
2	16	10.6200	1.2800
3	16	10.6250	1.2820

Grand mean $= (\text{mean } 1+2+3)/3 = 10.6250$

$$SS_{\text{between groups}} = 16(10.6300 - 10.6250)^2 + 16(10.6200 - 10.6250)^2 + 16(10.6250$$
$$- 10.6250)^2$$
$$= 0.000625 \text{ for 3 groups meaning } 3-1 = 2 \text{ degrees freedom}$$

$$MS_{\text{between groups}} = 0.000625 / 2 = 0.0003125$$

$$SS_{\text{within groups}} = 15 \times 1.2840^2 + 15 \times 1.2800^2 + 15 \times 1.2820^2$$
$$= 24.730 + 14.746 + 23.009 = 62.485 \text{ for } 15 + 9 + 14$$
$$= 38 \text{ degrees of freedom}$$

$$MS_{\text{within groups}} = 62.485 / 38 = 1.644$$

Table 12.3 F-values with unusually high p-values

| Degrees of freedom of the numerator | | | | | | | | | | | | | | | |
1	2	3	4	5	6	7	8	9	10	15	20	30	50	100	1000
Degrees of freedom denominator															
1 0.0062	0.054	0.099	0.13	0.15	0.17	0.18	0.19	0.20	0.20	0.22	0.23	0.23	0.25	0.25	0.26
2 0.0050	0.053	0.10	0.14	0.17	0.19	0.21	0.22	0.23	0.24	0.27	0.29	0.30	0.31	0.32	0.33
3 0.0046	0.052	0.11	0.15	0.18	0.21	0.23	0.25	0.26	0.27	0.30	0.32	0.34	0.36	0.37	0.38
4 0.0045	0.052	0.11	0.16	0.19	0.22	0.24	0.26	0.28	0.29	0.33	0.35	0.37	0.39	0.41	0.42
5 0.0043	0.052	0.11	0.16	0.20	0.23	0.25	0.27	0.29	0.30	0.34	0.37	0.40	0.42	0.43	0.45
6 0.0043	0.052	0.11	0.16	0.20	0.23	0.26	0.28	0.30	0.31	0.36	0.38	0.41	0.44	0.46	0.47
7 0.0042	0.052	0.11	0.16	0.20	0.24	0.26	0.29	0.30	0.32	0.37	0.40	0.43	0.45	0.48	0.50
8 0.0042	0.052	0.11	0.17	0.21	0.24	0.27	0.29	0.31	0.33	0.39	0.41	0.44	0.47	0.49	0.51
9 0.0041	0.052	0.11	0.17	0.21	0.24	0.27	0.29	0.31	0.33	0.39	0.42	0.45	0.48	0.51	0.53
10 0.0041	0.052	0.11	0.17	0.21	0.24	0.27	0.30	0.32	0.34	0.39	0.43	0.46	0.49	0.52	0.54
15 0.0041	0.052	0.11	0.17	0.22	0.25	0.28	0.31	0.33	0.35	0.42	0.45	0.50	0.53	0.56	0.60
20 0.0040	0.052	0.11	0.17	0.22	0.26	0.29	0.32	0.34	0.36	0.43	0.47	0.52	0.56	0.60	0.63
30 0.0040	0.051	0.12	0.17	0.22	0.26	0.30	0.32	0.35	0.37	0.44	0.49	0.54	0.59	0.64	0.68
50 0.0040	0.051	0.12	0.17	0.23	0.27	0.30	0.33	0.36	0.38	0.46	0.51	0.57	0.63	0.67	0.74
100 0.0040	0.051	0.12	0.18	0.23	0.27	0.31	0.34	0.36	0.39	0.47	0.52	0.59	0.66	0.72	0.79

$$F = MS_{between\ groups} / MS_{within\ groups} = 0.0003125 / 1.644 = 0.00019$$

According to the F-table (Table 12.3) for 2 and 38 degrees of freedom an F-value >0.051 means that p > 95%. The differences between the parallel groups are closer to zero than compatible with random sampling. We have a strong argument to believe that they are not completely random.

4   Additional Examples Simulating Real Practice, Multiple Comparisons

The issue of p-values >0.95 being not random is, of course, less true for studies testing multiple measurements. If you test many times, you are apt to find extreme p-values, either high or low, once in a while purely by chance. If the chance of finding an extreme p-value with a single test is equal to 0.05, then, according to the Bonferroni inequality, this chance increases to $1 - 0.95^k$ with k tests. However, the chance of finding multiple extreme p-values in this situation remains very small. E.g., the chance of finding k extreme p-values with k tests is equal to 0.05^k. If k = 5, then this chance = <0.000000. We should add that multiple comparisons/tests will not be independent in most cases. Therefore, the chance of finding extreme p-values will not be as dramatically small as implied by the above formula, but even with dependencies, this chance will soon get much smaller than the traditional 0.05, and unrandomness of data has to be accounted.

Table 12.4 gives examples of multiple comparisons/tests as commonly included in the reports of clinical drug trials/research. It show a remarkable similarity of (1) patient characteristics between two treatment groups, and (2) pharmacokinetic data between a brand name drug and its generic copy, (3) the virtual absence of time or carryover effect in a crossover study, and (4) virtually no difference in side effects between treatment and a placebo. All of these examples include multiple comparisons/tests in a single population, and these comparisons/tests can, therefore, not be expected to be independent of one another. The chance that these tables are unrandom is, therefore, not as small as implied by the above formula, but it is, certainly, smaller than 5% for each of the examples given.

Table 12.4 Examples of multiple comparisons/tests as commonly included in the reports of clinical drug trials/research

Example 1 Patient characteristics of a randomized controlled trial (*sds* = standard deviations)

	Treatment 1 (n = 5,000)	Treatment 2 (n = 5,000)	p-value
Females n (%)	979 (19.58)	974 (19.48)	>0.95
Age <60 years n (%)	1,882 (37.64)	1,877 (37.54)	>0.95
White n (%)	4,889 (97.78)	4,887 (97.74)	>0.99
Smokers n (%)	1,716 (34.32)	1,712 (34.32)	>0.95
Mean alcohol consumption (units, sds)	8.1(11.3)	8.0 (11.4)	>0.95
Mean systolic blood pressure (mmHg, sds)	164.2 (17.8)	164.2 (17.8)	1.00
Mean diastolic blood pressure (mmHg, sds)	95.0 (10.3)	95.0 (10.3)	1.00
Mean body mass index (kg/m², sds)	28.6 (4.7)	28.7 (4.6)	1.00
Mean total cholesterol (mmol/l, sds)	5.5 (0.8)	5.5 (0.8)	1.00
Mean triglycerides (mmol/l,sds)	1.74 (0.91)	1.73 (0.90)	> 0.99
Mean glucose (mmol/l, sds)	6.2 (2.1)	6.2 (2.1)	1.00

Example 2 Pharmacokinetic parameters

	Brand-name drug (n = 8)	Generic copy (n = 7)	p-value
Mean clearance (ml/h, sds)	158 (15)	158 (15)	1.00
Mean bio-availability (%, sds)	75 (7)	74 (7)	>0.95
Mean volume of distribution (ml)	9,300 (910)	9,296 (915)	>0.99
Mean elimination half life (h, sds)	41 (4)	40 (4)	>0.95
Mean area under curve (μg, h/ml)	547 (54)	543 (53)	>0.95

Example 3 Crossover study tested for treatment, carryover and time effects

	Period 1	Period 2
	Mean temperature (°C, sd)	
Group1	Treatment 1	Treatment 2
	Result 20.23 (4.12) *a*	Result 24.12 (4.21) *b*
Group2	Treatment 2	Treatment 1
	Result 24.11 (4.20) *c*	Result 20.22 (4.12) *d*

Treatment effect $a+d$ vs $b+c$ $p<0.001$

Carryover effect $a+c$ vs $b+d$ $p>0.95$

Time effect $a+b$ vs $c+d$ $p>0.95$

Example 4 Side effects of a parallel-group clinical trial

	Active treatment (n = 500)	Placebo (n = 500)	p-value
Nasal congestion (yes)	240	241	>0.99
Urine incontinence	44	45	>0.95
Impotence	50	52	>0.95
Depression	32	31	>0.95
Fatigue	99	98	>0.95
Palpitations	50	50	1.00
Dizziness	121	123	>0.95
Sleepiness	76	80	>0.95

5   Discussion

Main-endpoint results producing large p-values may not be entirely random. This issue has received little attention from the scientific community so far. Also statistical tables covering them are not in the statistical literature. Fortunately, current statistical software generally provides exact p-values. But, then, investigators, however excited to report how nicely their results match their prior expectations, are often reluctant to report the exact p-values, and confine themselves to the notion NS (not significant). The statistical tables as published in the current paper can be adequately used to test, a posteriori, such data. Whenever, p-values are >0.95, we have a strong argument that the data are not entirely random, and that they be interpreted with caution.

The current chapter is only a preliminary effort to assess randomness of clinical trial data. Other methods could include the more extensive use of population data for comparison, data transformations and non-parametric tests. We recommend that the scientific community develop guidelines for standard assessment of this issue. This is important to the body of evidence-based medicine, currently under pressure due to the conflicting results of recent trials producing different answers to similar questions (Julius 2003; Cleophas and Cleophas 2003). Many causes are mentioned. As long as the possibility of inappropriate data cleaning has not been addressed, this very possibility can not be excluded as potential cause of the obvious lack of homogeneity in current research.

6   Conclusions

A p-value of >0.95 literally means that we have >95% chance of finding a result less close to expectation, and, consequently, <5% chance of finding a result this close or closer. Using the traditional 5% decision level, this would mean, that we have a strong argument that such data are not completely random. The objective of this chapter was to facilitate the assessment of this issue. T-, chi-square-, and f-tables of unusually large p-values are given to calculate a posteriori p-values of study results closely matching their prior expectations. Simulated examples are given. Clinical trial data producing large p-values may not be completely random. The current chapter is a preliminary effort to assess randomness of clinical trial data.

References

Cleophas TJ (2004) Research data closer to expectation than compatible with random sampling. Stat Med 23:1015–1017

Cleophas TJ, Cleophas GM (2001) Sponsored research and continuing medical education. J Am Med Assoc 286:302–304

Cleophas GM, Cleophas TJ (2003) Clinical trials in jeopardy. Int J Clin Pharmacol Ther 41:51–56

Julius S (2003) The ALLHAT study: if you believe in evidence-based medicine, stick to it. J Hypertens 21:453–454

Chapter 13
Data Dispersion Issues

1   Introduction

Biological processes are full of variations, and so is clinical research. Statistics can give no certainties, only chances and, consequently, their results are often reported with a measure of dispersion, otherwise called uncertainty. Mostly, standard errors are calculated as a measure for dispersion in the data. For example, in a hypertension study a mean systolic blood pressure after active treatment of 125 mmHg compared to 135 mmHg after placebo treatment may indicate that either the treatment was clinically efficacious or that the difference observed is due to random variation. To answer this the standard errors of the mean results, 5 mmHg each, and a pooled standard error are calculated, $\sqrt{(5^2 + 5^2)} = 7.07$ mmHg. According to the Student's t-test this result is statistically insignificant: the t-value $= (135 - 125)/7.07 = 1.4$, and should have been larger than approximately 2. With such a result it is, usually, concluded that the treatment effect is not different from a placebo effect, and that the calculated mean difference is due to random variation, rather than a true treatment effect.

It is sometimes hard to assess complex estimators of clinical efficacy for standard errors. Consequently, they are reported, then, as mean results without further statistical test or p-value. For example, numbers needed to treat in clinical trials, reproducibility of quantitative diagnostic tests, sensitivity and specificity, Markov estimators, and risk profiles from multiple logistic models are routinely reported without measure of uncertainty. The predictions for general practice made from such estimators are not entirely in agreement with evidence-based medicine. As recommended by the STARD (Standards for the Reporting of Diagnostic Accuracy Studies) steering group (Bossuyt et al. 2003), ample efforts should be given to include a measure of uncertainty in any research result in order for predictions to be more accurate.

Another dispersion issue is the use of traditional standard errors in situations where the data are over-dispersed. Over-dispersion depicts the phenomenon that the spread in the data is wider than compatible with Gaussian modeling. This phenomenon is, particularly, common with logistic models, but can also occur with continuous real data samples (Tan 2003). Traditional statistical tests overestimate the precision of over-dispersed data, meaning that the calculated p-values are too small, and the conclusion of a significant effect is erroneously being made. To date statistical software programs do not routinely include tests for over-dispersion, and, so, investigators have to take care and make their own assessments prior to the analysis.

In the current paper we will review both the flaw of data without measure of dispersion and that of data with over-dispersion. As real data examples assessing these flaws are virtually missing in the medical literature, we will give hypothesized examples. Simple Gaussian distribution based methods for assessment are used, and most of them can be readily found in major statistical packages like SAS (www.sas.com), and special software programs for the calculation of confidence intervals like Confidence Interval Analysis (Gardner 1989).

2   Data Without Measure of Dispersion

2.1   Numbers Needed to Treat in Clinical Trials

In order to decide whether the results of a study are important for future patient care the numbers needed to treat (NNTs) are often calculated. As an example, in a clinical trial of beta-blocker versus placebo for the prevention of post-infarct arrhythmias the rate of post-infarct arrhythmias is significantly lower with the beta-blocker than with placebo, with 51/748 (proportion $=0.07$) in the beta-blocker group and 126/764 (proportion $=0.17$) in the placebo group (relative risk 2.4, 95% confidence interval 1.8–3.3). With this result, it is interesting to extrapolate these results to future populations. The number needed to treat in order to prevent one arrhythmic patient is often used for that purpose, and is calculated according to:

$$\text{number needed to treat } (NNT) = 1 / (0.168 - 0.068) = 1 / 0.1 = 10$$

We will need to treat ten patients with a beta-blocker in order to prevent one arrhythmic patient. This conclusion, however appealing to readerships of articles, is not justified, because it is based on the assumption that the proportions are 100% certain, but the proportions do have boundaries of uncertainty, the 95% (or 99%) confidence interval, which indicates that the number could considerably differ from 10.

Using the equation "proportion $\pm 2 \sqrt{[p(1-p)/n]}$", the 95% confidence intervals are calculated as follows:

0.068 is between 0.051 and 0.085
0.168 is between 0.126 and 0.210

If we include this uncertainty in the calculation of the NNTs, then we can be 95% sure that the numbers required to prevent one arrhythmic patient range between $1/(0.210 - 0.051) = 6.3$ and $1/(0.126 - 0.085) = 24.4$. If we consider to treat future populations, it is more adequate to think of NNTs between 6 and 25 instead of a NNT of 10 patients. We should add that the NNT can also be derived from the risk

Table 13.1 In a diagnostic study of patients with Raynaud's phenomenon the reliability of venous occlusion plethysmography is assessed by duplicate testing of six patients

Plethysmographic peripheral arterial flows (ml/min)			
Patient no.	Test 1	Test 2	Difference
1	1	11	−10
2	10	0	10
3	2	11	−9
4	12	2	10
5	11	1	10
6	1	12	−11
Mean difference			0

Table 13.2 More adequate for assessing reproducibility between tests are methods that assess the spread of differences between repeated measurements like for example the duplicate standard deviation

Plethysmographic peripheral arterial flows (ml/min)				
Patients no.	Test 1	Test 2	Difference (d)	(Difference)^2
1	1	11	−10	100
2	10	0	10	100
3	2	11	−9	81
4	12	2	10	100
5	11	1	10	100
6	1	12	−11	121
Averages	6.17	6.17	0	100.3

Duplicate standard deviation $= \sqrt{[\frac{1}{2} \Sigma d^2 / n]} = \sqrt{(1/2 \times 100.3)} = 7.08$

difference. The risk difference and its 95% confidence interval can be calculated in SAS (www.sas.com), Confidence Interval Analysis (Gardner 1989), and other software programs.

2.2 Reproducibility of Quantitative Diagnostic Tests

Reproducibility, otherwise called reliability, of diagnostic tests or questionnaires is an essential prerequisite for implementation. A routine but incorrect method for that purpose is the following. We calculate the mean value of the first set of tests, then from the second set of tests. If the difference is small, then we conclude, that the two tests are well-reproducible. As an example, in a diagnostic study of patients with Raynaud's phenomenon the reliability of venous occlusion plethysmography is assessed by duplicate testing of six patients (Table 13.1). The mean difference between the duplicate tests is as small as 0. Yet, the test is poorly reproducible, with a range of differences between two tests of no less than −11 to +10 ml/min.

The mean difference between two sets of tests is, obviously, not good enough for demonstrating a high level of reproducibility between tests. More adequate for that purpose are methods that assess the spread of differences between repeated measurements like, for example, the duplicate standard deviation (Table 13.2). For adequate reproducibility the magnitude of the duplicate standard deviation should equal 10–20% of the test-averages. Also adequate is the repeatability coefficient that is calculated by the standard deviation of the individual differences between the tests 1 and 2: a result equal to10–20% of the test averages is considered to be adequate.

2.3   Sensitivity and Specificity

In clinical research gold standard tests for making a diagnosis are often laborious and sometimes impossible. Instead, simple and non-invasive tests are used.

	Disease present (numbers of patients)	
	Yes	No
Test Positive	a	b
Negative	c	d

In the above 2×2 contingency table a = the number of truly positive patients in such a simple non-invasive test, b = the number false positive, c = the number false negative, and d = the number truly negative.

Validity of these kinds of tests is often assessed with sensitivity and specificity. Sensitivity = a/(a+c) = proportion in a sample of true positive patients, where the true positives are the patients with a positive test and the presence of disease; specificity = d/(d+b) = proportion in a sample of patients with a true negative test, where the true negatives are the patients with a negative test and without the presence of disease. A problem is, that most diagnostic tests have limited sensitivities and specificities. Levels around 0.5 (50%) means that no more information is given than flipping a coin. Levels substantially higher than 50% are, commonly, accepted as documented proof, that the diagnostic test is valid. However, sensitivity/specificity are estimates from experimental samples, and scientific rigor recommends that with experimental sampling amounts of uncertainty be included. Uncertainty is virtually never assessed in sensitivity/specificity evaluations of cardiovascular diagnostic tests. This is a pity, because calculated levels of uncertainty could be used for statistically testing whether the sensitivity/specificity are significantly larger than 0.5 or whether their 95% confidence intervals are between previously set validation boundaries. If not, then it is appropriate to reject the diagnostic test, because it is imprecise to predict the disease. As an example, a dimer test is used as a diagnostic test for the diagnosis of lung embolias.

	Lung embolia (numbers of patients)	
	Yes	No
Dimer test Positive	2	18
Negative	1	182

The sensitivity and specificity in the above example is calculated to be 0.6666 and 0.911 respectively. These results could be interpreted as acceptable, because they are much larger than 0.5. However, in order to conclude, that they are significantly larger than 0.5, their 95% confidence intervals should not cross the 50% boundary.

Sensitivity/specificity are proportions, and it is fairly straightforward to calculate standard errors from them (Levin et al. 2008). The equations are underneath:

$$\text{standard error sensitivity} = \sqrt{\left[ac / (a+c)^3 \right]}$$

$$\text{standard error specificity} = \sqrt{\left[db / (d+b)^3 \right]}$$

The 95% confidence intervals of sensitivity and specificity can be calculated from:

$$\text{95\% confidence interval} = \text{Sensitivity} \pm \text{its } 1.96 \times \text{standard error}$$

$$\text{95\% confidence interval} = \text{Specificity} \pm \text{its } 1.96 \times \text{standard error}$$

$$\text{sensitivity} = 0.666 \pm 1.96 \times 3.672 = \text{between} -5.4 \text{ and } 7.8.$$

$$\text{specificity} = 0.911 \pm 1.96 \times 0.286 = \text{between } 0.35 \text{ and } 1.47.$$

These intervals are very wide, and do not fall within the boundary 0.5–1.0 (50–100%). Validity of the above test is, thus, not demonstrated.

2.4   Markov Predictors

Regression models are only valid within observed range x-values. The Markov model goes one step further. It predicts beyond that range, and, in addition, it does so without accounting uncertainty. As an example, in an observational study, the presence of heart failure defined as a B natriuretic peptide test above 100 pg/ml is assessed in a group of 500 patients. At time 0 year 0/500 patients met the criterion. At the time point 1 year, however, 50/500 ($=10\%$) did. An exponential-pattern is assumed. It is concluded that, if after 1 year 90% had no heart failure, then

after 2 years $90\% \times 90\% = 81\%$ will have no heart failure

after 3 years $90\% \times 90\% \times 90\% = 73\%$ will have no heart failure

after 6.7 years $= 50\%$ will have no heart failure

Markov models are very popular for making predictions from health statistics or observational population-based studies like the Framingham studies. It is obvious that such models would better predict, if uncertainty were included. However, few studies have been published so far.

Table 13.3 Multiple logistic regression of an observational study of myocardial infarction in females treated with estrogenes. The dependent variable is the myocardial infarction (yes/no), estrogene use (yes/no), and the other underneath predictors are included in the model

Risk factors heart infarct	Regression coefficient (b)	Standard error	p-value	Odds ratio (or)
1. Estrogenes	2.60	0.25	<0.0001	13.5
2. Cholesterol	0.81	0.21	0.0001	2.2
3. Obesity	0.50	0.25	0.04	1.6
4. Hypertension	0.42	0.21	0.05	1.5
5. Nicotine	0.53	0.53	ns	

Markov models use multiplication of proportions and standard errors of them can be calculated using a logarithmic transformation (Cleophas and Zwinderman 2009a). The natural logarithm of a proportion is given by ln [a/(a+b)]. We recommend that the standard error be approached from the equation (ln = natural logarithm):

$$\text{standard error } \ln\left[a / (a+b) \right] = 1/a - 1/(a+b)$$

From the previously described example the 95% confidence of the proportion of patients who will have no failure after 6.7 years could be calculated according to (6.7 in superscript means here "to the power 6.7"):

$$\ln\left[a / (a+b) \right]^{6.7} = 6.7 \ln\left[a / (a+b) \right]$$

The standard error of ln [a/(a+b)]$^{6.7}$ = 6.7 standard error [a/(a+b)] = 6.7 [1/a − 1/(a+b)].

The logarithmic transformed 95% confidence interval

$$= 6.7 \ln\left[a / (a+b) \right] \pm 1.96 \times 6.7 \left[1/a - 1/(a+b) \right].$$

The true 95% confidence interval is found by taking the antilogarithm.

Along this line uncertainty can be included in Markov modelling, and more precise predictions can be made from this clinical estimator (Cleophas and Zwinderman 2009a).

2.5   Risk Profiles from Multiple Logistic Models

Logistic models are often applied for determining individual and population risk profiles. As an example we will use an observational study of myocardial infarction in females treated with estrogenes. Additional risk factors are included (Table 13.3). The odds of myocardial infarct in patients with estrogene is 13.5 times that of patients without. As four of the risk factors are significant, we remove factor 5 and assume that all of the remaining 4 factors independently predict an increased risk, and that, together, they predict the following risk:

the odds ratio (OR) of myocardial infarct with factors $1-4 =$

$$OR_1 \times OR_2 \times OR_3 \times OR_4 = 75.9$$

For an individual or a group of persons carrying all four risk factors the odds of obtaining myocardial infarct is 76 times that of the individual/group devoid of the risk factors. But is this true? Should we not include a boundary of uncertainty here. The standard error of each of the risk factors is given in the Table 13.3, and needs to be incorporated in the final result for the purpose of accuracy and precision.

Logistic models for determining risk profiles use multiplications of odds ratios. If only significant predictors are included, we may assume that they are independent of one another and a fairly straightforward method is available for calculating the pooled 95% confidence interval of the multiplication products. The above example is used once more.

The pooled standard error of the natural logarithms of the odds ratio of cancer with the factors 1–4 ($\ln OR_{factors\ 1-4}$) is given by (ln means natural logarithm):

standard error of $\ln OR_{factors\ 1-4}$
$= \sqrt{(\text{standard error}_1{}^2 + \text{standard error}_2{}^2 + \text{standard error}_3{}^2 + \text{standard error}_4{}^2)}$

The logarithmic transformed 95% confidence interval is found by taking:
$\ln OR_{factors\ 1-4} \pm 1.96 \times \text{pooled standard error of } \ln OR_{factors\ 1-4}$

In this manner uncertainty can be implied in the risk profile, and better precision for predictions from data can be given.

3   Data with Over-Dispersion

Over-dispersion depicts the phenomenon that the spread in the data is wider than compatible with Gaussian modelling. This phenomenon is, particularly, common with logistic models, but can also occur with continuous real data samples (Tan 2003). Over-dispersion can be detected by goodness of fit tests, for example the Pearson's chi-square goodness of fit test or the Kolmogorov-Smirnov test (Cleophas and Zwinderman 2009b). To date statistical software programs do not routinely include tests for over-dispersion, and, so, investigators have to make their own assessments prior to the analysis.

Table 13.4 shows a hypothesized example of a 2×2 multi-centre factorial clinical trial of the effect of a beta-blocker and a calcium channel blocker on hypertension. The analysis requires the binary logistic model (ln = natural logarithm):

$\ln$ odds of responding $= a + b_1\ x_1 + b_2\ x_2 + b_3\ x_1\ x_2$
$x_1 = $ beta-blocker
$x_2 = $ calcium channel blocker

Table 13.4 A hypothesized example of a 2×2 multi-centre factorial clinical trial of the effect of a beta-blocker and a calcium channel blocker on hypertension

| | Calcium channel blocker | | | | Dummy calcium channel blocker | | | |
| | Dummy b-b | | Beta-blocker | | Dummy b-b | | Beta blocker | |
Center	Resp	Total	Resp	Total	Resp	Total	Resp	Total
1	10	39	5	6	8	16	3	12
2	23	62	53	74	10	30	22	41
3	23	81	55	72	8	28	15	30
3	26	51	32	51	23	45	32	51
4	17	39	46	79	0	4	3	7
5			10	13				
Mean proportion per treatment combination								
	0.364		0.681		0.249		0.532	

b-b beta-blocker, *resp* number of responders (a mean blood pressure under 107 mmHg), *total* total number of patients with specific treatment combination per centre

Table 13.5 The Pearson goodness of fit test of the data of Table 13.4

$$\text{chi - square} = \sum \frac{\left(\text{observed numbers responders} - \text{expected numbers responders}\right)^2}{\text{expected numbers responders}}$$

The calculation per treatment combination per centre is as follows

1.	$(10-39 \times 0.364)/39 \times (10/39 - (1 - 10/39))$	$= 2.2$
2.		$= 0.0$
3.		$= 2.2$
4.		$= 4.5$
5.		$= 1.1+$
		$= 10.0$

There is a strong difference in the total numbers of observations per centre: between 4 and 81. This could lead to over-dispersion. The Pearson goodness of fit test can be used to assess the presence of it. The calculation is given in Table 13.5. If we add up the other three treatment combination results to 10.0, we will end up with a chi-square value of $10.0 + \ldots = 32$. This chi-square value should be approximately equal to its degrees of freedom for the logistic model to hold. We have, however, 21 (cells) – 4 (treatment combinations) = 17 degrees of freedom. This would mean that the data are over-dispersed. A solution recommended by Hojsgaard and Halekoh is used (Hojsgaard and Halekoh 2005). The magnitude of the dispersion can be estimated by the ratio:

$$\text{chi - square number / degrees of freedom} = 32 / 17 = 1.9$$

The square root of this ratio (here $\sqrt{1.9}$), sometimes called the variance inflating factor can, subsequently, be used to adjust the standard errors in the study. ln odds of responding $= a + b_1 \, x_1 + b_2 \, x_2 + b_3 \, x_1 \, x_2$ (ln = natural logarithm). The calculation is given in Table 13.6.

The probability of responding to a dummy beta-blocker and calcium channel blocker equals 0.36. This is unchanged after adjustment for dispersion. However, the

95% confidence of this probability changes from 0.31–0.42 to 0.28–0.45. In conclusion, with over-dispersion the parameter estimates are not affected, but their standard errors are likely to be underestimated, and should be adjusted for that flaw.

4 Discussion

This chapter is far from complete, many more examples can be given. Data without measure of dispersion also include pharmacokinetic/-dynamic parameters in simulated and real-data drug trials, diagnostic odds ratios in diagnostic meta-analyses (Moses et al. 1993), node impurities with binary partitioning (Lesterhuis and Cleophas 2009), propensity scores for data matching (Wasson et al. 1985). Also data with over-dispersion are very common with current multicenter and international clinical trials, though rarely assessed for that purpose (Tan 2003).

Conclusions from data without measure of dispersion should be interpreted with caution, because statistically insignificant differences may be interpreted as real differences while they are just a result of random fluctuations. Random fluctuations should never be the basis for new treatments. The STARD (Standards for Reporting Diagnostic Accuracy) working party recently advised "to include in the estimates of diagnostic accuracy adequate measures of uncertainty, e.g., 95%-confidence intervals" (Bossuyt et al. 2003), and rightly so, because the problem is not sporadically encountered, but can be almost routinely observed in research reports. For example, even in a journal like the Journal of the International Federation of Clinical chemistry and Laboratory Medicine out of 17 original papers addressing novel chemistry methods 16 communicated the above-mentioned flawed reproducibility assessments while the correct methods were used in only one (Imbert-Bismut et al. 2004).

What solutions can be given. First, calculating standard errors or confidence intervals is often possible. If not, alternative confidence intervals may be a possibility, for example, those based on Monte Carlo methods like bootstrap confidence intervals. Second, sometimes, the choice is deliberately made not to use the data fully, but to skip the standard errors, and to use the summary measures only. NNTs can be considered as such summary measures. The problem with this approach is that without accounting the uncertainty of the summary measure the overall results may produce inflated results, because the dispersion in the data is artificially minimized by removing this uncertainty. This limitation should be recognized in research reports.

Conclusions from data with over-dispersion should equally be interpreted with caution, because the calculated confidence intervals and p-values are too small and the conclusion of a significant effect may erroneously be made. Particularly, if a strong difference in numbers of responders or magnitudes of responses is in the data, the presence of over-dispersion should be assessed. Goodness of fit tests are available for that purpose. The advantage of the Pearson chi-square goodness of fit test, is, that, in addition to detecting over-dispersion, it enables to adjust for it. The adjusted mean of the data remains unchanged, while the measures of dispersion in the data, including variances and co-variances, log – likelihoods,

Table 13.6 The calculation
of a standard error adjusted
for over-dispersion

		SE	p	SE$_{adust}$	p
a	−0.41	0.18	0.025	0.25	0.119
b$_1$	0.54	0.25	0.031	0.34	0.132
b$_2$	−0.15	0.22	0.513	0.30	0.638
b$_3$	0.78	0.31	0.011	0.42	0.080

SE$_{adjust}$ = SE adjusted for over - dispersion = $\sqrt{1.9} \times$ SE.

Wald – intervals etc are, simply, multiplied by the square root of the ratio of the chi-square value and its degrees of freedom (variance inflating factor = chi-square/degrees of freedom).

In conclusion, we recommend that analytical methods in clinical research should always try and include a measure of dispersion in the data. Often standard errors or 95% confidence intervals can be used for the purpose. With large differences in the data, the presence of over-dispersion should be assessed and adjusted.

We should add that also the delta method (explained in the appendix of Chapter 47) is very helpful to provide measures of dispersion.

5   Conclusions

Biological processes are full of variations, and so is clinical research. Estimators of clinical efficacy are, therefore, usually reported with a measure of uncertainty, otherwise called dispersion.

The objective of this chapter was to review both the flaws of data reports without measure of dispersion, and those with over-dispersion.

Examples of estimators commonly reported without measure of dispersion include:

1. numbers needed to treat,
2. reproducibility of quantitative diagnostic tests,
3. sensitivity/specificity,
4. Markov predictors,
5. Risk profiles predicted from multiple logistic models.

Data with large differences between response magnitudes can be assessed for over-dispersion by goodness of fit tests. The chi-square goodness of fit test enables to adjust the over-dispersion.

For most clinical estimators the calculation of standard errors or confidence intervals is possible. Sometimes, the choice is deliberately made not to use the data fully, but to skip the standard errors, and to use the summary measures only. The problem with this approach is that the overall results may produce inflated results. We recommend that analytical methods in clinical research should always try and include a measure of dispersion in the data. With large differences in the data, the presence of over-dispersion should be assessed and adjusted.

References

Bossuyt PM, Reitsma JB, Bruns DE, Gatsonis CA, Glasziou PP, Irwig JG, Moher D, Rennie D, De Vet HC, for the STARD steering group (2003) Education and debate. Towards complete and accurate reporting of studies of diagnostic accuracy: the STARD initiative. BMJ 326:41–44

Cleophas TJ, Zwinderman AH (2009a) Markow modeling. In: Statistics applied to clinical trials, 4th edn. Springer, Dordrecht, pp 212–213

Cleophas TJ, Zwinderman AH (2009b) Testing clinical trials for randomness. In: Statistics applied to clinical trials, 4th edn. Springer, Dordrecht, pp 355–366

Gardner MJ (1989) Confidence interval analysis. BMJ Productions, London

Hojsgaard S, Halekoh U (2005) Overdispersion. Danish Institute of Agricultural Sciences, Copenhagen. http://gbi.agrsci.dk/statistics/courses

Imbert-Bismut F, Messous D, Thibaut V et al (2004) Intra-laboratory analytical variability of biochemical markers of fibrosis and activity and reference ranges in healthy blood donors. Clin Chem Lab Med 42:323–333

Lesterhuis W, Cleophas TJ (2009) Cardiovascular research: decision analysis using binary partitioning. Perfusion 22:88–91

Levin MD, Van de Bos E, Van Ouwerkerk BM, Cleophas TJ (2008) Uncertainty of diagnostic tests. Perfusion 21:42–48

Moses LE, Shapiro D, Littenberg B (1993) Combining independent studies of a diagnostic test into a summary ROC curve: data-analytic approaches and some additional considerations. Stat Med 12:1293–1316

Tan M (2003) Describing data, variability and over-dispersion in medical research. In: Lu Y, Fang J (eds) Advanced medical statistics. World Scientific, River Edge, pp 319–332

Wasson JH, Sox HC, Neff RK, Goldman L (1985) Clinical prediction rules: applications and methodologic standards. N Engl J Med 313:793–799

Chapter 14
Linear Regression, Basic Approach

1 Introduction

In the past chapters we discussed different statistical methods to test statistically experimental data from clinical trials. We did not emphasize correlation and regression analysis. The point is that correlation and regression analysis test correlations, rather than causal relationships. Two samples may be strongly correlated e.g., two different diagnostic tests for assessment of the same phenomenon. This does, however, not mean that one diagnostic test causes the other. In testing the data from clinical trials we are mainly interested in causal relationships. When such assessments were statistically analyzed through correlation analyses mainly, we would probably be less convinced of a causal relationship than we are while using prospective hypothesis testing. So, this is the main reason we so far did not address correlation testing extensively. With epidemiological observational research things are essentially different: data are obtained from the observation of populations or the retrospective observation of patients selected because of a particular condition or illness. Conclusions are limited to the establishment of relationships, causal or not. We currently believe that relationships in medical research between a factor and an outcome can only be proven to be causal if the factor is introduced, and, subsequently, gives rise to the outcome. We are more convinced when such is tested in the form of a controlled clinical trial. A problem with multiple regression and logistic regression analysis as method for analyzing multiple samples in clinical trials is closely related to this point. There is always an air of uncertainty about such regression data. Interventional trials usually use hypothesis-testing and 95% confidence intervals (CIs) of the data to describe and analyze data. They use multiple regression for secondary analyses, thus enhancing the substance of the research, and making the readership more willing to read the report, rather than proving the primary endpoints. Regression analysis may not be so important to randomized clinical trials, it is important to one particular study design, the crossover study, where every patient is given in random order test-treatment and standard treatment (or placebo). Figure 14.1 gives three hypothesized examples of crossover trials. It can be observed

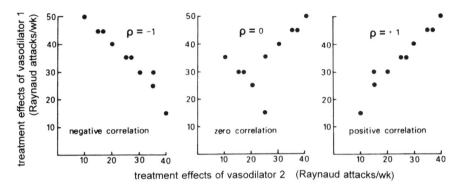

Fig. 14.1 Example of three crossover studies of two treatments in patients with Raynaud's phenomenon. The (Pearson's) correlation coefficient ρ varies between −1 and +1

from the plots that in the left and right graph there seems to be a linear relationship between treatment one and two. The strength of relationship is expressed as r (=correlation coefficient) which varies between −1 and +1. The strongest association is given by either −1 or +1 (all data exactly on the line), the weakest association 0 (all data are parallel either to x-axis or to y-axis, or half one direction, half the other). A positive correlation in a crossover study is observed if two drugs from one class are compared. The patients responding well to the first drug are more likely to respond well to the second. In contrast, in crossover studies comparing drugs from different classes a negative correlation may be observed: patients not responding well to one class are more likely to respond well to the other.

2   More on Paired Observations

Table 14.1 gives the real data of a crossover study comparing a new laxative versus a standard laxative, bisacodyl. Days with stool are used as primary endpoint. The table shows that the new drug is more efficacious than bisacodyl, but the figure (Fig. 14.2) shows something else: there is a positive correlation between the two treatments: those responding well to bisacodyl are more likely to respond well to the novel laxative.

A regression line can be calculated from the data according to the equation

$$y = a + bx$$

The line drawn from this linear function provides the best fit for the data given, where y=socalled dependent, and x=independent variable, b=regression coefficient.

a and b from the equation $y = a + bx$ can be calculated.

	New treatment (y-variables)	Bisacodyl (x-variables)
Patient no.	(days with stool)	(days of stool)
1	24	8
2	30	13
3	25	15
4	35	10
5	39	9
6	30	10
7	27	8
8	14	5
9	39	13
10	42	15
11	41	11
12	38	11
13	39	12
14	37	10
15	47	18
16	30	13
17	36	12
18	12	4
19	26	10
20	20	8
21	43	16
22	31	15
23	40	14
24	31	7
25	36	12
26	21	6
27	44	19
28	11	5
29	27	8
30	24	9
31	40	15
32	32	7
33	10	6
34	37	14
35	19	7

Table 14.1 Example of a crossover trial comparing efficacy of a new laxative versus bisacodyl

$$b = \text{regression coefficient} = \frac{\sum (x - \overline{x})(y - \overline{y})}{\sum (x - \overline{x})^2}$$

$$a = \text{intercept} = \overline{y} - b\overline{x}$$

$r =$ correlation coefficient $=$ another important determinant and looks a lot like b.

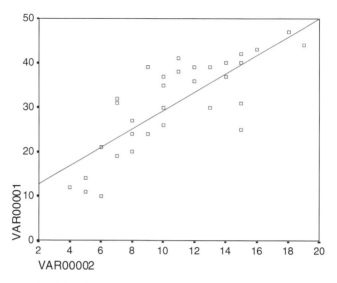

Fig. 14.2 Scatterplot of data from Table 14.1 with regression line

$$r = \frac{\sum (x - \overline{x})(y - \overline{y})}{\sqrt{\sum (x - \overline{x})^2 \sum (y - \overline{y})^2}}$$

r = measure for the strength of association between y and x-data. The stronger the association, the better y predicts x.

3   Using Statistical Software for Simple Linear Regression

Regression analysis without software is laborious. We may use a computer pro-gram, e.g., **SPSS Statistical Software**, to do the job for us. We command our soft-ware: **Statistics; Regression; Linear**. Excel files can be entered simply cutting and pasting.

The software calculates the values b and a and r so as to minimize the sum of the squared vertical distances of the points from the line (least squares fit). **SPSS for windows** provides us with three tables (Table 14.2): **(1) Model Summary, (2) ANOVA, (3) coefficients.**

1. **Model Summary** gives information on correlation coefficient (r) and its square (r^2) the coefficient of determination. A coefficient of determination of 0.63 indi-cates that 63% of the variation in the y variable is explained by variation in the x variable. The better the effect of bisacodyl the better the novel laxative is going to work. Adjusted r square is important for small samples only while std error of the estimate tells us something about the residue (variance not explained by the regression) and is equal to the square root of the Residual Mean Square.

Table 14.2   Three tables provided by SPSS for regression analysis

Model summary

Model	R	R square	Adjusted R square	Std. error of the estimate
1	.794[a]	.630	.618	6.1590

ANOVA[b]

Model		Sum of squares	df	Mean square	F	Sig.
1	Regression	2,128.393	1	2,128.393	56.110	.000[a]
	Residual	1,251.779	33	37.933		
	Total	3,380.171	34			

Coefficients[b]

Model		Unstandardized coefficients		Standardized coefficients		
		B	Std. error	Beta	t	Sig.
1	(Constant)	8.647	3.132		2.761	.009
	VAR00002	2.065	.276	.794	7.491	.000

[a]Predictors: (Constant), VAR00002
[b]Dependent Variable: VAR00001

At this point it is important to consider the following. Before doing any regression analysis we have to make the assumptions that our y – data are normally distributed and that variances in y-variable do not show a lot of difference, otherwise called heteroscedasticity (heteroscedasticity literally means "different standard deviations (SDs)").

White's Test is a simple method to check for this. Chi-square table is used for that purpose.

if n $r^2 < \chi^2 \cdot (n)$ we don't have to worry about heteroscedasticity.
n = sample size
r = correlation coefficient
$\chi^2(n)$ = the value for n degrees of freedom.
    In our example $35 \cdot (0.630) = 22.05$ while $\chi^2 \cdot (35) = 56.70$ (no heteroscedasticity)

2. **ANOVA (analysis of variance)** shows how the paired data can be assessed in the form of analysis of variance. Variations are expressed as sums of squares. The total variation in the regression is divided into sum of squares (SS) regression, or variances explained by the regression, and SS residual, variances unexplained by the regression.

$$ r^2 = \frac{\left(\sum (x - \bar{x})(y - \bar{y})^2\right)}{\sum (x - \bar{x})^2 \sum (y - \bar{y})^2} = \frac{SP^2 x \cdot y}{SSx \cdot SSy} $$

where SP = sum of products x·y
SS regression = SP^2 xy/SSx = 2128.393
SS total = SS y
SS regression/SS total = 2128.393/SS total = 0.63 (= r square (Model Summary))

As explained above this means that 63% of the variation in the y-variable is explained by the variation in the x-variable. This interpretation may be hard to understand, but it is helpful to imagine:

$r^2 = 0$ indicating no correlation at all,

$r^2 = 1.00$ indicating 100% correlation, each y-datum is exactly on the line,

$r^2 = 0.50$ indicating 50% certainty about a corresponding y – value if we know the x-value.

The strength of association of x- and y-values is dependent not only on the magnitude of the r^2 – value, but, in addition, on the sample size. For example, if we have a sample of $n = 3$ exactly on the line, then no accurate predictions can be made. However, if $n = 100$, then we are more convinced of the accuracy of the line as a predictor of y-values from given x-values. Therefore, in addition to calculating the magnitude of the r^2 – value, we have to include the sample size in our statistical work-up. For that purpose ANOVA is used. It tests whether r^2 is significantly larger than 0.00. The table shows that, indeed $p < 0.000$, and that the we, thus have a significant highly significant association between the x- and y-variables.

SPSS uses R (upper case), other software uses r (lower case) for expressing the correlation coefficient.

3. **Coefficients** shows the regression equation. The intercept is named "(constant)" and is given in the column under B and equals 8.647. The b-value in the linear regression equation is 2.065.

The regression equation is thus as follows.

$$Y = 8.647 + 2.065. \; x$$
$$\text{new laxative} = 8.647 + 2.065. \; \text{bisacodyl}$$

In addition to unstandardized coefficients, standardized coefficients are given. For that purpose SSy is defined to be 1. Then, $r = b$. Instead of testing that r is significantly larger than 0.00, we can now test that b is significantly larger than 0.000, and use for that purpose the t-test. The meaning of the two tests is very similar, and so is their result. The t-value of $7.491 = \sqrt{F} = \sqrt{56.110}$. This t-value is, obviously, equal to the square root of the F-value from the ANOVA-test.

4   Multiple Linear Regression

Linear regression would have never been so popular if only the inclusion of a single x-variable had been possible. We will now assess models with more than a single x-variable.

Obviously, there is a significant positive correlation between the x- and y-values in Fig. 14.3 (the above laxative-study). Maybe, there is also a positive correlation between the new laxative and patient age. If so, then the new laxative might be better, e.g.,

1. the better the bisacodyl,
2. the older the patient.

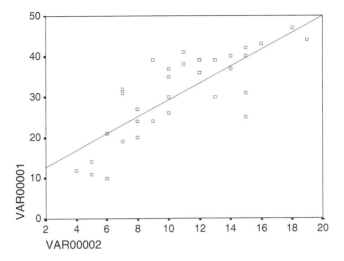

Fig. 14.3 Scatterplot of data from Table 14.1 with regression line

In this case we have, thus, 3 observations in 1 person

1. efficacy datum new laxative
2. efficacy datum bisacodyl
3. age.

In order to test possible correlations, we can define variables as follows

y variable presents new laxative data
x_1 variable bisacodyl data
x_2 variable age data.

Linear regression uses formula $y = a + bx$, where the y-variable = new laxative data, the x-variable = bisacodyl data. For example, if we fill out

$$x \text{ - value} = 0 \Rightarrow \text{then formula turns into } y = a$$

$$x \text{ - value} = 1 \Rightarrow \text{then formula turns into } y = a + b$$

$$x \text{ - value} = 2 \Rightarrow \text{then formula turns into } y = a + 2b$$

For each x-value the formula produces the best predictable y-value, all y-values constitute a line, the regression line (Fig. 14.4) which can be interpreted as the *best fit* line for data (the line with shortest distances from the y-values).

For multiple regression with three variables the regression formula $y = a + b_1 x_1 + b_2 x_2$ is being used. In order to visualize the model used, we can apply a three-axes-model with y-axis, x_1-axis and x_2-axis (Fig. 14.5). If we fill out

$$x_1 = 0, \text{ then the formula turns into } y = a + b_2 x_2$$

$$x_1 = 1, \text{then the formula turns into } y = a + b_1 + b_2 x_2$$

Fig. 14.4 Linear regression model gives best predictable y-value for the x-value given

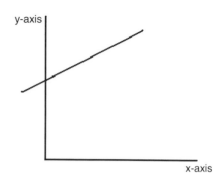

Fig. 14.5 Three axes model to illustrate multiple linear regression model with two x-variables

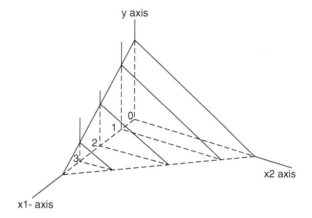

$$x_1 = 2, \text{then the formula turns into } y = a + 2b_1 + b_2 x_2$$
$$x_1 = 3, \text{then the formula turns into } y = a + 3b_1 + b_2 x_2.$$

Each x_1 –value has its own regression line, all of the regression-lines constitute a regression plane which is interpreted as the best fit plane for the data (the plane with the shortest distances to the y-values).

5   Multiple Linear Regression, Example

We may be interested to know if age is an independent contributor to the effect of the new laxative. For that purpose a simple regression equation has to be extended as follows

$$y = a + b_1 x_1 + b_2 x_2$$

b_1 are called partial regression coefficients. Just like simple linear regression, multiple linear regression can give us the best fit for the data given. The calculations of a, b_1 and b_2 are given underneath.

$$\Sigma y = na + b_1\Sigma x_1 + b_2\Sigma x_2$$

$$\Sigma x_1 y = a\Sigma x_1 + b_1 \Sigma x_1^2 + b_2 \Sigma x_1 x^2$$

$$\Sigma x_2 y = a\Sigma x_2 + b_1\Sigma x_1 x_2 + b_2\Sigma x_2^2$$

r between x_1, x_2 en y calculate from the equation

$$R = \sqrt{(b_1 r\, x_1 + b_2 r\, x_2)}$$

The calculations are hard without a computer. Also, it is hard to display the correlations in a figure. Table 14.3 gives the data from Table 14.1 extended by the variable age.

The Table 14.3 shows too many data to allow any conclusions. We use for assessment of these data the same SPSS program called linear regression and command again: **Statistics; Regression; Linear**. The software **SPSS for windows** provides us with the following three subtables: **(1) Model Summary, (2) ANOVA, (3) coefficients** (Table 14.4).

1. **Model Summary** shows r, here called the multiple r, The corresponding "multiple r square", otherwise called coefficient of determination, of 0.719 indicates that 71.9% of the variation in the y variable is explained by variation in the two x variables. Interestingly, the multiple r square is a bit larger than the simple r square (0.719 and 0.618). Information is thus given about the perfection of the model. After the first step 61.8% of variation is explained by the regression model, after the second no less than 71.9% is explained by it. The addition of age to the model produces 71.9% − 63% = 8.9% extra explanation of the variance in the y variable, the effect of the new laxative. The interpretation of the r^2 – value is similar to that in simple linear regression. If $r^2 = 0$, then no correlation exists, the x-values determines the y-values no way. If $r^2 = 1$, then the correlation is 100%, we are absolutely sure about the y-value if we know the x-values. If $r^2 = 0.5$, the 50% correlation exists. In our case $r^2 = 0.719 = 72\%$. The x-values determine the y-values by 72% certainty. We have 28% uncertainty = noise = (SE of $r^2 = 1 - r^2$).

Before going further we have to consider the hazard of collinearity, which is the situation where two x variables are highly correlated. One naive though common way in which collinearity is introduced into the data, is through inclusion of x variables that are actually the same measures under different names. This is, obviously, not so with bisacodyl effect and age. Nonetheless, we measure the presence of collinearity by calculating the simple correlation coefficient between the x variables before doing anything more. In our case r between x_1 variables and x_2 variables is 0.425, and so we don't have to worry about (multi)collinearity (r > 0.90).

Table 14.3 Example of a crossover trial comparing efficacy of a new laxative versus bisacodyl

Patient no.	New treatment y – variables (days with stool)	Bisacodyl x_1 – variables (days with stool)	Age x_2 – variables (years)
1	24	8	23
2	30	13	32
3	25	15	25
4	35	10	36
5	39	9	37
6	30	10	31
7	27	8	28
8	14	5	26
9	39	13	20
10	42	15	35
11	41	11	42
12	38	11	40
13	39	12	32
14	37	10	33
15	47	18	45
16	30	13	30
17	36	12	29
18	12	4	28
19	26	10	24
20	20	8	18
21	43	16	37
22	31	15	27
23	40	14	39
24	31	7	34
25	36	12	48
26	21	6	37
27	44	19	44
28	11	5	23
29	27	8	29
30	24	9	38
31	40	15	41
32	32	7	39
33	10	6	27
34	37	14	48
35	19	7	33

2. **ANOVA** is used to test whether r is significantly larger than 0.00. Again SS regression (by regression explained variance) is divided by SS residual (unexplained variance), the total variance being SS regression + SS residual. The division sum "304.570/SS total" yields 0.719 = r square, Called R square by SPSS. If r^2 is significantly different from the 0, then a regression plane like the one from Fig. 14.5 is no accident. If r^2 is significantly larger than 0 like here, then the data are closer to the regression plane than could happen by accident.

Table 14.4 Three tables provided by SPSS for regression analysis

Model summary

Model	R	R square	Adjusted R square	Std. error of the estimate
1	.848[a]	.719	.701	5.4498

ANOVA[b]

Model		Sum of squares	df	Mean square	F	Sig.
1	Regression	2429.764	2	1214.882	40.905	.000[a]
	Residual	950.407	32	29.700		
	Total	3380.171	34			

Coefficients[b]

Model		Unstandardized coefficients		Standardized coefficients		
		B	Std. error	Beta	t	Sig.
1	(Constant)	−1.547	4.233		−.366	.717
	VAR00002	1.701	.269	.653	6.312	.000
	VAR00003	.426	.134	.330	3.185	.003

[a]Predictors: (Constant), VAR00003, VAR00002
[b]Dependent Variable: VAR00001

3. **Coefficients** again shows the real regression equation. The intercept a is given by the (constant). The b values are the unstandardized regression coefficients of the x_1 and x_2 variables.

The regression equation is thus as follows

$$y = -1.547 + 1.701.x_1 + 0.426.x_2$$

$$\text{new laxative} = -1.547 + 1.701. \text{ bisacodyl} + 0.426 \cdot \text{age}$$

In addition to unstandardized coefficients, standardized coefficients are given. For that purpose SS y is taken to be 1. Then $r = b$. Instead of testing the null hypothesis that $r = 0$ we can now test that various $b_i = 0$, and use for that purpose t-test. As both bisacodyl and age are significantly correlated with the y variable (the efficacy of the new laxative), both x variables are independent predictors of the efficacy of the new laxative.

6 Purposes of Linear Regression Analysis

In summary, multiple regression-analysis with three variables and the equation formula $y = a + b_1 x_1 + b_2 x_2$, can be illustrated by a regression plane, the best fit plane for the scattered data (Fig. 14.6). A p-value <0.0001 means that the data are a lot closer to the regression plane than could happen by accident. If more than three variables are in the model, then the model becomes multidimensional, and a graph is impossible, but the principle remains the same.

Fig. 14.6 Regression plane

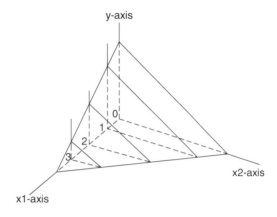

Multiple linear regression analysis is used for different purposes (see also the next chapter). The above example of two x-variables is an example where multiple linear regression is used in a controlled clinical crossover trial in order to provide more *precision* in the data. With a single x-variable the R^2-value $= 63\%$, with two x-variables the R^2-value $= 72\%$. Obviously, the level of certainty for making prediction about the y-variable increases by $72\% - 63\% = 9\%$, if a second x-variable is added to the data. Chapter 18 will give additional examples of this purpose. Another common purpose for its use is *exploratory* purposes. We search for significant predictors = independent determinants of the y-variable, and include multiple x-variables in the model. Subsequently, we asses which of the x-variables included are the statistically significant predictors of the y-variable according to the model

$$y = a + b_1 \, x_1 + b_2 \, x_2 + \ldots \ldots \ldots b_{10} \, x_{10}$$

The b-values are the partial correlation coefficients, and are used to test the strength of the correlation. If b_1 t/m b_{10} are significantly $</> 0$, then the corresponding x-variable is a significant predictor of the y-variable. The different x-variables can be added to the model one by one (stepwise, step-up), or all together. If added all together, we remove the insignificant ones starting with the one with the largest p-value (stepwise, step down). In practice the step-up and step-down method will produce rather similar results. If none of the x-variables produces a significant b-value, but the overall R^2-value is significantly different from 0, we have to conclude that none of the x-variables is an independent determinant of the y-variable, yet the y-value is significantly dependent on all of the x-variables.

Two more purposes of linear regression are the assessment of *confounding* and *interaction*. These purposes will be discussed as an introduction in the next chapter, and more fully in the Chaps. 19 and 20.

7   Another Real Data Example of Multiple Linear Regression (Exploratory Purpose)

We want to study "Independent determinants of quality of life of patients with angina pectoris". Note this is an observational rather than interventional study. We give the example because these kinds of data are often obtained as secondary data from interventional studies.

y-variable = index of quality of life of patients with stable angina pectoris
x-variables = 1. Age
              2. Gender
              3. Rhythm disturbances
              4. Peripheral vascular disease
              5. Concomitant calcium channel blockers
              6. Concomitant beta blockers
              7. NYHA-classification
              8. Smoking
              9. body mass index
              10. hypercholesterolemia
              11. hypertension
              12. diabetes mellitus
Index of quality of life $= a + b_1$ (age) $+ b_2$ (gender) $+ \ldots\ldots b_{12}$ (diabetes)

Correlation between independent variables may be correlated but not too closely: e.g. body mass index, body weight, body length should not be included all three. We used single linear regression for assessing this correlation, otherwise called multi-collinearity (Table 14.5).

Table 14.5 Correlation matrix in order to test multicollinearity in the regression analysis, p-values are given

	Age	Gender	Rhythm	vasc dis	ccb	bb	NYHA	Smoking	bmi	chol	hypt
Gender	0.19	1.00									
Rhythm	0.12	ns	1.00								
vasc dis	0.14	ns	ns	1.00							
ccb	0.24	ns	0.07	ns	1.00						
bb	0.33	ns	ns	ns	0.07	1.00					
NYHA	0.22	ns	ns	0.07	0.07	ns	1.00				
Smoking	−0.12	ns	0.09	0.07	0.08	ns	0.50	1.00			
bmi	0.13	ns	ns	ns	ns	0.10	−0.07	0.62	1.00		
chol	0.15	ns	ns	0.12	0.09	ns	0.08	0.09	ns	1.00	
hypt	0.09	ns	0.08	ns	0.10	0.09	0.09	0.09	0.07	0.41	1.00
Diabetes	0.12	ns	0.09	0.10	ns	0.08	ns	0.11	0.12	0.10	0.11

vasc dis peripheral vascular disease, *ccb* calcium channel blocker therapy, *bb* beta-blocker therapy, *bmi* body mass index, *hypt* hypertension, *ns* not statistically significantly correlated (Pearson's correlation p-value > 0.05)

Table 14.6 B-values used to test correlation, step down method

x-variable	Regression coefficient (B)	Standard error	Test (T)	Significance level (p-value)
Age	−0.03	0.04	0.8	0.39
Gender	0.01	0.05	0.5	0.72
Rhythm disturbances	−0.04	0.04	1.0	0.28
Peripheral vascular disease	−0.00	0.01	0.1	0.97
Calcium channel blockers	0.00	0.01	0.1	0.99
Beta blockers	0.03	0.04	0.7	0.43

Table 14.7 B-values to test correlation, step down method

x-variable	Regression coefficient (B)	Standard error	Test stat (t)	Significance level (p-value)
NYHA-classification	−0.08	0.03	2.3	0.02
Smoking	−0.06	0.04	1.6	0.08
Body mass index	−0.07	0.03	2.1	0.04
Hypercholesterolemia	0.07	0.03	2.2	0.03
Hypertension	−0.08	0.03	2.3	0.02
Diabetes mellitus	0.06	0.03	2.0	0.05

NYHA New York Heart Association

Table 14.6 shows the b-values that are not significantly different from 0. They are removed from the model. This procedure is called the step-down method (the step-up method includes the variables one by one, while removing those with an insignificant b-value). Table 14.7 summarizes the significant b-values. Conclusions: The higher the NYHA class the lower quality of life (Figs. 14.7 and 14.8). Smokers, obese subjects, and patients with concomitant hypertension have lower quality of life. Patients with hypercholesterolemia or diabetes mellitus have better quality of life. The latter two categories may have early endothelial dysfunction and may have significant angina pectoris with fairly intact coronary arteries. An alternative interpretation is that they have better quality of life because they better enjoy life despite a not so healthy lifestyle. This uncertainty about the cause of relationship established illustrates uncertainties produced by regression analyses. Regression analyses often establish relationships that are not causal, but rather induced by some unknown common factor.

8   It May Be Hard to Define What Is Determined by What, Multiple and Multivariate Regression

It may be sometimes hard in a linear regression to define what is determined by what, or, in other words, what are the dependent (y-values) and the independent variables (x-values). Generally, it is helpful to consider as independent determinants "causal – factors" determining the result, while the result is the dependent variable,

Fig. 14.7 A negative b-value
indicates: if x >, then y <

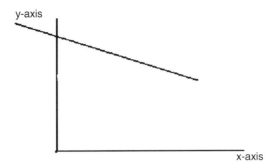

Fig. 14.8 A positive b-value
indicates: if x > then y >

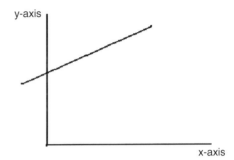

otherwise called outcome variable. Independent variables are currently often called exposure variables or indicator variables. In regression analyses of clinical trials the treatments modalities, in addition to patients' characteristics, are often independent variables. As examples we give two patient series with multiple variables:

1. Type operation
2. Type surgeon
3. Complications yes/no
4. Gender patients
5. Age patients
6. Required time for recovery,

(2) may determine (1),(3), and (6), but not (4) and (5),
(4) and (5) maybe (1),
(1) does not determine (4) and (5).

In another patient series the variables are:

1. Two types of anesthesia
2. Pain scores
3. Complications yes/no
4. Gender patients
5. Age patients

6. Comorbidity preoperatively
7. Quality of life after surgery

(1) determines (2) and maybe (3) and (7), but not (4), (5), and (6),
(4), (5), and (6) may determine (1) and maybe also (2), (3), and (7).
Regression can be nonsense and still produce significant results, e.g., if you let (1) determine (4), (5), and (6).

Mostly, a single y-variable and multiple x-variables are included in a regression analysis, and this is what we call a multiple regression analysis. In the reports the term multivariate analysis is often erroneously used for these models. The term multivariate analysis refers to models that include more than a single y-variable and the analysis is then called multivariate analysis of variance (MANOVA). A correct alternative term for multiple regression analysis is, thus, univariate analyses with multiple x-variables (independent variables). This subject will be elaborated on in Chap. 25.

9   Limitations of Linear Regression

The limitations of multiple regressions are reviewed in the above text, but a summary is given:

1. The risk of multicollinearity.
2. The requirement of homoscedasticity.
3. The spread around the y-values is in the form of equal Gaussian curves, if not then Rank correlation according to Spearman should be performed.
4. A linear correlation between x and y exists.
5. The risk of confounding.
6. The risk of interaction.

10   Conclusions

If the above information is too much, don't be disappointed: multiple linear regression analysis and its extensions like logistic regression and Cox's proportional hazard model are not as important for clinical trials as it is for observational research:

1. Regression analysis assesses associations not causalities.
2. Clinical trials assess causal relationships.
3. We believe in causality if factor is introduced and gives rise to a particular outcome.
4. Always air of uncertainty with regression analysis

Multiple linear regression is interesting, but, in the context of clinical trials mostly just exploratory.

Chapter 15
Linear Regression for Assessing Precision, Confounding, Interaction, Basic Approach

1 Introduction

When the size of the study permits, important demographic or baseline value-defined subgroups of patients can be studied for unusually large or small efficacy responses; e.g. comparison of effects by age, sex; by severity or prognostic groups. Naturally, such analyses are not intended to "salvage" an otherwise negative study, but may be helpful in refining patient or dose selection for subsequent studies (Department of Health and Human Services, Food and Drug Administration 1998).

Most studies have insufficient size to assess efficacy meaningfully in subgroups of patients. Instead a regression model for the primary or secondary efficacy-variables can be used to evaluate whether specific variables are confounders for the treatment effect, and whether the treatment effect interacts with specific covariates. The particular (statistical) regression model chosen, depends on the nature of the efficacy variables, and the covariates to be considered should be meaningful according to the current state of knowledge. In particular, when studying interactions, the results of the regression analysis are more valid when complemented by additional exploratory analyses within relevant subgroups of patients or within strata defined by the covariates.

In this chapter we will discuss the multiple linear regression model which is appropriate, for continuous efficacy variables, such as blood pressures or lipid levels (as discussed in Chap. 2). Regression models for dichotomous efficacy variables (logistic regression (Hosmer and Lemeshow 1989)), and for survival data (Cox regression (Cox 1999)) will not be assessed here. However, the principles underlying all of these models are to some extent equivalent. This chapter is just a brief introduction. Various subjects will be explained more explicitly in the Chaps. 18, 28, and 30,

T.J. Cleophas and A.H. Zwinderman, *Statistics Applied to Clinical Studies*,
DOI 10.1007/978-94-007-2863-9_15, © Springer Science+Business Media B.V. 2012

2   Example

As an example of the use of a regression model we consider trials such as those conducted to evaluate the efficacy of statins (HMG-CoA reductase inhibitors) to lower lipid levels in patients with atherosclerosis (Jukema et al. 1995). In unselected populations statins were extremely effective in lowering LDL cholesterol (LDL), but the question whether the efficacy depended on baseline LDL level was unanswered. Of course this could be answered by comparing efficacy in selected subgroups of patients with baseline *low*, *intermediate*, and *high* LDL levels, but a regression model could be used as well, and sometimes provides better sensitivity.

Consider a randomized clinical trial such as Regress (Jukema et al. 1995). In this trial 884 patients with documented coronary atherosclerosis and total cholesterol between 4 and 8 mmol/L were randomized to either 2-year pravastatin or placebo treatment. Efficacy of treatment was assessed by the fall in LDL cholesterol after 2 year treatment. In the $n_1 = 438$ patients who received pravastatin mean LDL cholesterol fell by $\bar{x}_1 = 1.2324$ mmol/L (standard deviation, $S_1 = 0.68$). In the $n_0 = 422$ available patients who received placebo, the mean LDL cholesterol fell by $\bar{x}_0 = -0.0376$ mmol/L ($S_0 = 0.589$). Consequently, the efficacy of pravastatin was $1.2324 - 0.0376 = 1.2700$ mmol/L LDL-decrease in 2 years with standard error (SE) 0.043 mmol/L, and the 95% confidence interval (ci) of the efficacy quantification ran from 1.185 to 1.355.

In a random patient with coronary atherosclerosis and total cholesterol in between 4 and 8 mmol/L, pravastatin produces a better reduction in LDL cholesterol than does placebo by 1.27 mmol/L. However, a patient with 8 mmol/L total cholesterol level may better benefit than a patient with 4 mmol/L at baseline may do. Multiple linear regression can be applied to assess this question.

3   Model

We first introduce some notation: the dependent variable Y_i is the amount of LDL decrease observed in patient i (i = 1, ... , 884), and the independent variable or covariate X_{1i} is an indicator variable, indicating whether patient i received pravastatin ($X_{1i} = 1$) or not ($X_{1i} = 0$). We define the linear regression model (Fig. 15.1):

$$Y_i = \beta_0 + \beta_1 X_{1i} + e_i, \tag{15.1}$$

where β_0 is the intercept, and β_1 the slope of the regression line and e_i is a residual variation term, which is assumed to be normally distributed with variance σ_e^2.

When X_{1i} is either zero or one, the usual estimates b_0, b_1, and S_e^2 of β_0, β_1, and δ_e^2 are:

$$b_0 = \bar{x}_0 = -0.0376, \quad b_1 = \bar{x}_1 - \bar{x}_0 = 1.2700, \quad \text{and}$$

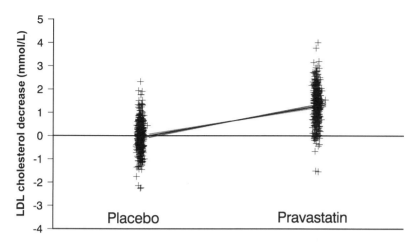

Fig. 15.1 The linear regression line is illustrated

$$S_e^2 = \frac{(n_1 - 1)S_1^2 + (n_0 - 1)S_0^2}{n_1 + n_2 - 2} = 0.4058,$$

which are exactly the same statistics as used in the t-test procedure one would normally employ in this situation. The quantification of the efficacy is thus given by b_1 and it has the same value and the same standard error and confidence interval as above. In Fig. 15.1 the linear regression line is illustrated.

Note: b and s are the best estimates, otherwise called best fits, of β and σ.

By using this regression model the following assumptions are made.

1. The relation between Y and X is linear. When X can attain only two values, this assumption is naturally valid, but, otherwise, this is not necessarily so.
2. The distribution of the residual term e_i is normal with mean zero and variance σ^2_e.
3. The variance of the distribution of e, σ^2_e, is the same for $X_1 = 0$ and for $X_1 = 1$: homoscedasticity.
4. The residual term e_i is independent of X_{1i}.

The object of regression modeling in clinical trials is to evaluate whether the efficacy quantification b_1 (I.) can be made more precise by taking covariates into consideration, (II.) is confounded by covariates, and (III.) interacts with covariates (synergism).

Increased precision (I.) is attained, and confounding (II.) can be studied by extending the regression model with a second independent variable X_2:

$$Y_i = \beta_0 + \beta_1 X_{1i} + \beta_2 X_{2i} + e_i, \tag{15.2}$$

This multiple regression model has the same underlying assumptions as the above linear regression model (15.1) except for the assumption that e_i is independent not only of X_1 but also of X_2. There is no need to assume that X_1 and X_2 are strictly independent, but the association must not be too strong (multicollinearity).

4   (I.) Increased Precision of Efficacy

When X_2 is independent of X_1 and is associated with Y (thus $b_2 \neq 0$), the estimate b_1 of the model in Eq. 15.2 will be the same as the estimate b_1 of the model in Eq. 15.1, but its precision will be increased, as indicated by a smaller standard error (Fig. 15.2).

This is a common case in randomized clinical trials. The randomization will ensure that no imbalances exist between the two treatment groups with respect to covariates such as X_2, and consequently X_2 will be independent of the treatment variable X_1. There are often many candidates for inclusion as covariates in the multiple regression model, but the choice should be made a priori and specified in the protocol. When the dependent variable is a change score, as in our example, the baseline level is the first candidate to consider because it is almost surely associated with the change score Y. Figure 15.2 shows the relationship between result of treatment and baseline values as demonstrated by scatterplots and linear regression lines for each treatment separately. The multiple linear regression model in Eq. 15.2 is appropriate for testing the contribution of baseline variability to the overall variability in the data.

Since X_2 is independent of X_1, inclusion of X_2 in the model must lead to a decreased variance S_e^2: some differences between patients with respect to the LDL decrease, are attributed to baseline LDL levels. Thus there will be less residual variation. Since the standard error of b_1 is a monotonic positive function of S_e^2, a decrease of S_e^2 leads to a smaller standard error of b_1. Thus by including baseline LDL levels in the

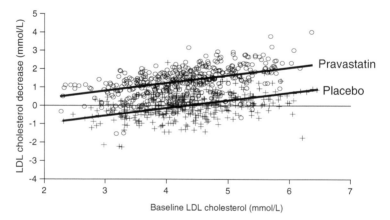

Fig. 15.2 Scatterplots and linear regression lines of baseline LDL cholesterol and LDL cholesterol decrease after treatment, separately for placebo and for pravastatin treatments

regression model, the efficacy of pravastatin lowering is estimated more precisely. This rule, however, only applies to large data-sets. With every additional covariate in the model an extra regression weight must be estimated, and since S_e^2 is an inverse function of the number of covariates in the model, too many covariates in the model will lead to decreased precision.

In our example the mean baseline LDL levels (X_2) were 4.32 (SD 0.78) and 4.29 (SD 0.78) in the placebo and pravastatin treatment groups (X_1) (p=0.60); hence X_1 and X_2 were independent. The baseline LDL levels were, however, associated with the LDL-changes (Y): $b_2=0.41$ (SE 0.024), p<0.0001. Consequently, the estimated efficacy was (almost) the same as before, but it had a somewhat smaller standard error, and is, thus, more precise:

with baseline LDL cholesterol levels: $b_1 = 1.27\,(\text{SE }0.037)$
without baseline LDL cholesterol levels: $b_1 = 1.27\,(\text{SE }0.043)$

Additional examples of regression modelling for improved precision are given in Chap. 15.

Note: In contrast to the linear regression models the efficacy estimates of non-linear regression models (e.g. logistic (Hosmer and Lemeshow 1989) and Cox regression (Cox 1999)) do not remain the same in this case. When using logistic or Cox regression it is, therefore, imperative to report the log odds ratio or log hazard ratio of treatments compared, together with the covariates in the model.

5 (II.) Confounding

In randomized clinical trials confounding plays a minor role in the data. The randomization will ensure that no covariate of the efficacy variable will also be associated with the randomized treatment. If, however, the randomization fails for a particular variable, which is already known to be an important covariate of the efficacy variable, such a variable is a confounder and adjustment of the efficacy estimate should be attempted. This is done by using the same (linear) regression model as given in Eq. 15.2. The adjusted efficacy estimate may become smaller or larger than the unadjusted estimate, depending on the direction of the associations of the confounder with the randomized treatment and the efficacy variable. Let b_1 and b_1^* denote the unadjusted and the adjusted efficacy estimate, and let r_{xz} and r_{yz} be the correlations of the confounder (z) with the randomized treatment (x) and the efficacy variable (y), then the following will hold:

$$\text{if } \quad r_{xz} > 0 \text{ and } r_{yz} > 0 \quad \text{then} \quad \left|b_1^*\right| < \left|b_1\right|,$$

$$\text{if } \quad r_{xz} > 0 \text{ and } r_{yz} < 0 \quad \text{then} \quad \left|b_1^*\right| > \left|b_1\right|,$$

$$\text{if } \quad r_{xz} < 0 \text{ and } r_{yz} < 0 \quad \text{then} \quad \left|b_1^*\right| < \left|b_1\right|,$$

$$\text{if } \quad r_{xz} < 0 \text{ and } r_{yz} > 0 \quad \text{then} \quad \left|b_1^*\right| > \left|b_1\right|,$$

Notice the possibility that the unadjusted efficacy estimate b_1 is zero whereas the adjusted estimate b_1^* is unequal to zero: an efficacy-difference between treatments may be masked by confounding.

In clinical trials it is sensible to check the balance between treatment groups of all known covariates of the efficacy variable. In most trials there are many more covariates and one should be careful to consider as a confounder a covariate which was not reported in the literature before.

6 (III.) Interaction and Synergism

A special kind of covariate is the interaction of the randomized treatment with some other covariate. This interaction is, by definition, associated with the randomized treatment, and possibly with the efficacy variable if the efficacy differs between treatments. In contrast to the discussion above, the focus of the statistical analysis is not on the change of b_1 by including an interaction in the model, but the regression weight of the interaction variable itself. When this regression weight is unequal to zero, this points to the existence of patient-subgroups for which the efficacy of treatment differs significantly.

An example is again provided by the Regress trial (Jukema et al. 1995). The primary effect variable was the decrease of the average diameter of the coronary arteries after 2 years of treatment. The average decrease was 0.057 mm (standard deviation (SD) 0.194) in the pravastatin group, and it was 0.117 mm (SD 0.212) in the placebo group (t-test: significance of difference at $p < 0.001$); thus the efficacy estimate b_1 was 0.060 (standard error SE = 0.016). Calcium channel blockers (CCB) were given to 60% of the placebo patients, and 59% of the pravastatin patients (chi-square: $p = 0.84$): thus CCB treatment was not a confounder variable. Also, CCB medication was not associated with diameter decrease ($p = 0.62$). In the patients who did not receive concomitant CCB medication, the diameter decreases were 0.097 (SD 0.20) and 0.088 (SD 0.19) in patients receiving placebo and pravastatin, respectively ($p = 0.71$). In patients who did receive CCB medication, the diameter decreases were 0.130 (SD 0.22) and 0.035 (SD 0.19), respectively ($p < 0.001$). Thus, pravastatin-efficacy was, on average, $0.097 - 0.088 = 0.009$ mm in patients without CCB medication, and $0.130 - 0.035 = 0.095$ in patients with CCB medication.

This difference was statistically significant (interaction test: $p = 0.011$). We used the following linear regression model for this test. Let $X_{1i} = 1$ denote that patient i received pravastatin ($X_{1i} = 0$, if not), let $X_{2i} = 1$ denote that patient i received CCB medication ($X_{2i} = 0$, if not), and let $X_{3i} = X_{1i} \times X_{2i}$:

$$Y_i = \beta_0 + \beta_1 X_{1i} + \beta_2 X_{2i} + \beta_3 X_{3i} + e_i.$$

The estimates were: $b_3 = 0.085$ (SE 0.033), $b_2 = -0.033$ (SE 0.023), and $b_1 = 0.009$ (SE 0.026). Notice that b_1 changed dramatically by including the interaction term X_3 in the linear model; this is a general feature of regression models with interaction terms: the corresponding main-effects (b_1 and b_2) cannot be interpreted independently of the interaction term. Another consequence is that the efficacy estimate no longer exists, but several estimates do exist: in our case there are different efficacy-estimates for patients with $(b_1 + b_3 = 0.009 + 0.085 = 0.094)$ and without CCB medication $(b_1 = 0.009)$. In the practice of clinical trials interactions are usually investigated in an exploratory fashion. When interaction is demonstrated in this way, its existence should be confirmed in a novel prospective clinical trial. Additional examples of regression modeling for interaction effects are given in Chap. 18.

7 Estimation, and Hypothesis Testing

Standard statistical computer programs like SPSS and SAS (and many others) contain modules that perform regression analysis for linear and many non-linear models such as logistic and Cox regression. The standard method to estimate the linear regression weights (and the residual standard deviation σ_e) is to minimize the squared distances between the data and the estimated regression line: the least squares method. For non-linear models, the maximum likelihood method is employed, but these are equivalent methods. The output of these estimation methods are the estimated regression weights (and the residual standard deviation σ_e) and their standard errors. It is important that the correlations between the covariates in the model are not too large (i.e. multicollinearity), but if these are too large, this will become clear by absurd regression weights, and very large standard errors. If this occurs, one or more covariates must be removed from the model.

Under the null hypothesis that β equals zero, the ratio of the estimated regression weight b and its standard error is distributed as a student's t statistic in the linear model, and this can be used to derive the p-value or the 95% confidence interval in the usual way. For non-linear models, the squared ratio of b and its standard error is called the Wald statistic which is chi-squared distributed. Alternatives for the Wald statistic are the score and likelihood ratio statistics (Rao 1973), but these give the same results except in highly unusual circumstances; if they differ, the score and likelihood statistics are better than the Wald statistic.

The power of these statistical tests is a sensitive function of the number of patients in the trial. Naturally, there is less opportunity for modeling in a small trial than in a large trial. There is no general rule about which sample sizes are required for sensible regression modeling, but one rule-of-thumb is that at least ten times as many patients are required as the number of covariates in the model.

8 Goodness-of-Fit

For the linear model the central assumptions are (1) the assumed linearity of the relation between Y and X, and (2) the normal distribution of the residual term e independent of all covariates and with homogeneous variance. The first step in checking these assumptions is by looking at the data. The linearity of the relation between Y and X, for instance, can be inspected by looking at the scatter-plot between Y and X. A nonlinear relation between Y and X will show itself as systematic deviation from a straight line. When the relation is non linear, either Y or X or both may be transformed appropriately; most often used are the logarithmic transformation $X* = \ln(X)$ and the power transformation $X* = X^p$ (e.g. the squared root transformation where $p = 0.5$). At this stage subjective judgments necessarily enter the statistical analysis, because the decision about the appropriate transformation is not well founded on statistical arguments. A few tools that may help, are the following.

1. The optimal power-transformation (X^p) may be estimated using the Box-Cox algorithm (Cox 1999). This may yield, however, difficult and unpractical power-transforms.
2. A 'better' model produces better correlations. When one compares two different models, the better of the two leads to a smaller residual variance (S_e^2) or higher multiple correlation coefficient (R): $S_e^2 = [(n-1)/(n-k)](1-R^2).S_y^2$, where k is the number of covariates in the model, n = sample size, S_y^2 = variance dependent variable.
3. Choosing an appropriate transformation may be enhanced by modelling the relation between Y and X as a polynomial function of X: $Y = b_0 + b_1X + b_2X^2 + b_3X^3 + .$ When the relation is strictly linear then $b_2 = b_3 = \ldots = 0$, and this can be tested statistically in the usual way. Obviously, the order of the polynomial function is unknown, but one rarely needs to investigate fourth or higher orders.
4. Finally, there exists the possibility to model the association between Y and X nonparametrically using various modern smoothing techniques (see Chap. 24).

The assumed normal distribution of the residual term can be checked by inspecting the histogram of e. The estimation method and the hypothesis testing are quite robust against skewed distributions of the residual term, but it is sensible to check for extreme skewness and the occurrence of important outlying data-points. Visual inspection is usually sufficient but one may check the distribution statistically with the Kolmogorov-Smirnov test (see also Chap. 42).

More important is the assumption of homogeneity of the residual variance S_e^2: this entails that the variation of e is more or less the same for all values of X. One may check this visually by inspecting the scatterplot of e (or Y) versus X. If heterogeneity is present, again an appropriate transformation of Y may help. If the ratio of S_e / y is equal for various levels of X, the logarithmic transformation $Y* = \ln(Y)$ may help, and if S_e^2 / y^2 is equal for various levels of X, the square-root transformation is appropriate: $Y* = (Y)^{0.5}$. The independence of the residual term e of all covariates X in the model can be tested with the Durbin-Watson test.

In the logistic regression model the most important underlying assumption is the assumed logistic form of the function linking the covariates to the binary efficacy variable. If not all relevant covariates are in the model, it can be shown that the link-function is not logistic. One way to statistically test this, is by using the Hosmer-Lemeshow test (Hosmer and Lemeshow 1989). But if the logistic regression model does not fit, this is of little consequence, because this usually points to missing covariates, and these are often not available. In Cox regression, the cardinal underlying assumption is the assumed proportionality of the hazard rates. There are several statistical tests for testing this assumption; if proportionality does not hold, accelerated failure time models can be used, or the time axis may be partitioned into several periods, otherwise called splines, in which proportionality does hold. Several of these non linear regression models will be reviewed more explicitly in the Chaps. 16, 17, 19, and 24.

9 Selection Procedures

In clinical trials usually many variables are sampled, and often many of these are candidates for inclusion in the regression model. A major problem is the selection of a subset of variables to include in the regression model. By far preferable is to select a (small) set of candidate variables on clinical and theoretical grounds, but if that is not possible a few rules are helpful in the selection process.

1. If the number of covariates is not too large, it is best not to use any selection at all, but simply include all candidates in the regression model. Often it is necessary to shrink the regression weights, using, for instance, a penalty function.
2. If the number of covariates is very large, backward selection methods are preferable to forward selection models. This is usually done according to the p-value or the size of the test-statistic-value.
3. Since the overriding interest of the regression modelling is the estimation of the efficacy of the randomized treatments, the safest course is to be liberal about including covariates in the model: use a p-value of 0.10 or even 0.20 to include covariates in the model.

10 Main Conclusions

The regular statistical analysis of the data of clinical trials should be extended by (exploratory) analysis if the existence of subgroups of patients for which the efficacy estimate differs, is suspected. An efficient way of doing this is by the use of regression analysis. If such subgroups are identified, the exploratory nature of the regression analysis should be emphasized and the subgroup issue should be further assessed in subsequent independent and prospective data-sets.

References

Cox B (1999) Statistical software. University Leyden, Leyden
Department of Health and Human Services, Food and Drug Administration (1998) International conference on harmonisation; guidance on statistical principles for clinical trials availability. Fed Regist 63(179):49583–49598

Hosmer DW, Lemeshow S (1989) Applied logistic regression. Wiley, New York
Jukema AJ, Zwinderman AH, et al for the REGRESS study group (1995) Effects of lipid lowering
    by pravastatin on progression and regression of coronary artery disease in symptomatic men
    with normal to moderately elevated serum cholesterol levels. The Regression Growth Evaluation
    Statin Study (REGRESS). Circulation 91:2528-2540
Rao CR (1973) Linear statistical inference and its applications. Wiley, New York

Chapter 16
Curvilinear Regression

1 Introduction

Polynomial analysis is an extension of simple linear regression, where a model is used to allow for the existence of a systematic dependence of the dependent y variable (blood pressure) on the independent x variable (time) different from a linear dependence. Polynomial extension from the basic model can be done as follows:

$y = a + bx$	(first order) linear relationship
$y = a + bx + cx^2$	(second order) parabolic relationship
$y = a + bx + cx^2 + dx^3$	(third order) hyperbolic relationship
$y = a + bx + cx^2 + dx^3 + ex^4$	(fourth order) sinusoidal relationship

where a is the intercept and b, c, d, and e are the partial regression coefficients. Statistical software can be used to calculate for the data the regression line that provides the best fit for the data. In addition, regression lines of higher than four orders can be calculated. Fourier analysis is a more traditional way of analyzing these types of data, and is given by the function

$$f(x) = p + q_1 \cos(x) + .. + q_n \cos n(x) + r_1 \sin(x) + .. + r_n \sin n(x)$$

with $p, q_1 ... q_n$, and $r_1 ... r_n$ = constants for the best fit of the given data.

As an example, ambulatory blood pressure monitoring (ABPM) using light weight automated portable equipment is given. ABPM has greatly contributed to our understanding of the circadian patterns of blood pressures in individual patients (Owens et al. 1998) as well as to the study of effects of antihypertensive drugs in groups of patients (Zanchetti 1997). However, a problem is that ABPM data using mean values of arbitrarily separated daytime hours are poorly reproducible (Omboni et al. 1998; Bleniaszewski et al. 1997), undermining the validity of this diagnostic tool. Previous studies have demonstrated that both in normo- (Van de Luit et al. 1998a) and in

T.J. Cleophas and A.H. Zwinderman, *Statistics Applied to Clinical Studies*,
DOI 10.1007/978-94-007-2863-9_16, © Springer Science+Business Media B.V. 2012

hypertensive groups (Van de Luit et al. 1998b) time is a more powerful source of variation in 24 h ABPM data than were other sources of variation (between P<0.01 and <0.001 versus between not significant and <0.01). This reflects the importance of the circadian rhythm in the interpretation of ABPM data, and the need for an assessment that accounts for this very rhythm more adequately than does the means of separated daytime hours. We also demonstrated that polynomial curves can be produced of ABPM data from both normo- (Van de Luit et al. 1998a) and hypertensive (Van de Luit et al. 1998b) groups, and that these polynomial curves are within the 95% confidence intervals of the sample means. However, intra-individual reproducibility of this approach has not been assessed, and is a prerequisite for further implementing this approach.

In this chapter we describe polynomial analysis of ABPM data, and test the hypothesis that it is better reproducible and that this is so, not only with means of populations, but also with individual data. For the estimate of reproducibility duplicate standard deviations as well as intra-class correlations are calculated of ABPM data from untreated mildly hypertensive patients who underwent ABPM for 24 h twice, 1 week interval.

2   Methods, Statistical Model

Ten patients, six females and four males, who had given their informed consent, participated in the study. Each patient had been examined at our outpatient clinic. Age varied from 33 to 52 years of age (mean 42 years), body mass index from 20 to 31 kg/m (mean 29 kg/m). Patients were either housewife or actively employed throughout the study and had no other diseases. Previously treated patients had a washout period of at least 8 weeks before they were included in the study. All patients were included if untreated diastolic blood pressure was repeatedly between 90 and 100 mmHg and systolic blood pressure less than 170 mmHg.

In all of the patients ABPM consisted of measurements every 60 min for 24 h with a validated (O'Brien et al. 1995) light weight automated portable equipment (Space Lab Medical Inc, Redmond WA, model 90207). In the meantime patients performed their usual daily activities.

We define the dependent variable, the blood pressure recording at hour t, and, subsequently, model it as a function of hour t, hour t squared, hour t to the power 3, hour t to the power 4, and so on. The a- and b-values are constants for the best fit of the given data, and are also called the regression weights.

$$\text{Blood pressure at hour t} = a + b_1(\text{hour t}) + b_2(\text{hour t})^2 + b_3(\text{hour t})^3$$
$$+ b_4(\text{hour t})^4 + \dots.$$

If we use Fourier analysis instead the equation is

Blood pressure at hour t $= p + q_1 \cos(\text{hour t}) + .. + q_n \cos n(\text{hour t})$

$+ r_1 \sin(\text{hour t}) + .. + r_n \sin n(\text{hour t})$

with p, q_{1-n} and r_{1-n} being constants for the best fit of the given data.

Reproducibility of ABPM was studied in the ten patients by performing 24 h ABPM in each of them twice, intervals at least 1 week. Reproducibility of the duplicate data, as obtained, were assessed both by quantifying reproducibility of means of the population, and of the individual data.

2.1 Reproducibility of Means of the Population

For this purpose we used duplicate standards deviation (Duplicate SD) and intra-class correlation (ρ_1) (Hays 1988).

Duplicate SD was calculated according to Duplicate $SD = \sqrt{\dfrac{\sum(x_1 - x_2)^2}{2n}}$,

where x_1 and x_2 are individual data during 1st and 2nd tests, and $n = 240$ (ten times 24 duplicate observations).

Intra-class correlation (ρ_1) is another approach for the estimate of replicability of repeated measures in one subject, and is calculated according to

$$\rho_1 = \frac{\sigma^2 \overline{x}_1 - \sigma^2 \overline{x}_2 / \overline{x}_1}{\sigma^2 \overline{x}_1}$$

where $\overline{x}_1$ and $\overline{x}_2$ are the means of the 240 values during test 1 and test 2 respectively, and $\sigma^2 \overline{x}_2 / \overline{x}_1$ is the variance of $\overline{x}_2$ given $\overline{x}_1$, and

$$\sigma^2 \frac{\overline{x}_2}{\overline{x}_1} = \sigma^2 \overline{x}_1 - \frac{(\overline{x}_1 - \overline{x}_2)^2}{4}.$$

A slightly different method to calculate intraclass correlations is described in Chap. 26.

Note: Greek symbols like σ instead of s and ρ instead of r are often used in statistics. They are used to indicate population parameters instead of sample parameters.

2.2 Reproducibility of Individual Data

For this purpose we similarly used duplicate standards deviation (SD) and intra-class correlation (ρ).

Duplicate SD was calculated according $SD = \sqrt{\dfrac{\sum (x_1 - x_2)^2}{2n}}$ \where x_1 and x_2 are individual data during 1st and 2nd tests, and $n = 24$ (24 duplicate observations per patient).

Intra-class correlation (ρ_1) was calculated according to

$$\rho_1 = \frac{\sigma^2 \overline{x}_1 - \sigma^2 \overline{x}_2 / \overline{x}_1}{\sigma^2 \overline{x}_1}$$

where $\overline{x}_1$ and $\overline{x}_2$ are the means of the 24 values during test 1 and test 2 respectively, and $\sigma^2\, \overline{x}_2 / \overline{x}_{1,}$ is the variance of $\overline{x}_2$ given $\overline{x}_1$, and

$$\sigma^2 \frac{\overline{x}_2}{\overline{x}_1} = \sigma^2 \overline{x}_1 - \frac{(\overline{x}_1 - \overline{x}_2)^2}{4}$$

Calculations were performed using SPSS statistical software, polynomial curves were drawn using Harvard Graphics 3 (SPSS 2002; Harvard Graphics-3 2001). Under the assumption of standard deviations of 25% and intraclass correlations of +0.7, at least 240 duplicate observations had to be included to obtain a regression analysis with a statistical power of 80% and a 5% significance level. And so, it seemed appropriate to include hourly data of at least ten patients tested twice for 24 h. Paired means, Duplicate SDs and intraclass correlations were statistically tested by t-tests, F tests, or McNemar's chi-square tests, whenever appropriate.

3   Results

3.1   *Reproducibility of Means of Population*

Figure 16.1 shows mean values of ABPM of ten untreated patients and their SDs, recorded twice, one week in-between. Obviously, there is an enormous variance in the data both between-subject and within-subject as demonstrated respectively by the large SDs and the considerable differences between means. Figures 16.2 and 16.3 give polynomes of corresponding data from Fig. 16.1, reflecting a clear circa-dian rhythm in systolic blood pressures. Figure 16.4 shows that the two polynomes are, obviously, very much similar. Within-subject tests for reproducibility are given in Table 16.1. Duplicate SDs of means versus zero and versus grand mean were 15.9 and 7.2, while of polynomes they were only 1.86 (differences in Duplicate SDs significant at a $P < 0.001$ level). Intra-class correlations (ρ_1s) of means versus zero and versus grand mean were 0.46 and 0.75, while of polynomes they were 0.986 (differences in levels of correlation significant at a $P < 0.001$). Obviously, polynomes of ABPM data of means of populations produce significantly better reproducibility than do the actual data.

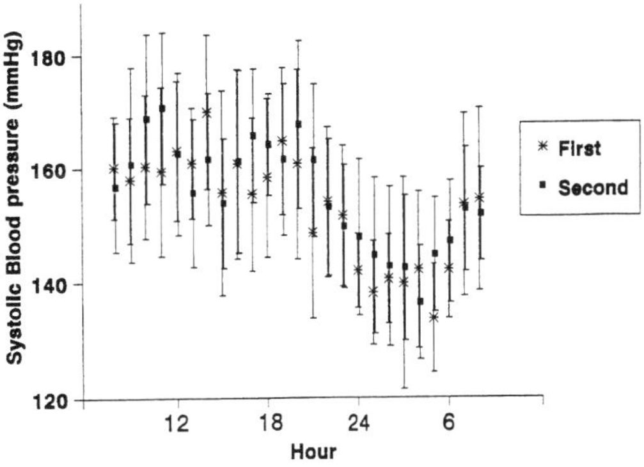

Fig. 16.1 Mean values of
ABPM data of ten untreated
patients with mild
hypertension and their SDs,
recorded twice, 1 week
in-between

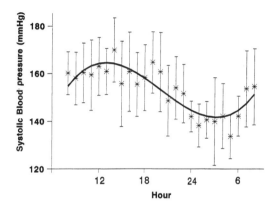

Fig. 16.2 Polynome of
corresponding ABPM
recording (*first one*) from
Fig. 16.1, reflecting a clear
circadian rhythm of systolic
blood pressures

Fig. 16.3 Polynome of
corresponding ABPM
recording (*second one*) from
Fig. 16.1, again reflecting a
clear circadian rhythm of
systolic blood pressures

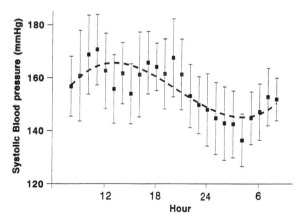

Polynomes are, obviously, very much similar. Within-subject tests for reproducibility are given in Table 16.1. Duplicate SDs of means versus zero and versus grand
mean were 15.9 and 7.2, while of polynomes they were only 1.86 (differences in
Duplicate SDs significant at a $P < 0.001$ level). Intra-class correlations (ρs) of means

Fig. 16.4 The two polynomes from Figs. 16.2 and 16.3 are, obviously, very much similar

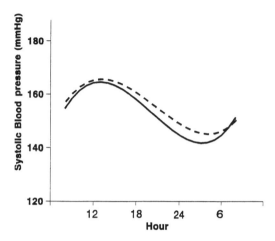

Table 16.1 Twenty-four hour ambulatory blood pressure measurements in a group of ten patients with untreated mild hypertension tested twice: reproducibility of means of population (*vs* versus)

	Mean values variations vs zero	Mean values variations vs grand mean	Polynomes
Means (mmHg) (test 1/test 2)	153.1/155.4	153.1/155.4	–
SD (σ) (mmHg) (test 1/test 2)	21.9/21.1	15.7/13.8	–
95% CIs[a] (mmHg) (test 1/test 2)	139.4–166.8/142.2–168.6	143.3–163.9/146.8–164.0	–
Differences between means (SD, σ) (mmHg)	−2.4 (22.4)	−2.3 (10.5)	–
P values differences between results tests 1 and 2	0.61	0.51	0.44
Duplicate SDs[b] (mmHg)	15.9	7.2	1.86
Relative Duplicate SDs[c] (%)	66	31	7
Intra-class correlations[d] (ρ_Is)	0.46	0.75	0.986
95% CIs	0.35–0.55	0.26–0.93	0.972–0.999
Proportion total variance responsible for between-patient variance (%)	46	75	99
95% CIs (%)	35–55	26–93	97–100

[a]CIs = confidence intervals

[b]Duplicate SDs calculated according to Duplicate $SD = \sqrt{\dfrac{\sum (x_1 - x_2)^2}{2n}}$, where x_1 and x_2 are individual data during 1st and 2nd test, and n = 240 (ten times 24 duplicate observations)

[c]Calculated as 100% × [Duplicate SD/(overall mean − 130 mmHg)]

[d]Intra-class correlations (ρ_I s) calculated according to $\rho_I = \dfrac{\sigma^2 \overline{x}_1 - \sigma^2 \overline{x}_2 / \overline{x}_1}{\sigma^2 \overline{x}_1}$

where $\overline{x}_1$ and $\overline{x}_2$ are the means of the 240 values during test 1 and test 2 respectively, and $\sigma^2 \overline{x}_2 / \overline{x}_1$ is the variance of $\overline{x}_2$ given $\overline{x}_1$, and $\sigma^2 \dfrac{\overline{x}_2}{\overline{x}_1} = \sigma^2 \overline{x}_1 - \dfrac{(\overline{x}_1 - \overline{x}_2)^2}{4}$

Table 16.2 Twenty-four hour ambulatory blood pressure measurements in ten patients with untreated mild hypertension tested twice: reproducibility of individual data

Patient	Mean (mmHg) Test 1/test 2	SD (mmHg) Test 1/test 2	Duplicate SDs (mmHg)[a] Raw data	Polynomes	Intraclass Raw data	Correlations[b] Polynomes
1	160/157	14/18	17.7	2.1	0.07	0.58
2	158/161	17/27	17.6	9.0	0.27	0.53
3	160/169	20/29	19.7	2.6	−0.23	0.03
4	159/171	23/21	19.1	7.2	0.11	0.29
5	163/163	19/23	19.7	9.9	0.10	0.20
6	161/156	15/20	21.4	6.4	0.03	0.10
7	170/162	21/18	10.1	8.2	0.57	0.70
8	156/154	28/18	6.3	6.7	0.26	0.24
9	161/161	26/25	18.2	13.5	0.60	0.81
10	155/166	21/19	11.9	6.6	0.53	0.96
Pooled data						
	153.1/155.4	21.9/21.1	16.2(5.0)[c]	7.2(3.3)	0.26(0.26)	0.42(0.34)
			_P<0.001_		_P=0.009_	

[a]Duplicate SDs calculated according to $SD = \sqrt{\dfrac{\sum (x_1 - x_2)^2}{2n}}$, where x_1 and x_2 are individual

data during 1st and 2nd test, and $n=24$ (24 duplicate observations per patient)

[b]Intra-class correlations (ρs) calculated according to $\rho_1 = \dfrac{\sigma^2 \overline{x}_1 - \sigma^2 \overline{x}_2 / \overline{x}_1}{\sigma^2 \overline{x}_1}$

where $\overline{x}_1$ and $\overline{x}_2$ are the means of the 24 values during test 1 and test 2 respectively, and $\sigma^2 \overline{x}_2 / \overline{x}_1$

is the variance of $\overline{x}_2$ given $\overline{x}_1$, and $\sigma^2 \dfrac{\overline{x}_2}{\overline{x}_1} = \sigma^2 \overline{x}_1 - \dfrac{(\overline{x}_1 - \overline{x}_2)^2}{4}$

[c]SDs between the brackets

versus zero and versus grand mean were 0.46 and 0.75, while of polynomes they were 0.986 (differences in levels of correlation significant at a P<0.001). Obviously, polynomes of ABPM data of means of populations produce significantly better reproducibility, than do the actual data.

3.2 Reproducibility of Individual Data

Figure 16.5 gives an example of the individual data of patient no. 1 during the first and second test and also shows his corresponding polynomes of test 1 and test 2. Although, again, there is enormous variability in the data, the polynomes have rather similar patterns. Table 16.2 gives an overview of assessments of reproducibility for each patient separately. Duplicate SDs of raw data were generally more than twice the size of those of the polynomes, while intraclass correlations of the actual data were accordingly generally almost half the size of those of the polynomes with

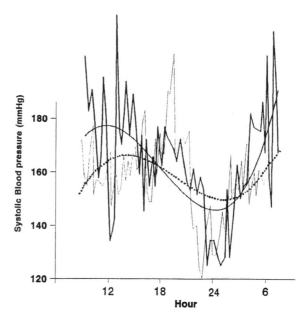

Fig. 16.5 Individual data from patient 1 (Table 16.2) during first ABPM (*fat line*) and second ABPM recording (*thin line*). The corresponding polynomes of the two recordings (*continuous* and *dotted* curves respectively) are somewhat more different from each other than are the differences between the group data polynomes (Fig. 16.4). Yet, they offer much better similarity than do the actual data

median values of 0.26 and 0.38 and ranges between −0.23 and 0.60 and between 0.03 and 0.96 respectively. Pooled differences were highly significant both for the Duplicate SDs, and for the intraclass correlations ($P < 0.001$ and $P = 0.009$ respectively, Table 16.2).

4   Discussion

In this chapter we demonstrate that ABPM systolic blood pressures in untreated mildly hypertensive patients can be readily assessed by polynomial analysis and that this approach unlike the actual data analysis is highly reproducible. Similar results were obtained when instead of systolic blood pressures diastolic or mean pressures were analyzed. It may be argued from a mathematical-statistical point of view that the better reproducibility is a direct consequence of the procedure where variability is reduced by taking means of a population rather than individual values. However, when we compared polynomial and actual data for each subject separately, although the overall level of reproducibility fell, the former approach still performed better than did the latter. This indicates that the better reproducibility may at least in part be connected with mechanisms other than the mathematical necessity of reducing variability by taking the polynomial modeling of the actual data. Particularly, polynomes may be better reproducible, because they are a better estimate of the circadian rhythm of blood pressure than the actual data, which are of course influenced by a variety of exogenous factors including daily activities, meals and breaks, psychological effects. A polynome would be a more accurate estimate of the true endogenous circadian rhythm, where the mathematical procedure takes care that exogenous factors are largely removed. This would explain the high reproducibility not only of polynomial analyses of population data but also of individual patient data.

Polynomial analysis has been validated in chronobiology, as a reproducible method for the study of circadian rhythms in normotensive subjects, and is, actually, routinely used for that purpose in the Department of Chronobiology of our academic hospital (Scheidel et al. 1990; Lemmer et al. 1991). So far, however, it has received little attention in the clinical assessment of patients with hypertension. The current chapter suggests, that the method would be a reliable instrument for that purpose.

Polynomial analysis, could, e.g., be used to identify circadian patterns of blood pressure in individual patients. Figure 16.6 gives an example of five such patterns readily demonstrable by polynomes. These polynomes were drawn from ABPM data from our own outpatient clinic database. Figure 16.7 gives another example of how polynomes can be helpful in clinical assessments. The polynomes present the mean results of a recent study by our group, comparing the short term effects of different blood pressure reducing agents in mildly hypertensive patients ($n = 10$) (Van de Luit et al. 1998b). All of the polynomes were within 95% CIs of the mean data of our samples. Differences between the data in this study, as assessed by two-way analysis of variance, established that on enalapril, and amlodipine, unlike beta-blockers carvedilol and celiprolol, time effect was a major source of variability. The polynomes visualized that this was so, because beta-blockers did not reduce night-time blood pressures. So, polynomial analysis was helpful in interpreting the results of this study.

Polynomial analysis of ABPM data, unlike actual data analysis, is highly reproducible in patients with mild hypertension, and this is so not only with population means but also with individual data. It is, therefore, a valid approach for the clinical assessment of hypertensive patients, and may, thus, be helpful for a variety of purposes, e.g., for identifying circadian patterns of blood pressure in individual patients, and for the study of antihypertensive drugs in groups of patients. The goodness of fit of polynomial models estimated by levels of correlation between observed and modelled data, is very good, and sometimes even better than the real sine-like function derived from the Fourier analysis. Particularly, the regression lines of the 4th and 7th order generally provide the best fit for typical sinusoidal patterns. In the above example the 7th order polynome provided a slightly better fit than did the 4th order polynome.

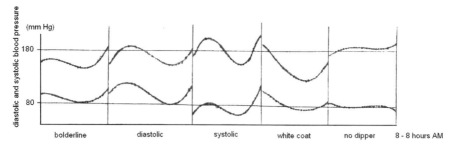

Fig. 16.6 Polynomial analysis can be used to identify circadian patterns of blood pressure in individual patients

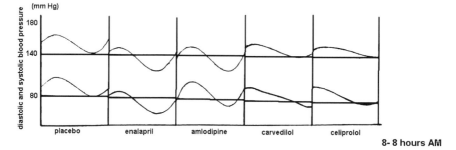

Fig. 16.7 Polynomial analysis can be used to study the effects of antihypertensive drugs in groups of patients

5   Conclusions

Polynomial analysis is an extension of simple linear regression, where a power model is used to allow for the existence of a systematic, though not linear, dependence of the independent y variable on the dependent x variable, often a time variable. Particularly, fourth and seventh order polynomes are adequate to assess sinusoidal relationships, like circadian rhythms of hemodynamic and hormonal estimators.

References

Bleniaszewski L, Staessen JA, Byttebier G, De Leeuw PW, Van Hedent T, Fagard R (1997) Trough-to-peak versus surface ration in the assessment of antihypertensive agents. Blood Press 4:350–357

Harvard Graphics-3 (2001) Statistical software. Harvard, Inc, Boston

Hays WL (1988) Curvilinear regression. In: Hays WL (ed) Statistics, 4th edn. Holt, Rinehart and Winston, Inc, Chicago, pp 698–716

Lemmer B, Scheidel B, Behne S (1991) Chronopharmacokinetics and chronopharmacodynamics of cardiovascular active drugs: propranolol, organic nitrates, nifedipine. Ann N Y Acad Sci 618:166–171

O'Brien E, Atkins N, Staessen J (1995) State of the market, a review of ambulatory blood pressure-monitoring devices. Hypertension 26:835–842

Omboni S, Parati G, Palatini P, Vanasia A, Muiesan ML, Cuspidi C, Mancia G (1998) Reproducibility and clinical value of nocturnal hypotension: prospective evidence from the SAMPLE study. J Hypertens 16:733–738

Owens P, Lyons S, O'Brien E (1998) Ambulatory blood pressure in hypertensive population: patterns and prevalence of hypertensive subforms. J Hypertens 16:1735–1745

Scheidel B, Lemmer B, Blume H (1990) Influence of time of day on pharmacokinetics and hemodynamic effects of beta-blockers. In: Clinical chronopharmacology, vol 6. Zuckschwerdt Verlag, Munich, pp 75–79

SPSS (2002) Statistical software. Professional statistics. Chicago

Van de Luit L, Van der Meulen J, Cleophas TJ, Zwinderman AH (1998a) Amplified amplitudes of circadian rhythms and nighttime hypotension in patients with chronic fatigue syndrome; improvement by inopamil but not by melatonin. Eur J Intern Med 9:99–103

Van de Luit L, Cleophas TJ, Van der Meulen J, Zwinderman AH (1998b) Nighttime hypotension in mildly hypertensive patients prevented by beta-blockers but not by ACE-inhibitors or calcium channel blockers. Eur J Intern Med 9:251–256

Zanchetti A (1997) Twenty-four-hour ambulatory blood pressure evaluation of antihypertensive agents. J Hypertens 15:S21–S25

Chapter 17
Logistic and Cox Regression, Markov Models, Laplace Transformations

1 Introduction

Data modeling can be applied for improving precision of clinical studies. Multiple regression modeling is often used for that purpose. Relevant papers on this topic have recently been published (Breithaupt-Grogler et al. 1997; Debord et al. 1998; Kato et al. 1994; Mahmood and Mahayni 1999; Sabot et al. 1995; Ulrich et al. 2003; Vrecer et al. 2003). Although multiple regression modeling, generally, does not influence the magnitude of the treatment effect versus control, it may reduce overall variances in the treatment comparison and thus increase sensitivity or power of statistical testing. It tries to fit experimental data in a mathematical model, and, subsequently, tests how far distant the data are from the model. A statistically significant correlation indicates that the data are closer to the model than will happen with random sampling. The very model-principle is at the same time its largest limitation. biological processes are full of variations and will not allow for a perfect fit. In addition, the decision about the appropriate model is not well founded on statistical arguments. The current chapter assesses uncertainties and risks of misinterpretations commonly encountered with regression analyses and rarely communicated in research papers. Simple regression models and real data examples are used for assessment.

2 Linear Regression

Multiple linear regression for increasing precision of clinical trials assumes that a covariate like a baseline characteristic of the patients is an independent determinant of the treatment efficacy, and that the best fit for the treatment and control data is given by two separate regression lines with identical regression coefficients. The assumption may be too strong, and introduce important bias in the interpretation of the data, even if the variable seems to fit the model.

As an example is again taken the Regression Growth Evaluation Statin Study (REGRESS) (Jukema et al. 1995), a randomized parallel-group trial comparing placebo and pravastatin treatment in 434 and 438 patients, respectively. Primary endpoint was change in coronary artery diameter, secondary endpoint change in LDL (low density lipoprotein) cholesterol, as measured before and after 2 years of treatment. The average decreases of LDL cholesterol are

$$\text{statin} : \quad 1.23 \left(\text{standard deviation } (SD) 0.68\right) \text{mmol}/\text{l}$$

$$\text{placebo} : \quad -0.04 \left(SD\ 0.59\right) \text{mmol}/\text{l}$$

Obviously, LDL decrease varies considerably in both treatment groups but, on average, treatment efficacy can be quantified as $1.23 - (-0.04) = 1.27$ mmol/l. Since the patients in the two parallel groups are independent of each other, the standard error (SE) of this estimate equals

$$\sqrt{\frac{0.68^2}{438} + \frac{0.59^2}{434}} = 0.043 \text{ mmol}/\text{l}.$$

The same results can be obtained by drawing the best fit for the data in the form of a regression line according to the equation:

$$y = a + bx,$$

where

y = the dependent variable representing the LDL cholesterol decrease of the patients,

x = the independent variable representing treatment modality, 1 if a patient receives statin, and 0 if placebo.

The term a is the intercept of the regression line with the y-axis and b is the regression coefficient (= direction coefficient of the regression line) which must be estimated.

Figure 17.1 gives the linear regression line in graph. It yields an estimate of b of 1.27 with SE 0.043; hence, completely equal to the above analysis.

We wish to adjust these data for baseline LDL cholesterol. First, we draw a scatter plot of the individual baseline LDL cholesterol values and LDL cholesterol decreases (Fig. 17.2a). Both on placebo and on active treatment a positive linear correlationship is suggested between LDL cholesterol decrease and baseline LDL cholesterol: the larger the baseline LDL cholesterol the better the LDL cholesterol-decrease. Figure 17.2b shows that the overall linear correlation between these two variables is, indeed, significant at $p < 0.001$. Baseline LDL cholesterol is thus an independent determinant of LDL cholesterol decrease.

Fig. 17.1 The linear
regression line is illustrated
(b=regression coefficient,
SE=standard error)

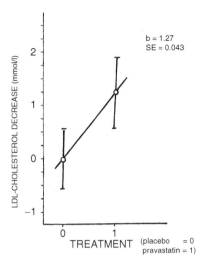

To test whether this significant independence remains after adding the variable treatment modality to the regression, we use the following (multiple) linear regression model:

$$y \; = \; a + b_1 x_1 + b_2 x_2$$

where

y = the dependent variable representing the LDL cholesterol decrease of the patients,

x_1 = the independent variable representing treatment modality, 1 if a patient receives statin, and 0 if placebo,

x_2 = a second independent variable, baseline LDL cholesterol.

An Excel data file, entered into SPSS Statistical Software, produces the following results:

$$b_2 = 0.41 \; (SE \; = 0.024, \; p < 0.0001),$$
$$b_1 = 1.27 \; (SE \; = 0.037, \; p < 0.0001).$$

Figure 17.2c shows how the model works. It assesses whether the data are significantly closer to two regression lines with identical regression coefficients (=direction coefficients) than compatible with random sampling.

With placebo ($x_1 = 0$) the best fit for the data is given by the formula

$$y \; = \; a + b_2 x_2,$$

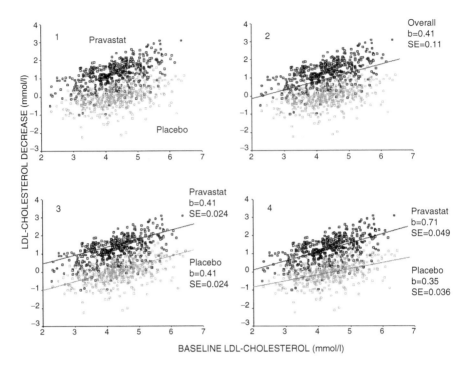

Fig. 17.2 (**a**) Both on placebo and on active treatment there seems to be a positive correlation between LDL cholesterol decrease and baseline LDL cholesterol: the larger the baseline LDL cholesterol the better the LDL cholesterol decrease. (**b**) Overall correlation is significant at p < 0.001, baseline LDL cholesterol is thus an independent determinant of LDL cholesterol decrease. (**c**) The multiple linear regression model assesses whether the data are significantly closer to two regression lines with identical regression coefficients (= direction coefficients) than compatible with random sampling. (**d**) The separately calculated regression lines are not parallel (regression coefficients 0.71 (SE 0.049, p < 0.0001) and 0.35 (0.036, p < 0.0001, difference in slope 0.36 (SE 0.06, p < 0.0001)); (b = regression coefficient, SE = standard error)

With pravastatin ($x_1 = 1$) the best fit for the data is given by the formula

$$y = a + b_1 + b_2 x_2.$$

The estimated treatment effect, b1, is 1.27, the same as in the simple linear regression from Fig. 17.1, but its SE is lowered from 0.043 to 0.037. This means that, indeed, increased precision has been obtained by the multiple regression modeling. The difference between the two regression lines represents the treatment efficacy of pravastatin versus placebo: for each point on the x-axis (baseline LDL cholesterol) the average LDL cholesterol decrease is 1.27 mmol/l larger in the statin (grey) group than in the placebo (black) group. The positive linear correlation between LDL cholesterol decrease and baseline LDL cholesterol (the larger the baseline LDL cholesterol the better the LDL cholesterol decrease) in either of the groups could be explained by a regression-to-the-mean-like-phenomenon: the patients scoring low the first time are more likely to score higher the second time vice versa. However, why should the best fit regression lines of the pravastatin data and of the placebo data produce exactly the same regression coefficients. In order to assess this question regression lines for either of the groups can be calculated separately. Figure 17.2d shows the results. In contrast with the multiple linear regression lines, the separately calculated regression lines are not parallel. Their regression coefficients are 0.71 (SE=0.049, p<0.0001) and 0.35 (SE=0.036, p<0.0001). The difference in slope is significant with a difference in regression of 0.36 (SE=0.06, p<0.0001). Obviously, there is no homogeneity of regression for the groups.

If the parallel regression lines from Fig. 17.2c are interpreted as a homogeneous regression-to-the-mean-like-phenomenon in either of the two treatment groups, then the appropriate implication will be that pravastatin's efficacy is independent of baseline LDL cholesterol. However, the true regression lines from Fig. 17.2d indicate that there is a significant difference in slope. This difference in slope can only be interpreted as a dependency of pravastatin's efficacy on baseline LDL cholesterol: the higher the baseline-cholesterol the better the efficacy of treatment. In clinical terms, based on the multiple regression analysis all patients no matter their baseline LDL cholesterol would qualify for pravastatin treatment equally well, while based on the true regression lines patients would qualify better the higher their baseline LDL cholesterol.

3 Logistic Regression

3.1 Logistic Regression Analysis for Predicting the Probability of an Event

The odds of an infarction is given by the equation

$$\text{odds infarct in a group} = \frac{\text{number of patients with infarct}}{\text{number of patients without}}$$

The odds of an infarction in a group is correlated with age, the older the patient the larger the odds

According to Fig. 17.3 the odds of infarction is correlated with age, but we may ask how?

According to Fig. 17.4 the relationship is not linear, but after transformation of the odds values on the y-axis into log odds values the relationship is suddenly linear.

We will, therefore, transform the linear equation

$$y = a + bx$$

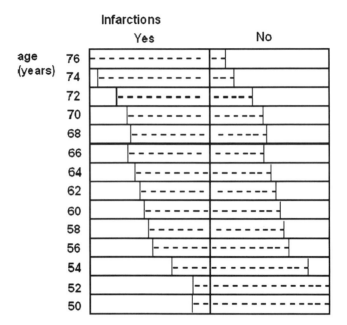

Fig. 17.3 In a group of multiple ages the numbers of patients at risk of infarction is given by the *dotted line*

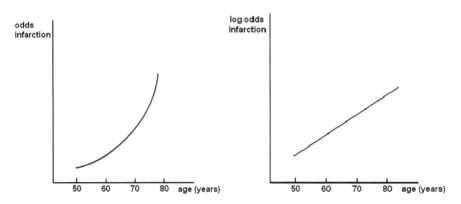

Fig. 17.4 Relationships between the odds of infarction and age

into a log linear equation (ln = natural logarithm)

$$\ln \text{odds} = a + b \times (x = \text{age})$$

Our group consists of 1,000 subjects of different ages that have been observed for 10 years for myocardial infarctions. Using SPSS statistical software, we command binary logistic regression

dependent variable infarction yes/no (0/1)
independent variable age

The program produces a regression equation:

$$\ln \text{odds} = \ln \frac{\text{pts with infarctions}}{\text{pts without}} = a + bx$$

a = −9.2
b = 0.1 (SE = 0.04; p < 0.05)

The age is, thus, a significant determinant of odds infarction (which can be used as surrogate for risk of infarction).

Then, we can use the equation to predict the odds of infarction from a patient's age:

$$\text{Ln odds} \, 55 \, \text{years} = -9.2 + 0.1{\cdot}55 = -4.82265$$
$$\text{odds} = 0.008 = 8 / 1000$$

$$\text{Ln odds} \, 75 \, \text{years} = -9.2 + 0.1{\cdot}75 = -1.3635$$
$$\text{odds} = 0.256 = 256 / 1000$$

Odds of infarction can, of course, more reliably be predicted from multiple x-variables. As an example, 10,000 pts are followed for 10 years, while infarctions and baseline-characteristics are registered during that period.

Dependent variable	Infarction yes/no
Independent variables	Gender
Predictors	Age
	Bmi (body mass index)
	Systolic blood pressure
	Cholesterol
	Heart rate
	Diabetes
	Antihypertensives
	Previous heart infarct
	Smoker

The data are entered in SPSS, and it produces b-values (predictors of infarctions)

	b-value	p-value
1. Gender	0.6583	<0.05
2. Age	0.1044	"
3. Bmi	−0.0405	"
4. Systolic blood pressure	0.0070	"
5. Cholesterol	0.0008	"
6. Heart rate	0.0053	"
7. Diabetes	1.2509	<0.10
8. Antihypertensives	0.3175	<0.050
9. Previous heart infarct	0.8659	<0.10
10. Smoker	0.0234	<0.05
a-value	−9.1935	"

It is decided to exclude predictors that have a p-value>0.10.
The regression equation is used

$$\text{"ln odds infarct} = a + b_1x_1 + b_2x_2 + b_3x_3 + ...\text{"}$$

to calculate the best predictable y-value from every single combination of x-values.
For instance, for a subject

- Male (x_1)
- 55 years of age (x_2)
- cholesterol 6.4 mmol/l (x_3)
- systolic blood pressure 165 mmHg (x_4)
- antihypertensives (x_5)
- dm (x_6)
- 15 cigarettes/day (x_7)
- heart rate 85 beats/min (x_8)
- Bmi 28.7 (x_9)
- smoker (x_{10})

the calculated odds of having an infarction in the next 10 years is the following:

	b-values	x-values	
Gender	0.6583	1 (0 or 1)	=0.6583
Age	0.1044	55	=5.742
BMI	−0.0405	28.7	=..
Blood pressure	0.0070	165	=
Cholesterol	0.0008	6.4	=
Heart rate	0.0053	85	=
Diabetes	1.2509	1	=
Antihypertensives	0.3175	1	=
Previous heart infarct	0.8659	0	=
Smoker	0.0234	15	=
a-value			=−9.1935 +
		Ln odds infarct	=−0.5522
		Odds infarct	=0.58=58/100

The odds is often interpreted as risk. However, the true risk is a bit smaller than
the odds, and can be found by the equation

$$\text{risk event} = 1/(1+1/\text{odds})$$

If odds of infarction=0.58, then the true risk of infarction=0. 37.
The above methodology is currently an important way to determine, with limited
health care sources, what individuals will be:

1. operated.
2. given expensive medications.
3. given the assignment to be treated or not.
4. given the "do not resuscitate sticker".
5. etc.

Table 17.1 Examples of predictive models where multiple logistic regression has been applied

Dependent variable (odds of event)	Independent variables (predictors)
1. TIMI risk score (Antman et al. 2000)	
Odds of infarction	Age, comorbidity, comedication, riskfactors
2. Car producer (Strategic Management Research) (Hoetner 2007)	
Odds of successful car	Cost, size, horse power, ancillary properties
3. Item response modeling (Rasch models for computer adapted tests) (Rudner 1998)	
Odds of correct answer to three questions of different difficulty	Correct answer to three previous questions

We need a large data base to obtain accurate b-values. This logistic model for turning the information from predicting variables into probability of events in individual subjects is being widely used in medicine, and was, for example, the basis for the TIMI (Thrombolysis In Myocardial Infarction) prognostication risk score. However, not only in medicine, also in strategic management research, psychological tests like computer adapted tests, and many more fields it is increasingly observed (Table 17.1). With linear regression it is common to provide a measure of how well the model fits the data, and the squared correlation coefficient r^2 is mostly applied for that purpose. Unfortunately, no direct equivalent to r^2 exists for logistic, otherwise called loglinear, models. However, pseudo-R2 or R2-like measures for estimating the strength of association between predictor and event have been developed.

3.2 Logistic Regression for Efficacy Data Analysis

Logistic regression is often used for comparing proportions of responders to different treatments. As an example, we have two parallel groups treated with different treatment modalities.

	Responders	Non-responders
New treatment (group 1)	17 (A)	4 (B)
Control treatment (group 2)	19 (C)	28 (D)

The odds of responding is given by A/B and C/D, and the odds ratio by $\dfrac{A/B}{C/D}$.

It has been well-established that no linear relationship exists between treatment modalities and odds of responding, but that there is a close-to-linear relationship between treatment modalities and the logarithm of the odds. The natural logarithm (ln) even better fits such assessments. And so, for the purpose of the logistic regression we assume that the usual linear regression formula

$$y = a + bx$$

is transformed into

$$\ln \text{odds} = a + bx,$$

where

ln odds = the dependent variable,
x = the independent variable representing treatment modality, 1 if a patient receives new treatment, and 0 if control treatment.

The term a is the intercept of the regression line, and b is the regression coefficient (direction coefficient of the regression line).

$$\text{Instead of } \ln \text{odds} = a + bx$$

the equation can also be described as

$$\text{odds} = e^{a+bx}$$
$$\text{odds}_{\text{new treatment}} = e^{a+b} \text{ because } x = 1$$
$$\text{odds}_{\text{control treatment}} = e^{a} \text{ because } x = 0$$
$$\text{odds ratio} = e^{a+b} / e^{a} = e^{b}$$

The new treatment is significantly different from the control treatment if the odds ratio of the two treatments is significantly different from 1. If b=0, then the odds ratio = e^0 = 1, which means no difference between new and control treatment. If b is significantly > 0, then the odds ratio is significantly > 1, which means a significant difference between new and control treatment.

SPSS Statistical Software produces the best fit b and a for the data:

$$a = -1.95 \text{ (SE} = 0.53)$$
$$b = 1.83 \text{ (SE} = 0.63, \ p = 0.004).$$

The estimated b is significantly different from 0 at p=0.004, and so we conclude that new and control treatment are significantly different from one another. A similar result could have been obtained by the usual chi-square test. However, the logistic model can adjust the results for relevant subgroups variables like age, gender, and concomitant illnesses. In our case, the data are divided into two age groups

	>50 years		<50 years	
	Responders	Non-responders	Responders	Non-responders
Group 1	4	2	13	2
Group 2	9	16	10	12

The underlying assumptions are that the chance of response may differ between the subgroups, but that the odds ratio does not. SPSS Statistical Software calculates the best fit b- and a-values for data:

$$a_{>50 \text{ years}} = -2.37 \text{ (SE} = 0.65)$$
$$a_{<50 \text{ years}} = -1.54 \text{ (SE} = 0.59)$$
$$b = 1.83 \text{ (SE} = 0.67, \ p = 0.007)$$

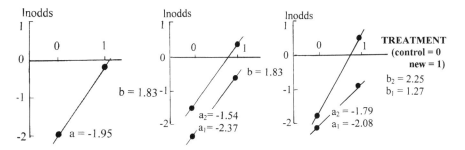

Fig. 17.5 Left graph shows a linear correlation between ln odds of responding and treatment modalities (b = 1.83, SE = 0.63, p = 0.004). The logistic model (*middle graph*) assesses whether the data are closer to two regression lines with identical direction coefficients than compatible with random sampling. The separately calculated regression lines (*right graph*) are not parallel (regression coefficients 2.25 (SE = 0.38, p < 0.001) and 1.27 (SE = 0.48, p < 0.001), difference in slope 0.98 (SE = 0.60, p < 0.05); (b = regression coefficient, a = intercept, SE = standard error)

The estimated b is significantly different from 0 also after age-adjustment. Figure 17.5 shows how the model works. Like with the linear regression model it assesses whether the data are closer to two regression lines with identical regression coefficients than compatible with random. However, why should the best fit regression lines of the different age groups produce exactly the same regression coefficients? Regression lines for either group can be calculated separately to answer this question. In contrast to the logistic regression lines the separately calculated regression lines are not parallel. Their regression coefficients are 1.27 (SE = 0.39, p < 0.001) and 2.25 (SE = 0.48 p < 0.001). The difference in slope is significant, with a difference in regression of 0.98 (SE = 0.60, p < 0.05). Obviously, there is no parallelism between the groups. Younger patients not only respond better, but also benefit more from the new than from the control treatment. This latter mechanism of action is clinically very relevant but remains unobserved in the logistic regression analysis.

4 Cox Regression

Cox regression is based on the assumption that per time unit approximately the same percentage of subjects at risk will have an event, either deadly or not. This exponential model is suitable for mosquitoes whose risk of death is determined by a single factor, i.e., the numbers of collisions, but less so for human beings whose deaths are, essentially, multicausal. Yet, it is widely applied for the comparison of two Kaplan-Meier curves in human beings. Figure 17.6 shows that after 1 day 50% is alive, while after the second day 25% is, etc.

The formula for the proportion of survivors is given by:

$$\text{proportion survivors} = 1 / 2^t = 2^{-t}$$

Fig. 17.6 Hypothesized
example of the exponential
surviving pattern of
mosquitoes

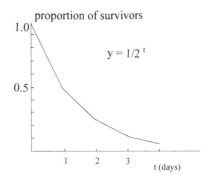

In true biology "e (=2.71828)" instead of "2" better fits the observed data, while k is dependent on the species:

$$\text{proportion survivors } = e^{-kt}$$

The Cox regression formula for the comparison of exponential survival curves is given by:

proportion survivors $= e^{-kt - bx}$,
x = binary variable (only 0 or 1; 0 means treatment-1, and 1 means treatment-2),
b = regression coefficient,
proportion survivors treatment-1 $= e^{-kt}$ because x = 0,
proportion survivors treatment-2 $= e^{-kt - b}$ because x = 1,
relative risk of surviving $= e^{-kt - b}/e^{-kt} = e^{-b}$,
relative risk of death = hazard ratio $= e^{b}$.

Figure 17.7 shows two Kaplan-Meier curves. Although an exponential pattern is hard to prove from the curves (or from their logarithmic transformations), the Cox model seems reasonable, and SPSS software is used to calculate the best b for the given data.

If b is significantly larger than 0, the hazard ratio will be significantly larger than 1, and there will, thus, be a significant difference between treatment-1 and treatment-2. The following results are obtained:

b = 1.1 with a standard error of 0.41
hazard ratio = 3.0
p = 0.01 (t-test)

The Cox regression provides a p-value of 0.01, and, so, it is less sensitive than the traditional summary chi-square test (p-value of 0.002). However, the Cox model has the advantage that it enables to adjust the data for relevant prognostic factors like disease stage and presence of b-symptoms. The model is extended accordingly:

$$\text{hazard ratio } = e^{b_1 x_1 + b_2 x_2 + b_3 x_3}$$

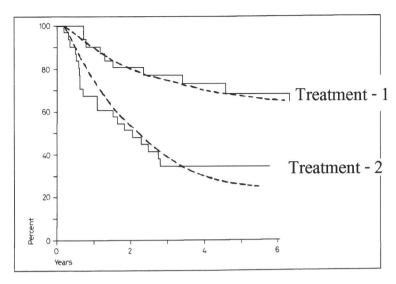

Fig. 17.7 Two Kaplan-Meier curves estimating effect on survival of treatment 1 and 2 in two parallel groups of patients with malignancies (33 and 31 patients respectively). The *dotted curves* present the modeled curves produced by the Cox regression model

$x_1 = 0$ (treatment-1); $x_1 = 1$ (treatment-2)
$x_2 = 0$ (disease stage I-III); $x_2 = 1$ (disease stage IV)
$x_3 = 0$ (A symptoms); $x_3 = 1$ (B symptoms)

The test for multicollinearity is negative (Pearson correlation coefficient between disease stage and B symptoms <0.85), and, so, the model is deemed appropriate. SPSS produces the following result:

$b_1 = 1.10$ with a standard error of 0.41

$b_2 = 1.38$ with a standard error of 0.55

$b_3 = 1.74$ with a standard error of 0.69

unadjusted hazard ratio = 3.0

adjusted hazard ratio = 68.0

Treatment-2 after adjustment for advanced disease and b-symptoms raises a 68 higher mortality than treatment-1 without adjustments. This Cox regression analysis, despite prior examination of the appropriateness of the model, is hardly adequate for at least three reasons. First, the method is less sensitive than the usual chi-square summary test, probably because the regression does not fit the data well enough. Second, Cox regression tests the null-hypothesis that treatment-2 is not significantly different from the treatment-1, and it assumes for that purpose that the hazard ratio is constant over time. Figure 17.5 gives the modeled treatment-curves (dotted curves), in addition to the true treatment-curves. It can be observed in the modeled curve that few patients died in the first 8 months, while, in reality, 34% of the patients in group 2 died, probably, due to the toxicity of the treatment-2. Also it can be observed in the modeled curves that patients continued to die after 2 1/2 years, while, in reality, they stopped dying in group 2, because they actually went into a complete remission. Obviously, this Cox regression analysis gives rise to some serious misinterpretations of the data. Third, a final problem with the above Cox analysis is raised by the adjustment-procedure. An adjusted hazard ratio as large as 68 is clinically unrealistic. Probably, the true adjusted hazard ratio is less than 10. From a clinical point of view, the x_2 and x_3 variables must be strongly dependent on one another as they are actually different measures for estimating the same. And so, despite the negative test for multicollinearity, they should not have been included in the model.

Note: Cox regression can be used for other exponential time relationships like pharmacokinetic data. Limitations similar to ones described above apply to such analyses.

5 Markov Models

Regression models are only valid within the range of the x-values. Markov modeling goes one step further, and aims at predicting outside the range of x-values. Like with Cox regression it assumes an exponential-pattern in the data which may be a strong assumption.

As an example, in patients with diabetes mellitus type II, sulfonureas are highly efficacious, but they will, eventually, induce beta-cell failure. Beta-cell failure is sometimes defined as a fasting plasma glucose >7.0 mmol/l. The question is, does the severity of diabetes and/or the potency of the sulfonurea-compound influence the induction of beta-cell failure?

This was studied in 500 patients with diabetes type II:

> at time 0 year   0 / 500 patients   had beta - cell failure
>
> at time 1 year   50 / 500 patients (= 10%)   had beta - cell failure.

As after 1 year 90% had no beta-cell failure, it is appropriate according to the Markow model to extrapolate:

> after 2 years 90% × 90%   = 81% no beta - cell failure
>
> after 3 years 90% × 90% × 90% = 73% no beta - cell failure
>
> after 6.7 years   = 50% nobeta - cell failure.

A second question was, does the severity of diabetes mellitus type II influence induction of beta-cell failure. A cut-off level for severity often applied is a fasting plasma glucose >10 mmol/l. According to the Markov modeling approach the question can be answered as follows:

250 patients had fasting plasma glucose <10 mmol/l at diagnosis (Group-1)
250 patients had fasting plasma glucose >10 mmol/l at diagnosis (Group-2)

If after 1 year sulfonureas (su) treatment 10/250 of the patients from Group-1 had b-cell failure, and 40/250 of the patients from Group-2, which is significantly different by $p < 0.01$, then we can again extrapolate:

In Group-1 it takes 12 years before 50% of the patients develop beta-cell failure.
In Group-2 it takes 2 years before 4% of the patients develop beta-cell failure.

The next question is, does potency of su-compound influence induction of b-cell failure?

250 patients started on amaryl (potent sulfonurea) at diagnosis (Group-A)
250 patients started on artosin (non-potent sulfonurea) at diagnosis (Group-B)

If after 1 year 25/250 of Group-A had beta-cell failure, and 25/250 of the group-B, it is appropriate according to the Markov model to conclude that a non-potent does not prevent beta-cell failure. Note Markov modeling is highly speculative, because nature does not routinely follow mathematical models.

6   Regression-Analysis with Laplace Transformations

There is an increasing trend towards the use of non linear mixed effect models (commonly called population pharmacokinetics and pharmacodynamics) for describing the pharmacokinetics and pharmacodynamics of drugs in humans. The term mixed effect models refers to the random effect statistical regression model applied. These models allow for sparse sampling and at the same time can account for multiple effect associated variables and even account for errors in sampling (Boeckman et al. 1992; Davidian and Giltinan 1995; Lindstrom and Bates 1990). These new modelling approaches are increasingly becoming a very important part of the drug approval process. They routinely make use of multi-exponential models, according to equations like for example the one underneath:

$$f(t) = D / V (e^{-at} + e^{-bt} + e^{-ct} ....)$$

D = dose drug
V = volume of distribution
a = elimination constant compartment 1
b = elimination constant compartment 2
c = elimination constant compartment 3
t = time

As logarithmic transformations only allow for mono-exponential equations, generally Laplace transformations, based on second differentiations, are used:

$$f(t) = C(t) = C(0)(e^{-at} + e^{-bt})$$

$C(t)$ = concentration at time t, $C(0)$ = concentration at time 0.

is transformed into

$$F(s) = C(0) / (s+a)(s+b)$$

s = unit Laplace-functions = unit amount-of-drug/time (time thus disappears from the equation).

The final data are then transformed back to their initial equations.

The advantage of the exponential modeling in pharmacokinetics is, that it is very easy to calculate the keystone pharmacokinetic parameters according to which compounds are currently registered: plasma-half-life, volume of distribution, plasma-clearance rate etc.

Exponential pharmacokinetic models assume first order kinetics, and it may be true that many drugs at the therapeutically given concentrations would follow first order kinetics. However, zero order patterns are followed for example by ethyl-alcohol, acetyl-salicylic-acid, and by any drug at higher dosages, while second order elimination-patterns are followed for example by drugs that are hydrolyzed or conjugated before excretion (Keusch 2003). The simplest equations and curves for zero, first, and second order kinetics are given (Fig. 17.8).

1. Zero order $C(t) = C(0) - kt$ linear pattern

2. First order $C(t) = C(0) \cdot e^{-kt}$ exponential pattern

3. Second order $1 / C(t) = 1 / C(0) - kt$ hyperbolic pattern

k = elimination constant

As shown in the example of Fig. 17.9, there may be a wide spread in the data of a pharmacokinetic study. The 95% confidence intervals calculated with the NON-MEM software (Boeckman et al. 1992), which uses the Laplace transformations, assumes a first order pharmacokinetic. In fact both a zero and a second order pattern provided a better fit in this example. However, a problem with either of them is, that it is impossible to derive plasma-half-life and other pharmacokinetic parameters from them. As can be observed only in Eq. 2 plasma-half-life is not dependent on $C(0)$. With Eqs. 1 and 3 we have many plasma-half-lifes, with Eq. 2 we have only one. This is a very elegant property of first order kinetics, but it should not mean that the best fit data models are sacrificed for the purpose of unreliable pharmacokinetic parameters. A second problem with the Laplace models is that they assume independence of confounders. In pharmacology confounders like gender, age, body mass, renal function, notoriously interact with the treatment modalities.

Fig. 17.8 Examples of
hypothesized time-
concentration curve following
zero-, first-, and second order
pharmacokinetics

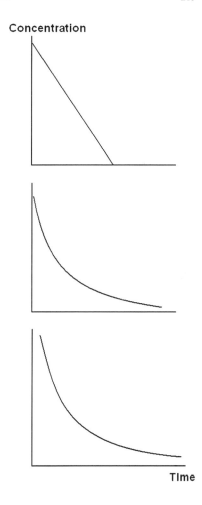

Fig. 17.9 Example of an
exponentially modeled
time-concentration
relationship with wide 95%
confidence intervals

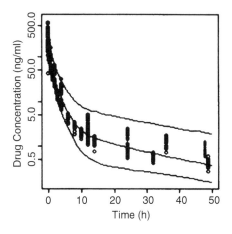

7   Discussion

In randomized controlled trials regression analysis of possibly confounding variables is, traditionally, not emphasized, because the randomization ensures that such variables are equally distributed among the treatment groups. Also, regression analysis tests correlations rather than causal relationships. In testing the data from clinical trials we are mainly interested in causal relationships. When such assessments were statistically analyzed through correlation analyses, we would probably be less convinced of a causal relationship than we are while using prospective hypothesis testing. In the past few years, however, regression analyses have increasingly entered the stage of primary data analysis. For example, of 28 randomized controlled trials published in the Lancet in the 2003 Volume 362, 20 (71%) used regression models for primary data analysis, including linear regression twice, logistic regression 5 times, and Cox regression 12 times.

Obviously, regression analyses are increasingly used for the primary data analysis of clinical trials. The current paper assesses problems of this new development. More uncertainties are added to the data in the form of subjective judgments and uncertainty about the appropriate transformation of the data. Regression analyses may also give rise to serious misinterpretations of the data:

1. The assumption that baseline characteristics are independent of treatment efficacies may be wrong.
2. Sensitivity of testing is jeopardized if the models do not fit the data well enough.
3. Relevant clinical phenomena like unexpected toxicity effects and complete remissions can go unobserved.
4. The inclusion of multiple variables in regression models raises the risk of clinically unrealistic results.

Markov modeling is an exponential regression model like Cox regression that aims at predicting outside the range of observed observations. It is, therefore even more at risk of unrealistic results. As an example, many suggestions from the famous Framingham studies are based on Markov modeling. Current trials and observations confirm that some of these are true, some not. Regression modeling, although a very good tool for exploratory research, is not adequately reliable for randomized clinical trials. This is, of course, different with exploratory research like observational studies. For example, a cohort of postmenopausal women is assessed for exploratory purposes. The main question is: what are the determinants of endometrial cancer in this category of females. Logistic regression is excellent for the purpose of this exploratory research. The following logistic model is used:

y-variable = ln odds endometrial cancer
x_1 = estrogene consumption short term
x_2 = estrogene consumption long term
x_3 = low fertility index

x_4 = obesity
x_5 = hypertension
x_6 = early menopause

ln odds endometrial cancer = $a + b_1$ estrogene data + $b_2 ... + b_6$ early menopause data

The odds ratios for different x-variables are defined, e.g., for:

x_1 = chance cancer in consumers of estrogene/non-consumers
x_3 = chance cancer in patients with low fertility/their counterparts
x_4 = chance cancer in obese patients/their counterparts etc.

Risk factors	Regression coefficient(b)	Standard error	p-value	Odds ratio (e^b)
1. Estrogenes short	1.37	0.24	<0.0001	3.9
2. Estrogenes long	2.60	0.25	<0.0001	13.5
3. Low fertility	0.81	0.21	0.0001	2.2
4. Obesity	0.50	0.25	0.04	1.6
5. Hypertension	0.42	0.21	0.05	1.5
6. Early menopause	0.53	0.53	ns	1.7

The data are entered in the software program, which provides us with the best fit b-values. The model not only shows a greatly increased risk of cancer in several categories, but also allows us to consider that the chance of cancer if patients consume estrogens, suffer from low fertility, obesity, and hypertension might have an increased risk as large as = $e^{b2+b3+b4+b5}$ = 75.9 = 76 fold. This huge chance is, of course, clinically unrealistic! We must take into account that some of these variables must be heavily correlated with one another, and the results are, therefore, largely inflated. In conclusion, regression modeling is an adequate tool for exploratory research, the conclusions of which must be interpreted with caution, although they often provide scientifically highly interesting questions. Such questions are, then, a sound basis for confirmation by prospective randomized research. Regression modelling is not adequately reliable for the analysis of the primary data of randomized controlled trials. Of course, regression analysis is also fully in place for the exploratory post-hoc analyses of randomized controlled trials (Chaps. 17, 18, and 19).

8   Conclusions

Data modeling can be applied for improving precision of clinical studies. Multiple regression modeling is increasingly used for that purpose. The objective of this chapter was to assess uncertainties and risks of misinterpretations commonly encountered with regression analyses and rarely communicated in research papers.

Regression analyses add uncertainties to the data in the form of subjective judgments and uncertainty about the appropriate transformation of the data. Additional flaws include: (1) the assumption that baseline characteristics are independent of treatment efficacies; (2) the loss of sensitivity of testing if the models do not fit the data well enough; (3) the risk that clinical phenomena like toxicity effects and complete remissions go unobserved; (4) the risk of clinically unrealistic results if multiple variables are included. Regression analyses, although a very good tool for exploratory research, are not adequately reliable for randomized controlled trials.

References

Antman EM, Cohen M, Bernink P, McGabe CH, Horacek T, Papuches G, Mautner B, Corbalan R, Radley D, Braunwald E (2000) The TIMI Risk score for unstable angina pectors, a method for prognostication and therapeutic decision making. J Am Med Assoc 284:835–842

Boeckman AJ, Sheiner LB, Beal SL (1992) NONMEM user's guide. NONMEM Project Group, University California, San Francisco

Breithaupt-Grogler K, Maleczyk C, Belz GG, Butzer R, Herrman V, Stass H, Wensing G (1997) Pharmacodynamic and pharmacokinetic properties of an angiotensin II receptor antagonist – characterization by use of Schild regression techniques in man. Int J Clin Pharmacol Ther 35:434–441

Davidian M, Giltinan DM (1995) Nonlinear models for repeated measurements data. Chapman and Hall, New York

Debord J, Carpentier N, Sabot C, Bertin P, Marquet P, Treves R, Merle I, Lachatre G (1998) Influence of biological variables upon pharmacokinetic parameters of intramuscular methotrexate in rheumatoid arthritis. Int J Clin Pharmacol Ther 36:227–230

Hoetner G (2007) The use of logit and probit models in strategic management research. Strateg Manage J 28:331–343

Jukema JW, Bruschke AV, Van Boven AJ, Reiber JH, Bal ET, Zwinderman AH, Jansen H, Boerma GJ, Van Rappard FM, Lie KI (1995) Effects of lipid lowering by pravastatin on progression and regression of coronary artery disease in symptomatic men with normal to moderately elevated serum cholesterol levels (REGRESS Trial). Circulation 91:2528–2540

Kato Z, Fukutomi O, Yamazaki M, Kondo N, Imaeda N, Orii T (1994) Prediction of steady-state serum theophylline concentration in children by first-order and zero -order absorption models. Int J Clin Pharmacol Ther 32:231–234

Keusch P (2003) Chemical kinetics, rate laws, Arrhenius equation-experiments. http://www.uniregensburg.de/Fakultaeten/nat_Fak_IV/Organische_Chemie/Didaktik.html.

Lindstrom MJ, Bates BM (1990) Nonlinear mixed effects models for repeated measures data. Biometrics 46:673–678

Mahmood I, Mahayni H (1999) A limited sampling approach in bioequivalence studies: application to low half-life drugs and replicate design studies. Int J Clin Pharmacol Ther 37:275–281

Rudner LM (1998) Computer adaptive testing. http://edres.org/scripts/cat/catdemo.htm

Sabot C, Debord J, Roullet B, Marquet P, Merle L, Lachatre G (1995) Comparison of 2- and 3-compartment models for the Bayesian estimation of methotrexate pharmacokinetics. Int J Clin Pharmacol Ther 33:164–169

Ulrich S, Baumann B, Wolf R, Lehmann D, Peters B, Bogerts B (2003) Therapeutic drug monitoring of clozapine and relapse – a retrospective study of routine clinical data. Int J Clin Pharmacol Ther 41:3–13

Vrecer M, Turk S, Drinovec J, Mrhar A (2003) Use of statins in primary and secondary prevention of coronary heart disease and ischemic stroke. Meta-analysis of randomized trials. Int J Clin Pharmacol Ther 41:567–577

Chapter 18
Regression Modeling for Improved Precision

1 Introduction

Small precision of clinical trials is defined as a large spread in the data. Repeated observations have a central tendency, but also a tendency to depart from the central tendency. If the latter is large compared to the former, the data are imprecise. This means that p-values are large, and reliable predictions cannot be made. Often a Gaussian pattern is in the data. The central tendency can, then, be adequately described using mean values as point estimates. However, if the data can be fitted to a different pattern like a linear or a curvilinear pattern, the central tendency can also be described using the best fit lines or curves of the data instead of mean values. This method is called data modeling, and may under the right circumstances reduce the spread in the data and improve the precision of the trial. Extensive research on the impact of data modeling on the analysis of pharmacodynamic/pharmacokinetic data has been presented over the past 10 years. The underlying mechanism for improved precision was explained by the late Lewis Sheiner: "Modeling turns noise into signals" (Sheiner and Steimer 1984; Fuseau and Sheiner 1984). In fact, instead of treating variability as an "error noise", modeling uses the variability in the data as a signal explaining outcome. If regression models are used for such purpose, an additional advantage is the relative ease with which covariates can be included in the analysis. So far, data modeling has not been emphasized in the analysis of prospective randomized clinical trials, and special statistical techniques need to be applied including the transformation of parallel-group data into regression data. In the current chapter we demonstrate two regression models that can be used for such purpose. Both real and hypothesized examples are given.

T.J. Cleophas and A.H. Zwinderman, *Statistics Applied to Clinical Studies*,
DOI 10.1007/978-94-007-2863-9_15, © Springer Science+Business Media B.V. 2012

2   Regression Modeling for Improved Precision of Clinical Trials, the Underlying Mechanism

The better the model fits the data, the better precision is obtained. Regression modeling is, essentially, an attempt to fit experimental data to specific patterns, and, subsequently, to test how far distant the data are from the best fit pattern. A statistically significant correlation indicates that the data are closer to the best fit pattern than could happen by random sampling. As an example, the simple linear regression analysis of a parallel-group study of the effects on LDL-cholesterol on pravastatin versus placebo in 884 patients, also used in the Chaps. 14 and 15, is given (Cleophas 2003). The overall spread in the data is estimated by a standard error of 0.11 mmol/l around the regression line (Fig. 18.1 upper graph). A smaller standard error (0.024 mmol/l), and, thus, less spread in the data is provided by a multiple regression model, using two regression lines instead of one (Fig. 18.1, lower graph). Obviously, this multiple regression pattern provided an overall shorter distance to the data than did the simple linear regression pattern. Or, in other words, it better fitted the data than did the simple linear regression. In the next few sections we give additional examples.

3   Regression Model for Parallel-Group Trials with Continuous Efficacy Data

Table 18.1 shows the data of a parallel-group trial comparing efficacy of a new laxative versus control laxative. The mean difference in response between new treatment and control $= 9.824$ stools per 4 weeks (Se $= 2.965$). The t-test produces a t-value of $9.824/2.965 = 3.313$, and the t-table gives a p-value of <0.01.

A linear regression according to

$$y = a + bx$$

with y $=$ response and x $=$ treatment modalities ($0 =$ new treatment, $1 =$ control), a $=$ intercept, and b $=$ regression coefficient,

produces a similar result

$b = 9.824$
$se_b = 2.965$
$t = 3.313$
p-value <0.01.

Improved precision of this data analysis is a possibility if we extend the regression model by including a second x-variable $=$ baseline stool frequency according to

$$y = a + b_1 x_1 + b_2 x_2$$

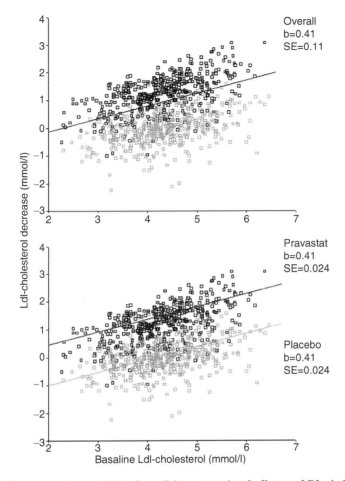

Fig. 18.1 Linear regression analysis of parallel-group study of effect on LDL-cholesterol of pravastatin versus placebo in 872 patients. The overall spread in the data is estimated by a standard error of 0.11 mmol/l around the regression line (*upper graph*). The multiple regression model using two regression lines, instead of one, leads to a standard error of only 0.024 mmol/l (*lower graph*)

with x_1 = treatment modalities (0 = new treatment, 1 = control),
x_2 = baseline stool frequencies, and b-values are partial regression coefficients.

This produces the following results

$b_1 = 6.852$
$se_{b1} = 1.792$
$t = 3.823$
p-value < 0.001.

After adjustment for the baseline stool frequencies an improved precision to test the efficacy of treatment is obtained as demonstrated by a larger t-value and a smaller p-value.

Table 18.1 A parallel-group trial comparing a new laxative versus control

Patient no.	Treatment modality (new = 0, control = 1)	Response = stool frequency after treatment (4 week stools)	Baseline stool frequency (4 week stools)
1	0	24	8
2	0	30	13
3	0	25	15
4	1	35	10
5	1	39	9
6	0	30	10
7	0	27	8
8	0	14	5
9	1	39	13
10	1	42	15
11	1	41	11
12	1	38	11
13	1	39	12
14	1	37	10
15	1	47	18
16	0	30	13
17	1	36	12
18	0	12	4
19	0	26	10
20	1	20	8
21	0	43	16
22	0	31	15
23	1	40	14
24	0	31	7
25	1	36	12
26	0	21	6
27	0	44	19
28	1	11	5
29	0	27	8
30	0	24	9
31	1	40	15
32	1	32	7
33	0	10	6
34	1	37	14
35	0	19	7

4   Regression Model for Parallel-Group Trials with Proportions or Odds as Efficacy Data

Consider the underneath two by two contingency table.

	Numbers responders	Numbers non-responders
Treatment 1	30 a	45 b
Treatment 2	45 c	30 d

The odds-ratio-of-responding equals $\dfrac{a/b}{c/d} = \dfrac{30/45}{45/30} = 0.444$. The natural loga-rithmic (ln) transformation of this odds ratio equal -0.8110. The standard error of this logarithmic transformation is given by $\sqrt{\dfrac{1}{a} + \dfrac{1}{b} + \dfrac{1}{c} + \dfrac{1}{d}} = \sqrt{\dfrac{1}{30} + \dfrac{1}{45} + \dfrac{1}{30} + \dfrac{1}{45}} = 0.333$.

A t-test of these data produces a t-value of $0.8110/0.333 = 2.435$. According to the t-table this odds-ratio is significantly different from an odds ratio of 1.0 with a p-value of 0.015.

Logistic regression according to the model

ln odds-of-responding $= a + bx$
with $x =$ treatment modality (0 or 1),
$a =$ intercept, and $b =$ regression coefficient,

produces the same result:

$b = 0.8110$
$Se_b = 0.333$
t-value $= 2.435$
p-value $= 0.015$

The patients can be divided into two age classes:

	Over 50 years		Under 50 years	
	Responders	Non-responders	Responders	Non-responders
Treatment 1	16	22	9	28
Treatment 2	34	4	16	21

Improved precision of the statistical analysis is a possibility if we control for age groups using the underneath multiple logistic regression model

ln odds-of-responding $= a + b_1 x_1 + b_2 x_2$
with $x_1 =$ treatment modalities ($0 =$ treatment 1, $1 =$ treatment 2)
$x_2 =$ age classes ($1 = {<}50$ years, $2 => 50$ years)
b-values are regression coefficients.

The following results are obtained:

$b_1 = 1.044$
$Se_{b1} = 0.387$
t-value $= 2.697$
p-value $= 0.007$

After adjustment for age class improved precision to test the efficacy of treatment is obtained as demonstrated by a larger t-value and smaller p-value.

5   Discussion

Multiple regression analysis of confounding variables, although routinely used in retrospective observational studies, is not emphasized in prospective randomized clinical trials (RCTs). The randomization process ensures that such potential confounders are equally distributed among the treatment groups. If not, the result of the study is flawed, and regression analysis is sometimes used in a post hoc attempt to salvage the data, but there is always an air of uncertainty about such data. Multiple regression can, however, be used in prospective RCTs for a different purpose. Certain patient characteristics in RCTs may cause substantial spread in the data even if they are equally distributed, and, thus, independent of the treatment groups. Including such data in the efficacy analysis may reduce the overall spread in the data, and reduce the level of uncertainty in the data analysis. Regression models are also adequate for such purpose, although rarely applied so far.

Regression modeling is a very sophisticated statistical technique which needs to be applied carefully and under the right circumstances. Therefore, when using regression analysis for the purpose of improving precision of RCTs a number of potential problems have to be accounted. They have been recently published by us (Cleophas 2005), are reviewed in the previous chapter.

1. The sensitivity of testing is jeopardized if the linear or exponential models do not fit the data well enough. This can be checked for example by scatter-plots and histograms.
2. Relevant clinical phenomena like unexpected toxicity effects and complete remissions can go unobserved by the use of a regression model to assess the data.
3. The inclusion of multiple variables in regression models raises the risk of clinically unrealistic results.

Nonetheless, if certain patient characteristics are largely independent of the treatment modality, they can be included in the data analysis, in order to reduce the overall spread in the data. We should emphasize that it has to be decided prior to the trial and stated explicitly in the trial protocol whether a regression model will be applied, because post hoc decisions regarding regression modeling like any other post hoc change in the protocol raises the risk of statistical bias due to multiple testing. Naturally, there is less opportunity for modeling in a small trial than in a large trial. There is no general rule about which sample sizes are required for sensible regression modeling, but one rule-of-thumb is that at least ten times as many patients are required as the number of variables in the model. This would mean that a data set of at least 30 is required if we wish to include a single covariate in the model for the purpose of improving precision. With every additional covariate in the model an extra regression weight must be estimated, which may lead to a decreased rather than improved precision. Regression analysis can be adequately used for improving precision of efficacy analysis. Application of these models is very easy since many computer programs are available. For a successful application the fit of the regression models should, however, always be checked, and the covariate selection should be sparse.

6   Conclusions

Small precision of clinical trials is defined as a large spread in the data. Certain patient characteristics of randomized controlled trials may cause substantial spread in the data even if they are equally distributed among the treatment groups. The objective of this chapter was to assess whether improved precision of the analysis can be obtained by transforming the parallel-group data into regression data, and, subsequently, including patient characteristics in the analysis.

In a 35 patient parallel-group trial with continuous efficacy data, after adjustment of the efficacy scores for baseline scores, the test-statistic rose from $t = 3.313$ to $t = 3.823$, while the p-value fell from < 0.01 to < 0.001. In a 150 patient parallel-group trial with odds as efficacy variable, after adjustment of the efficacy variable for age class, the test statistic rose from $t = 2.435$ to $t = 2.697$, while the p-value fell from 0.015 to 0.007.

We conclude that regression analysis can be adequately applied for improving precision of efficacy data of parallel-group trials. We caution that, although application of these models is very easy with computer programs widely available, the fit of the regression models should always be carefully checked, and the covariate selection should be sparse.

References

Cleophas TJ (2003) The sense and non-sense of regression modeling for increasing precision of clinical trials. Clin Pharmacol Ther 74:295–297

Cleophas TJ (2005) Problems in regression modeling of randomized clinical trials. Int J Clin Pharmacol Ther 43:5–12

Fuseau E, Sheiner LB (1984) Simultaneous modeling of pharmacokinetics and pharmacodynamics with a nonparametric pharmacodynamic model. Clin Pharmacol Ther 35:733–741

Sheiner LB, Steimer JL (1984) Pharmacokinetic/pharmacodynamic modeling and drug development. Clin Pharmacol Ther 35:733–741

Chapter 19
Post-hoc Analyses in Clinical Trials, A Case for Logistic Regression Analysis

1 Multiple Variables Methods

Multiple variables methods are used to adjust asymmetries in the patient characteristics in a trial (see page 171 for a discussion of the difference between multivariate and multiple variables methods). It can also be used for a subsequent purpose. In many trials simple primary hypotheses in terms of efficacy and safety expectations, are tested through their respective outcome variables as described in the protocol. However, sometimes it is decided already at the design stage that post hoc analyses will be performed for the purpose of testing secondary hypotheses. For example, suppose we first want to know whether a novel beta-blocker is better than a standard beta-blocker, and second, if so, whether this better effect is due to a vaso-dilatory property of the novel compound. The first hypothesis is assessed in the primary analysis. For the second hypothesis, we can simply adjust the two treatment groups for difference in vasodilation by multiple regression analysis and see whether differences in treatment effects otherwise are affected by this procedure. However, with small data power is lost by such procedure. More power is provided by the following approach. We could assign all of the patients to two new groups: patients who actually have improvement in the primary outcome variable and those who have not, irrespective of the type of beta-blocker. We, then, can perform a regression analysis of the two new groups trying to find independent determinants of this improvement. If the dependent determinant is binary, which is generally so, our choice of test is logistic regression analysis. Testing the second hypothesis is, of course, of lower validity than testing the first one, because it is post-hoc and makes use of a regression analysis which does not differentiate between causal relationships and relationships due to an unknown common factor.

T.J. Cleophas and A.H. Zwinderman, *Statistics Applied to Clinical Studies*,
DOI 10.1007/978-94-007-2863-9_19, © Springer Science+Business Media B.V. 2012

2   Examples

In a double-blind randomized study of the new beta-blocker celiprolol for patients with angina pectoris the main outcome variable was anginal attack rate. Additional outcome variables include systolic and diastolic blood pressure, heart rate, rate pressure product, peripheral vascular resistance. Although this study measures several outcomes, the various outcomes to some degree measure the same thing, and this may be particularly so with blood pressure, heart rate and pressure rate product since they are assumed to represent oxygen demand to the heart, which is jeopardized during anginal attacks. The new beta-blocker has been demonstrated preclinically not only to reduce rate pressure product like any other beta-blocker but also to reduce peripheral vascular resistance. The novel beta-blocker indeed performed significantly better than the latter (persistent angina pectoris at the completion of the trial 17 versus 33%, $P < 0.01$, $1 - \beta = \pm 80\%$), and this was accompanied by a significantly better reduction of systolic blood pressure and reduction of peripheral resistance. A problem with multiple variables analysis is its relatively small power with usual sample sizes. For the purpose of better power patients may be divided into new groups according to their main outcome. In order to determine the most important determinants of the better clinical benefit, the patients were, therefore, divided into two new groups: they were assigned to "no-angina-pectoris" at the completion of the trial or "persistent-angina-pectoris" (Table 19.1). The univariable analysis of these two new groups showed that most of the additional outcome variables including treatment assignment were significantly different between the two groups.

Table 19.1 Angina pectoris and odds ratios of persistent angina pectoris in the celiprolol (novel compound) and propranolol (reference compound) group adjusted for independent variables

	No angina pectoris (n = 23)		Persistent angina pectoris (n = 30)
	Mean ± SD	P	Mean ± SD
Systolic blood pressure(mmHg)	134 ± 17	<0.001	155 ± 19
Diastolic blood pressure (mmHg)	77 ± 13	<0.02	84 ± 9
Heart rate (beat/min)	65 ± 9	<0.09	69 ± 9
Rate pressure product (mmHg·beats/ min·10^{-3})	8.6 ± 11	<0.001	10.7 ± 14
Fore arm blood flow (ml/100 ml tissue·min)	8.8 ± 10.8	<0.02	4.1 ± 2.2
Treatment assignment (celiprolol/ propanolol)	18/5	<0.001	8/22

	Odds ratio of persistent angina	95% CIs	P-value
Unadjusted	0.38	0.25–0.52	<0.002
Adjusted for rate pressure product	0.13	0.05–0.22	<0.0005
Adjusted for systolic pressure plus heart rate	0.12	0.04–0.20	<0.0005

Data from Cleophas et al. (1996)
Odds ratio = odds of persistent angina pectoris in the celiprolol group/odds of persistent angina pectoris in the propranolol group. Means ± SDs are given
CI confidence interval, *SD* standard deviation

Table 19.2 Mean data (*SDs*) after assignment of patients according to whether (responders) or not (non-responders) their ischemia-onset-time increased after treatment with calcium channel blockers, and odds ratios of mibefradil or diltiazem versus amlodipine for responding, unadjusted and after adjustment for difference of heart rate

	Responders (n=239)	Non-responders (n=61)	
	Mean (SD)	Mean (SD)	P-value
At rest			
Systolic blood pressure (mmHg)	−5 (19)	−1 (23)	0.27
Diastolic blood pressure (mmHg)	−5 (10)	−3 (10)	0.13
Heart rate (beats/min)	−5 (11.0)	1.1 (9.6)	<0.001
Rate pressure product (mmHg·beats/ min·10^{-3})	−1.0 (1.9)	0.1 (2.1)	<0.001
At maximal workload			
Systolic blood pressure (mmHg)	−1 (21)	−2 (27)	0.68
Diastolic blood pressure (mmHg)	−4 (11)	−4 (11)	0.97
Heart rate (beats/min)	−12 (17)	−6 (15)	0.010
Rate pressure product (mmHg·beats/ min·10^{-3})	−2.3 (4.5)	−1.2 (4.5)	0.090
Treatment assignment (n, %)			
Amlodipine	76 (32%)	27 (44%)	
Diltiazem	75 (31%)	26 (43%)	
Mibefradil	88 (37%)	8 (13%)	

	Unadjusted odds ratio (95% CIs) odds ratio adjusted for change in heart rate (95% CIs)	Odds ratio adjusted for change in heart rate (95% CIs)
Amlodipine	1 (−)	1(−)
Diltiazem	1.02 (0.55–1.92)	0.86 (0.45–1.66)
Mibefradil	3.91 (1.68–9.11)	2.26 (0.86–5.97)

Van der Vring et al. (1999)
Odds ratio=odds of responding on mibefradil or diltiazem or amlodipine/odds of responding on amlodipine
CI confidence interval, *SD* standard deviation.

These variables were entered in the logistic regression analysis: the variables double product, systolic blood pressure and heart rate were independent of treatment assignment, while fore arm blood flow (=1/peripheral vascular resistance) was not. After adjustment for fore arm blood flow the difference in treatment assignment was lost. This suggests that celiprolol exerted its beneficial effect to a large extent through its peripheral vasodilatory property.

As a second example is given a double-blind randomized parallel-group study comparing chronotropic (mibefradil ands diltiazem) and non-chronotropic calcium channel blockers (amlodipine) in patients with angina pectoris. Although all of the calcium channel blockers improved exercise tolerance as estimated by % increased time to onset ischemia during bicycle ergometry, mibefradil and diltiazem performed better than amlodipine (20.8 and 12.4 s versus 9.9 s, P<0.01 and<0.001). In order to determine the most important determinants of this better clinical benefit, patients were divided into two new groups: they were assigned to non-responders if their change in ischemic onset time was zero or less, and to responders if it was larger than zero (Table 19.2). Univariable analysis of these two groups showed that many variables including treatment assignment tended to be different between the two groups.

These variables were entered into the logistic regression analysis: the difference in treatment assignment between the two groups was lost after adjustment for heart rates. This suggests that the beneficial effect of calcium channel blockers in this category of patients is largely dependent upon their effect on heart rate.

It is important to recognize that in the first study there is a positive correlation between peripheral flow and clinical benefit (when peripheral flow increases benefit gets better), whereas in the second study there is a negative correlation between heart rate and clinical benefit (when heart increases benefit gets worse). Multiple variables analysis only measures dependencies but makes no differences between a positive and negative correlation. So, we must not forget to look at the trend in the data before interpretations can be made.

3   Logistic Regression Equation

Logistic regression is similar to linear regression the main equation of which is explained in Chap. 11:

$$y = a + b_1 x_1 + b_2 x_2 + \dots b_n x_n$$

Linear regression software finds for you an equation that best predicts the outcome y from one or more x variables. Continuous data are measured. Y is assumed to be the expected value of a normal distribution. With y being a binary (yes/no) variable, the proportion of, e.g., "yes" data (p in the underneath example) lies between 0 and 1, and this is too small a range of values for the expression of a summary of multiple variables like $a + b_1 x_1 + b_2 x_2 + \dots b_n x_n$. The range of y-responses can be broadened to 0 to ∞ if we take $p/(1-p)$ as y-variable, and even to $-\infty$ to $+\infty$ if we take $\ln p/(1-p)$. The simplest logistic regression model using only a single x-variable can be presented in a contingency table of proportional data:

	High	Low leucocyte count
Transplant rejections	p_1	$1-p_1$
No transplant rejections	p_0	$1-p_0$

$$\ln \frac{p_1}{1-p_1} = bx + a$$

$$\text{If } x = 1 \rightarrow \ln \frac{p_1}{1-p_1} = b + a$$

$$\text{If } x = 0 \rightarrow \ln \frac{p_0}{1-p_0} = a$$

$$\ln \frac{\dfrac{p_1}{1-p_1}}{\dfrac{p_0}{1-p_0}} = b$$

Odds ratio $= e^b$

$p/(1-p) =$ the odds of finding yes-data. The regression coefficient value (b-value) in the logistic regression equation can be best understood as the natural logarithm of the odds ratio of finding $p_1/(1-p_1)$ given $p_0/(1-p_0)$. Although with multiple-variables logistic regression becomes a formidable technique, it is straightforward to understand, and logistic regression increasingly finds its way into the secondary analysis of trial data.

4   Conclusions

Sometimes it is decided already at the design stage of a clinical trial to perform post-hoc analyses in order to test secondary hypotheses. For the purpose of power we may make two new groups: those who have improvement and those who have not, irrespective of the type of treatment. We, then, can perform a regression analysis of the two new groups trying to find independent determinants of improvement. If one or more determinants for adjustment are binary, which is generally so, our choice of test is logistic regression analysis. This procedure does of course provide no proof. However, it may give strong support for the presence of particular underlying mechanisms in the data. Also, it gives you odds ratios presenting the relative presence of a beneficial outcome in a treatment group as compared to that in a control group.

References

Cleophas TJ, Remmert HP, Kauw FH (1996) Celiprolol versus propranolol in unstable angina pectoris. Clin Pharmacol Ther 45:476–473
Van der Vring AF, Cleophas TJ, Zwinderman AH et al (1999) Different classes of calcium channel blockers in addition beta-blockers for exercise induced angina pectoris. Br J Clin Pharmacol 50:545–560

Chapter 20
Multistage Regression

1 Introduction

The basic idea of multistage regression goes back to the early thirtieth when Sewal Wright, professor of economics at the University of Chicago, described direct and indirect predictors (Wright 1928). If you want to predict the price of vegetables, then the weather-reports seemed to be a better predictor than problematic information about the crops (Wright 1928). Indirect predictors are defined as instrumental variables that come from a detailed knowledge of the underlying mechanisms determining both the predictor and the outcome (Angrist and Krueger 2001). They are widely applied in economics, but in the past years a few studies on health statistics have been published: cigarette tax, counselling, proximity of health facility better predicted health outcomes than did direct causal factors (Evans and Ringel 1999; Permutt and Hebel 1989; McClellan et al. 1994).

In clinical pharmacology multistage regression is rarely used: searching Pubmed, we found four molecular biology studies (O'Reilly et al. 2009; Morris 2010; Gibbons et al. 1986; Steiner et al. 1985), and two toxicological studies (Qiu 2007; Eyler et al. 2009), and only three drug efficacy studies (Meltzer et al. 2000; Tollefson and Sanger 1997; Barone et al. 2010). This is remarkable, given the multistage patterns of many medical conditions. We have to add that modern analytical models like linear, logistic, and Cox regression, although they allow for multiple predictors, only assess single step relationships to the outcome variable. With multistage regression the predictors are supposed to produce not only direct effects on the outcome variable, but also indirect effects through concomitant predictors. This chapter uses a simple evaluation study of a new treatment to assess whether multistage regression better predicts the efficacy of a new treatment than does the standard methodology. We hope that this chapter will stimulate researchers analyzing efficacy data of new treatments to more often apply multistage regression.

T.J. Cleophas and A.H. Zwinderman, *Statistics Applied to Clinical Studies*,
DOI 10.1007/978-94-007-2863-9_20, © Springer Science+Business Media B.V. 2012

2   An Example, Usual Linear Regression Modeling

Patients' non-compliance is a factor notoriously affecting the estimation of drug efficacy. An example is given of a simple evaluation study that assesses the effect of non-compliance on the efficacy of a novel laxative, with numbers of stools in a month as efficacy estimator, (the y-variable) and "pills not used" as non-compliance variable and predictor (the x-variable). The data are in Table 20.1. We use linear regression for data analysis. The magnitude of the regression coefficient (b-value) and of the correlation coefficient (r-value) are used for estimating the strength of association between the predictor and outcome variable. Significant b- and r-values indicate that the association is better than a zero-association is, and, thus, that the data are closer to the regression line than could happen by the play of chance. With simple linear regression the "pills not used" was a significant predictor of "treatment efficacy" with a p-value of 0.005, a b-value of 0.70, and an r-square value of 0.18. This means that non-compliance predicted treatment efficacy only by 18%, and that 82% was unexplained. Two x-variables generally give more precision than a single one to determine the y-variable (outcome variable). Therefore, a second x-variable was included in the model, the numbers of counselling events per patient, and a multiple linear regression was performed. Indeed, the overall r-square value rose from 0.18 to 0.66: non-compliance and counselling together predicted the outcome by 66% (p=0.0001). However, non-compliance was not very significant anymore (b=0.29, p=0.09) with a decrease of the b-value by 58.6%.

3   Path Analysis

We might be able to do better, if we take into account, that non-compliant patients not only use fewer drugs, but also tend to attend fewer counselling events. This may contribute, indirectly, to their non-compliant behavior. In order to account for this possible indirect effect of counselling path analysis can be adequately used. The requirements for a path analysis include

(1). a significant effect of the predictors variables on the outcome variable in the
      multiple linear regression, and
(2). a significant correlation between the predictor variables.

Using the p<0.10 as level for significance, both requirement (1) and (2) were met, with p-values of 0.0001, 0.09, and 0.024 (Fig. 20.1).

Essentially, path analysis assumes two effects, (1) the effect of non-compliance on efficacy and (2) the effect of non-compliance through counselling on efficacy. These two effects can be, simply, added up, and can be used to cover the joint effect of non-compliance on the efficacy.

With path analysis usual regression coefficients cannot be used, because they have the same unit as the outcome variable, i.e., stools per months in our example.

Table 20.1 Example of a study of the effects of counselling and non-compliance on the efficacy of a novel laxative drug

Pt	Instrumental variable Frequency counselling	Problematic predictor Pills not used	Outcome Efficacy estimator of new laxative (stools/month)	Improved values of problematic predictor Pills not used	Quality of life score
1.	8	25	24	27.68	69
2.	13	30	30	30.98	110
3.	15	25	25	32.30	78
4.	14	31	35	29.00	103
5.	9	36	39	28.34	103
6.	10	33	30	29.00	102
7.	8	22	27	27.68	76
8.	5	18	14	25.70	75
9.	13	14	39	30.98	99
10.	15	30	42	32.30	107
11.	11	36	41	29.66	112
12.	11	30	38	29.66	99
13.	12	27	39	30.32	86
14.	10	38	37	29.00	107
15.	15	40	47	32.30	108
16.	13	31	30	30.98	95
17.	12	25	36	30.32	88
18.	4	24	12	25.04	67
19.	10	27	26	29.00	112
20.	8	20	20	27.68	87
21.	16	35	43	32.96	115
22.	15	29	31	32.30	93
23.	14	32	40	31.64	92
24.	7	30	31	27.02	78
25.	12	40	36	30.32	112
26.	6	31	21	26.36	69
27.	19	41	44	34.94	66
28.	5	26	11	25.70	75
29.	8	24	27	27.68	85
30.	9	30	24	28.34	87
31.	15	20	40	32.30	89
32.	7	31	32	27.02	89
33.	6	29	10	26.36	65
34.	14	43	37	31.64	121
35.	7	30	19	27.02	74

Counselling has a unit different from that of efficacy, namely frequency of counselling events. If we want to add up the effects of both variables, their units will have to be the same. Standardizing the data is the solution. For that purpose both the values and their variance are divided by their own variance.

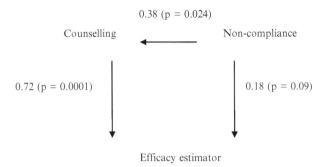

Fig. 20.1 Path diagram of study assessing the direct and indirect effects of non-compliance on efficacy of a new laxative

$$\text{Values} \quad (\text{variance of values})$$

$$\frac{\text{Values}}{\text{variance}} \quad \left(\frac{\text{variance of values}}{\text{variance}}\right)$$

The "values/variance" terms are called the standardized values. They have a variance of 1, which is very convenient for the calculations. In the analysis all regressions are performed on standardized values, giving rise to standardized regression coefficients, which can be simply added up, since they now have the same unit, while variances (equalling 1) no longer have to be taken into account. The standardized regression coefficients are calculated by many software programs. SPSS statistical software (Barone et al. 2010) routinely reports the standardized regression coefficients together with the usual regression coefficients. With simple linear regression the standardized regression coefficient is equal to the r-value. A path diagram must be constructed with arrows for indicating supposed causal effect paths. Figure 20.1 summarizes the supposed effects for our example: (a) non-compliance causes an effect on efficacy, and (b) non-compliance causes an additional effect on efficacy though counselling. The standardized regression coefficients are added to the arrows (Fig. 20.1). Then, they are added up according to:

$$0.18 + 0.38 \times 0.72 = 0.18 + 0.27 = 0.45.$$

This result is expressed as the path statistic, and equals the sum of the standardized regression coefficients. Its magnitude is sometimes interpreted similarly to the overall r-square value of a multiple regression, but this is not entirely correct. Unlike r-square values, standardized regression coefficients and their sums can be somewhat larger than 1.0. Also negative indirect factors are sometimes produced, reducing the magnitude of the add-up sums. Yet, the interpretation is much the same. The larger the result of your path statistic, the better the independent variable predicts the dependent one. And, so, the two-path statistic of 0.45 is a lot better than the single-path statistic of 0.18 with an increase of 60.0% (Fig. 20.1).

4 Multistage Least Squares Method

Instead of path analysis multistage least square is another possibility for the analysis of the above study. Also this method requires both a significant correlation between the predictors and the outcome in the multiple regression, and a significant correlation between the predictors. The simplest version, called 2 stage least squares (2SLS), is available in the regression module of SPSS (2011), and is adequate for most data files. The analysis can also be performed applying the usual linear regression commands without the 2SLS commands. Its theoretical basis is slightly different from that of path analysis. Path analysis assumes causal pathways. The 2SLS method assumes that in a linear regression the independent variable (x-variable), here traditionally called the exogenous variable, is problematic. Problematic means that it is somewhat uncertain. Basically, the method of linear regression does not allow for uncertainty of the x-variable: the x-values are measured with 100% certainty. However, in practice there are many situations where this assumption is not warranted. For example, non-compliant patients are not very helpful to make the assessment for non-compliance 100% certain. If an additional variable can be argued to provide additional information about a problematic variable, it may be worthwhile to include it in the analysis. The variable counselling in the above example may, indeed, cause improvement of patients' compliance and, thus, also, indirectly improve the outcome variable. In the 2SLS model counselling is, thus, used as an instrumental variable, for the purpose of reducing the uncertainty of the problematic variable non-compliance.

The analysis consists of two stages.

1st stage
A simple linear regression is performed with non-compliance as outcome and counselling as independent variable. For convenience the independent variable is here called the z-variable.

The result shows a significant correlation with a p-value of 0.024 and the following equation:

$$x - values = intercept + regression\ coefficient * z - values$$
$$= 22.4 + 0.66 * z - values$$
$$(* = sign\ of\ multiplication).$$

With the help of the above equation, modified (and improved) x-values are calculated, e.g. for patient no 1

$$x = 22.4 + 0.66 * 8$$
$$= 27.68$$

In Table 20.1 the improved x-values are given in column 4.

2nd stage

A simple linear regression is performed with efficacy as outcome and the improved x-values as predictor. The result shows a very significant correlation with a p-value of 0.0001 and the following equation (* = sign of multiplication):

$$y - value = intercept + regression\ coefficient * improved\ x - values$$
$$= -117.7 + 6.99 * improved\ x - values$$

The r-square value = 0.54. This would mean that knowing the improved x-values we can predict with 54% certainty the efficacy of the novel laxative. Using the problematic x-variable the result produced a significant effect with p = 0.011. However, the r-square value was a lot smaller, 0.18 compared to the 0.54, with an increase of 66.7%.

5   Bivariate Analysis Using Path Analysis

Not only frequency of stools, but also quality of life may be considered an important outcome variable of drug efficacy. The addition of such an outcome variable may enable to make even better use from our predicting variables. For that purpose a multivariate regression with two rather than one outcome variable would be an interesting option. However, this option is not available in SPSS (Barone et al. 2010) and many other software programs. A pleasant thing about path analysis is that it can, indeed, be used as an alternative approach to multivariate regression, with a result similar to that of the more complex mathematical approach. As an example, we extend the data from the above study with quality of life scores of the patients. We assume that counselling and non-compliance not only affect the efficacy of the drug but also the patients' quality of life. First, we have to check that the relationship of either of the two predictors with the outcome quality of life is significant in the usual regression model: they were so with p-values of 0.03 and 0.02. Then, a path diagram with standardized regression coefficients is constructed (Fig. 20.2). The standardized regression coefficients of the residual effects are obtained by taking the square root of $(1 - r^2)$. The standardized regression coefficient of one residual effect versus another can be assumed to equal 1.00.

We now find the overall correlation between the two outcome variables as follows:

1. Direct effect of counselling	
$0.72 \times 0.31 =$	0.22
2. Direct effect of non-compliance	
$0.32 \times 0.18 =$	0.06
3. Indirect effect of counselling and non-compliance	
$0.72 \times 0.38 \times 0.32 + 0.18 \times 0.38 \times 0.31 =$	0.11
4. Residual effects	
$1.00 \times 0.58 \times 0.83 =$	0.48 +
Total	0.85

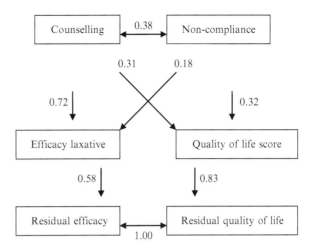

Fig. 20.2 Decomposition of correlation between efficacy laxative and quality of life score, all of the correlations in the above example were statistically significant at $p < 0.10$

A path statistic of 0.85 is considerably larger than that of the single outcome model: 0.85 versus 0.45 (47.1% larger). Obviously, two outcome variables make better use of the predictors in our data than does a single one. An advantage of this nonmathematical approach to multivariate regression is that it nicely summarizes all relationships in the model, and it does so in a quantitative way (Fig. 20.2).

6   Discussion

The present chapter uses data of an efficacy study of a new treatment to explain path analysis and multistage least squares. Both are multistep statistical methods that are adequate for simultaneous assessment of direct and indirect effects. They are very successful in economics, but rarely used in clinical research. The current chapter shows that they can be readily applied to efficacy studies, and enable to make better predictions from your data than does usual linear regression.

This possible benefit may be extended to studies of more general health issues. A problem with such studies is that they frequently have to make use of rather uncertain predictor variables, for example levels of arteriosclerosis, and inflammation may predict cardiovascular death and severity of infections respectively, but such levels are difficult to measure. Table 20.2 gives some more examples. The performance of multistep statistics with these examples has not been tested, but the results of the simple efficacy study in this paper supports benefits similar to those of economical studies as widely published (Wright 1928; Angrist and Krueger 2001).

A pleasant thing about path analysis is that it can be used for a nonmathematical approach of multivariate regression. We should emphasize that the term multivariate regression is often erroneously applied, when multiple independent and

Table 20.2 Example of possible instrumental variables for studies with problematic predictors

Instrumental variable	Problematic predictor	Outcome
Assignment to small school classes	School class size	Achievement score
Alcohol tax	Use of alcoholic beverages	Liver disease
Regulatory measures	Use of hard drugs	Death
Hours of TV	Home work	Achievement score
C-reactive protein	Level of inflammation	Severity of infection
Cholesterol levels	Level arteriosclerosis	Cardiovascular death

just a single dependent variable are in the data. Strictly, multivariate regression regards models with more than a single dependent variable (y-variable). The main aim is to quantify reasons for the correlation between two or more dependent variables. In our hands the multivariate model of our data with two instead of one outcome variables made even better use of the predictors than did the single outcome model.

Some limitations of multistep regression have to be mentioned. First, instrumental variables may be weak predictors. In order to exclude weak predictors multistage regression should always be preceded by the usual multiple regression: only relatively strong predictor variables significantly predicting the outcome variables can be included. Second, also significant correlations between the predictor variables are required. At the same time, however, they must not be too strong. An r-value > 0.85 indicates the presence of collinearity, which is an important validity criterion of multiple regression.

We conclude that

1. multistep regression methods, as used in the present paper produced much better predictions about the drug efficacy than did standard linear regression;
2. the inclusion of additional outcome variables enables to make still better use of the predicting variables;
3. multistage regression must always be preceded by usual linear regression in order to exclude weak predictors.

7   Conclusions

Multistage regression is rarely used in therapeutic research despite the multistage pattern of many medical conditions.

Using an example of an efficacy study of a new laxative, path analysis and the two stage least square method were compared with standard linear regression.

Standard linear regression showed a significant effect of the predictor "noncompliance" on drug efficacy at $p = 0.005$. However, after adjustment for the covariate "counselling", the magnitude of the regression coefficient fell from 0.70 to 0.29, and the p – value rose to 0.10.

Path analysis was valid, given the significant correlation between the two predictors ($p = 0.024$), and produced an increase of the regression coefficient between "non-compliance" and "drug efficacy" by 60.0%. The two stage least squares method, using "counselling" as instrumental variable, produced, similarly, an increase of the overall correlation by 66.7%.

A bivariate path analysis with "quality of life" as second outcome variable increased the magnitude of the path statistic further by 47.1%, and, thus, enabled to make still better use of the predicting variables.

We conclude that

1. multistage regression methods, as used in the present paper produced much better predictions about the drug efficacy than did standard linear regression;
2. the inclusion of additional outcome variables enables to make still better use of the predicting variables;
3. multistage regression must always be preceded by usual linear regression in order to exclude weak predictors.

We recommend that researchers analyzing efficacy data of new treatments more often apply multistage regression.

References

Angrist JD, Krueger AB (2001) Instrumental variables and the search for identification: from supply and demand to natural experiments. J Econ Perspect 15:69–85

Barone P, Poewe W, Albrecht S, Debleuve C, Massey D, Rascol O, Tolosa E, Weintraub D (2010) Pramipexole for the treatments of depressive symptoms in patients with Parkinson's disease: a double blind placebo controlled trial. Lancet Neurol 9:573–580

Evans W, Ringel J (1999) Can higher cigarette taxes improve birth outcomes? J Public Econ 72:135–154

Eyler FD, Warner TD, Behnke M, Hou W, Wobie K, Wilson GC (2009) Executive functioning at ages 5 and 7 years in children with prenatal cocaine exposure. Dev Neurosci 31:121–136

Gibbons RD, Maas JW, Davis JM, Swann AC, Redmond DE, Casper RC, Hanin I, Bowden CL, Kocsis J, Stokes PE (1986) Path analysis of psychopharmacological data: catecholamine breakdown in man. Psychiatr Res 18:89–105

McClellan M, McNeil B, Newhouse JP (1994) Does more intensive treatment of acute myocardial infarction in the elderly reduce mortality? JAMA 272:859–866

Meltzer H, Arato M, Connor O (2000) Path analysis of the ZEUS study provides evidence of direct effect of ziprasidone on primary negative symptoms in chronic stable schizophrenia. Schizophr Res 41(Special Iss 1):B 91

Morris MS (2010) Opioid modulation of oxytocin release. J Clin Pharmacol 50:1112–1117

O'Reilly KC, Shumake J, Bailey SJ, Gonzalez-Lima F, Lane MA (2009) Chronic 13-cis-retinoid acid administration disrupts network interactions between the raphne nuclei and the hippocampal system in young adult mice. Eur J Pharmacol 605:68–77

Permutt T, Hebel JR (1989) Simultaneous estimation in a clinical trial of the effect of smoking on birth weight. Biometrics 45:619–622

Qiu L (2007) Path analysis of biomarkers of exposure and early biologic effects among coke-oven workers exposed to polycyclic aromatic hydrocarbons. Cancer Epidemiol Biomark Rev 16:1193–1199

SPSS statistical software. www.SPSS.com. Accessed 14 Dec 2011

Steiner E, Iselius L, Alvan G, Lindsten J, Sjoqvist F (1985) A family study of genetic and environmental factors determining polymorphic hydroxylation of debrisoquin. Clin Pharmacol Ther
38:394–401

Tollefson GD, Sanger TM (1997) Negative symptoms: a path analysis approach to a double
Blind placebo and haloperidol controlled clinical trial with olanzapine. Am J Psychiatr
154:466–474

Wright S (1928) Appendix. In: Wright PC (ed) The tariff on animal and vegetable oils. Macmillan,
New York

Chapter 21
Categorical Data

1 Introduction

A major objective of clinical research is to improve the effectiveness of individual therapies by studying treatment effects and health effects in subgroups of patients, for example age-groups, races, genders etc. Sometimes, the use of continuous or binary variables are possible for the purpose. However, races, numbers of co-medications, co-morbidities and many more variables in clinical research have stepping functions with a limited number of values, e.g., *four* races, *zero to eight* co-medications etc. If such stepping functions are analyzed using continuous variables in a linear or logistic regression model, we assume that the outcome variable will rise linearly, but this needs not necessarily be so. This assumption raises the risk of underestimating the effects. In the given situation, it may be more safe to recode the stepping variables into the form of categorical variables.

Until the late 1990s the proper handling of categories received little attention from the scientific community. In 1996 Nichols polled statistical software users, and found out that the proper use of categorical variables was of major concern to them (Nichols 1996). In the past few years adequate methods for coding categorical variables have been published (Williams 2006; Long and Freese 2006; Anonymous 2010a, b; Skrondal and Rabe-Hesketh 2005). Unfortunately, statistical software programs, to date, do not routinely allow for recoding stepping variables into categorical ones. For example, with linear regression analysis in SPSS (SPSS statistical software 2011) categorical variables have to be created. In contrast, logistic regression in SPSS provides a special dialog box for the purpose.

In the current chapter we will demonstrate from examples how recoding works. The examples show that the stepping functions, if used as continuous variables, do not produce significant effects, whereas they produce very significant effects after recoding. We hope this explanatory chapter will be helpful to researchers assessing categories.

T.J. Cleophas and A.H. Zwinderman, *Statistics Applied to Clinical Studies*,
DOI 10.1007/978-94-007-2863-9_21, © Springer Science+Business Media B.V. 2012

2   Races as a Categorical Variable

In the first example the effects of race on physical strength are studied. Physical strength scores are assessed in four groups of each 15 subjects with different races (hispanics, blacks, asians and whites). The data are in Table 21.1. The effects of gender and age on physical strength are pretty predictable, but those of races are rather uncertain (White 1972). Yet, we decided to analyze the effect of race together with the factors gender and age in a multiple linear regression model with physical strength as outcome variable. The races hispanics, blacks, asians, and whites were given the numbers of respectively 1–4. The result of the analysis is shown in Table 21.2.

Table 21.1 The effects on physical strength (scores 0–100) are assessed in 60 subjects of different races (hispanics (1), blacks (2), asians (3), and whites (4)), ages (years), and genders (0=female, 1=male)

Patient number	Physical strength	Race	Age	Gender
1	70,00	1,00	35,00	1,00
2	77,00	1,00	55,00	0,00
3	66,00	1,00	70,00	1,00
4	59,00	1,00	55,00	0,00
5	71,00	1,00	45,00	1,00
6	72,00	1,00	47,00	1,00
7	45,00	1,00	75,00	0,00
8	85,00	1,00	83,00	1,00
9	70,00	1,00	35,00	1,00
10	77,00	1,00	49,00	1,00
11	63,00	1,00	74,00	0,00
12	72,00	1,00	49,00	1,00
13	78,00	1,00	54,00	1,00
14	62,00	1,00	46,00	0,00
15	69,00	1,00	34,00	1,00
16	90,00	2,00	25,00	1,00
17	98,00	2,00	46,00	1,00
18	82,00	2,00	35,00	1,00
19	83,00	2,00	50,00	1,00
20	90,00	2,00	52,00	1,00
21	86,00	2,00	46,00	1,00
22	59,00	2,00	53,00	0,00
23	99,00	2,00	44,00	1,00
24	87,00	2,00	30,00	0,00
25	78,00	2,00	80,00	1,00
26	96,00	2,00	56,00	1,00
27	97,00	2,00	55,00	0,00
28	89,00	2,00	35,00	1,00
29	90,00	2,00	58,00	1,00

(continued)

Table 21.1 (continued)

Patient number	Physical strength	Race	Age	Gender
30	91,00	2,00	57,00	0,00
31	60,00	3,00	65,00	1,00
32	61,00	3,00	45,00	1,00
33	66,00	3,00	51,00	0,00
34	54,00	3,00	55,00	0,00
35	53,00	3,00	82,00	0,00
36	57,00	3,00	64,00	0,00
37	63,00	3,00	40,00	0,00
38	70,00	3,00	36,00	1,00
39	59,00	3,00	64,00	0,00
40	62,00	3,00	55,00	0,00
41	65,00	3,00	50,00	1,00
42	67,00	3,00	53,00	0,00
43	53,00	3,00	73,00	0,00
44	69,00	3,00	34,00	1,00
45	51,00	3,00	55,00	0,00
46	54,00	4,00	59,00	0,00
47	68,00	4,00	64,00	1,00
48	69,00	4,00	45,00	0,00
49	70,00	4,00	36,00	1,00
50	90,00	4,00	43,00	0,00
51	90,00	4,00	23,00	1,00
52	89,00	4,00	44,00	1,00
53	82,00	4,00	83,00	0,00
54	85,00	4,00	40,00	1,00
55	87,00	4,00	42,00	1,00
56	86,00	4,00	32,00	0,00
57	83,00	4,00	43,00	1,00
58	80,00	4,00	35,00	1,00
59	81,00	4,00	34,00	0,00
60	82,00	4,00	33,00	1,00

Table 21.2 Linear regression analysis with physical strength score as dependent and race, age, and gender as independent variable (p-values <0.10 are defined statistically significant)

Coefficients[a]

Model		Unstandardized coefficients		Standardized coefficients		
		B	Std. error	Beta	t	Sig.
1	(Constant)	79,528	8,657		9,186	,000
	Race	,511	1,454	,042	,351	,727
	Age	−,242	,117	−,260	−2,071	,043
	Gender	9,575	3,417	,349	2,802	,007

[a]Dependent Variable: strengthscore

Obviously, race is not a significant predictor of physical strength, suggesting that physical strength scores are not significantly different between different races. However, this linear regression model looked at the linear effect of race, which was, actually, not what we intended to do. We intended to look at any differences between the races, and the linear model was a wrong model for that purpose. For assessing any differences between the races it is more adequate to analyze the races as categories. In order to assess the effects of races on strength scores, we manually recode the variable in such a way that all information about the four races is given in the model. For that purpose four new variables are created. Table 21.3 shows how it works.

For the analysis we use, otherwise, the same multiple linear regression model as that of Table 21.1, and, in addition, three of the four new variables as additional independent variables. Table 21.4 gives the result of the analysis. Race is now a very significant predictor of physical strength. The result shown in Table 21.4 can be interpreted as follows.

The underneath regression equation is used:

$$y = a + b_1 x_1 + b_2 x_2 + b_3 x_3 + b_4 x_4 + b_5 x_5$$

a = intercept
b_1 = regression coefficient for blacks (0 = no, 1 = yes),
b_2 = regression coefficient for asians
b_3 = regression coefficient for whites
b_4 = regression coefficient for age
b_5 = regression coefficient for gender

Table 21.3 The race variable from Table 21.1 is recoded into four binary variables, one for each race (1 = presence of race, 0 = absence of race)

Patient number	Physical strength	Race	Age	Gender	Race 1 Hispanics	Race 2 Blacks	Race 3 Asians	Race 4 Whites
1	70,00	1,00	35,00	1,00	1,00	0,00	0,00	0,00
2	77,00	1,00	55,00	0,00	1,00	0,00	0,00	0,00
3	66,00	1,00	70,00	1,00	1,00	0,00	0,00	0,00
4	59,00	1,00	55,00	0,00	1,00	0,00	0,00	0,00
5	71,00	1,00	45,00	1,00	1,00	0,00	0,00	0,00
6	72,00	1,00	47,00	1,00	1,00	0,00	0,00	0,00
7	45,00	1,00	75,00	0,00	1,00	0,00	0,00	0,00
8	85,00	1,00	83,00	1,00	1,00	0,00	0,00	0,00
9	70,00	1,00	35,00	1,00	1,00	0,00	0,00	0,00
10	77,00	1,00	49,00	1,00	1,00	0,00	0,00	0,00
11	63,00	1,00	74,00	0,00	1,00	0,00	0,00	0,00
12	72,00	1,00	49,00	1,00	1,00	0,00	0,00	0,00
13	78,00	1,00	54,00	1,00	1,00	0,00	0,00	0,00
14	62,00	1,00	46,00	0,00	1,00	0,00	0,00	0,00
15	69,00	1,00	34,00	1,00	1,00	0,00	0,00	0,00

(continued)

Table 21.3 (continued)

Patient number	Physical strength	Race	Age	Gender	Race 1 Hispanics	Race 2 Blacks	Race 3 Asians	Race 4 Whites
16	90,00	2,00	25,00	1,00	0,00	1,00	0,00	0,00
17	98,00	2,00	46,00	1,00	0,00	1,00	0,00	0,00
18	82,00	2,00	35,00	1,00	0,00	1,00	0,00	0,00
19	83,00	2,00	50,00	1,00	0,00	1,00	0,00	0,00
20	90,00	2,00	52,00	1,00	0,00	1,00	0,00	0,00
21	86,00	2,00	46,00	1,00	0,00	1,00	0,00	0,00
22	59,00	2,00	53,00	0,00	0,00	1,00	0,00	0,00
23	99,00	2,00	44,00	1,00	0,00	1,00	0,00	0,00
24	87,00	2,00	30,00	0,00	0,00	1,00	0,00	0,00
25	78,00	2,00	80,00	1,00	0,00	1,00	0,00	0,00
26	96,00	2,00	56,00	1,00	0,00	1,00	0,00	0,00
27	97,00	2,00	55,00	0,00	0,00	1,00	0,00	0,00
28	89,00	2,00	35,00	1,00	0,00	1,00	0,00	0,00
29	90,00	2,00	58,00	1,00	0,00	1,00	0,00	0,00
30	91,00	2,00	57,00	0,00	0,00	1,00	0,00	0,00
31	60,00	3,00	65,00	1,00	0,00	0,00	1,00	0,00
32	61,00	3,00	45,00	1,00	0,00	0,00	1,00	0,00
33	66,00	3,00	51,00	0,00	0,00	0,00	1,00	0,00
34	54,00	3,00	55,00	0,00	0,00	0,00	1,00	0,00
35	53,00	3,00	82,00	0,00	0,00	0,00	1,00	0,00
36	57,00	3,00	64,00	0,00	0,00	0,00	1,00	0,00
37	63,00	3,00	40,00	0,00	0,00	0,00	1,00	0,00
38	70,00	3,00	36,00	1,00	0,00	0,00	1,00	0,00
39	59,00	3,00	64,00	0,00	0,00	0,00	1,00	0,00
40	62,00	3,00	55,00	0,00	0,00	0,00	1,00	0,00
41	65,00	3,00	50,00	1,00	0,00	0,00	1,00	0,00
42	67,00	3,00	53,00	0,00	0,00	0,00	1,00	0,00
43	53,00	3,00	73,00	0,00	0,00	0,00	1,00	0,00
44	69,00	3,00	34,00	1,00	0,00	0,00	1,00	0,00
45	51,00	3,00	55,00	0,00	0,00	0,00	1,00	0,00
46	54,00	4,00	59,00	0,00	0,00	0,00	0,00	1,00
47	68,00	4,00	64,00	1,00	0,00	0,00	0,00	1,00
48	69,00	4,00	45,00	0,00	0,00	0,00	0,00	1,00
49	70,00	4,00	36,00	1,00	0,00	0,00	0,00	1,00
50	90,00	4,00	43,00	0,00	0,00	0,00	0,00	1,00
51	90,00	4,00	23,00	1,00	0,00	0,00	0,00	1,00
52	89,00	4,00	44,00	1,00	0,00	0,00	0,00	1,00
53	82,00	4,00	83,00	0,00	0,00	0,00	0,00	1,00
54	85,00	4,00	40,00	1,00	0,00	0,00	0,00	1,00
55	87,00	4,00	42,00	1,00	0,00	0,00	0,00	1,00
56	86,00	4,00	32,00	0,00	0,00	0,00	0,00	1,00
57	83,00	4,00	43,00	1,00	0,00	0,00	0,00	1,00
58	80,00	4,00	35,00	1,00	0,00	0,00	0,00	1,00
59	81,00	4,00	34,00	0,00	0,00	0,00	0,00	1,00
60	82,00	4,00	33,00	1,00	0,00	0,00	0,00	1,00

Table 21.4 Linear regression analysis with physical strength score as dependent and the presence of race 2 (blacks), race 3 (asians), and race 4 (whites), age, and gender as independent variables (p-values <0.10 are defined statistically significant)

Coefficients[a]

Model		Unstandardized coefficients		Standardized coefficients		
		B	Std. error	Beta	t	Sig.
1	(Constant)	72,650	5,528		13,143	,000
	Race 2	17,424	3,074	,559	5,668	,000
	Race 3	−6,286	3,141	−,202	−2,001	,050
	Race 4	9,661	3,166	,310	3,051	,004
	Age	−,140	,081	−,150	−1,716	,092
	Gender	5,893	2,403	,215	2,452	,017

[a]Dependent Variables: strengthscore

If an individual is hispanic (race 1), then x_1, x_2, and x_3 will turn into 0, and the regression equation becomes $y = a + b_4 x_4 + b_5 x_5$.

$$\text{If black, } y = a + b_1 + b_4 x_4 + b_5 x_5$$
$$\text{If asian, } y = a + b_2 + b_4 x_4 + b_5 x_5$$
$$\text{If white, } y = a + b_3 + b_4 x_4 + b_5 x_5$$

So, e.g., the best predicted physical strength score of a white male of 25 years of age would equal

$y = 72.65 + 9.66 − 0.14 * 25 + 5.89 * 1 = 84.7$ (on a linear scale from 0 to 100), (* = sign of multiplication).

Compared to the presence of the hispanic race, the black and white races are significant positive predictors of physical strength (p=0.0001 and 0.004 respectively), the asian race is a significant negative predictor (p=0.050). All of these results are adjusted for age and gender.

3   Numbers of Co-medications as a Categorical Variable

Numbers of co-medications may be positively correlated with admissions to hospital due to adverse drug effects. In the second example we use the data from a recently published cohort study from our group (Atiqi et al. 2010) about adverse-drug-effect-admissions to assess this question.

In a logistic regression with numbers of co-medications (zero to eight) as independent and adverse-drug-effect-admission as dependent variable the correlation was, indeed, very significant at p=0.0001. However, after adjustment for age, gender, and presence of co-morbidity this significant correlation was lost, suggesting the presence of confounding rather than a true effect. The results of the analysis are in Table 21.5. This negative finding did not at all agree with our prior expectations.

Table 21.5 Multiple binary logistic regression analysis of 2,000 admissions to hospital with the odds of iatrogenic admission as dependent variable and age (variable 1), gender (variable 2), presence of co-morbidity (variable 9, yes = 0, no = 1), and number of co-medications (variable 10, zero to eight co-medications) as independent variables (p-values <0.10 are defined statistically significant)

Variables in the equation							
		B	S.E.	Wald	df	Sig.	Exp (B)
Step 1[a]	VAR00001	−,023	,004	32,062	1	,000	,977
	VAR00002	,089	,116	,580	1	,446	1,093
	VAR00010	,004	,072	,003	1	,953	1,004
	VAR00009	,095	,073	1,672	1	,196	1,099
	Constant	43,752	8,077	29,345	1	,000	1,003E19

[a]Variable(s) entered on step 1: VAR00001, VAR00002, VAR00010, VAR00009

Table 21.6 The same data as those from Table 21.5. Co-medication has been recoded from a continuous into a categorical variable with nine categories (zero to eight co-medications), (p-values <0.10 are defined statistically significant)

Variables in the equation							
		B	S.E.	Wald	df	Sig.	Exp (B)
Step 1[a]	VAR00001	−,024	,004	32,859	1	,000	,976
	VAR00002	,080	,117	,470	1	,493	1,084
	VAR00010			22,241	8	,004	
	VAR00010(1)	18,900	40199,059	,000	1	1,000	1,615E8
	VAR00010(2)	19,490	40199,059	,000	1	1,000	2,914E8
	VAR00010(3)	18,923	40199,059	,000	1	1,000	1,653E8
	VAR00010(4)	19,342	40199,059	,000	1	1,000	2,514E8
	VAR00010(5)	18,820	40199,059	,000	1	1,000	1,491E8
	VAR00010(6)	19,122	40199,059	,000	1	1,000	2,017E8
	VAR00010(7)	17,932	40199,059	,000	1	1,000	6,133E7
	VAR00010(8)	−1,109	56845,749	,000	1	1,000	,330
	VAR00009	,109	,076	2,047	1	,152	1,115
	Constant	25,804	40199,060	,000	1	,999	1,609E11

[a]Variable(s) entered on step 1:VAR00001, VAR00002, VAR00010, VAR00009.

The problem is, that, if scores "zero to eight" are used as a linear covariate in a logistic model, then we assume that the risk of adverse-drug effect-admissions rises linearly, but this needs not to be so. If the relationship is a stepping function, like with categories, and, if we assume a linear relationship, then we are at risk of severely underestimating effects. In order to escape this risk, it is more appropriate to transform a quantitative estimator used as continuous variable into a categorical one. Using logistic regression in SPSS is convenient for the purpose, we need not manually transform the quantitative estimator. For the analysis we apply the usual commands: analyze – regression – binary logistic – enter dependent variable – enter independent variables. Then, open dialog box labelled categorical variables, select co-medication and transfer it into the box categorical variables, then click continue. Co-medication is now transformed into a categorical variable. Click OK. The Table 21.6 gives the results. The number of co-medications has become a very significant predictor of the risk of admissions due to adverse drug effects with a p-value of 0.004. Obviously, the numbers of co-medications is an independent predictor of adverse-drug-effect-admissions, although not strictly in a linear way. This predictor remains statistically significant even after adjustment for age, gender, and presence co-morbidity (Table 21.6).

4   Discussion

Categories are widely applied in clinical research. For example, in hypertension, cholesterol, and other consensuses for cardiovascular risk management treatment recommendations are given category-wise. Clinical trials are classified in categories, otherwise called phases. The NYHA (New York Heart Association) classifications of heart failure and angina pectoris into four categories are applied worldwide. In spite of this, categorical variables are rarely analyzed in a proper way. Mostly they are analyzed in the form of continuous variables. However, this approach does not always fit the data patterns well causing imprecise and negative results, as demonstrated in the examples of this chapter. We recommend to use the process of recoding such variables into multiple dummy variables as also demonstrated in this chapter.

However, there are other possibilities. For example with a single independent categorical variable ANOVA (analysis of variance) according to general linear models (Anonymous 2010b) or generalized linear models (Skrondal and Rabe-Hesketh 2005) can be used with the categorical variable as independent variable. The benefit of this approach is that manually creating dummy variables is not needed, and the result is statistically similar. Instead of dummy coding other codings are possible, and may better fit your data. With dummy coding one of the group becomes the reference group and all of the other groups are compared to that group. As an alternative we can create a variable comparing category 1 with 2 and another variable comparing category 2 with 3. We, thus, create coefficients that compare successive categories with one another. Other possibilities include: comparing categories with the mean of the previous or the mean of the subsequent categories, or coding categories with deviations from the mean (Williams 2006; Long and Freese 2006; Anonymous 2010a, b; Skrondal and Rabe-Hesketh 2005). Also, multiple categorical variables can be entered into regression models, and the interaction and confounding of such variables can be assessed. (Anonymous 2010b; Skrondal and Rabe-Hesketh 2005).

Finally one or two caveats are in place. Manually constructing the best fit codings for your categorical variables can be tedious and error prone. Also the more complex the models the more loss of statistical power. If you want to prove much with small data, you are at risk of proving nothing at all.

Categorical variables are rarely analyzed in a proper way. Mostly they are analyzed in the form of continuous variables. However, this approach does not always fit the data patterns well causing imprecise and negative results, as demonstrated in the examples of this chapter. We recommend to use the process of recoding such variables into multiple dummy variables.

4.1   Multinomial Logistic Regression

We should add that this chapter only addressed the analysis of categorical exposure variables, otherwise called predictor variables. However, in research it is not uncommon that outcome variables are categorical, e.g., the choice of food, treatment modality, type of doctor etc. If such outcome variables are binary then binary logistic regression is appropriate. If, however, we have three or more alternatives, then multinomial logistic regression must be used. This is available in SPSS (SPSS Statistical Software 2011) and other software programs. It works, essentially, similarly to the above recoding procedure, and can in this way be considered a multivariate technique, because the dependent variable is recoded from a single categorical variable into multiple dummy variables. More on multivariate techniques will be reviewed in Chap. 25. Multinomial logistic regression should not be confounded with ordered logistic regression which is used in case the outcome variable consists of categories that can be ordered in a meaningful way, e.g., anginal class or quality of life class. Also ordered logistic regression is readily available in most software programs.

5   Conclusions

A major objective of clinical research is to study outcome effects in subgroups. Such effects generally have stepping functions that are not strictly linear. Analyzing stepping functions in linear models, thus, raises the risk of underestimating the effects. In the past few years recoding subgroup properties from continuous variables into categorical ones has been recommended as a solution for the problem.

The objective of this chapter was to demonstrate from examples how recoding works. To show that stepping functions, if used as continuous variables, do not produce significant effects, whereas they produce very significant effects after recoding.

In the first example the effects on physical strength were assessed in 60 subjects of different races. A linear regression in SPSS with race as independent and physical strength score as dependent variable showed that race was not a significant predictor of physical strength. Using the process of recoding the variable race into categorical dummy variables showed that compared to the presence of a hispanic race, the black and white races were significant positive predictors ($p = 0.0001$ and 0.004 respectively), the asian race is a significant negative predictor ($p = 0.050$).

In the second example the effects of numbers of co-medications on admissions to hospital due to adverse drug effects were assessed. A logistic regression in SPSS with numbers of co-medications as independent variable showed that co-medications was not a significant predictor of iatrogenic admission. Using again the process of recoding for categorical dummy variables showed that co-medication was a very significant predictor of iatrogenic admission with $p = 0.004$.

Categorical variables are currently rarely analyzed in a proper way. Mostly they are analyzed in the form of continuous variables. This approach does not always fit the data patterns causing negative results, as demonstrated in the examples of this paper. We recommend that such variables be recoded into categorical dummy variables.

References

Anonymous (2010a) Regression with SPSS, regression with categorical predictors, pp 1–42. www.ats.ucla.edu/stat/spss. Accessed 14 Dec 2011

Anonymous (2010b) Regression with SAS, additional coding systems for categorical variables in regression analysis, pp 1–18. www.ats.ucla.edu/stat/sas. Accessed 14 Dec 2011

Atiqi R, Van Bommel E, Cleophas TJ, Zwinderman AH (2010) Prevalence of iatrogenic admissions to the departments of medicine, cardiology, pulmonology in a 1250 beds general hospital. Int J Clin Pharmacol Ther 48:517–525

Long JS, Freese J (2006) Regression models for categorical dependent variables, 2nd edn. Stata Press, NY

Nichols DP (1996) Using categorical variables in regression. SPSS Keywords 56:1–4

Skrondal A, Rabe-Hesketh S (2005) Structural equation modeling: categorical variables. Entry for the Encyclopedia of statistics in behavioral sciences. Wiley, London, pp 1–8

SPSS Statistical Software. www.spss.com. Accessed 14 Dec 2011

White G (1972) Muscle strength, appearance, and race. Am J Physiol Anthropol 10:31–64

Williams R (2006) Revision of regression models for categorical dependent variables. Stata J 6:273–278

Chapter 22
Missing Data

1 Introduction

The imputation of missing data using mean values or values of the "closest neighbor observed", has been routinely carried out on demographic data files since 1960 (Anonymous 2011). The appointment of congressional seats and other political decisions have been partly based on it (Anonymous 2011), and president Obama is having the White House use it again in its 2010 census (Anonymous). Also in clinical research missing data are common, but compared to demographics, clinical research produces generally smaller files, making a few missing data more of a problem than it is with demographic files. As an example, a 35 patient data file of 3 variables consists of $3 \times 35 = 105$ values if the data are complete. With only 5 values missing (1 value missing per patient) 5 patients will not have complete data, and are rather useless for the analysis. This is not 5% but 15% of this small study population of 35 patients. An analysis of the remaining 85% patients is likely not to be powerful to demonstrate the effects we wished to assess. This illustrates the necessity of data imputation. Apart from the above two methods for data imputation regression-substitution has been employed in clinical research. In principle, the blanks are replaced with the best predicted values from a multiple linear regression-equation obtained from the data available.

Imputed values are, of course, not real data, but constructed values that should increase the sensitivity of testing the data by increasing their fit to some analytical model chosen. Sensitivity is often expressed as the magnitude of the test statistic "mean value/SE (its standard error)". If a few values are imputed in a sample, then the SE will generally decrease, while the mean value might increase or decrease depending on the fit of the constructed values. Regression-substitution may be a bit more sensitive than the other two methods, because the relationship with all of the other values from the file is more closely taken into account. Yet, simple linear regressions often did not provide a better sensitivity of testing in the past (Haitovsky 1968). Nowadays, with the advent of the computer *multiple* instead of *simple* linear regression enables to include multiple independent variables rather than a single one, and this may improve its sensitivity. Also, we can think of measures like prior limitation of the acceptable number of missing data, and prior requirements regarding the strength of association, in order to improve the quality of the method.

The current chapter was written to compare different methods for handling missing data with a type of regression-substitution that uses multiple linear regression and quality measures. We hope that the measures proposed in this chapter will be helpful to researchers assessing data files with missing data.

2   Current Methods for Missing Data Imputation

Three methods of data imputation commonly used are compared. The first one, a very old procedure, is to substitute the missing data of a variable with the mean value from that same variable. The problem with this approach is that no new information is given (the overall mean will remain unchanged after the imputations), but the standard error is reduced, and, thus, precision is overstated. The second method is often called the closest neighbour datum substitution. This method is, otherwise, called hot deck imputation, a term dating back to the storage of data on punched cards. The closest neighbour observation is found by subtracting the data of the patients with the missing data from those without the missing data one by one. The add-up sums of the smallest differences will unmask the closest neighbour. The problem with this approach is that both the patient and his/her closest neighbour may be outliers, and not provide the best fit for the data. As a third method, regression-substitution is possible. The incomplete data are used to calculate the best fit equation. For example, the best fit equation may look like:

$$y = 14 + 1.8 \, x$$

If in a particular case the x-value is missing, then we can use the y-value to find the best fit x value. With $y = 42$, x should equal 16. Then we can imputate the value 16 at the place of the missing datum. This method has the advantage, compared to the mean method, that the imputed datum is in some way connected with information from all of the other data. However, this conclusion is only true if the regression coefficient, the b-value, is statistically significant.

3   A Proposed Novel Approach to Regression-Substitution

The history of regression analysis for imputating missing data started long before the era of the computer. Fisher and Yates in 1933 and Chakrabarti in 1962 used simple linear regressions for calculating auxiliary values to be used in an analysis in place of missing observations (Feingold 1982). However, the method's popularity grew with the advent of the computer facilitating multiple regression analyses. From the very start it was recognized that the sums of squares obtained were biased, and it was recommended to add artificially some error to the imputed data (Kshirsagar and Deo 1989), and current software like the SPSS add-on module for missing data is still doing this. However, this procedure is rather arbitrary, and a better approach may be to use some requirements for making the quality of the regression-substitution such that addition of artificial error is not needed. We propose the following requirements/recommendations.

(a) At least two independent variables are required for regression-substitution. This is, because in the past studies with a single independent variable did not produce a lot of sensitivity (Haitovsky 1968).
(b) With more than one missing datum in a single subject delete the subject entirely. This is because a linear regression equation can only be adequately used to find a single missing datum.
(c) The number of missing data in a data file must not be larger than 5%. This is because it can be statistically tested that any percentage <5% is not statistically different from a percentage of 0%. A percentage large than 5% can, correspondingly, be considered not to be due to chance but to some systematic mechanism, such as disease progression or cumulative drug toxicity. Finding the mechanism is, then, generally of greater importance to the interpretation of the data than imputating the missing data.
(d) If the percentage is larger than 5%, and no particular mechanism is found, e.g., 8%., then 3% could be deleted, and the remaining sample could be treated using regression-imputation.
(e) Variables with a statistically insignificant regression coefficient (b-value) should not be included in the analysis, because in this situation no relationship between the variable and the rest of the data is obvious, and, thus, no prediction about the value of the missing datum can be made from the rest of the data. With regression modeling p-values larger than 0.05 are often defined significant. We recommend that the p-values should be smaller than 0.15 at most, and that with a p-value > 0.15 the variable must be removed from the regression model.
(f) Provided that all of the above criteria are met, correction of the standard error of the imputed data file may no longer be needed.

4 Example

Thirty-five patients with constitutional constipation are treated in a crossover study with a standard laxative bisacodyl and a new compound using the numbers of stool within 1 month time as the main outcome variable. We wish to determine whether the efficacy of the standard laxative is a significant predictor of the efficacy of the new compound, and, also, whether age is a significant concomitant predictor. SPSS 17.0 (IBM SPSS 2011) was used for the linear regression analysis. Table 22.1 shows the data file, and Table 22.6 gives the results of a multiple linear regression analysis: both the standard laxative and the age are significant predictors with p-values of 0.0001 and 0.048. Table 22.2 gives the data file after randomly removing five values. This reduces the sensitivity of testing. The t-value of bisacodyl (B_1) fell from 6.3 to 5.9 (p-value 0.0001–0.0001), of age (B_2) from 2.0 to 1.7 (p-value from 0.048 to 0.101).

Table 22.1 Complete data file of 35 patients, the first and second variable indicate respectively numbers of stool on a new and on a standard laxative (bisacodyl), the third variable indicates the patients' ages

New lax	Bisacodyl	Age
24,00	8,00	25,00
30,00	13,00	30,00
25,00	15,00	25,00
35,00	10,00	31,00
39,00	9,00	36,00
30,00	10,00	33,00
27,00	8,00	22,00
14,00	5,00	18,00
39,00	13,00	14,00
42,00	15,00	30,00
41,00	11,00	36,00
38,00	11,00	30,00
39,00	12,00	27,00
37,00	10,00	38,00
47,00	18,00	40,00
30,00	13,00	31,00
36,00	12,00	25,00
12,00	4,00	24,00
26,00	10,00	27,00
20,00	8,00	20,00
43,00	16,00	35,00
31,00	15,00	29,00
40,00	14,00	32,00
31,00	7,00	30,00
36,00	12,00	40,00
21,00	6,00	31,00
44,00	19,00	41,00
11,00	5,00	26,00
27,00	8,00	24,00
24,00	9,00	30,00
40,00	15,00	20,00
32,00	7,00	31,00
10,00	6,00	23,00
37,00	14,00	43,00
19,00	7,00	30,00

lax laxative

The Tables 22.3, 22.4, and 22.5 show the effects of (1) mean imputation, (2) hot deck imputation, and (3) regression-substitution for handling the missing data. The magnitude of the r-square values is a measure for the strength of association between all variables, and is, obviously, larger with regression-substitution than with mean imputation and hot deck imputation, 0.73 vs 0.65 and 0.66. The magnitude of the F-value is a somewhat better estimate of sensitivity than the r-square value, because it is adjusted for sample size. It acts similar, 44.1 vs 29.4 and 31.0. This F-value is (much) larger with the regression substitution. The t-values are estimators of the strength of association of the separate x-variables with the y-variable, and their magnitudes are,

Table 22.2 The data file
from Table 22.1 with 22.5
data randomly removed

New lax	Bisacodyl	Age
24,00	8,00	25,00
30,00	13,00	30,00
25,00	15,00	25,00
35,00	10,00	31,00
39,00	9,00	
30,00	10,00	33,00
27,00	8,00	22,00
14,00	5,00	18,00
39,00	13,00	14,00
42,00		30,00
41,00	11,00	36,00
38,00	11,00	30,00
39,00	12,00	27,00
37,00	10,00	38,00
47,00	18,00	40,00
	13,00	31,00
36,00	12,00	25,00
12,00	4,00	24,00
26,00	10,00	27,00
20,00	8,00	20,00
43,00	16,00	35,00
31,00	15,00	29,00
40,00	14,00	32,00
31,00		30,00
36,00	12,00	40,00
21,00	6,00	31,00
44,00	19,00	41,00
11,00	5,00	26,00
27,00	8,00	24,00
24,00	9,00	30,00
40,00	15,00	
32,00	7,00	31,00
10,00	6,00	23,00
37,00	14,00	43,00
19,00	7,00	30,00

lax laxative

similarly, much larger for the regression-substitution than for the other two methods
of imputating missing data, 7.6 vs 5.6 and 5.7, and 3.0 vs 1.7 and 1.8.

Just like mean imputation and hot deck imputation, regression-substitution
considerably changed both the B and the SE values of the data's regression equation.
In the given example it can be observed, however, that the t-values of regression-
substitution equation were larger than those of the full data's equation, 7.6 and 3.0
vs 6.3 and 2.0. In other words, with regression-substitution, unlike with mean imputation and hot deck imputation, the sensitivity of testing is larger than that of the full
data, with overstatement of sensitivity. Artificially changing the error as implemented

Table 22.3 Mean values of the variable are imputed in the missing data from Table 22.2

New lax	Bisacodyl	Age
24,00	8,00	25,00
30,00	13,00	30,00
25,00	15,00	25,00
35,00	10,00	31,00
39,00	9,00	*29,00*
30,00	10,00	33,00
27,00	8,00	22,00
14,00	5,00	18,00
39,00	13,00	14,00
42,00	*11,00*	30,00
41,00	11,00	36,00
38,00	11,00	30,00
39,00	12,00	27,00
37,00	10,00	38,00
47,00	18,00	40,00
30,00	13,00	31,00
36,00	12,00	25,00
12,00	4,00	24,00
26,00	10,00	27,00
20,00	8,00	20,00
43,00	16,00	35,00
31,00	15,00	29,00
40,00	14,00	32,00
31,00	*11,00*	30,00
36,00	12,00	40,00
21,00	6,00	31,00
44,00	19,00	41,00
11,00	5,00	26,00
27,00	8,00	24,00
24,00	9,00	30,00
40,00	15,00	*29,00*
32,00	7,00	31,00
10,00	6,00	23,00
37,00	14,00	43,00
19,00	7,00	30,00

The imputed data are in italics
lax laxative

by the add-on module Missing Value Analysis of SPSS (IBM SPSS 2011) may be needed in this situation (see Appendix).

5 Discussion

The current chapter suggests that for limited and incidentally occurring missing data, multiple regression-substitution, that uses regression equations with statistically significant predictors, may be the best sensitive method of data imputation.

Table 22.4 The closest
neighbor data were imputed
in the missing data from
Table 22.2

New lax	Bisacodyl	Age
24,00	8,00	25,00
30,00	13,00	30,00
25,00	15,00	25,00
35,00	10,00	31,00
39,00	9,00	_30,00_
30,00	10,00	33,00
27,00	8,00	22,00
14,00	5,00	18,00
39,00	13,00	14,00
42,00	_14,00_	30,00
41,00	11,00	36,00
38,00	11,00	30,00
39,00	12,00	27,00
37,00	10,00	38,00
47,00	18,00	40,00
_30,00_	13,00	31,00
36,00	12,00	25,00
12,00	4,00	24,00
26,00	10,00	27,00
20,00	8,00	20,00
43,00	16,00	35,00
31,00	15,00	29,00
40,00	14,00	32,00
31,00	_15,00_	30,00
36,00	12,00	40,00
21,00	6,00	31,00
44,00	19,00	41,00
11,00	5,00	26,00
27,00	8,00	24,00
24,00	9,00	30,00
40,00	15,00	_32,00_
32,00	7,00	31,00
10,00	6,00	23,00
37,00	14,00	43,00
19,00	7,00	30,00

lax laxative

The International Conference of Harmonisation Guidance on General Considerations for Clinical Trials recognized a special case of missing data being the loss of patients due to progression of disease, death, or cumulative drug toxicity. The so-called LOCF (Chi et al. 2003) method (last observation carried forward) was recommended in this situation. An intention to treat analysis can, then, be performed on all of the data with the argument that the last observation may be the best possible prediction of what the observation would have been, had the patient been followed. This solution may be appropriate for its purpose, but not for incidentally occurring missing data during a trial due, e.g., to equipment dysfunction or the patients' inclination not to report at some moment.

Table 22.5 The best
predicted values from a
multiple linear regression
equation ($y = 0.98 + 1.89$
$x_1 + 0.31 x_2$, variable 1
dependent) are imputed in the
missing data from Table 22.2

New lax	Bisacodyl	Age
24,00	8,00	25,00
30,00	13,00	30,00
25,00	15,00	25,00
35,00	10,00	31,00
39,00	9,00	*69,00*
30,00	10,00	33,00
27,00	8,00	22,00
14,00	5,00	18,00
39,00	13,00	14,00
42,00	*17,00*	30,00
41,00	11,00	36,00
38,00	11,00	30,00
39,00	12,00	27,00
37,00	10,00	38,00
47,00	18,00	40,00
35,00	13,00	31,00
36,00	12,00	25,00
12,00	4,00	24,00
26,00	10,00	27,00
20,00	8,00	20,00
43,00	16,00	35,00
31,00	15,00	29,00
40,00	14,00	32,00
31,00	*11,00*	30,00
36,00	12,00	40,00
21,00	6,00	31,00
44,00	19,00	41,00
11,00	5,00	26,00
27,00	8,00	24,00
24,00	9,00	30,00
40,00	15,00	*35,00*
32,00	7,00	31,00
10,00	6,00	23,00
37,00	14,00	43,00
19,00	7,00	30,00

The imputed data are in italics
lax laxative

Logistic and Cox regression cannot be applied for regression-imputation, because the dependent variable, here, is not a real response value, but, rather, respectively the odds and hazard of responding. However, most data files consist of at least one continuous variable that can be used instead as dependent variable for regression-substitution.

With larger percentages of missing data than approximately 5%, either entire deletion of the patients with missing data is required or treating them as a separate subgroup. Multiple groups ANOVAs (analysis of variance) can, subsequently, be used to assess whether there is a significant difference between the missing and

Table 22.6 Data-analysis of the data files from the Tables 22.1, 22.2, 22.3, 22.4, and 22.5

R square	F	Sig	B_1	SE_1	t	Sig	B_2	SE_2	t	Sig
Table 22.1 (full data)										
0.67	32.9	0.0001	1.82	0.29	6.3	0.0001	0.34	0.16	2.0	0.048
Table 22.2 (5% missing data)										
0.71	32.4	0.0001	1.89	0.32	5.9	0.0001	0.31	0.19	1.7	0.101
Table 22.3 (means imputated)										
0.65	29.4	0.0001	1.82	0.33	5.6	0.0001	0.33	0.19	1.7	0.094
Table 22.4 (hot deck imputation)										
0.66	31.0	0.0001	1.77	0.31	5.7	0.0001	0.34	0.18	1.8	0.074
Table 22.5 (regression-equation imputation)										
0.73	44.1	0.0001	1.89	0.25	7.6	0.0001	0.31	0.10	3.0	0.005

F F-value, *Sig* significance level, *B* regression coefficient, *SE* standard error

non-missing patients. No significance difference supports the robustness of the data, and supports that the result with or without missing data will be rather similar.

Instead of the three methods discussed in this paper, two more modern methods for data imputation are possible. The first one is the maximum likelihood approach using log likelihood ratio tests, that are based, just like linear regression, on normal distributions, and are a bit more sensitive than conventional t- or ANOVA tests as applied in linear regression. SPSS statistical software has it in its add-on module Missing Value Analysis (IBM SPSS 2011). SPSS adds here a bit of random error to each substitution, a rather arbitrary procedure. The second one is multiple imputations. For that purpose Little and Rubin applied multiple hot deck imputations instead of a single one, and used the pooled result of them for final data analysis (Little and Rubin 1987). This method may provide better sensitivity than single hot deck imputation. Monte Carlo Markov simulation models are used for data generation (see Chap. 57 for the description of the principles as applied) (Scheuren 2005). The multiple imputation models are rather complex, and, again, bits of random error are added. These procedures may be defensible. But they are, at the same time, kind of black box models, hard to check. The appendix gives an example.

We conclude that regression-substitution is a very sensitive method to imputate missing data provided the following measures are taken into account:

(a) At least two independent variables in the equation.
(b) With more than 1 missing datum in a single subject delete the subject entirely.
(c) The number of missing data in a data file must not be larger than 5%.
(d) If the percentage is larger than 5%, and no particular mechanism is found, then 5% could be randomly chosen to be treated using regression-imputation, while the remainder should be deleted.
(e) Variables with a statistically insignificant regression coefficient should not be included in the analysis. We recommend that the p-values should be smaller than 0.15 at most, and that, with a p-value > 0.15, the variable must be removed from the regression model.
(f) Adjustment of the standard errors of the imputed data is not needed.

6 Conclusions

In clinical research missing data are common. Imputed data are not real data, but constructed values that should increase the sensitivity of testing. Regression-substitution for the purpose of data imputation did not always provide a better sensitivity than did other methods. This chapter compares different methods of missing data imputation with that of regression-substitution taking into account particular quality measures. A real data example with a 105 value file was used. After randomly removing five values from the file, mean imputation and hot deck imputation were compared with regression-substitution, taking account of the following requirements:

(a) at least two independent variables in the equation,
(b) no more than 1 missing datum per patient,
(c) no more than 5% missing data,
(d) with more than 5% missing data after randomly choosing 5% for regression-substitution deletion of the remainder,
(e) only statistically significant variables in the regression model,
(f) no addition of random errors to the imputed data.

The test statistics after regression-substitution were much better than those after the other two methods with F-values of 44.1 vs 29.4 and 31.0, and t-values of 7.6 vs 5.6 and 5.7, and 3.0 vs 1.7 and 1.8.

We conclude that regression-substitution is a very sensitive method for imputating missing data under the provision that particular quality measures are taken into account.

Appendix

In order to perform the multiple imputation method the SPSS add-on module "Missing Values" is suitable. For explanation the example of the constipation study is used once more. First, the pattern of the missing data must be checked using the command "analyze pattern". If the missing data are equally distributed and no "islands" of missing data exist, the model will be appropriate.

The following commands are needed:

Transform…random number generators…
    Analyze…multiple imputations…impute missing data… (the imputed data file must be given a new name e.g. "study name imputed").

Five or more times a file is produced by the software program in which the missing values are replaced with simulated versions using the Monte Carlo method (Table 22.7, see also Chap. 57). In our example the variables are continuous and, thus, need no transformation. If you run a usual linear regression of the summary of your "imputed" data files, then the software will automatically produce pooled

Table 22.7 Missing data file and 5 imputed data files (35 patients) produced by the SPSS add-on module "Missing Vales" using the command multiple imputations

File 1			File 2			File 3			File 4			File 5			File 6		
New lax	Bisacodyl	Age	New lax	Bisacodyl	Age	New lax	Bisacodyl	Age	New lax	Bisacodyl	Age	New lax	Bisacodyl	Age	New lax	Bisacodyl	Age
24,00	8,00	25,00	24,00	8,00	25,00	24,00	8,00	25,00	24,00	8,00	25,00	24,00	8,00	25,00	24,00	8,00	25,00
30,00	13,00	30,00	30,00	13,00	30,00	30,00	13,00	30,00	30,00	13,00	30,00	30,00	13,00	30,00	30,00	13,00	30,00
25,00	15,00	25,00	25,00	15,00	25,00	25,00	15,00	25,00	25,00	15,00	25,00	25,00	15,00	25,00	25,00	15,00	25,00
35,00	10,00	31,00	35,00	10,00	31,00	35,00	10,00	31,00	35,00	10,00	31,00	35,00	10,00	31,00	35,00	10,00	31,00
39,00	9,00		39,00	9,00	33,77	39,00	9,00	21,49	39,00	9,00	31,22	39,00	9,00	31,22	39,00	9,00	34,89
30,00	10,00	33,00	30,00	10,00	33,00	30,00	10,00	33,00	30,00	10,00	33,00	30,00	10,00	33,00	30,00	10,00	33,00
27,00	8,00	22,00	27,00	8,00	22,00	27,00	8,00	22,00	27,00	8,00	22,00	27,00	8,00	22,00	27,00	8,00	22,00
14,00	5,00	18,00	14,00	5,00	18,00	14,00	5,00	18,00	14,00	5,00	18,00	14,00	5,00	18,00	14,00	5,00	18,00
39,00	13,00	14,00	39,00	13,00	14,00	39,00	13,00	14,00	39,00	13,00	14,00	39,00	13,00	14,00	39,00	13,00	14,00
42,00		30,00	42,00	15,10	30,00	42,00	15,99	30,00	42,00	15,07	30,00	42,00	17,00	30,00	42,00	18,04	30,00
41,00	11,00	36,00	41,00	11,00	36,00	41,00	11,00	36,00	41,00	11,00	36,00	41,00	11,00	36,00	41,00	11,00	36,00
38,00	11,00	30,00	38,00	11,00	30,00	38,00	11,00	30,00	38,00	11,00	30,00	38,00	11,00	30,00	38,00	11,00	30,00
39,00	12,00	27,00	39,00	12,00	27,00	39,00	12,00	27,00	39,00	12,00	27,00	39,00	12,00	27,00	39,00	12,00	27,00
37,00	10,00	38,00	37,00	10,00	38,00	37,00	10,00	38,00	37,00	10,00	38,00	37,00	10,00	38,00	37,00	10,00	38,00
47,00	18,00	40,00	47,00	18,00	40,00	47,00	18,00	40,00	47,00	18,00	40,00	47,00	18,00	40,00	47,00	18,00	40,00
	13,00	31,00	23,86	13,00	31,00	39,02	13,00	31,00	31,51	13,00	31,00	34,53	13,00	31,00	48,42	13,00	31,00
36,00	12,00	25,00	36,00	12,00	25,00	36,00	12,00	25,00	36,00	12,00	25,00	36,00	12,00	25,00	36,00	12,00	25,00
12,00	4,00	24,00	12,00	4,00	24,00	12,00	4,00	24,00	12,00	4,00	24,00	12,00	4,00	24,00	12,00	4,00	24,00
26,00	10,00	27,00	26,00	10,00	27,00	26,00	10,00	27,00	26,00	10,00	27,00	26,00	10,00	27,00	26,00	10,00	27,00
20,00	8,00	20,00	20,00	8,00	20,00	20,00	8,00	20,00	20,00	8,00	20,00	20,00	8,00	20,00	20,00	8,00	20,00
43,00	16,00	35,00	43,00	16,00	35,00	43,00	16,00	35,00	43,00	16,00	35,00	43,00	16,00	35,00	43,00	16,00	35,00
31,00	15,00	29,00	31,00	15,00	29,00	31,00	15,00	29,00	31,00	15,00	29,00	31,00	15,00	29,00	31,00	15,00	29,00
40,00	14,00	32,00	40,00	14,00	32,00	40,00	14,00	32,00	40,00	14,00	32,00	40,00	14,00	32,00	40,00	14,00	32,00

(continued)

Table 22.7 (continued)

File 1			File 2			File 3			File 4			File 5			File 6		
New lax	Bisacodyl	Age	New lax	Bisacodyl	Age	New lax	Bisacodyl	Age	New lax	Bisacodyl	Age	New lax	Bisacodyl	Age	New lax	Bisacodyl	Age
31,00		30,00	31,00	13,60	30,00	31,00	10,37	30,00	31,00	8,20	30,00	31,00	12,92	30,00	31,00	11,83	30,00
36,00	12,00	40,00	36,00	12,00	40,00	36,00	12,00	40,00	36,00	12,00	40,00	36,00	12,00	40,00	36,00	12,00	40,00
21,00	6,00	31,00	21,00	6,00	31,00	21,00	6,00	31,00	21,00	6,00	31,00	21,00	6,00	31,00	21,00	6,00	31,00
44,00	19,00	41,00	44,00	19,00	41,00	44,00	19,00	41,00	44,00	19,00	41,00	44,00	19,00	41,00	44,00	19,00	41,00
11,00	5,00	26,00	11,00	5,00	26,00	11,00	5,00	26,00	11,00	5,00	26,00	11,00	5,00	26,00	11,00	5,00	26,00
27,00	8,00	24,00	27,00	8,00	24,00	27,00	8,00	24,00	27,00	8,00	24,00	27,00	8,00	24,00	27,00	8,00	24,00
24,00	9,00	30,00	24,00	9,00	30,00	24,00	9,00	30,00	24,00	9,00	30,00	24,00	9,00	30,00	24,00	9,00	30,00
40,00	15,00		40,00	15,00	27,38	40,00	15,00	33,62	40,00	15,00	33,20	40,00	15,00	31,69	40,00	15,00	34,93
32,00	7,00	31,00	32,00	7,00	31,00	32,00	7,00	31,00	32,00	7,00	31,00	32,00	7,00	31,00	32,00	7,00	31,00
10,00	6,00	23,00	10,00	6,00	23,00	10,00	6,00	23,00	10,00	6,00	23,00	10,00	6,00	23,00	10,00	6,00	23,00
37,00	14,00	43,00	37,00	14,00	43,00	37,00	14,00	43,00	37,00	14,00	43,00	37,00	14,00	43,00	37,00	14,00	43,00
19,00	7,00	30,00	19,00	7,00	30,00	19,00	7,00	30,00	19,00	7,00	30,00	19,00	7,00	30,00	19,00	7,00	30,00

Table 22.8 The regression coefficients and their p-values obtained using different methods of data imputation

	B$_1$ Bisacodyl	SE$_1$	t	Sig	B$_2$ Age	SE$_2$	t	Sig
Full data	1.82	0.29	6.3	0.0001	0.34	0.16	2.0	0.048
5% Missing data	1.89	0.32	5.9	0.0001	0.31	0.19	1.7	0.101
Means imputation	1.82	0.33	5.6	0.0001	0.33	0.19	1.7	0.094
Hot deck imputation	1.77	0.31	5.7	0.0001	0.34	0.18	1.8	0.074
Regression imputation	1.89	0.25	7.6	0.0001	0.31	0.10	3.0	0.005
Multiple imputations	1.84	0.31	5.9	0.0001	0.32	0.19	1.7	0.097

regression coefficients instead of the usual regression coefficients. In our example the multiple imputation method produced a much larger p-value for the predictor age than the regression imputation did, and the result was, thus, less overstated than it was with regression imputation. Actually, the result was rather similar to that of mean and hot deck imputation, and statistical significance at $p < 0.05$ was not obtained (Table 22.8). Why then do it anyway. The argument is that, with the multiple imputation method, the imputed values are not used as constructed real values, but rather as a device for representing missing data uncertainty. This approach is a safe and probably, scientifically, better alternative to the standard methods. In the given example, unlike regression imputation, it did not seem to overstate the sensitivity of testing (Table 22.8, p-values regression imputation versus multiple imputation 0.005 versus 0.097).

References

Anonymous. Hot deck imputation. http://www.convervapedia.com/Hot-Deck_Imputation. Accessed 15 Dec 2011
Anonymous (2001) Utah v Evans, 182 F. supp. 2d 1165
Chi GY, Jin K, Chen G (2003) Some statistical issues of relevance to confirmatory trials; statistical bias. In: Lu Y, Fang J (eds) Advanced medical statistics. World Scientific, Hackensack, pp 523–579
Feingold M (1982) Missing data in linear models with correlated errors. Comm Stat 11:2831–2833
Haitovsky Y (1968) Missing data in regression analysis. J R Stat Soc 3:2–3
IBM SPSS Missing values. www.spss.com/software/statistics/missing-values/. Accessed 14 Dec 2011
IBM SPSS Statistics 17.0. www.spss.com/software/statistics/chnages.htm. Accessed 14 Dec 2011
Kshirsagar AM, Deo S (1989) Distribution of the biased hypothesis sum of squares in linear models with missing observations. Commun Stat 18:2747–2754
Little RJ, Rubin DB (1987) Statistical analysis with missing data. Wiley, New York
Scheuren F (2005) Multiple imputation: how it began and continues. Am Stat 59:315–319

Chapter 23
Poisson Regression

1   Introduction

In 1837 the French mathematician Simeon Poisson published a mathematical model for the analysis of events (Poisson 1837). It was based on regression with the dependent variable "events per time unit" logarithmically transformed to "log events per time unit". The model appeared to better fit the crime events data from Paris at that time, than did a usual linear model.

In clinical studies the outcome is often, similar to the count of crimes in Paris in 1837, a count within a length of observation time, for example, the numbers of episodes of paroxysmal atrial fibrillation in a subject within 1 month of observation, or the numbers of cardiac events of a study population within 10 years of observation. The causal factors of such outcomes are usually analyzed using linear and logistic regression. Poisson regression is applied if patients are followed for different periods of time. Currently, most cardiovascular studies include a single overall time of observation. It has been observed that Poisson regression can also produce valid results with such studies (www.spss.com). The current chapter uses examples to compare the performance of the traditional linear and logistic regression with that of Poisson regression for the analysis of such studies. We use SPSS Statistical Software (Campbell 2006) for data-analysis.

2   Example 1

Psychological and social scores may contribute to the occurrence of paroxysmal atrial fibrillation (PAF). In a one-month parallel-group study 316 patients were treated with either verapamil or metroprolol (Table 23.1). In addition to the treatment modality, the psychological and social scores were included as predictors of the outcome variable, the number of episodes of PAF. The data were first analyzed using linear regression. We command:

Table 23.1 Data file of a parallel-group study of 316 patients treated with either verapamil or metoprolol for paroxysmal atrial fibrillation

Var 1	Var 2	Var 3	Var 4	Var 1	Var 2	Var 3	Var 4	Var 1	Var 2	Var 3	Var 4	Var 1	Var 2	Var 3	Var 4
4	56.99	42.45	1	5	45.21	48.94	0	8	46.82	42.45	0	0	38.35	55.34	0
4	37.09	46.82	1	3	56.99	65.56	0	1	46.82	52.65	1	14	46.29	55.34	1
2	32.28	43.57	0	30	41.31	48.94	0	2	66.98	86.87	0	2	65.56	51.06	0
3	29.06	43.57	0	16	47.35	46.82	0	3	32.28	51.06	0	2	51.59	65.56	0
3	6.75	27.25	0	15	38.35	43.01	0	4	29.06	29.06	0	2	46.82	68.49	0
13	61.65	48.41	0	12	10.39	6.75	0	2	98.99	42.45	0	0	50.53	43.01	1
11	56.99	40.74	0	1	41.89	36.45	1	4	61.65	84.64	0	1	59.26	55.34	1
7	10.39	15.36	0	1	40.15	38.96	1	7	47.88	37.09	1	19	49.47	43.01	1
10	50.53	52.12	0	7	33.74	35.8	1	0	53.71	56.99	0	2	43.01	46.82	0
9	49.47	42.45	0	1	68.49	52.65	0	1	59.26	51.59	1	11	58.11	71.83	1
4	39.56	36.45	0	45	98.99	64.2	0	1	73.72	93.25	0	0	46.29	70.94	1
5	33.74	13.13	0	10	62.91	43.01	0	0	61.04	51.59	0	5	48.94	53.71	0
5	62.91	62.27	0	3	60.44	36.45	1	13	33.02	45.21	0	13	98.99	56.99	0
3	65.56	44.66	0	27	37.09	10.39	0	1	39.56	41.31	0	0	41.31	50.53	0
1	23.01	25.25	1	2	26.28	33.02	0	0	56.99	62.27	1	5	73.72	82.74	1
0	75.83	61.04	0	13	64.87	53.71	0	1	46.82	47.88	0	3	64.2	65.56	1
1	41.31	49.47	0	2	18.92	29.06	0	0	41.31	44.66	1	2	53.71	51.59	0
0	41.89	65.56	0	5	54.79	47.88	1	1	65.56	71.83	0	2	55.88	98.99	1
2	65.56	46.82	1	5	38.35	38.96	0	0	82.74	98.99	0	5	62.91	56.99	1
24	13.13	6.75	1	4	53.71	52.12	0	1	45.21	44.12	0	0	61.04	71.83	0
2	33.02	42.45	0	3	46.82	51.59	0	0	59.26	61.04	0	3	98.99	98.99	0
0	55.88	64.87	1	20	51.59	71.83	0	2	55.88	56.99	0	0	62.91	54.79	1
1	45.21	55.34	1	12	34.44	40.15	0	0	69.28	79.59	1	0	58.69	60.44	1
0	56.99	44.66	1	31	38.35	44.66	0	1	56.99	59.26	0	1	53.71	35.13	1
8	31.51	38.35	0	6	44.66	40.74	1	0	56.99	47.35	1	9	65.56	44.12	1
3	52.65	50	1	14	49.47	31.51	1	4	65.56	62.27	1	1	51.59	40.15	1
7	17.26	6.75	1	13	43.57	46.82	0	3	47.88	51.06	0	0	62.91	62.27	1
0	33.02	40.15	0	6	39.56	49.47	1	1	20.41	40.15	1	1	70.94	58.11	1

2	61.04	57.55	1	5	86.87	86.87	1	12	33.02	47.35	0	0	55.88	81.08	0	12	70.09	48.41	1
0	66.98	71.83	1	26	61.04	64.2	0	12	20.41	29.06	1	1	61.65	60.44	0	3	65.56	62.27	0
0	1.01	45.21	1	7	23.01	6.75	0	0	43.01	34.44	1	4	58.11	68.49	0	0	46.82	65.56	1
1	38.35	35.13	0	1	27.25	35.13	1	1	51.59	43.57	1	1	45.21	47.35	0	1	66.98	51.59	0
3	44.66	46.82	1	9	32.28	46.82	1	4	39.56	50.53	1	9	29.06	32.28	1	5	51.59	59.26	1
0	44.12	46.82	1	11	24.17	17.26	1	0	53.71	1.01	1	0	33.74	59.85	0	1	46.29	64.2	0
0	59.85	46.29	1	18	45.75	50	1	0	53.71	38.96	1	4	53.71	40.15	1	1	47.88	58.69	1
28	32.28	47.35	0	12	6.75	13.13	1	2	54.79	64.2	0	8	50.53	53.71	0	7	41.89	58.11	0
8	23.01	49.47	1	3	35.13	27.25	1	1	38.35	54.79	0	13	63.55	54.25	1	6	56.99	59.85	0
5	70.94	61.04	1	0	43.01	28.17	1	2	45.21	71.83	1	0	45.21	48.94	1	0	64.2	81.08	0
2	1.01	1.01	1	4	26.28	13.13	1	0	61.65	58.69	0	0	73.72	56.43	1	8	70.94	58.69	0
27	41.89	52.12	0	10	10.39	29.06	1	0	54.79	50	1	0	59.26	49.47	0	0	45.21	57.55	1
5	40.15	35.13	0	16	61.04	66.26	1	0	61.65	54.79	1	0	98.99	69.28	0	1	40.15	48.41	0
18	41.31	38.35	0	1	37.09	51.59	0	7	61.04	58.69	0	2	56.99	74.75	0	0	25.25	13.13	1
19	44.66	58.69	0	9	1.01	1.01	0	2	65.56	66.26	1	5	58.11	58.11	0	4	55.88	86.87	1
9	38.35	42.45	1	3	55.88	45.21	0	9	61.04	71.83	0	1	61.65	86.87	0	17	98.99	93.25	0
9	32.28	1.01	1	0	46.82	38.35	1	6	73.72	55.34	0	0	65.56	66.98	1	6	59.26	44.12	1
4	37.09	32.28	0	9	41.89	56.99	1	4	54.79	51.59	1	0	59.26	56.99	0	0	41.89	41.31	1
2	63.55	57.55	1	14	66.26	35.8	1	7	58.11	58.11	1	1	66.98	63.55	0	0	61.04	56.99	0
3	43.57	41.31	1	7	10.39	38.96	0	0	37.73	46.82	0	2	32.28	50	0	1	73.72	70.94	0
9	33.02	24.17	1	3	33.02	40.15	1	0	65.56	70.09	1	1	70.94	73.72	1	3	61.04	47.88	1
20	68.49	59.26	0	10	36.45	20.41	1	5	58.11	68.49	1	5	37.73	37.73	1	1	53.71	61.04	1
6	29.06	21.76	1	12	46.82	65.56	1	4	62.91	71.83	0	3	32.28	29.91	0	2	46.82	59.26	1
0	54.79	54.79	1	6	48.41	34.44	0	2	98.99	55.34	1	1	36.45	32.28	1	2	36.45	46.82	0
27	48.94	51.59	1	35	41.89	41.89	0	0	53.71	66.98	0	3	64.2	71.83	0	2	56.99	61.04	1
12	52.65	50.53	0	13	20.41	25.25	0	4	65.56	50	0	6	56.99	71.83	0	5	20.41	15.36	0
34	13.13	32.28	0	3	73.72	74.75	0	2	53.71	65.56	0	8	44.12	24.17	1	41	47.88	54.79	0

(continued)

Table 23.1 (continued)

Var 1	Var 2	Var 3	Var 4	Var 1	Var 2	Var 3	Var 4	Var 1	Var 2	Var 3	Var 4	Var 1	Var 2	Var 3	Var 4	Var 1	Var 2	Var 3	Var 4
1	53.71	41.89	1	10	10.39	40.15	1	18	48.41	29.06	0	21	40.15	40.15	1	3	56.99	43.01	1
25	15.36	32.28	1	6	17.26	20.41	1	1	35.13	52.12	0	1	28.17	30.72	0	7	54.79	71.83	0
5	10.39	17.26	1	0	75.83	64.87	1	0	70.94	70.94	1	7	52.65	79.59	0	1	47.88	69.28	0
3	34.44	38.35	0	2	26.28	23.01	1	1	62.91	65.56	0	5	40.15	44.66	1	1	36.45	47.88	1
2	41.89	42.45	0	6	70.94	82.74	1	16	68.49	58.69	1	1	41.31	40.15	0	3	66.98	68.49	0
1	40.74	55.34	1	5	76.99	68.49	1	6	51.06	41.31	0	1	59.26	89.61	0	0	54.79	53.18	0
7	37.09	52.65	0	13	61.65	58.11	0	16	64.2	67.72	0	0	45.21	46.82	0	0	76.99	69.28	0
4	26.28	26.28	1	4	28.17	6.75	0	0	58.11	78.24	1	4	45.21	53.18	1	2	65.56	70.94	0
8	47.88	36.45	1																

Var 1 = Variable 1 = numbers of episodes of paroxysmal atrial fibrillation

Var 2 = Variable 2 = psychological score

Var 3 = Variable 3 = social score

Var 4 = Variable 4 = treatment modality (0 = verapamil, 1 = metoprolol)

Table 23.2 Results of multiple linear regression of the data from Table 23.1

Coefficients[a]

Model		Unstandardized coefficients		Standardized coefficients		
		B	Std. error	Beta	t	Sig.
1	(Constant)	11.564	1.411		8.194	.000
	Social score	−.022	.032	−.053	−.697	.487
	Psychological score	−.071	.032	−.171	−.2.224	.027
	Treat	−2.291	.832	−.154	−.2.753	.006

[a]Dependent variable: paf

Table 23.3 Results of Poisson regression of the data from Table 23.1

Parameter estimates

Parameter	B	Std. error	95% Wald confidence interval		Hypothesis test		
			Lower	Upper	Wald chi-square	df	Sig.
(Intercept)	2.688	.0727	2.545	2.830	1368.563	1	.000
Social	−.004	.0018	−.007	4.656E-5	3.742	1	.053
Psychological	−.012	.0018	−.016	−.009	43.865	1	.000
Treat	−.401	.0484	−.496	−.306	68.582	1	.000
(Scale)	1[a]						

Dependent variable: paf

Model: (Intercept), social, psychological, treat

[a]Fixed at the displayed value

Analyze – regression – linear – dependent = numbers of episodes of PAF – independent = psychological score and social score and treatment modality – OK.

Table 23.2 shows the main results of the linear regression. Treatment modality is a significant predictor of numbers of episodes of PAF at p=0.006, and psychological score is an independent covariate with a p-value of 0.027. Social score has no effect. The data are subsequently analyzed using Poisson regression. We command:

Generalized linear models – mark: custom – Distribution: Poisson – Link function: log – Response: dependent variable: numbers of episodes of PAF – Predictors: main effect: treatment modality and psychological score and social score – Model: main effects: treatment modality and psychological score and social score – Estimation: mark: model-based estimation – OK.

Table 23.3 shows the main results of the Poisson regression. The treatment modality is again a significant predictor of the numbers of episodes of PAF but at a lower level of significance (p=0.0001 versus 0.006). Also the independent covariate psychological score performs better than with linear regression (p=0.0001 versus 0.027). Finally, social score while insignificant with linear regression has a tendency to significance here (p=0.053 versus 0.487).

Obviously, the Poisson regression produces much better levels of significance than does the traditional linear regression in the given example.

3   Example 2

During two treatment regimens the numbers of patients with torsade de pointes were assessed. Table 23.4 gives the entire data file. The data are summarized in the underneath 2×2 contingency table.

Number of patient with torsade de pointes		
	Yes	No
Treatment regimen 1	17	15
Treatment regimen 2	5	15

Binary logistic regression was first applied to assess the effect of the treatment regimens on the numbers of patients with torsade de pointes. We command:

Analyze – regression – binary logistic – Dependent: torsade – Covariates: treatment – OK.

Table 23.4 Data file of study of two regimens for the treatment of torsades de pointe

Variable 1	Variable 2	Variable 1	Variable 2
0	1	0	0
0	1	0	0
0	1	0	0
0	1	0	0
0	1	0	0
0	1	0	0
0	1	1	1
0	1	1	1
0	1	1	1
0	1	1	1
0	1	1	1
0	1	1	1
0	1	1	1
0	1	1	1
0	1	1	1
0	0	1	1
0	0	1	1
0	0	1	1
0	0	1	1
0	0	1	1
0	0	1	1
0	0	1	0
0	0	1	0
0	0	1	0
0	0	1	0
0	0	1	0

Variable 1 = treatment modality
Variable 2 = presence of torsade de pointes (1 = yes, 0 = no)

Table 23.5 Results of logistic regression of the data from Table 23.4

Variables in the equation		B	S.E.	Wald	df	Sig.	Exp (B)
Step 1[a]	VAR00001	1.224	.626	3.819	1	.051	3.400
	Constant	−.125	.354	.125	1	.724	.882

[a]Variable(s) entered on step 1: VAR00001

Table 23.6 Results of Poisson regression of the data from Table 23.4

Parameter estimates			95% Wald confidence interval		Hypothesis test		
Parameter	B	Std. error	Lower	Upper	Wald chi-square	df	Sig.
(Intercept)	−.758	.1882	−1.127	−.389	16.210	1	.000
VAR00001	.470	.2282	.023	.917	4.241	1	.039
(Scale)	1[a]						

Dependent variable: torsade
Model: (Intercept), VAR00001
[a]Fixed at the displayed value

Table 23.5 gives the main result of the logistic regression. The treatment modality (VAR00001) does not seem to be a significant predictor of number of patients with torsade de pointes ($p = 0.051$). Subsequently, a Poisson regression is performed. We command:

Generalized linear models – mark: custom – Distribution: Poisson – Identity: log – response: dependent variable: torsade – predictors: main effect: VAR00001 – Estimation: mark: robust estimation – OK.

Table 23.6 gives the main result of the Poisson regression. Unlike with logistic regression, here a significant effect is observed at $p = 0.039$. According to the Poisson model the treatment modality is a significant predictor of torsade de pointes. One treatment regimen is better than the other.

4   Discussion

The general principle of regression analysis is, that it calculates the best fit line or curve (with the shortest distance to the data), and then tests how far distant from curve the data are. A significant correlation between y- and x-data indicates that the y-data are closer to the model than will happen with random sampling. For testing simple t-tests or analysis of variance are usually applied. The "model-principle", however essential to regression modeling, is at the same time its largest limitation: it is, generally, no use forcing nature into a model. Data are massaged by regression modeling, and never fit perfectly. Moreover, the regression models are, generally, more appropriate for the description of events in simple creatures, like, e.g., mosquito collisions than that of multicausal events in humans. Nonetheless, regression models have been helpful for making sensible predictions about future events and other clinical effects.

Underneath are the mathematical equations of the regression models as used in the current chapter.

Linear regression
$$\text{Events} = a + b_1\, x_1 + b_2\, x_2 + b_3\, x_3$$

Logistic regression
$$\text{Log odds events} = a + b_1\, x_1 + b_2\, x_2 + b_3\, x_3$$

Poisson regression
$$\text{Log events} = a + b_1\, x_1 + b_2\, x_2 + b_3\, x_3$$

Poisson regression uses an exponential rather than linear relationship between the predictors, the x-values, and the outcome variable. In the examples given Poisson regression provided better p-values than did the other two. Based on these results one may infer that Poisson regression is more appropriate for the analysis of cardiovascular count data than linear/logistic regression. Unfortunately, it is little used so far. We recommend that in future clinical data-analyses linear/logistic models be more often replaced with Poisson regression. This is, particularly, important, if the former models do not produce statistically significant results.

5   Conclusions

In clinical studies the outcome is often the number of events within a length of observation time. This chapter was written to compare the performance of the traditional linear and logistic regression with that of Poisson regression for the analysis of such studies. Examples of cardiovascular event studies are used. SPSS Statistical Software is used for analysis.

In a 316 patient parallel-group study of predictors for paroxysmal atrial fibrillation Poisson regression provided better p-values than did linear regression: p-values of 0.0001 versus 0.006, 0.0001 versus 0.027, and 0.055 versus 0.487 for treatment modality, psychological score, and social score respectively. In a 52 patient study of two treatment regimens for patients with torsade de pointes the Poisson regression, unlike the logistic regression, provided a significant result: p-values 0.039 versus 0.051.

In the examples given Poisson regression provides better p-values than did linear or logistic regression. We recommend that in future clinical event studies linear/logistic models be more often replaced with Poisson regression. This is, particularly, important, if the former models do not produce statistically significant results.

References

Campbell MJ (2006) Poisson regression used to estimate relative risks from a 2×2 table. In: Campbell MJ (ed) Statistics at square two, 2nd edn. BMJ Books, Blackwell Publishing, Oxford, pp 88–9

Poisson SD (1837) Recherches sur la probabilité de jugements en matières criminelles civile. Memoir. Ecole Polytechnique, Paris

Chapter 24
More on Non Linear Relationships, Splines

1 Introduction

The general principle of regression analysis is that the best fit line/exponential-curve/curvilinear-curve etc is calculated, i.e., the one with the shortest distances to the data, and it is, subsequently, tested how far the data are from the curve. A significant correlation between the y (outcome data) and the x (exposure data) means that the data are closer to the model than will happen purely by chance. The level of significance is usually tested, simply, with t-tests or analysis of variance. The initial regression model is almost always a linear model.

The model-principle of regression analysis is the basis but at the same time its largest limitation, because it is often hard forcing nature into a mathematical model. In the past, non linear relationships like the smooth shapes of airplanes, boats, and motor cars were constructed from scale models using stretched thin wooden strips, producing smooth curves, assuming a minimum of strain in the materials used. With the advent of the computer it became possible to replace it with statistical modeling for the purpose: already in 1964 it was introduced by Boeing (Ferguson 1964) and General Motors (Birkhof and De Boor 1965). Mechanical spline methods were replaced with their mathematical counterparts. More complex regression models were required, and they were often laborious so that even modern computers had difficulty to process them. Software packages currently make use of a technique called iterations: five or more regression curves are estimated ("guesstimated") and the one with the best fit is chosen. With large data samples the calculation time may, nonetheless be hours or days, and modern software will automatically proceed to use Monte Carlo calculations (Chap. 57) in order to reduce the calculation times. Nowadays, many non linear data patterns can be developed mathematically, and this chapter reviews some of them.

A first step with any data analysis is to assess the data pattern is a scatter plot (Fig. 24.1). Sometimes a better fit of the data is obtained by drawing y versus x instead of the reverse or residuals of y versus x with or without adjustments for other x-values are helpful for finding a recognizable data pattern. Statistically we test for

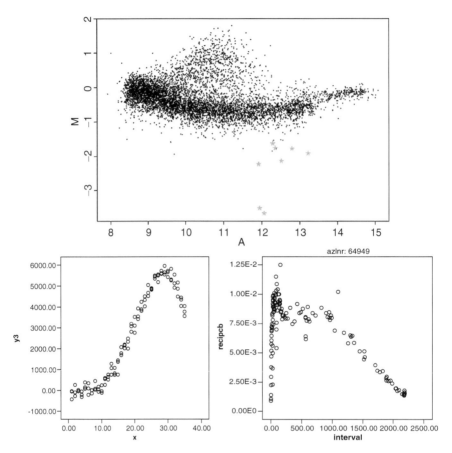

Fig. 24.1 Examples of non linear data sets

linearity by adding a non linear term of x to the model, particularly x squared or square root x. If the squared correlation coefficient r (Birkhof and De Boor 1965) gets smaller by this action, then the pattern is, obviously, not linear.

In this chapter several mathematical models for modeling non linear data are reviewed. The mathematical equations of all of these models are summarized in the appendix. They are helpful to make you understand the assumed nature of the relationships between the dependent and independent variables of the models used, but can be disregarded for those not fond on maths.

2   Logit or Probit Transformation

If linear regression (in SPSS (2011) covered by the general linear model) produces a non-significant effect, then other regression functions can be chosen and may provide a better fit for your data. The following methods are possible. Following

Fig. 24.2 Example of non linear relationship that is linear after log transformation (Michaelis-Menten relationship between substrate concentration and enzymatic reaction rate)

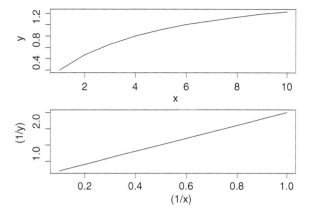

Fig. 24.3 Another example of a non linear relationship that is linear after logarithmic transformation

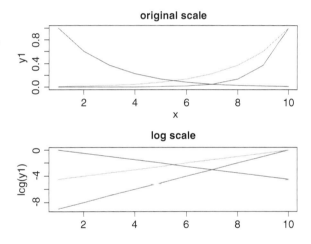

logit (=logistic) or probit ($\approx \pi\sqrt{3} \times$ logit) transformation a linear model is produced. Binary and multinomial logistic regression (Chaps. 17, 19, and 21), Cox regression (Chaps. 17 and 31), Poisson regression (Chap. 23), Markov modeling (Chap. 17), and various bivariate and probit regressions not covered in this chapter (Chap. 25) are examples. SPSS statistical software (SPSS 2011) provides most of these methods in its module "Generalized linear methods". There are examples of datasets where we have prior knowledge that they are, definitely, linear after a known transformation (Figs. 24.2 and 24.3). As a particular caveat we should add here that many examples can be given, but beware!!! Most models in biomedicine have considerable residual scatter around the regression line.

For example, if the model applied is the following (e = random variation)

$$y_i = \alpha\, e^{\beta x} + e_i,$$

then

$$\ln(y_i) \neq \ln(\alpha) + \beta x + e_i.$$

The smaller the e_i term, the better the fit of the model applied.

3　"Trial and Error" Method, Box Cox Transformation, ACE/AVAS Packages

If logit or probit transformation does not work, then additional transformation techniques may be helpful. How do you find the best transformations? First, prior knowledge about the patterns to be expected is helpful. If this is not available, then the "trial and error" method can be recommended, particularly, logarithmically transforming either x- or y-axis or both of them (Fig. 24.4).

$$\log(y) \text{ vs } x,\; y \text{ vs } \log(x),\; \log(y) \text{ vs } \log(x).$$

The above methods can be performed by hand (vs = versus), Box Cox transformation (Box Cox normality plot 2011), additive regression using ACE

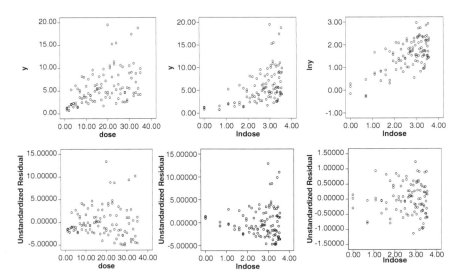

Fig. 24.4 Trial and error methods used to find recognizable data patterns

(alternating conditional expectations), and AVAS (additive and variance stabilization). ACE or AVAS (2011) packages contain modern non-parametric methods, otherwise closely related to the "trial and error" method. They can also be used for the purpose. They are largely empirical techniques to normalize non normal data that can, subsequently, be easily modeled, and they are also available in virtually all modern software programs.

4 Curvilinear Data

If the data plot looks, obviously, sinusoidal, then curvilinear regression models including polynomial regression and Fourier analysis could be adequate (Chap. 16). Figure 24.5 gives an example of polynomial models with increasing orders. If an adequate fit is not obtained using these models, non linear regression may be possible using multi-exponential modeling with Laplace transformations (Chap. 17). Non linear mixed effect modeling of two-compartment pharmacokinetic studies is an example (Fig. 24.6). The data plot show that data spread is wide and, so, accurate predictions can not be made in the given example. Nonetheless, the method is helpful to give an idea about some pharmacokinetic parameters like drug plasma half life and distribution volume. Additional explanations are given in the Chaps. 16 and 17.

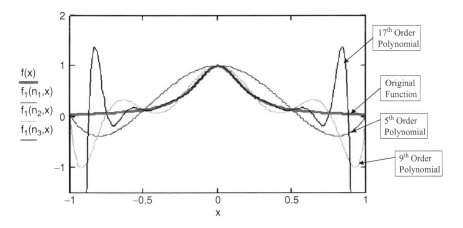

Fig. 24.5 Example of polynomial regression models to describe the data

Fig. 24.6 Example of non linear mixed effect multi-exponential model to describe pharmacokinetic data

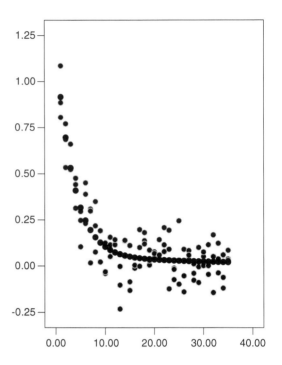

5   Spline Modeling

If all of the above models do not adequately fit your data, you may use a method called spline regression. It stems from the thin flexible wooden splines formerly used by shipbuilders and car designers to produce smooth shapes (Ferguson 1964; Birkhof and De Boor 1965). Spline modeling will be, particularly, suitable for smoothing data patterns, if the data plot leaves you with no idea of the relationship between the y- and x-values.

Figure 24.7 gives an example of non linear dataset suitable for spline modeling.

Technically, the method of local smoothing, categorizing the x-values is used. It means that, if you have no idea about the shape of the relation between the y-values and the x-values of a two dimensional data plot, you may try and divide the x-values into a (small) number of categories, where θ-values are the cutt-offs of categories of x-values otherwise called the knots of the spline model.

- cat. 1: min $\leq x < \theta_1$
- cat. 2: $\theta_1 \leq x < \theta_2$
- ...
- cat. k: $\theta_{k-1} \leq x < \max$.

Fig. 24.7 Example of a non linear dataset suitable for spline modeling

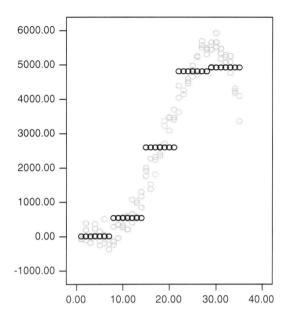

Then, estimate y as the mean of all values within each category. Prerequisites and primary assumptions include

- the y-value is more or less constant within categories of the x-values,
- categories should have a decent number of observations,
- preferably, category boundaries should have some meaning.

A linear regression of the categories is possible, but the linear regression lines are not necessarily connected (Fig. 24.8). Instead of linear regression lines a better fit for the data is provided by separate low-order polynomial regression lines for all of the intervals between two subsequent knots, where knots are x-values that connect one x-category with a subsequent one. Usually, cubic polynomial regression, otherwise called third order polynomial regression, is convenient. It has as simplest equation $y = a + b \cdot x^3$. Eventually, the separate lines are joined at the knots.

Even with knots as few as 2, cubic regression may provide an adequate fit for the data.

In computer graphics spline models are popular curves, because of their accuracy and capacity to fit complex data patterns. So far, they are not yet routinely used in clinical research for making predictions from response patterns, but this is a matter of time. Excel provides free cubic spline function software (Cubic Spline for Excel 2011). The spline model can be checked for its smoothness and fit using lambda-calculus (Lambda calculus 2011), and generalized additive models (Hastie and Tibshirani 1990; Generalized additive model 2011). Unfortunately, multidimensional smoothing using spline modeling is difficult. Instead you may perform separate procedures for each covariate (Figs. 24.9 and 24.10).

Fig. 24.8 Multiple linear regression lines from the data from Fig. 24.7

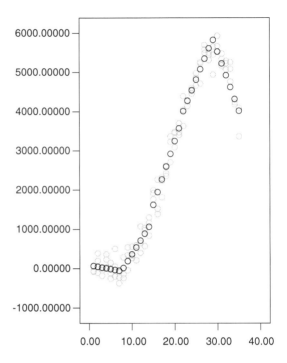

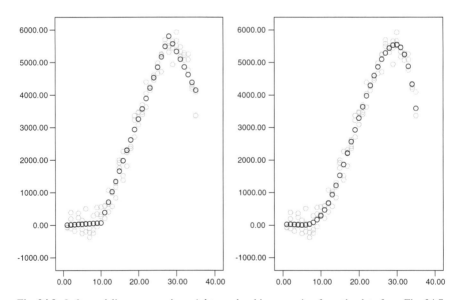

Fig. 24.9 *Left graph* linear regression, *right graph* cubic regression from the data from Fig. 24.7

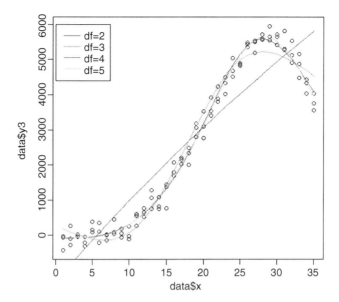

Fig. 24.10 Cubic regression of the data from Fig. 24.7 with increasing numbers of knots

6 Discussion

Many tools are available for developing non linear models for characterizing data sets and making predictions from them. Sometimes it is difficult to choose the degree of smoothness of such models:

- polynomial regression: which order?
- spline: how many knots, which locations, lambda?

Another method is kernel frequency distribution modeling which unless histograms consists of multiple similarly sized Gaussian curves rather than multiple bins of different length. In order to perform kernel modeling the bandwidth (span) of the Gaussian curves has to be selected which may be a difficult but important factor of the potential fit of a particular kernel method.

Maybe, the best fit for many types on non linear data is offered by still another novel regression method called LOESS (locally weighted scatter plot smoothing) (Local regression 2011). This computationally very intensive program. calculates the best fit polynomials from subsets of your data set in order to eventually find out the best fit curve for the overall data set, and is related to Monte Carlo modeling.

Irrespective of the smoothing method applied, there are some problems: smoothing

- introduces bias,
- and reduces variance.

The Akaike information criterion (AIC 2011) is a measure of the relative goodness of fit of a mathematical model for describing data patterns. It can be used to describe the tradeoff between bias and variance in model construction, and to assess the accuracy of the regression model used. However, the AIC, as it is a relative measure, will not be helpful to confirm a poor result, if all of the regression models fit the data set equally poorly.

7   Conclusions

Background:

The pattern of clinical research data is often non linear. Novel mathematical models are being developed for describing those patterns for the benefit of making predictions from them.

Objective:

This chapter was written to review some of the modern models successfully applied for the purpose.

Methods and results:

1. Logit and probit transformation can sometimes be used to mimick a linear model. Binary and multinomial logistic regression, Cox regression, Poisson regression, and Markow modeling are examples of logit transformation.
2. Either the x- or y-axis or both of them can be logarithmically transformed. Also Box Cox transformation equation and ACE (alternating conditional expectations) or AVAS (additive and variance stabilization for regression) packages are simple empirical methods often successful for linearly remodeling non linear data.
3. Data that are, obviously, curvilinear, can, generally, be successfully modeled using polynomial regression and bi-exponential modeling.
4. Spline modeling is, particularly, suitable for smoothing data patterns, if the data plot leaves you with no idea of the relationship between the y- and x-values.

Conclusion:

One of the important goals of statistical analyses is making inferences, i.e., predicting future outcomes from the current data pattern. When a predictor is linearly related to an outcome variable, linear regression is a beautiful method for that purpose. If not, various ways of non linear are available. Some of them are reviewed in this chapter.

Appendix

In this appendix the mathematical equations of the non linear models as reviewed are given. They are, particularly, helpful for those trying to understand the assumed relationships between the dependent and independent variables, but can be disregarded by those without affection to maths (ln = natural logarithm).

$y = a + b_1x_1 + b_2x_2 + \ldots\ldots\ldots b_{10}x_{10}$ linear

$y = a + bx + cx^2 + dx^3 + \ldots$ polynomial

$y = a + sinus\ x + cosinus\ x + \ldots$ Fourier

$Ln\ odds = a + b_1x_1 + b_2x_2 + \ldots\ldots\ldots b_{10}x_{10}$ logistic

$Ln\ multinomial\ odds = a + b_1x_1 + b_2x_2 + \ldots\ldots\ldots b_{10}x_{10}$ multinomial logistic

$Ln\ hazard = a + b_1x_1 + b_2x_2 + \ldots\ldots\ldots b_{10}x_{10}$ Cox

$Ln\ rate = a + b_1x_1 + b_2x_2 + \ldots\ldots\ldots b_{10}x_{10}$ Poisson

Instead of ln odds (= logit) also probit ($\approx \pi\sqrt{3}$ x logit) is often used for transforming binomial data.

                                                                                    probit

$\log y = a + b_1x_1 + b_2x_2 + \ldots\ldots\ldots b_{10}x_{10}$ logarithmic
or

$y = a + b_1\ \log x_1 + b_2x_2 + \ldots\ldots\ldots b_{10}x_{10}etc$ "trial and error"

transformation function of $y = (y^\lambda - 1)/\lambda$ with λ as power   Box-Cox
    parameter

$y = (transformation\ function^{-1})\ a + b_1\ \log x_1 + b_2\ x_2 + \ldots$ ACE modeling

$y = e^{x_1 x_2\ \sin x_3}$ etc   AVAS modeling

$y = a + e^{b_1\ x_1} + e^{b_2\ x_2}$ multi-exponential modeling

θ = magnitude of x-value (example)

$\theta_1 < x < \theta_2$ $y = a_1 + b_1x^3$ spline modeling

$\theta_2 < x < \theta_3$ $y = a_2 + b_2x^3$

$\theta_3 < x < \theta_4$ $y = a_3 + b_3x^3$

References

Additive regression and transformation using ACE or AVAS. http://pinard.progiciels-bpi.ca/LibR/library/Hmisc/html/transace.html. Accessed 15 Dec 2011

Akaike information criterion. http://en.wikipedia.org/wiki/Akaike_information_criterion. Accessed 15 Dec 2011

Birkhof F, De Boor R (1965) Piecewise polynomial interpretation and approximation. In: Proceedings of general motors symposium of 1964, pp 164–190

Box-Cox normality plot. http://itl.nist.gov/div898/handbook/eda/section3/eda336.htm. Accessed 15 Dec 2011

Cubic Spline for Excel. www.srs1software.com/download.htm#pline. Accessed 15 Dec 2011

Ferguson JC (1964) Multi-variable curve interpolation. JACM 11:221–228

Generalized additive model. http://en.wikipedia.org/wiki/generalized_additive_model. Accessed 15 Dec 2011

Hastie and Tibshirani (1990) Generalized additive models. Chapman & Hall, London

Lambda-calculus. http://en.wikipedia.org/wiki/lambda_calculus. Accessed 15 Dec 2011

Local regression. http://en.wikidepia.org/wiki/Local_regression. Accessed 15 Dec 2011

SPSS. www.spss.com. Accessed 15 Dec 2011

Chapter 25
Multivariate Analysis

1 Introduction

In the preceding chapters only data analyses with a single outcome variable (y-variable) have been addressed. Linear, logistic, Cox regressions are examples. If these methods included multiple predictors variables (otherwise called exposure variables or x-variables), they are sometimes erroneously called multivariate methods. However, this is not correct, because the term multivariate analysis refers to the simultaneous analysis of more than one *outcome* variable. An more adequate term for the analysis of multiple predictors variables is "multivariable or multiple variables analysis".

In clinical research often multiple outcomes variables are being assessed. For example, in a study of the efficacy of a novel laxative an important outcome may be the frequency of stools. However, an improved quality of life score may be considered another and maybe even more important outcome. In order to assess two outcomes, simply, two ANOVAs can be performed, but this assessment does not account and adjust the possible relationship between the two outcomes. Also the type I error is inflated. Another nice thing about multivariate analyses is that weak predictors may not be able to significantly predict a single outcome, but it may significantly predict two outcomes that point in the same direction.

In order to assess the two outcome variables simultaneously an analysis with two, rather than a single outcome variable, would be an interesting option for the purpose. For continuous outcome variables both path analysis and MANOVA (multiple ANOVA) is adequate, for binary outcome variables probit analysis is adequate.

In the current chapter the following multivariate methods are reviewed:

1. path analysis (see also Chap. 20),
2. multiple analysis of variance (MANOVA),
3. probit regression modeling.

T.J. Cleophas and A.H. Zwinderman, *Statistics Applied to Clinical Studies*, DOI 10.1007/978-94-007-2863-9_25, © Springer Science+Business Media B.V. 2012

2   Multivariate Regression Analysis Using Path Analysis

In a self-controlled study in 35 patients with constitutional constipation the outcome variables were improvements of frequency of stools and quality of life scores. The predictor variables were compliance with counselling and compliance with drug treatment (Var = variable). The data file is given underneath.

Var 1 (y_1) Improvement frequency stools	Var 2 (y_2) Improved quality life score	Var 3 (x_1) Compliance with drug treatment	Var 4 (x_2) Compliance with counselling
24,00	69,00	25,00	8,00
30,00	110,00	30,00	13,00
25,00	78,00	25,00	15,00
35,00	103,00	31,00	14,00
39,00	103,00	36,00	9,00
30,00	102,00	33,00	10,00
27,00	76,00	22,00	8,00
14,00	75,00	18,00	5,00
39,00	99,00	14,00	13,00
42,00	107,00	30,00	15,00
41,00	112,00	36,00	11,00
38,00	99,00	30,00	11,00
39,00	86,00	27,00	12,00
37,00	107,00	38,00	10,00
47,00	108,00	40,00	15,00
30,00	95,00	31,00	13,00
36,00	88,00	25,00	12,00
12,00	67,00	24,00	4,00
26,00	112,00	27,00	10,00
20,00	87,00	20,00	8,00
43,00	115,00	35,00	16,00
31,00	93,00	29,00	15,00
40,00	92,00	32,00	14,00
31,00	78,00	30,00	7,00
36,00	112,00	40,00	12,00
21,00	69,00	31,00	6,00
44,00	66,00	41,00	19,00
11,00	75,00	26,00	5,00
27,00	85,00	24,00	8,00
24,00	87,00	30,00	9,00
40,00	89,00	20,00	15,00
32,00	89,00	31,00	7,00
10,00	65,00	29,00	6,00
37,00	121,00	43,00	14,00
19,00	74,00	30,00	7,00

Fig. 25.1 Decomposition of correlation between efficacy laxative and quality of life score, all of the correlations in the above example were statistically significant at p<0.10

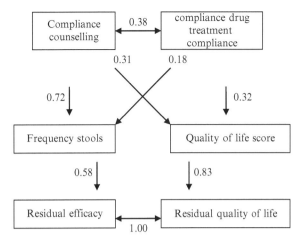

A pleasant thing about path analysis is that it can, indeed, be used as an alternative approach to multivariate regression, with a result similar to that of the more complex mathematical approach. An example is given above. We assume that compliance with counselling and drug compliance not only affect the efficacy of the drug but also the patients' quality of life. First, we have to check that the relationship of either of the two predictors with the outcome quality of life is significant in the usual linear regression model: they were so with p-values of 0.03 and 0.02. Then, a path diagram with standardized regression coefficients is constructed (Fig. 25.1). The standardized regression coefficients of the residual effects are obtained by taking the square root of $(1-r^2)$. The standardized regression coefficient of one residual effect versus another can be assumed to equal 1.00.

We now find the overall correlation between the two outcome variables as follows:

1. Direct effect of counselling	
$0.72 \times 0.31 =$	0.22
2. Direct effect of non-compliance	
$0.32 \times 0.18 =$	0.06
3. Indirect effect of counseling and non-compliance	
$0.72 \times 0.38 \times 0.32 + 0.18 \times 0.38 \times 0.31 =$	0.11
4. Residual effects	
$1.00 \times 0.58 \times 0.83 =$	0.48 +
Total	0.85

A path statistic of 0.85 is considerably larger than that of the single outcome model: 0.85 versus 0.45 (Chap. 20, 47.1% larger). Obviously, two outcome variables make better use of the predictors in our data than does a single one. An advantage of this nonmathematical approach to multivariate regression is that it nicely summarizes all relationships in the model, and it does so in a quantitative way (Fig. 25.1).

3 Multiple Analysis of Variance, First Example

The example from the above section will be used once more. We will first assess whether compliance with counselling is a significant predictor of both improvement of frequency of stools and improved quality of life. We will use SPSS 17.0 (SPSS 2011) for data analysis. Command: Analyze...General Linear Model... Multivariate...in dialog box multivariate transfer y_1 and y_2 to dependent variables and x_1 to the fixed factors, and...ok.

The Table 25.1 shows that even MANOVA can be considered a regression model with intercepts and regression coefficients. Just like ANOVA it is based on normal distributions and homogeneity of the variables. SPSS has checked the assumptions, and the results as given indicate that the model is adequate for the data. Generally Pillai's method gives the best robustness and Roy's the best p-values. We can conclude that counselling is a strong predictor of both improvement of stools and improved quality of life.

In order to find out which of the two outcomes is the most important one, two ANOVAs with each of the outcomes separately must be performed. We command: Analyze...General Linear Model...Univariate...in dialog box univariate transfer y_1 to dependent variables and x_1 to the fixed factors, and...ok. Do the same for variable y_2.

Compliance with counselling is an important predictor of not only improved frequency of stools but also of improved quality of life (Table 25.2).

In order to find out whether the compliance of drug treatment is a contributory predicting factor in this multivariate model, MANOVA with two predictors and two outcomes is performed. Instead of x_1 both x_1 and x_2 are transferred to fixed factors. Table 25.3 shows the results.

The Table 25.3 shows that after including a second predictor variable the MANOVA is not significant anymore. Probably, the second predictor is a confounder of the first one. The analysis of this model stops here.

Table 25.1 MANOVA test statistics of the above data. All of the test statistics show that compliance with counselling is a strong predictor of both improvement of frequency of stools and improved quality of life

Multivariate tests[a]

Effect		Value	F	Hypothesis df	Error df	Sig.
Intercept	Pillai's trace	,992	1185,131[b]	2,000	19,000	,000
	Wilks' lambda	,008	1185,131[b]	2,000	19,000	,000
	Hotelling's trace	124,751	1185,131[b]	2,000	19,000	,000
	Roy's largest root	124,751	1185,131[b]	2,000	19,000	,000
VAR00004	Pillai's trace	1,426	3,547	28,000	40,000	,000
	Wilks' lambda	,067	3,894[b]	28,000	38,000	,000
	Hotelling's trace	6,598	4,242	28,000	36,000	,000
	Roy's largest root	5,172	7,389[c]	14,000	20,000	,000

[a]Design: Intercept + VAR00004
[b]Exact statistic
[c]The statistic is an upper bound on F that yields a lower bound on the significance level.

Table 25.2 ANOVAs of the data from Table 25.1. Also in ANOVA compliance with counselling is a strong predictor of not only improvement of frequency of stools but also improved quality of life

Test of between-subjects effects

Dependent variable:improv freq stool

Source	Type III sum of squares	df	Mean square	F	Sig.
Corrected model	2733,005[a]	14	195,215	6,033	,000
Intercept	26985,054	1	26985,054	833,944	,000
VAR00004	2733,005	14	195,215	6,033	,000
Error	647,167	20	32,358		
Total	36521,000	35			
Corrected total	3380,171	34			

Tests of between-subjects effects

Dependent variable:improv gol

Source	Type III sum of squares	df	Mean square	F	Sig.
Corrected model	6833,671[b]	14	488,119	4,875	,001
Intercept	223864,364	1	223864,364	2235,849	,000
VAR00004	6833,671	14	488,119	4,875	,001
Error	2002,500	20	100,125		
Total	300129,000	35			
Corrected total	8836,171	34			

improv freq stool improvement of frequency of stools, *improve qol* improved quality of life scores
[a]R Squared=,809 (Adjusted R Squared=,675)
[b]R Squared=,733 (Adjusted R Squared=,615)

Table 25.3 MANOVA of the above data with two predictor (x_1 and x_2) and two outcome variables (y_1 and y_2)

Multivariate tests[a]

Effect		Value	F	Hypothesis df	Error df	Sig.
Intercept	Pillai's trace	1,000	29052,980[b]	1,000	1,000	,004
	Wilks' lambda	,000	29052,980[b]	1,000	1,000	,004
	Hotelling's trace	29052,980	29052,980[b]	1,000	1,000	,004
	Roy's largest root	29052,980	29052,980[b]	1,000	1,000	,004
VAR00004	Pillai's trace	,996	27,121[b]	10,000	1,000	,148
	Wilks' lambda	,004	27,121[b]	10,000	1,000	,148
	Hotelling's trace	271,209	27,121[b]	10,000	1,000	,148
	Roy's largest root	271,209	27,121[b]	10,000	1,000	,148
VAR00003	Pillai's trace	,995	13,514[b]	14,000	1,000	,210
	Wilks' lambda	,005	13,514[b]	14,000	1,000	,210
	Hotelling's trace	189,198	13,514[b]	14,000	1,000	,210
	Roy's largest root	189,198	13,514[b]	14,000	1,000	,210
VAR00004* VAR00003	Pillai's trace	,985	12,884[b]	5,000	1,000	,208
	Wilks' lambda	,015	12,884[b]	5,000	1,000	,208
	Hotelling's trace	64,418	12,884[b]	5,000	1,000	,208
	Roy's largest root	64,418	12,884[b]	5,000	1,000	,208

[a]Design: Intercept + VAR00004 + VAR00003 + VAR00004 * VAR00003
[b]Exact statistic

4 Multiple Analysis of Variance, Second Example

As a second example we use the data from Field (2005) on the effect of three treatment modalities on compulsive behaviour disorder estimated by two scores, a thought-score and an action-score (Var = variable).

| Var 1 (y_1) | Var 2 (x) | Var 3 (y_2) |
Action	Treatment	Thought
5,00	1,00	14,00
5,00	1,00	11,00
4,00	1,00	16,00
4,00	1,00	13,00
5,00	1,00	12,00
3,00	1,00	14,00
7,00	1,00	12,00
6,00	1,00	15,00
6,00	1,00	16,00
4,00	2,00	14,00
4,00	2,00	15,00
1,00	2,00	13,00
1,00	2,00	14,00
4,00	2,00	15,00
6,00	2,00	19,00
5,00	2,00	13,00
5,00	2,00	18,00
2,00	2,00	14,00
5,00	2,00	17,00
4,00	3,00	13,00
5,00	3,00	15,00
5,00	3,00	14,00
4,00	3,00	14,00
6,00	3,00	13,00
4,00	3,00	20,00
7,00	3,00	13,00
4,00	3,00	16,00
6,00	3,00	14,00
5,00	3,00	18,00

Command: Analyze...General Linear Model...Multivariate...in dialog box multivariate transfer y_1 and y_2 to dependent variables and x_1 to the fixed factors, and...ok.

The Pillai test shows that the predictor (treatment modality) has a significant effect on both thoughts and actions at p = 0.049. Roy's test being less robust gives an even better p-value of 0.020 (Table 25.4).

We will use ANOVAs to find out which of the two outcomes are more important.

Table 25.4 MANOVA test statistics of the above data. The Pillai test shows that the predictor (treatment modality) has a significant effect on both thoughts and actions at p=0.049. Roy's test being less robust gives an even better p-value of 0.020

Multivariate tests[a]

Effect		Value	F	Hypothesis df	Error df	Sig.
Intercept	Pillai's trace	,983	745,230[b]	2,000	26,000	,000
	Wilks' lambda	,017	745,230[b]	2,000	26,000	,000
	Hotelling's trace	57,325	745,230[b]	2,000	26,000	,000
	Roy's largest root	57,325	745,230[b]	2,000	26,000	,000
VAR00002	Pillai's trace	,318	2,557	4,000	54,000	0,49
	Wilks' lambda	,699	2,555[b]	4,000	52,000	,050
	Hotelling's trace	,407	2,546	4,000	50,000	0,51
	Roy's largest root	,335	4,520[c]	2,000	27,000	,020

[a]Design: Intercept + VAR00002
[b]Exact statistic
[c]The statistic is an upper bound on F that yields a lower bound on the significance level

Table 25.5 ANOVAs of the data from Table 25.4. In ANOVA nor actions nor thought are significant outcomes from the predictor treatment modality

ANOVA[b]

Model		Sum of squares	df	Mean square	F	Sig.
1	Regression	,050	1	,050	,023	,881[a]
	Residual	61,417	28	2,193		
	Total	61,467	29			

[a]Predictors: (Constant), cog/beh/notreat
[b]Dependent Variable: actions

ANOVA[b]

Model		Sum of squares	df	Mean square	F	Sig.
1	Regression	12,800	1	12,800	2,785	,106[a]
	Residual	128,667	28	4,595		
	Total	141,467	29			

[a]Predictors: (Constant), cog/beh/notreat
[b]Dependent Variable: thoughts

Command: Analyze…General Linear Model…Univariate…in dialog box univariate transfer y_1 to dependent variables and x to the fixed factors, and…ok. Do the same for variable y_2.

Table 25.5 shows that in the ANOVAs nor thoughts nor actions are significant outcomes of treatment modality anymore. This would mean that the treatment modality is a rather weak predictor of either of the outcomes, and that it is not able to significantly predict a single outcome, but that it significantly predicts two outcomes pointing into a similar direction.

5   Multivariate Probit Regression

For univariate analyses with binary outcome variables logistic regression is adequate. A problem with logistic regression with multiple outcome variables is that after iteration (=computer program for finding the largest log likelihood ratio (see Chap. 4) for fitting the data) the results often do not converse, i.e., a best log likelihood ratio is not established. This is due to insufficient data size, inadequate data, or non-quadratic data patterns. A better alternative for that purpose is probit modeling. This may sound incomprehensible, but the dependent variable of logistic regression (the log odds of responding) is closely related to log probit (probit is the z-value corresponding to its area under curve value of the normal distribution). It can be shown that log odds of responding = logit $\approx (\pi \sqrt{3}) \times$ probit. Multivariate probit analysis is not available in SPSS and we will use the statistical software of the program Stata (STATA 10) (Stata 2011). An example is given of the effect of the physicians' age (x) on their inclination to prescribe life style treatments (1) non smoking advise (0 = no, 1 = yes) and (2) weight reduction advise (0 = no, 1 = yes), (y and z), (Var = variable).

Var(x)	Var (y)	Var (z)
42.7	0	0
47.6	0	0
36.4	0	0
49.0	0	0
49.0	0	1
55.3	0	1
57.4	0	1
63.0	0	1
27.3	0	1
53.2	1	0
54.6	1	0
32.9	1	0

We can quickly input the data with the commands:

Input x y z…input values…end…List…Statistics…binary outcomes…Bivariate probit regression…dependent variable 1 y…dependent variable 2 z….independent variables x… ok.

Table 25.6 shows that physicians' age is significant predictor of both prescribing non smoking and weight reduction advise. In order to find out which is the most significant outcome, simple logistic regression can be performed using physicians' ages as predictor and the non drug treatments as separate outcomes (see Chap. 17).

Table 25.6 According to the underneath analysis the probit regression shows that indeed physicians' age is significant predictor of both prescribing non smoking and weight reduction advise

STATA
Probit var 3 var 2 var 1
Fitting comparison equation 1:
Iteration 0: log likelihood = −8.3177662
Fitting comparison equation 2:
Iteration 0: log likelihood = −8.3177662
Comparison: log likelihood = −16.635532
Fitting full model:
Iteration 0: log likelihood = −16.635532
Iteration 1: log likelihood = −15.9573
Iteration 2: log likelihood = −15.955936
Iteration 3: log likelihood = −15.955936
Bivariate probit regression   number of observations = 12
Wald chi2 (2) = 0.00
Log likelihood = −15.955936   Prob > chi2 = 1.0000
2 log likelihood ratio = 31.911872
$P < 0.000$

6 Discussion

A number of advantages of multivariate analysis instead of multiple univariate analyses are summarized:

1. It prevents the type I error from being inflated.
2. It looks at interactions between dependent variables.
3. It can detect subgroup properties and includes them in the analysis.
4. It can demonstrate otherwise underpowered effects

Multivariate analysis should not be used for explorative purposes and data dredging, but should be based on sound clinical arguments. In this chapter three methods are reviewed and explained with examples.

A pleasant thing about path analysis (see also Chap. 20) is that it can be used as a nonmathematical approach to multivariate regression. We should emphasize once more that the term multivariate regression is often erroneously applied, when multiple independent and just a single dependent variable are in the data. Strictly, multivariate regression regards models with more than a single dependent variable (y-variable). The main aim is to quantify reasons for the correlation between two or more dependent variables. In the example given the multivariate model of our data with two instead of one outcome variables made even better use of the predictors than did the single outcome model.

If you read articles you will find that it is not uncommon for researchers to perform multiple ANOVAs instead of a single MANOVA. There are problems with this approach. First you have to perform multiple tests, which means that the risk of type I errors is enhanced (see also the Chaps. 8 and 9). In the first MANOVA example it would therefore be appropriate to perform a Bonferroni adjustment of the ANOVAs meaning that the p-values should be doubled. Another problem is that of weak outcomes. The second MANOVA example is an example of weak outcomes: the MANOVA was statistically significant, while the ANOVAs of the same data were not. Another method for post hoc analysis of a positive MANOVA is socalled discriminant analysis using normally distributed eigenvectors which assess the correlation of the outcome variables using scatterplots in the form of ellipses. The advantage of this method which is readily provided by SPSS is, that it does not need Bonferroni adjustment and gives somewhat more quantitative result about underlying mechanisms than ANOVA does.

Multivariate probit regression is a more safe alternative for multivariate logistic regression, and it is available in Stata and other software programs. In case of a significant multivariate probit regression, post hoc analysis can be performed in the usual way by binary logistic models to find out which of the outcome is more important.

7   Conclusions

The term multivariate analysis refers to the simultaneous analysis of more than one *outcome* variable.

This chapter reviews multivariate methods suitable to analyze data files with multiple outcome variables

For the analysis of continuous outcome variables path analysis and multiple analysis of variance (MANOVA) are suitable, for the analysis of binary outcome variables probit analysis is recommended.

We conclude that multivariate methods have multiple advantages compared to univariate methods.

1. It prevents the type I error from being inflated.
2. It looks at interactions between dependent variables.
3. It can detect subgroup properties and includes them in the analysis.
4. It can demonstrate otherwise underpowered effects

Multivariate analysis should not be used for explorative purposes and data dredging, but should be based on sound clinical arguments. In this chapter three methods are reviewed and explained with examples.

References

Field A (2005) Discovering statistics using SPSS, 2nd edn. Sage Publications, London, pp 571–618

SPSS. www.spss.com. Accessed 15 Dec 2011

Stata. www.stata.com. Accessed 15 Dec 2011

Chapter 26
Bhattacharya Modeling

1 Introduction

In 1967 Bhattacharya, a biologist from India, presented a method for identifying juvenile-fish subgroups from random samples (Bhattacharya 1967). By now this test, based on Gaussian curves, has become a key-method for the analysis and sustainability of this important resource in the eco-system, and is recommended by the Food and Agricultural Organization of the United Nations Guidelines (FAO 2011). As Gaussian curves are the mainstream not only with fish population research, but also with clinical data, it is peculiar that, so far, this method has not been widely applied in clinical research. When searching Pub Med we only found a few clinical-laboratory studies (Guerin et al. 1992; Watson et al. 1999; Pottel et al. 2008; Baadenhuijsen and Smit 1985), epidemiological (Metz et al. 2002; Zhang et al. 2004) and genetic studies (Miescke and Musea 1994; Evans et al. 1983), and not a single cardiovascular study. In clinical research data-files are, usually, summarized by their means and standards deviations (SDs). Standard deviations are a convenient way of estimating the spread in your data, but they are only valid if your data can be assumed to follow a clock-like Gaussian curve. Under this assumption the mean $\pm 1.96 \times$ SDs covers 95% of the data. Of course, many cardiovascular data samples are not perfectly Gaussian-like. Mean and SDs are, therefore, just approximations. There may be better methods to find the best fit Gaussian curves for your data. Instead of the mean, the mode or median can be used, and instead of histograms consistent of bins, more refined Kernel histograms consistent of multiple similarly sized small Gaussian curves can be drawn (Metz et al. 2002). Also, distribution-free statistical methods like non-parametric tests can be applied to "quasi-gaussianize" the data. However, all of these methods massage the data. Bhattacharya modeling does not massage the data, but, instead, unmasks Gaussian curves, as truly present in the data, and removes outlier frequencies. In clinical research it could be used (1) for unmasking normal values of diagnostic tests, (2) for improving the p-values of data testing, and (3) for objectively searching subsets in your data. The current chapter uses as examples simulated vascular lab scores to investigate

the performance of Bhattacharya modeling as compared to standards methods, and
was written to acquaint the clinical research community with this novel method.

2 Unmasking Normal Values

Vascular laboratories often define their estimators of peripheral vascular disease
according to add-up scores of ankle, thigh, calf, and toe pressures. Figure 26.1 upper
graph and Table 26.1 left two columns give as an example the frequency distribution
of such scores in La Fontaine stage I patients. Normal values, otherwise called reference values, customarily present the central 95% of the values obtained from a
representative reference population. Consequently, 2.5% of the reference population will exceed the reference range and 2.5% will be below it. This central 95%,
otherwise called 95% confidence interval, is calculated from the equation

$$95\% \text{ confidence interval} = \text{mean} \pm 1.96 \times \text{sd}$$
$$= 13.236 \pm 1.96 \times 5.600 =$$
$$= \text{between } 2.260 \text{ and } 24.212.$$

Alternatively to the above standard procedure a Bhattacharya procedure can be
performed. Table 26.1 shows how it works. We logarithmically transform the frequencies, and then calculate the differences between two subsequent log-frequencies,
named the delta log values. Figure 26.2 shows a plot of the scores against these delta

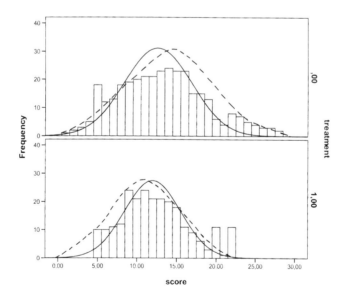

Fig. 26.1 The frequency distributions of the vascular lab scores of untreated (0,00), and treated
(1,00) La Fontaine stage I patients. The continuous Gaussian curves are calculated from the
mean ± standard deviation, the interrupted Gaussian curves from Bhattacharya modeling

Table 26.1 The frequency distribution of the vascular lab scores of 244 untreated La Fontaine stage I patients (treatment$_0$ patients of Fig. 26.1)

Score	Frequency	Log	Delta log
5	10	1.000	
6	10	1.000	0.000
7	11	1.041	0.041
8	12	1.079	0.038
9	24	1.380	0.301
10	21	1.322	−0.058
11	24	1.380	0.058
12	21	1.322	−0.058
13	21	1.322	0.000
14	20	1.301	−0.021
15	18	1.255	−0.046
16	11	1.041	−0.214
17	9	0.954	−0.087
18	6	0.778	−0.176
19	3	0.477	−0.301
20	21	1.322	0.845
21	1	0.000	−1.322
22	21	1.322	−1.322

The log and delta log terms are respectively log transformations of the frequencies and differences between two subsequent log transformations

log values. A straight line with a correlation coefficient as high as 1.000 is identified, and the equation of this line is used for unmasking the values of the Gaussian curve truly present in these data.

$$y = a + bx$$
$$a = \text{intercept}$$
$$b = \text{direction coefficient}$$

This line is used as the first derivative of a Gaussian curve with

$$\text{mean} = -a / b$$
$$\text{standard deviation} = \sqrt{(-1/b)}.$$

This procedure leads to a result different from that of the standard procedure.

$$95\% \text{ confidence interval} = \text{mean} \pm 1.96 \times \text{sd}$$
$$= 14.700 \pm 1.96 \times 7.390 =$$
$$= \text{between } 0.216 \text{ and } 29.184.$$

The Bhattacharya estimate is wider than the standard estimate, and it is not obvious from the graph which one will best fit the data. Figure 26.1 also shows the graphs of the standard and Bhattacharya Gaussian curves. When counting the tops of the bins cut by either of the curves, it seems that the Bhattacharya curve performs better: 15 cuts versus 9 cuts. And, so, the Bhattacharya 95% confidence interval produces a better data fit than does the standard 95% confidence interval as calculated directly from the mean and standard deviation.

3   Improving the p-Values of Data Testing

Figure 26.1 gives an example of frequency distributions of untreated and treated Fontaine stage I patients with vascular lab scores on the x-axis and "how often" on the y-axis. We wish to test whether the treatment is better than no treatment. The two sample t-test of these data produced a p-value of 0.051. The non-parametric test of the same data (the Mann–Whitney test) produced a p-value of 0.085. In order to test with improved sensitivity a t-test of the Bhattacharya Gaussian curves is performed. The first two columns of the Tables 26.1 and 26.2 present the x and y axes values of the histograms from Fig. 26.1. First, the y-axis variable is log transformed. Then the differences between two subsequent log transformed y-values are calculated (delta log terms):

$0.301-0=0.301$
$0.477-0.301=0.176$
$0.699-0.477=0.222$ etc

A plot of the vascular lab scores against the delta log terms is drawn, and we identify the points that will give you a straight line (Figs. 26.2 and 26.3). A straight line consistent of delta log terms means the presence of a Gaussian distribution in

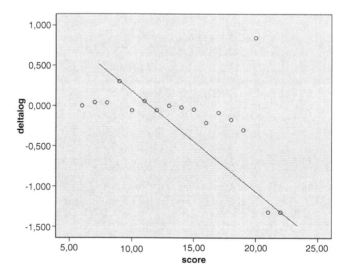

Fig. 26.2 The scores from Fig. 26.1 *upper graph* plotted against the delta log terms as calculated from the frequencies from Fig. 26.1

Table 26.2 The frequency distribution of the vascular lab scores of 331 treated La Fontaine stage I patients (treatment$_1$ patients of Fig. 26.1)

Score	Frequency	Log	Delta log
1	1	0.000	
2	2	0.301	0.301
3	3	0.477	0.176
4	5	0.699	0.222
5	18	1.255	0.556
6	12	1.079	−0.176
7	13	1.114	0.035
8	18	1.255	0.141
9	19	1.279	0.024
10	20	1.301	0.022
11	21	1.322	0.021
12	21	1.322	0.000
13	23	1.362	0.040
14	24	1.380	0.018
15	23	1.362	−0.018
16	23	1.362	0.000
17	15	1.176	−0.186
18	15	1.176	0.000
19	13	1.114	−0.036
20	6	0.778	−0.336
21	4	0.602	−0.176
22	8	0.903	0.301
23	7	0.845	−0.058
24	5	0.699	−0.146
25	4	0.602	−0.097
26	3	0.477	−0.125
27	3	0.477	0.000
28	2	0.301	−0.176

The log and delta log terms are respectively log transformations of the frequencies and differences between two subsequent log transformations

your data. It can be shown that a linear regression analysis of this line serves as the first derivative of a Gaussian curve and that it can be used for calculating the characteristics of this Gaussian distribution in a way that is unaffected by other distributions.

For the treatment$_0$-data we find

The correlation coefficient $R = 0.998$
The regression equation is given by $y = 0.269 - 0.0183 \, x$
The mean of our Gaussian distribution is given by $-0.2690 / -0.0183 = 14.70$
De squared standard deviation is given by $1/0.0183 = 54.60$
The standard deviation (SD) is $\sqrt{54.60} = 7.39$.

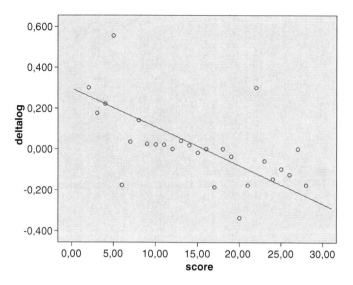

Fig. 26.3 The scores from Fig. 26.1 *lower graph* plotted against the delta log terms as calculated from the frequencies from Fig. 26.1

With $n = 331$, this would mean that the standard error (SE) of the Gaussian distribution is

$$SE = SD / \sqrt{n} = 0.406.$$

For the treatment$_1$-data we find

The correlation coefficient $R = 1.000$
The regression equation is given by $y = 1.418 - 0.137\,x$
The mean of our Gaussian distribution is given by $-1.418\,/-0.137 = 10.35$
De squared standard deviation is given by $1/0.137 = 7.299$
The standard deviation (SD) is $\sqrt{7.299} = 2.77$.

With $n = 244$, this would mean that the standard error (SE) of the Gaussian distribution is

$$SE = SD / \sqrt{n} = 0.173$$

An unpaired t-test of these two mean produces a t-value of t-value $= (14.70 - 10.35)/(0.173^2 + 0.406^2) = 9.86$ which means that the two Gaussian curve are largely different with $p = 0.0001$.

4   Objectively Searching Subsets in the Data

Figure 26.4 givens an example of the frequency distributions of vascular lab scores of a population of 787 patients at risk of peripheral vascular disease. Overall normal values of this population can be calculated from the mean and standard deviation:

Normal values = 95% confidence interval = $24.28 \pm 1.96 \times 11.68$ = between 1.38 and 47.17.

The pattern of the histogram is suggestive of certain subsets in this population. Bhattacharya modeling is used for objective searching the subset normal values. Table 26.3 left two columns give the scores and frequencies. The frequencies are log transformed (third column), and, then, the differences between two subsequent log transformed scores are calculated (fourth column). Figure 26.5 show the plot of the scores against the delta log terms. Three straight lines are identified. Linear regression analyses of these lines produces r-values of 0.980, 0.999, and 0.998.

1. The first regression equation is given by

$$y = 0.944 - 0.078 \, x$$

The mean of the corresponding Gaussian curve is given by $-0.944/-0.137 = 12.10$.
The squared standard deviation is given by $1/0.078 = 12.82$
The standard deviation (SD) is $\sqrt{12.82} = 3.58$
The normal values of this Gaussian curve is $12.10 \pm 1.96 \times 3.58$, and is between 5.08 and 19.12.

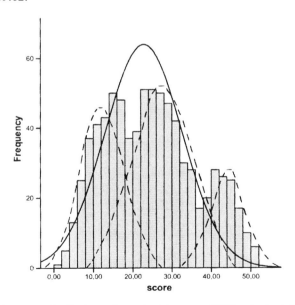

Fig. 26.4 The frequency distributions of vascular lab scores of 787 patients at risk of peripheral vascular disease. The continuous Gaussian curves are calculated from the mean ± standard deviation, the interrupted Gaussian curves from Bhattacharya modeling

Table 26.3 The frequency distribution of the vascular lab scores of 787 patients at risk of peripheral vascular disease (the data of Fig. 26.4)

Score	Frequency	Log	Delta log
2	1	0.000	0.000
4	5	0.699	0.699
6	13	1.114	0.415
8	25	1.398	0.284
10	37	1.568	0.170
12	41	1.613	0.045
14	43	1.633	0.020
16	50	1.699	−0.018
18	48	1.681	−0.111
20	37	1.570	0.021
22	39	1.591	0.117
24	51	1.708	0.000
26	51	1.708	−0.009
28	50	1.699	−0.027
30	47	1.672	−0.049
32	42	1.623	−0.146
34	30	1.477	−0.176
36	28	1.447	−0.030
38	16	1.204	−0.243
40	20	1.301	0.097
42	28	1.447	0.146
44	26	1.415	−0.032
46	25	1.398	−0.017
48	17	1.230	−0.168
50	10	1.000	−0.230
52	6	0.778	−0.222

The log and delta log terms are respectively log transformations of the frequencies and differences between two subsequent log transformations

2. The second regression equation is given by

$$y = 0.692 - 0.026\,x$$

The mean of the corresponding Gaussian curve is given by $-0.692/-0.026 = 26.62$
The squared standard deviation is given by $1/0.026 = 38.46$
The standard deviation (SD) is $\sqrt{38.46} = 6.20$
The normal values of this Gaussian curve is $26.62 \pm 1.96 \times 6.20$, and is between 14.47 and 38.77.

3. The third regression equation is given by

$$y = 2.166 - 0.048\,x$$

The mean of the corresponding Gaussian curve is given by $-2.166/-0.048 = 45.13$.
The squared standard deviation is given by $1/0.048 = 20.83$

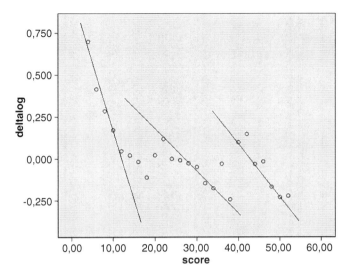

Fig. 26.5 The scores from Fig. 26.4 plotted against the delta log terms as calculated from the frequencies from Fig. 26.4

The standard deviation (SD) is $\sqrt{20.83} = 4.57$

The normal values of this Gaussian curve is $45.13 \pm 1.96 \times 4.57$, and is between 36.17 and 54.09.

In Fig. 26.4 the above three Gaussian curves are drawn as interrupted curves. When there are obviously subsets, to investigators, that is when thing first get very excited. A careful investigation of the potential causes has to be accomplished. The main focus should be on trying to understand any source of heterogeneity in the data. In practice, this may be not be very hard since investigators frequently noticed clinical differences already, and it thus becomes relatively easy to fit the results accordingly. Sometimes differences in age groups or genders are involved. Sometimes also morbidity stages or comorbidities are involved. In the given situation it was decided that the three subsets largely represented (1) stage I la Fontaine patients, (2) patients with risk factors including smoking, and (3) patients with risk factors excluding smoking.

5   Discussion

The current paper suggests that Bhattacharya modeling not only produces results different from those of the standard approach, but also provides additional benefits. First, it provided a better fit for the data. Second, a better precision as demonstrated by better p-values was obtained. Third, it enabled to better identify certain subgroups in the data.

The current paper using simulated examples of vascular lab scores has to be confirmed by larger data, but it suggests that Bhattacharya modeling for clinical data analysis tends to perform better than do standards methods.

An important condition for the method to be successful is the presence of Gaussian distributions in the data. In spite of numerous discussions in the literature the conformity of data obtained from patients to a Gaussian distribution is still believed to be of fundamental importance (Armitage and Berry 1994; Altman 1995; Feng et al. 1996), and data files including over one million values have been used to confirm this belief (Janecki 2008).

There are, of course, some problems. The first problem is that current clinical research often uses convenience samples from selected hospitals rather than random samples. Particularly, cut-off inclusion criteria like age, gender and laboratory value limits, raises the risk of non-Gaussian data (see also Chap. 43). The Figs. 26.1 and 26.2 in Chap. 43 give examples of non-normal data not suitable for Bhattacharya modeling. Goodness of fit tests can be used for checking normality. However, with small samples as commonly observed in clinical research these tests have little power, and a negative goodness of fit test does not exclude the possibility of non-normal data. Also, partly overlapping Gaussian distributions are often present. The method becomes invalid when such distributions are too close to one another, thereby preventing the recognition of the linear part in the first derivative function.

A second problem is that current clinical research often uses convenience samples from selected hospitals rather than random samples. Particularly, cut-off inclusion criteria like age, gender and laboratory value limits, raises the risk of non-Gaussian data. Goodness of fit tests can be used for checking normality. However, with small samples as commonly observed in clinical research these tests have little power, and a negative goodness of fit test does not exclude the possibility of non-normal data.

Third, the choice of the appropriate straight lines may sometimes be somewhat subjective: sometimes in a single interval of scores more than a single straight line is possible. For example, in Fig. 26.2 an almost horizontal line can be drawn though about six delta log terms. However, only lines with a clearly negative direction coefficient are suitable for Bhattacharya modeling

In spite of the above limitations, we believe that Bhattacharya modeling is a welcome help to clinical data analysis, and we recommend that it be used for the purpose of (1) unmasking normal values of diagnostic tests, (2) improving p-values of testing, and (3) objectively searching subsets in the data. Particularly, when standard data analyses do not produce the expected levels of sensitivity, Bhattacharya modeling is an adequate and more sensitive alternative.

6   Conclusions

Bhattacharya modeling is a Gaussian method recommended by the Food and Agricultural Organization of the United Nations Guidelines for analyzing the ecosystem. It is rarely used in clinical research. The objective of the current chapter was to investigate the performance of Bhattacharya modeling for clinical data analysis.

Using as examples vascular lab scores we assessed the performance of the Bhattacharya method. SPSS statistical software is used.

1. The Bhattacharya method better fitted the data from a single sample than did the usual Gaussian curve derived from the mean and standard deviation with 15 versus 9 cuts.
2. Bhattacharya models demonstrated a significant difference at $p < 0.0001$ between the data from two parallel-groups, while the usual t-test and Mann–Whitney test were insignificant at $p = 0.051$ and 0.085.
3. Bhattacharya modeling of a histogram suggestive of certain subsets identified three Gaussian curves.

We recommend that Bhattacharya modeling be more often considered in clinical research for the purpose of (1) unmasking normal values of diagnostic tests, (2) improving the p-values of data testing, and (3) objectively searching subsets in the data.

References

Altman DG (1995) Statistical notes: the normal distribution. BMJ 310:298

Armitage P, Berry G (1994) Statistical methods in medical research. Blackwell Scientific Publications, Oxford, pp 66–71

Baadenhuijsen H, Smit JC (1985) Indirect estimation of clinical chemical reference intervals from total hospital patient data. J Clin Chem Clin Biochem 23:829–839

Bhattacharya CG (1967) A simple solution of a distribution into Gaussian components. Biometrics 23:115–135

Evans DA, Harmer D, Downham DY, Whibley EJ, Idle JR, Ritchie J, Smith RL (1983) The genetic control of sparteine and debrisoquine metabolism in man with new methods of analysing bimodal distributions. J Med Genet 20:321–329

Feng Z, McLerran D, Grizzle J (1996) A comparison of statistical methods for clustered data analysis with Gaussian error. Stat Med 15:1793–1806

Food and Agricultural Organization of the United Nations (2011) Manuals and guides BOBP/MAG/14. Separating mixtures of normal distributions: basic programs for Bhattacharya's method and their applications to fish analysis. Copyright@fao.org. Accessed 15 Dec 2011

Guerin MD, Sikaris KA, Martin A (1992) Pathology informatics: an expanded role for laboratory information systems. Pathology 24:523–529

Janecki JM (2008) Application of statistical features of the Gaussian distribution hidden in sets of unselected medical laboratory results. Biocyb Biomed Eng 28:71–81

Metz J, Maxwell EL, Levin MD (2002) Changes in folate concentrations following voluntary food fortification in Australia. Med J Aust 176:90–91

Miescke KJ, Musea MN (1994) On mixtures of three normal populations caused by Monogenic inheritance: application to desipramine metabolism. J Psychiatry Neurosci 19:295–300

Pottel H, Vrydags N, Mahieu B, Vandewynckele E, Croes K, Martens F (2008) Establishing age/sex related serum creatinine reference intervals from hospital laboratory data based on different statistical methods. Clin Chim Acta 396:49–55

Watson N, Sikaris KA, Morris G, Mitchell DK (1999) Confirmation of age related rise in reference intervals for fasting glucose using the Bhattacharya method and patient data. Clin Biochem Rev 20:92–98

Zhang L, Liu C, Davis CJ (2004) A mixture model-based approach to the classification of habitats using forest inventory and analysis data. Can J For Res 34:1150–1156

Chapter 27
Trend-Testing

1 Introduction

Some 15 years ago serious statistical analyses of clinical trials were conducted by specialist statisticians using mainframe computers. Nowadays, there is ready access to statistical computing using personal computers, and this practice has changed boundaries between basic and more advanced statistical methods. Clinical researchers, currently, perform basic statistics without professional help from a statistician, including t-tests and chi-square tests for two treatment comparisons. Current clinical trials often involve more than two treatments or treatment modalities, e.g., dose–response and dose-finding trials, studies comparing multiple drugs from one class with different potencies, or different formulas from one drug with various bio-availabilities and other pharmacokinetic properties. In such situations small differences in efficacies are to be expected and we need, particularly, sensitive tests. A standard approach to the analysis of such data is multiple groups analysis of variance (ANOVA) and multiple groups chi-square tests, but a more sensitive, although so far little used, approach may be a trend-analysis. A trend means an association between the order of treatment and the magnitude of response. We should add that, within the context of a clinical trial, demonstrating trends, generally, provides more convincing evidence of causal treatment effects than do simple comparisons of treatment modalities (Kirkwood and Sterne 2003).

In the current chapter we review methods for trend-analysis in clinical trials that can be used by clinical investigators without the support of a statistician. We also demonstrate that trend-tests may be more sensitive to demonstrate statistically significant treatment effects than do the standard methods for treatment comparisons.

T.J. Cleophas and A.H. Zwinderman, *Statistics Applied to Clinical Studies*, DOI 10.1007/978-94-007-2863-9_27, © Springer Science+Business Media B.V. 2012

2 Binary Data, the Chi-Square-Test-for-Trends

For trend-analysis of binary data the chi-square-test–for-trends is adequate, although similar results can be obtained from logistic regression modeling. However, the former test is conceptually more straightforward and mathematically less complex. A real data example is given. In a hypertension trial responders were defined as patients with a blood pressure under 140/90 mmHg. The data (Table 27.1) were first analyzed using multiple groups chi-square test, and this analysis produced a chi-square value of 3.872 with two degrees of freedom. According to the chi-square table this would mean, that this result is not statistically significant ($p = 0.144$). We have a negative study, that does not enable to conclude anything else than "no treatment differences in these data". However, if we calculate the odds of responding (Table 27.1), we find incremental odds from treatment 0 to treatment 2, suggesting an association between the order of treatment and the magnitude of response, otherwise called a trend. The chi-square-test-for-trend can be used for assessment of this possible trend.

$$\Sigma d \quad = 10 \times 0 + 20 \times 1 + 27 \times 2 = 74$$

$$\Sigma n \quad = 25 \times 0 + 39 \times 1 + 42 \times 2 = 123$$

$$\Sigma(n^2) = 25 \times 0 + 39 \times 1 + 42 \times 4 = 207$$

$$O = 57 \quad T = 106 \quad T - O = 49$$

$$U = \Sigma d - (O / T \times \Sigma n) = 74 - (57 / 106 \times 123) = 8.0$$

$$V = \frac{O(T - O)}{T^2 \times (T - 1)} \times \left(T \times \Sigma(n^2) - (\Sigma n)^2\right) = \frac{57 \times 49}{106^2 \times 105} \times (106 \times 207 - 123^2) = 16.079$$

The chi-square-trend is calculated to be $U^2/V = 3.980$ with one degree of freedom. According to the chi-square table this would mean, that we have a significant trend at $p < 0.05$. There is evidence that the higher the number of the treatment the more efficacious the treatment is. Particularly, if we have clinical arguments, like with increasing potencies of otherwise similar treatments, this result provides the evidence. Interestingly, the trend-test is significant in spite of a negative overall test for differences in the data. Obviously, a trend-test is sometimes more sensitive than a standard overall test to find differences in the data. The test is provided by SPSS under the commands "Descriptive statistics – crosstabs – statistics – chi-square".

Table 27.1 In a hypertension trial responders were defined as patients with a blood pressure under 140/90 mm Hg

	Treatment 0	Treatment 1	Treatment 2	Total
Number responders (d)	10	20	27	57 (O)
Number non-responders	15	19	15	49
Total number patients (n)	25	39	42	106 (T)
Odds of responding	0.67 (10/15)	1.11 (20/19)	1.80 (27/15)	

The Linear-by–Linear Association in the table given has 1 degree of freedom and provides the chi-square value for trends plus an adequate p-value (see Cleophas and Zwinderman 2010).

3   Continuous Data, Linear-Regression-Test-for-Trends

For trend-analysis of continuous data linear-regression-modeling, is often used. As an example a hypertension trial with mean arterial blood pressures (MAPs) as efficacy variable is given (Table 27.2).

First the data are assessed by an overall test. Multiple groups ANOVA is used for that purpose, and provides an F-value of 2.035 with 2 and 27 degrees of freedom. This result means that we have a p-value of 0.150, and, thus, no significant difference between the three groups of patients. Also, as expected, the largest difference between the mean MAP of treatments 1 and 3 are not significant in the unpaired t-test:

$$t\text{ - value} = \frac{122 - 115}{\sqrt{\left(8.08^2 / 10 + 8.08^2 / 10\right)}} = 7 / 3.613 = 1.937$$

(with $20 - 2 = 18$ degrees of freedom, $0.05 < p < 0.10$.)

A linear-regression-test-for-trends using SPSS statistical software (2011) produces the following results. We first enter the data or a data-file, e.g., from Excel (Microsoft's Excel 2011). Then we command: Statistics; Regression; Linear; dependent = MAP values; independent = treatment modality; ok. Table 27.3 gives the results. The top-table calculates the correlation coefficient R and R^2.

Table 27.2 In a hypertension trial mean arterial blood pressures (MAPs) after treatment were assessed as efficacy variable

	Treatment 1	Treatment 2	Treatment 3
	Number of patients		
	10	10	10
MAP (mmHg)	122	118	115
	113	109	105
	131	127	125
	112	110	106
	132	126	124
	114	111	107
	130	125	123
	115	118	108
	129	124	115
	122	112	122
Mean	122	118	115
Standard deviation	8.08	7.15	8.08

Table 27.3 Results of statistical analysis using SPSS software of the data from Table 27.2

Model summary				
Model	R	R square	Adjusted R square	Std. error of the estimate
1	.361[a]	.130	.099	7.64775

ANOVA[b]						
Model		Sum of squares	df	Mean square	F	Sig.
1	Regression	245.000	1	245.000	4.189	.050[a]
	Residual	1637.667	28	58.488		
	Total	1882.667	29			

Coefficients[b]		Unstandardized coefficients		Standard coefficients		
Model		B	Std. error	Beta	t	Sig.
1	(Constant)	125.333	3.694		33.927	.000
	VAR00001	−3.500	1.710	−.361	−2.047	.050

The top-table gives the R-values, the middle-table tests with ANOVA whether R is significantly different from 0, the bottom-table provides the regression equation
ANOVA analysis of variance, *df* degree of freedom, *F* F-statistic, *sig.* level of signifi-
cance, *R* correlation coefficient, *B* regression coefficient, *t* t-statistic
[a]Predictors: (Constant), VAR00001
[b]Dependent variable: VAR00002

The middle-table gives the result of testing with ANOVA whether R^2 is significantly different from 0. If $R^2=0$, the order of the treatment determines the MAPs no way, there is no trend. In our situation $R^2=0.13$, and, thus, 13% of the MAP results are determined by the differences in treatment modalities: there is a significant trend at p=0.05. The bottom-table from Table 27.3 gives the regression equation that can be used to draw the best fit regression line for the data.

In spite of the negative ANOVA- and t-tests for treatment comparisons, there is a significant trend in the data. We are able to conclude that the order of the treatments is associated with the magnitude of efficacy. Like in the above example of a binary variable, the trend-test was more sensitive than the standard tests to find differences in the data.

4   Discussion

In this chapter only trend-tests for parallel-group data are reviewed. Although not commonly used in clinical trials and statistically somewhat more sophisticated, trend-tests are also available for repeated measurements in one subject or one group of patients. In the case of continuous data a linear mixed-model effect can be used, where the subjects are regarded as random variable, and the treatment as fixed effect variable. The presence of a significant treatment-by-subjects interaction is, then, considered as documented evidence of order-of-treatments-effect or trend. Analyses are available in SPSS (2011) and SAS (2011). Just like with parallel-group data a significant trend may be found in spite of a negative overall test for treatment differences. Repeated measurements with binary data are even less common in clinical research, and statistical software for trends is also less generally available, but some methods are presented in SAS proc nlmixed (SAS 2011). To assess trends of odds ratios we can make use of the assumed normal distribution of the regression coefficients, the b-values. Log likelihood ratio tests with the b-value as variable can be used for the purpose.

Why is trend-analysis often more sensitive than standard testing? We should add that with two treatments a trend-test and a standard test provide identical results. This is, because we have equal degrees of freedom. However, with three or more treatment modalities the degrees of freedom with a standard analysis rapidly increase, while with trend-analysis they do not, giving rise to smaller p-values.

The limitations of trend-analysis have to be accounted. First, if there is no trend in the data, then the standard method of analysis may be more sensitive than the trend-test. So, standard tests should be performed in addition to the trend tests. Second, trend-testing assumes a linear trend in response in the data with subsequent treatments. This means that, with continuous data the means of the treatment groups increase linearly, and with binary data, the odds of responding increase exponentially (or the logarithms of the odds increase linearly). The linear effect is a simplifying assumption that should be checked. With only three categories as dependent variable, linearity is easy to check from a graph or even from the tables of the data. However, with multiple categories linearity checking is less straightforward, and special methods have to be used. Assuming a quadratic relationship between dependent and independent variable, and, then, performing a regression analysis is an adequate approach for that purpose, because the quadratic relationship is mathematically the simplest relationship that comes next to the linear relationship. If a better p-value is provided by the quadratic model, then this relationship should be pursued, and the linear relationship has to be abandoned.

Clinical researchers, currently, perform basic statistics without professional help from a statistician, and current cardiovascular trials often involve more than two treatments or treatment modalities. Trend-tests may be more sensitive than standard methods for treatments comparisons. A trend means an association between the order of treatment and the magnitude of response. The chi-square-test-for-trends and the linear-regression-test-for-trends are adequate for the analysis of parallel-group data. Although not commonly used in clinical trials, trend-tests for repeated measurements in one subject or one group of patients are available in SPSS (2011), SAS (2011), and other major statistical software programs.

Limitations of trend-testing include: (1) trend-testing may be less sensitive than standard tests if a trend in the data is lacking, (2) trends may not be linear. We recommend that trend-testing be included more routinely in clinical trial-protocols in order to increase the sensitivity of data analysis of clinical trials.

5   Conclusions

Clinical investigators tend to perform basic statistics without professional help from a statistician, and current clinical trials often involve more than two treatments or treatment modalities. Trend-tests may be more sensitive than standard methods for treatments comparisons. This chapter reviews methods for trend-analysis of parallel-group data from clinical trials.

1. A trend means an association between the order of treatment and the magnitude of response.
2. The chi-square-test-for-trends and the linear-regression-test-for-trends are adequate for the analysis of parallel-group data.
3. Although not commonly used in cardiovascular trials, trend-tests for repeated measurements in one subject or one group of patients are available in SPSS, SAS, and other major statistical software programs.
4. Limitations of trend-testing include: (1) trend-tests may be less sensitive than standard tests if a trend in the data is lacking, (2) trends may not be linear.
5. We recommend that trend-testing be included more routinely in trial-protocols in order to increase the sensitivity of data analysis of clinical trials.

References

Cleophas TJ, Zwinderman AH (2010) SPSS for starters. Springer, Dordrecht, pp 43–45
Kirkwood BR, Sterne JAC (2003) Dose response relationships (trends). In: Medical statistics. Blackwell Science, Malden, pp 336–338
Microsoft's Excel. www.microsoft.com. Accessed 15 Dec 2011
SAS. http://www.prw.le.ac.uk/epidemiol/personal/ajs22/meta/macros.sas. Accessed 15 Dec 2011
SPSS Statistical Software. http://www.spss.com. Accessed 15 Dec 2011

Chapter 28
Confounding

1   Introduction

When published, a randomized parallel-group drug trial essentially includes a table listing all of the factors, otherwise called baseline characteristics, known possibly to influence outcome. E.g., in case of heart disease these will probably include apart from age and gender, the prevalence in each group of diabetes, hypertension, cholesterol levels, smoking history, other cardiovascular comorbidities, and concomitant medications. If the prevalence of such factors is similar in the two groups, then we can attribute any difference in outcome to the effect of test-treatment over reference-treatment. However, if this is not the case, we have a problem which can be illustrated by an example. Figure 28.1 shows the results of a study where the treatment effects are better in the males than they are in the females. This difference in efficacy does not influence the overall assessment as long as the numbers of males and females in the treatment comparison are equally distributed. If, however, many females received the new treatment, and many males received the control treatment, a peculiar effect on the overall data analysis is observed: the overall regression line is close to horizontal, giving rise to the erroneous conclusion that no difference in efficacy exists between treatment and control. This phenomenon is called confounding, and may have a profound effect on the outcome of a trial. In randomized controlled trials confounding is, traditionally, considered to play a minor role in the data. The randomization ensures that no covariate of the efficacy variable is associated with the randomized treatment (Cleophas et al. 2006a). However, the randomization may fail for one or more variables, making such variables confounders. Then, adjustment of the efficacy estimate should be attempted. Methods include subclassification (Cochran 1968), regression modeling (Cleophas et al. 2006a), and propensity scores (Rosenbaum and Rubin 1983; Rubin 1997). This chapter reviews these three methods and uses hypothesized and real data examples for that purpose.

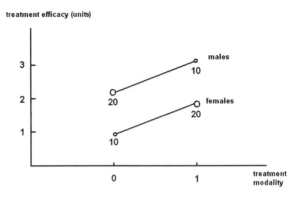

Fig. 28.1 Efficacy of control (*0*) and test treatment (*1*) in a trial where females and males are assessed separately. The magnitude of the circles corresponds to the size of the subclass samples

2   First Method for Adjustment of Confounders: Subclassification on One Confounder

Figure 28.2 gives an example of confounding on one variable, age. In a large database from Canada (Cochran 1968) the overall mortality from cigar smoking was significantly larger than that from cigarette smoking However, the cigar smokers were significantly older, and, therefore, hardly comparable (mean age 66 versus 51 years, p<0.05). How do we assess this inequality of age in the groups. One way of assessment is as follows: (1) we divide the population into age subclasses of approximately equal size, the younger, middle-ages, and older, then, (2) compare mortality per subclass, and, finally, (3) calculate a so-called weighted average. Figure 28.2 shows that in any of the three subclasses mortality from cigarettes was higher than from cigars, but differences were not statistically significant. The higher mortality from cigars in the overall assessment was caused by the fact that many youngsters smoked cigarettes, while many elderly, obviously, preferred cigars. The weighted average is calculated as

$$\frac{(R_{cigt} - R_{cig})_1 / variance_1 + (R_{cigt} - R_{cig})_2 / variance_2 + (R_{cigt} - R_{cig})_3 / variance_3}{1/variance_1 \quad + \quad 1/variance_2 \quad + \quad 1/variance_3}$$

where $(R_{cigt} - R_{cig})$ = difference in mortality rate (R) between cigarette and cigar smokers for subclass 1 (the younger), subclass 2 (the middle-ages), and subclass 3 (the elderly) respectively, variance are the variances of these difference-in-rates. For testing the significance of difference between cigarette and cigar smoking of the weighted averages a weighted variance is required which is calculated as add-up sum of the separate variances. Cochran used, among other examples, the above example and reasoned that as long as a reasonable number of persons are in each

mortality rates per 1000 person-years(%)

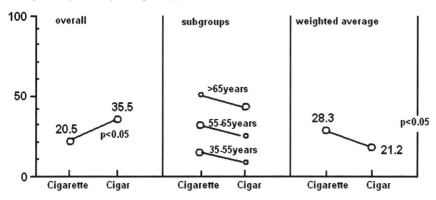

Fig. 28.2 Example of subclassification on one confounder (age). *Left graph*: overall mortality from cigar smoking is significantly larger than that from cigarette smoking; *middle graph*: if divided into three subclasses, the mortality from cigarettes is larger than that from cigars although the differences were not statistically significant; *right graph*: a weighted average from the comparisons from the middle graph shows that the mortality from cigarettes is significantly larger than from cigars

subclass this procedure removes up to 90% of the bias due to confounding (Cochran 1968). The advantages of subclassification over regression analysis for confounding include, first, that empty subclasses in the treatment comparisons are readily visualized, and, second, that subclassification does not rely on a linear or other regression model, and is, thus, universally applicable. The problem with subclassification is that, with multiple confounders, it is simply impossible to divide the population in subclasses. For that purpose multivariable regression analysis is required.

3   Second Method for Adjustment of Confounders: Regression Modeling

Instead of subclassification regression modeling can be applied to adjust a confounding variable (Cleophas et al. 2006a). An example is given in Fig. 28.1. The data of a parallel-group study produced a significant difference

Mean treatment 0	1.666	standard deviation 0.479	
Mean treatment 1	2.333	standard deviation 0.479	
Difference	0.666	standard error 0.214	$p < 0.001$

The same result is obtained using a linear regression model with treatment modality on the x-axis and treatment efficacy on the y-axis. The regression coefficient is the direction coefficient of the regression line and equals 0.666 (standard error 0.214), which is equal to the mean treatment efficacy as obtained in the above usual analysis. From the Fig. 28.1 it is concluded that gender is a confounding variable and the data are thus adjusted for gender by adding it as a second dependent variable (variable z) to the model. SPSS (2011) statistical software produces the following results after commanding: statistics; regression; linear;

	r^2	b	se	p-value
Unadjusted	0.333	0.666	0.214	<0.001
Adjusted	1.000	1.000	0.000	<0.00001

where r correlation coefficient, b regression coefficient, se standard error

The adjusted efficacy estimate b may become smaller or larger than the unadjusted estimate, depending on the direction of the associations of the confounder with the randomized treatment and the efficacy variable. Let b_1 and b_1^* denote the unadjusted and the adjusted efficacy estimate, and let r_{xz} and r_{yz} be the correlations of the confounder (z) with the randomized treatment (x) and the efficacy variable (y), then the following will hold:

$$\text{if } r_{xz} > 0 \text{ and } r_{yz} > 0 \quad \text{then} \quad \left|b_1^*\right| < \left|b_1\right|,$$

$$\text{if } r_{xz} > 0 \text{ and } r_{yz} < 0 \quad \text{then} \quad \left|b_1^*\right| > \left|b_1\right|,$$

$$\text{if } r_{xz} < 0 \text{ and } r_{yz} < 0 \quad \text{then} \quad \left|b_1^*\right| < \left|b_1\right|,$$

$$\text{if } r_{xz} < 0 \text{ and } r_{yz} > 0 \quad \text{then} \quad \left|b_1^*\right| > \left|b_1\right|,$$

Notice the possibility that the unadjusted efficacy estimate b_1 is zero whereas the adjusted estimate b_1^* is unequal to zero: an efficacy-difference between treatments may be masked by confounding. In clinical trials it is sensible to check the balance between treatment groups of all known covariates of the efficacy variable. In most trials there are many more covariates and one should be careful to consider as a confounder a covariate which was not reported in the literature before. The advantage of regression analysis compared to subclassification is that multiple variables can be added to the model in order to test whether they are independent determinants, and thus significant confounders of the dependent variable, treatment efficacy. The power of these tests is a sensitive function of the number of patients in the trial. Naturally, there is less opportunity for modeling in a small trial than there is in a large trial. There is no general rule about what sample sizes are required for sensible regression modeling, but a rule of thumb is that at least ten times as many patients are required as the number of covariates in the model. If these requirements are not met, the trial rapidly loses power, and a different approach is needed. Propensity scores have been recommended for that purpose.

4 Third Method for Adjustment of Confounders: Propensity Scores

The method of propensity scores is relatively new (Rosenbaum and Rubin 1983; Rubin 1997), but increasingly accepted in observational research, although its theoretical properties have not yet been entirely elucidated. Each patient is assigned a propensity score, which is his/her probability, based on his/her covariate value, of receiving a particular treatment modality. As an example, in a parallel group study of 100 versus 100 patients, 63 out of 100 patients in treatment group 1 were older than 65, while 76 were so in treatment group 2. The probability of receiving treatment 1 in patients older than 65 years can be calculated to be 63/76 / 37/24 = 0.54. This probability equals the odds of treatment 1 with the characteristic/odds of treatment 1 without the characteristic, otherwise called the odds ratio (OR) of the two. This odds ratio can, then, be applied as measure for adjustment the asymmetric prevalence of the patient characteristic between the treatment groups. Two alternative methods as described in the above sections are available, and propensity score are therefore rarely used for that purpose. Things are different when multiple confounding variables are in a treatment comparison. Subclassification is, then, impossible, and regression modeling gets powerless.

Propensity scores including more than 1 covariates can be calculated according to the following method (Table 28.1). For each patient the odds ratios of the covariates at risk of confounding are calculated. Statistically significant odds ratios are assumed to be significant confounders (Table 28.1 upper table), and are, subsequently, combined into one propensity per patient in the form of their product of multiplication (Table 28.1 lower table). The next step is to divide the patients into four or more subclasses dependent on their magnitude of propensity score. Then, calculate per subclass mean difference in treatment effect. In order to determine an adjusted overall treatment difference between the two treatment groups, a weighted average can be calculated using the same weighting procedure as that used with subclassification described in one of the previous sections. Figure 28.3 gives the results of this procedure. It is observed that the adjusted overall difference is larger than the unadjusted overall difference, and unlike the latter the former is statistically significantly different from a difference of zero. Obviously, the confounders masked a true treatment difference, which is being unmasked by the propensity procedure. As an alternative to the subclassification procedure, a regression model comparable with the regression, described in the above section, with treatment efficacy as independent, treatment modality as first dependent and propensity score as second dependent variable will produce a largely similar result.

Table 28.1 With propensity scores for each patient the odds ratios of the covariates at risk of confounding are calculated (odds ratio=odds of treatment 1 with confounder/odds without confounder) (upper table). Then the statistically significant odds ratios are assumed to be significant confounders and are combined into one propensity score per patient calculated as their product of multiplication (lower table)

Characteristic at risk of confounding	Treatment 1 n=100	Treatment 2 n=100	Odds treatment 1 with characteristic/odds without	p-value
1. Age >65 years	63	76	0.54 (63/76 / 37/24)	0.05
2. Age <65 years	37	24	1.85 (= 1/OR $_{Age >65 years}$)	0.05
3. Diabetes	20	33	0.51	0.10
4. No diabetes	80	67	1.96	0.10
5. Smoker	50	80	0.25	0.10
6. No smoker	50	20	4.00	0.10
7. Hypertension	60	65	0.81	ns
8. No hypertension	40	35	1.23	ns
9. Cholesterol	75	78	0.85	ns
10. No cholesterol	25	22	1.18	ns
11. Renal insufficiency	12	14	0.84	ns
12. No renal insufficiency	88	86	1.31	ns

Patient	Old y/n	dm y/n	Smoker y/n	Propensity score= $OR_1 \times OR_2 \times OR_3$
1	y	y	n	$0.54 \times 0.51 \times 4 = 1.10$
2	n	n	n	$1.85 \times 1.96 \times 4 = 14.5$
3	y	n	n	$0.54 \times 1.96 \times 4 = 3.14$
4	y	y	y	$0.54 \times 0.51 \times 0.25 = 0.06885$
5	n	n	y	
6	y	y	y	
7				

OR odds ratio, *y* yes, *n* no, *ns* not significant
p<0.01 =statistically significant here

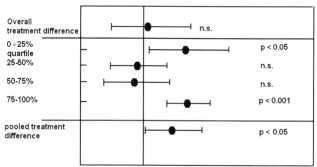

Treatment differences and their 95% confidence intervals

Fig. 28.3 A propensity score adjustment for confounding. The patients are divided into four quartiles according to the magnitude of their propensity scores. The weighted average (pooled treatment difference) is statistically significant different from zero, while the overall treatment difference (unadjusted for confounders) was not so

5 Discussion

In large randomized controlled trials a random imbalance of the covariates is mostly negligible. However, with smaller studies it may be substantial. In the latter situation assessment and adjustment for confounders is a requirement in order to reduce a biased assessment of the treatment comparison. In the current paper three methods for that purpose are reviewed.

We like to discuss the limitations of the three methods for the assessment of confounding. The subclassification assessment has the limitation that it can only be used for one confounder. With multiple confounders multivariable regression analysis is the method of choice. However, this method is limited by the sample size of the trial. We need at least ten times as many patients in our samples than numbers of variables in the analysis. This would mean that, with n = 100 in either of two subgroups, and the treatment efficacy and treatment modality as primary variables, we have only room for eight additional variables. For studies with binary efficacy variables or survival studies other regression models are adequate like multivariable logistic or multivariable Cox regression. However, such models often require additional primary variables like a variable for censored data, and even less room is left for additional variables for the purpose of confounding assessments. With multiple covariates at risk of confounding, propensity scores is an alternative possibility (Rosenbaum and Rubin 1983; Rubin 1997). However, also the method of propensity scores has major limitations. First, propensity score are entirely based upon odds ratios, and odds ratios are relative rather than absolute measures (Sobb et al. 2008). E.g., if one patient in treatment group 1 and two patients in treatment group 2 have a certain characteristic, the odds of treatment 1 with the characteristic/the odds of treatment 1 without the characteristic is 0.5, which is a huge odds ratio (OR) for an otherwise insignificant covariate. It has been advocated to include in confounding assessments any variable that is potentially causally related to the treatment response (Cleophas et al. 1996). However, technically, statistically insignificant ORs in a propensity score severely reduce the power of the method, and regression models may provide better sensitivity under these circumstances as demonstrated by Soledad Cepeda et al in a Monte Carlo simulation study (Soledad Cepeda et al. 2003). Second, very large and very small ORs are not reliable predictors of the chance of a patient being in a category. If such ORs are included in propensity scores a simulated atmosphere of certainty is created. Nonetheless, propensity scores that account the above limitations, and include a sensible series of covariates relevant to the treatment comparison according to previous knowledge, can be more reliable than multivariable regression modeling for adjustment of covariates, particularly if studies are not large.

Irrespective of the method of adjustment for confounders, the question is should we adjust or not. Wickramaratne and Holford (1987) gave an example in which identical results were obtained whether or not account was taken of the potential confounder. The variance estimated from the collapse table (ignoring the confounder) was lower than that from the stratified table. They concluded that precision can be lost by unnecessary adjusting for covariates. Studies at risk of this phenomenon are of course particularly those with small samples and wide variances in the subgroups. In addition, no major differences between the variances of the covariates included in the analysis is an important requirement for assessing causal effects as attempted in most clinical trials (Hullsiek and Louis 2002).

For the assessment of confounding the intention to treat population, unlike the completed protocol population, has the advantage that samples are larger. The problem is that treatment differences may be smaller and precision may be lost. Precision may be somewhat improved using the so-called least observation carried forward analysis under the assumption that the last observation is the best estimate for the missing data (Begg 2000). There are often many candidates for inclusion as covariates, but the choice should be made a priori and specified in the protocol. If subgroups are identified post-hoc, the exploratory nature of the subgroups analyses should be emphasized and the subgroup issue should be further assessed in subsequent independent and prospective data-sets.

Sometimes in clinical trials time-concentration relationships of new drugs are assessed. These assessments make use of multi-exponential rather linear regression models. As no direct methods for the analysis of exponential models are available, data have to be transformed and Laplace's transformations are often used for that purpose (Beal and Sheiner 1996). The Laplace transformed relationships are linear or quadratic and can be analyzed and adjusted for confounders using linear or polynomial regression analysis. Statistical software for that purpose includes S-plus SAS (2011) and the Non- mem (non-linear mixed effects models) Software (Boeckman et al. 1984).

We should add that all of the methods described in this paper can not be used for the assessment or adjustment of interacting factors. Unlike confounding where all of the treatments perform better in one subclass than in the other, interaction shows that one treatment outperforms in one subclass while the other treatment does so in the other. The presence of interaction can be statistically tested by comparing the effect sizes, e.g., by using odds ratios of treatment success in either subclass, or by mixed models analysis of variance (Cleophas et al. 2006b).

6   Conclusions

In large randomized controlled trials the risk of random imbalance of the covariates is mostly negligible. However, with smaller studies it may be substantial. In the latter situation assessment and adjustment for confounders is a requirement in order to reduce a biased assessment of the treatment comparison. The objective of this chapter is to review three methods for confounding assessment and adjustment for a nonmathematical readership.

First method, subclassification: the study population is divided into subclasses with the same subclass characteristic, then, treatment efficacy is assessed per subclass, and, finally, a weighted average is calculated.

Second method, regression modeling: in a multivariable regression model with treatment efficacy as independent and treatment modality as dependent variable, the covariates at risk of confounding are added as additional dependent variables to the model. An analysis adjusted for confounders is obtained by removing the covariates that are not statistically significant.

Third method, propensity scores: each patient is assigned several odds ratios (ORs), which are his/her probability, based on his/her covariate value of receiving a particular treatment modality. A propensity score per patient is calculated by multiplying all of the statistically significant ORs. These propensity scores are, then, applied for confounding adjustment using either subclassification or regression analysis.

The advantages of the first method include that empty subclasses in the treatment comparison are readily visualized, and that subclassification does not rely on a linear or any other regression model. A disadvantage is, that it can only be applied for a single confounder at a time. The advantage of the second method is, that multiple variables can be included in the model. However, the number of covariates is limited by the sample size of the trial. An advantage of the third method is, that it is generally more reliable and powerful with multiple covariates than regression modeling. However, irrelevant covariates and very large/small ORs reduce power and reliability of the assessment. The above methods can not be used for the assessment of interaction in the data.

References

Beal SL, Sheiner LB (1996) A note on the use of Laplace's approximations for non-linear mixed-effects models. Biometrika 83:447–452

Begg CB (2000) Commentary: ruminations on the intent to treat. Control Clin Trials 21:241–243

Boeckman AJ, Sheiner LB, Beal SL (1984) NONMEM user guide: part V. NONMEM Project Group, University of California, San Francisco

Cleophas TJ, Tuinenburg E, Van der Meulen J, Kauw FH (1996) Wine drinking and other dietary characteristics in males under 60 before and after acute myocardial infarction. Angiology 47:789–796

Cleophas TJ, Zwinderman AH, Cleophas AF (2006a) Statistics applied to clinical trials. Springer, New York, pp 141–150

Cleophas TJ, Zwinderman AH, Cleophas AF (2006b) Statistics applied to clinical trials. Springer, New York, pp 329–336

Cochran WG (1968) The effectiveness of adjustment by subclassification in removing bias in observational studies. Biometrics 24:295–313

Hullsiek KH, Louis TA (2002) Propensity scores modeling strategies for the causal analysis of observational data. Biostatistics 3:179–193

Rosenbaum P, Rubin DB (1983) The central role of the propensity score in observational studies for causal effects. Biometrika 70:41–55

Rubin DB (1997) Estimating causal effects from large data sets using propensity score. Ann Intern Med 127:757–763

SAS. http://www.prw.le.ac.uk/epidemiol/personal/ajs22/meta/macros.sas. Accessed 15 Dec 2011

Sobb M, Cleophas TJ, Hadj-Chaib A, Zwinderman AH (2008) Clinical trials: odds ratios, why to assess them, and how to do so. Am J Ther 15:44–53

Soledad Cepeda M, Boston R, Farrer JT, Strom BL (2003) Comparison of logistic regression versus propensity scores when the number of events is low and there are multiple confounders. Am J Epidemiol 158:280–287

SPSS Statistical Software. http:/www.spss.com. Accessed 15 Dec 2011

Wickramaratne PJ, Holford TR (1987) Confounding in epidemiological studies: the adequacy of the control groups as a measure of confounding. Biometrics 43:751–765

Chapter 29
Propensity Score Matching

1 Introduction

Propensity-scores and propensity-score-matching can be used respectively for adjusting covariates in a multiple regression analysis and for stratification/matching of asymmetric observational clinical data, and have recently been emphasized by Dr. D'Agostino in an invited paper in Circulation as a promising additional tool for analyzing such data (D'Agostino 2007). It was first described by Rosenbaum and Rubin in 1985 (Rosenbaum and Rubin 1985), as a method for adjusting confounding variables, otherwise called covariates, alternative to the usual subclassification and regression methods. In the pas few years its application has been extended to so-called propensity-score-matching, a method able to transform asymmetric into symmetric data that can be further analyzed like randomized controlled trials. Due to the increase of costs for randomized trials, more and more clinical investigators turn to observational studies as a method of research. The current chapter was written to familiarize the readership of this book with these relatively novel methods.

2 Calculation of Propensity-Scores

Suppose two parallel groups of 100 patients each are compared. The mean age of the treatment-2 group is significantly different from that of treatment-1 group. For adjustment of this asymmetry we calculate in the older group the odds of receiving the treatment-1:

Odds of receiving treatment-1 in the older patients =

$$\frac{\text{number receiving treatment - 1}}{\text{number not receiving treatment - 1}} = \frac{\text{number receiving treatment - 1}}{\text{number receiving treatment - 2}}$$

Odds of receiving treatment-1 in the older $= 63/76$

Similarly we calculate the odds of treatment-1 in the younger = 37/24

Thus the odds ratio (OR) = 63/76 / 37/24 = 0.54

This odds ratio is smaller than 1.00 with p < 0.05.

The propensity-score is defined as the risk ratio of receiving treatment-1 compared to treatment-2 if you are old in this study population =

$$\text{Propensity - score} = OR / (1 + OR) = 0.54 / (1 + 0.54) = 0.35$$

If we use p = 0.10 as criterion for statistical significance, then, in the underneath two group comparison, not a single, but multiple significant inequalities of characteristics are demonstrated (ns = not significant).

	Treatment-1 n = 100	Treatment-2 n = 100	Odds treatment-1/odds treatment-2 (OR)	p-value
1. Age >65	63	76	0.54 (63/76 / 37/24)	0.05
2. Age <65	37	24	1.85 (= $OR_2 = 1/OR_1$)	0.05
3. Diabetes	20	33	0.51	0.10
4. Not diabetes	80	67	1.96	0.10
5. Smoker	50	80	0.25	0.10
6. Not smoker	50	20	4.00	0.10
7. Hypertension	51	65	0.65	0.05
8. Not hypertension	49	35	1.78	0.05
9. Cholesterol	61	78	0.44	0.01
10. Not cholesterol	39	22	2.27	0.01
11. Renal failure	12	14	0.84	ns
12. Not renal failure	88	86	1.31	ns

Now, we can calculate a combined propensity-score for all of the inequal characteristics by multiplying the significant odds ratios and then calculating from this product the combined propensity-score = combined risk ratio (= combined OR/(1 + combined OR)), y = yes, n = no, combined $OR = OR_1 \times OR_3 \times OR_5 \times OR_7 \times OR_9$.

Patient	Old	Diabetes	Smoker	Hypertension	Cholesterol	Combined OR	Combined propensity score
1	y	y	n	y	y	7.99	0.889
2	n	n	n	y	y	105.27	0.991
3	y	n	n	y	y	22.80	0.958
4	y	y	y	y	y	0.4999	0.333
5	n	n	y				
6	y	y	y				
7							
8							

Each patient has his/her own propensity score based on and adjusted for the significantly larger chance of receiving one treatment versus the other. We should add that with large data samples and multiple predictors binary logistic regression provides a more rapid way of calculating the propensity scores. In the Appendix we summarize how it works.

3 Propensity-Scores for Adjusting Covariates

The above example is used again. Traditionally, asymmetry between treatment groups is adjusted by subclassification or regression analysis. Subclassification makes use of the underneath equation to calculate the treatment-effect separately for the subgroups −1 and −2 and, then a weighted average.

$$\frac{\text{difference - 1 / variance - 1} + \text{difference - 2 / variance - 2}}{\text{1 / variance - 1} \quad + \quad \text{1 / variance - 2}}$$

With more than a single confounder regression-analysis is employed where $y =$ the dependent variable, generally the treatment effect, and $x_1 =$ the treatment modality ($0 =$ new treatment, $1 =$ control treatment), and x_2, x_3 etc. are confounders.

$$y = b_1 x_1 + b_2 x_2 + b_3 x_3 + \ldots$$

If in a treatment comparison the number of confounders is larger than 3 the regression method soon becomes powerless, and propensity-scores are an better possibility for adjustment. The propensity scores have largely different sizes. Usually propensity-score adjustment of confounders is performed by dividing all patients into four or more subgroups. Then, the treatment effect is calculated per subgroup as shown in Fig. 29.1, and an overall weighted treatment effect is derived from the same weighting procedure as the one applied with subclassification described above. In Fig. 29.1 the overall weighted treatment effect is, obviously, larger than the unadjusted treatment effect. The weighted treatment effect gives a better picture of the real treatment effect, because between-group differences due to age, smoking, diabetes etc. have been removed from the treatment comparison.

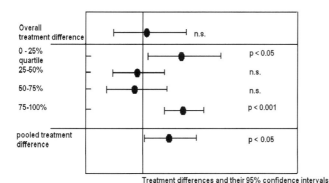

Treatment differences and their 95% confidence intervals

Fig. 29.1 Usually propensity-score adjustment of confounders is performed by dividing all patients into four or more subgroups. Then, the treatment effect is calculated per subgroup, and an overall pooled treatment effect is calculated using a weighting procedure. The overall pooled treatment effect is, obviously, larger than the unadjusted treatment effect. The pooled treatment effect gives a better picture of the real treatment effect, because between-group differences due to age, smoking, diabetes etc. have been removed from the treatment comparison

As an alternative approach, the propensity-score can be entered in a multiple regression model as a confounding x-variable, and then, an adjusted regression analysis can be performed similarly to the on top of this section described regression analysis for adjusting separate confounders.

4 Propensity-Scores for Matching

Propensity-scores are sometimes used to make observational data look more like randomized controlled trials. The problem with efficacy assessments of new treatments is that some patients in one of the treatment groups may be older, and, therefore, respond differently affecting the overall treatment comparison. With randomization this difference is, generally, washed out due to the randomization process. With observational data this is not so, and propensity-score-matching can be used as a method for removing such subgroup effects. In the above study of 200 patients each patient has his/her own propensity-score. We select for each patient in group 1 a patient from group 2 with the same propensity-score. Then we will end up sampling two new groups that are entirely symmetric on their subgroup variables, and can, thus, be simply analyzed as two groups in a randomized trial. Several assessments for matching are possible (Love 2003), including Caliper matching, Mahalanobis metric matching, stratification matching (5 quintiles are constructed and assessed with bootstraps), and Kernel matching. However, obviously, nearest neighbor watching is the simplest of all: in random order the first patient from group 1 is selected. Then he/she is matched to the patient of group 2 with the nearest propensity-score. We continue until there are no longer similar propensity-scores. The patients with dissimilar propensity-scores that can not be matched are removed from the data.

Figure 29.2 displays this method. Both treatment-2 users and treatment-1 users without match are removed from the data. In the example two matched groups of 71 patients each are left for comparison of the treatments. Underneath the patient characteristics (%) of the two treatment groups are summarized both unmatched and matched. Although 58 patients did not find an adequate match and had to be removed, the remaining two groups of 71 patients seem to be enough for making a sensible comparison. It can be observed that after matching the asymmetry has entirely gone.

	Unmatched (n = 200)			Matched (n = 142)		
	Treatment-1	Treatment-2	p-value	Treatment-1	Treatment-2	p-value
Gender	63	76	0.05	70	72	ns
Diabetes	37	24	0.10	15	15	ns
Smoker	50	80	0.10	26	27	ns
Hypertension	51	65	0.05	50	51	ns
Cholesterol	61	78	0.01	76	75	ns
Renal failure	12	14	ns	16	12	ns

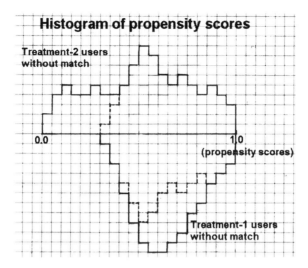

Fig. 29.2 The nearest neighbor watching method for matching patients with similar propensity scores. Each square represents one patient. In random order the first patient from group 1 is selected. Then, he/she is matched to the patient of group 2 with the nearest propensity score. We continue until there are no longer similar propensity scores. Group 1 is summarized above the x-axis, group 2 under it. The patients with dissimilar propensity scores that can not be matched, are removed from the analysis

We can now analyze the two groups of 71 patients as though they were two randomized groups from a randomized controlled trial, and we can do so, for example, using two group t-tests or chi-square tests without need to further account confounding anymore.

5   Discussion

Propensity-scores of observational data have witnessed a tremendous attention in recent years, particularly, in cardiovascular research, as a less expensive alternative for controlled trials. The first application, propensity-scores for adjusting covariates, is an excellent method to handle data with many confounders for which subclassification or regression analysis is impossible. The second application, propensity-score-matching may, sometimes, be hard to accept, as it generally makes the results of the analysis look quite different from the raw data.

Also, the approach is rather sophisticated sometimes giving rise to an air of uncertainty.

Another problem with propensity-scores is the fact, that irrelevant covariates although significant, are often included, reducing the power of this procedure. In this way a pseudo-certainty is created. Also, the mathematical basis of propensity methods are not fully recognized. We should add that only statistically significant confounders should be included, because insignificant differences in clinical research are due to chance rather than real effects.

We should emphasize that propensity scores are only for confounders, otherwise called covariates, but not for interactions between confounders. Many confounders in cardiovascular research, if not all, do not only confound, but also interact with one another. Propensity-scores do not protect against interactions, a major flaw of the approach.

Stratification matching requires a special multivariate final analysis which uses multiple dependent variables, a procedure that, generally, enhances the complexity of the model and increases the difficulty to understand what is going on.

It may not be correct to state that propensity-scores can make a randomized trial from your observational data. The adjustment of the original data can introduce new biases, e.g. loss of valuable observations, and increased interaction effects. Observational data have their own place in clinical research, because they are more adequate than clinical trial data to study unselected groups, to observe unexpected adverse effects, and to really show what is going on in clinical practice.

We recommend that propensity-scores can be helpful to better estimate the unbiased treatment effect in observational studies. However, in reports both adjusted and unadjusted results have to be reported, because the unadjusted data rather than the adjusted data picture what will happen with future unadjusted treatment groups in real clinical practice.

6 Conclusions

Propensity-scores and propensity-score-matching can be used respectively for adjusting covariates in a multiple regression analysis and for stratification/matching of asymmetric observational clinical data, and have received a growing attention in recent years, particularly, in clinical research.

This chapter was written to familiarize the clinical community with this important methodology.

An example is used to explain both propensity-based-regression and propensity-score-matching.

Propensity-scores are applied in observational treatment comparisons with unequal presence of risk factors in the treatment groups. They can be defined as the risk ratio of receiving treatment-1 compared to treatment-2 if you are suffering from the risk factor, for example, advanced age. Also multiple risk factors can be implemented in an overall propensity-score. Propensity-scores can be used for adjustment of the unequally distributed risk factors, and, with multiple risk factors, like commonly observed in cardiovascular research, they are better for that purpose than the usual subclassification or regression methods. With propensity-score-matching each patient in treatment-1 group is matched to the patient of treatment-2 group with the nearest propensity-score. After matching of all patients, some patients without match are left, and are no further used in the analysis. In this way propensity-score makes observational look like the data from a controlled trial, which can be analyzed in the usual way.

Propensity-scores is one of the few methods to handle data with many confounders, and works excellently for that purpose. Limitations are: (1) The methods is sometimes hard to accept because the results look entirely different from the raw data. (2) The method is rather sophisticated sometimes giving rise to an air of uncertainty. (3) Irrelevant and statistically insignificant confounders are often included reducing the power of the procedure. (4) Mathematically the method has not been entirely recognized. (5) Propensity-score are used for confounding risk factors only, they are not used to assess interactions between them.

Appendix

Binary logistic regression is based on the log-linear equation

$$\ln \text{odds} = a + bx$$

where ln means the natural logarithm, odds = the odds of receiving treatment-1, a = the intercept, b = the regression coefficient, and x = a binary predictor variable, for example for old age x = 1, for young age x = 0.

Instead of the above equation we can write:

$$\text{odds} = e^{a+bx}$$

if old, x = 1 $\text{odds} = e^{a+b}$

if young, x = 0 $\text{odds} = e^{a}$

the division sum = odds ratio $= e^{a+b} / e^{a} = e^{b}$

The odds ratio of treatment-1 compared to treatment-2, if you are old in this study population, thus, equals e^{b}. SPSS software (www.SPSS.com) requires to command binary logistic regression, then enter the treatment modality as dependent variable and the age category as independent variable, and analyze (ln = natural logarithm).

The calculated b for these variables = −0.62

$$e^{b} = \text{antiln } b = 0.54 = \text{OR}_{\text{for treatment - 1 vs treatment - 2}}.$$

In the same way additional predictors can be added to the same model. The software program produces a b-value for each x-variable added (b_1, b_2, b_3 etc), and the outcome variable equals

$$e^{b_1 + b_2 + b_3 + \cdots} = \text{OR}_1 \times \text{OR}_2 \times \text{OR}_3 \ldots$$

This result is similar to the that of the pocket calculator method described above, and from it the propensity scores can be similarly readily derived.

References

D'Agostino RB (2007) Propensity scores in cardiovascular research. Circulation 115:2340–2343
Love TE (2003) Propensity scores: what do they do, how should I use them and why should I care? www.chrp.org/love/ASACleveland, Accessed 15 Dec 2011
Rosenbaum PR, Rubin DB (1985) Constructing a control group using multivariate matched sampling methods that incorporate the propensity score. Am Stat 39:33–38

Chapter 30
Interaction

1 Introduction

In pharmaceutical research and development, multiple factors like age, gender, comorbidity, concomitant medication, genetic and environmental factors co-determine the efficacy of the new treatment. In statistical terms we say they interact with the treatment efficacy. It is impossible to estimate all of these factors. Instead, randomized controlled trials are used to ensure that no major imbalances exist regarding these factors, and an overall assessment is made. The limitation of this approach becomes obvious once the new medicine is applied in practice where benefits of new medicines are far less consistent than they are in the trials (Riegelman 2005). Despite this limitation, interaction effects, are not routinely assessed in clinical trials, probably because the statistical methods for identifying and integrating them into the data have low power. Moreover, if we introduce a large number of interaction terms in a regression analysis, the power to demonstrate a statistical significance for the primary endpoint will be reduced. Nonetheless, the assessment of a small number of interaction terms in clinical research can be an important part of the evaluation of new drugs, particularly, if it can be argued that the interaction terms make clinically sense. The current chapter gives some important factors that may interact with the treatment efficacy, and proposes some guidelines for implementing an interaction assessment in the analysis of clinical trials, in order to better predict the efficacy/safety of new medicines in future clinical treatment of individual patients.

2 What Exactly Is Interaction, a Hypothesized Example

The aim of clinical trials of new medicines is, generally, to use the estimated effects in forecasting the results of applying a new medicine to the general population. For that purpose a representative sample of subjects is treated with the new medicine or

T.J. Cleophas and A.H. Zwinderman, *Statistics Applied to Clinical Studies*,
DOI 10.1007/978-94-007-2863-9_30, © Springer Science+Business Media B.V. 2012

a control medicine. For example, in a parallel group study 400 patients are treated as follows:

	Patients who received new medicine (n = 200)	Control medicine (n = 200)	p-value
Successfully treated patients	130/200 (65%)	110/200 (55%)	<0.01

Based on this assessment the best bet about the difference between the two treatment modalities is given by the overall difference between the two treatment groups. We can expect that the new medicine performs 10% better than does the control medicine. If, however, we include the factor gender into our data, the results look slightly different:

	Patients who received new medicine (n = 200)	Control medicine (n = 200)	Accumulated data
Successfully treated females	55/100	65/100	120/200
Successfully treated males	75/100	45/100 +	120/200
	130/200	110/200	

The above result shows, that, although no difference between females and males exists in the accumulated data, the new medicine performs better in the males, while the control medicine does so in the females. The adequate interpretation of this result is, if you don't wish to account gender, then the new medicine performs better, while, if you include only females, the control medicine performs better. The treatment modalities interact with gender. Interaction effects usually involve situations like this. It is helpful to display interaction effects important to the interpretation of the data in a graph with treatment modality on the x-axis and subgroup results on the y-axis. If the lines drawn for each subgroup are parallel (Fig. 30.1 upper graph), no interaction is in the data. A different slope, and, particularly, crossing lines (Fig. 30.1, lower graph), suggest the presence of interaction effects between treatment efficacy and subgroups, in our example *treatment × gender interaction*. The new medicine is better in females than it is in males.

The medical concept of interaction is synonymous to the terms heterogeneity and synergism. Interaction must be distinguished from confounding. In a trial with interaction effects the parallel groups have similar characteristics. However, there are subsets of patients that have an unusually high or low response. With confounding things are different. For whatever reason the randomization has failed, the parallel groups have asymmetric characteristics. For example, in a placebo-controlled trial of two parallel-groups asymmetry of age may be a confounder. The control group is significantly older than the treatment group, and this can easily explain the treatment difference. Particularly, in survival studies differences in baseline age may be an important confounder as recently demonstrated by De Craen and Westendorp (2005).

Fig. 30.1 The effect of gender on a treatment comparison of two parallel groups treated with a new and a control medicine. *Upper graph*: the males respond better to both of the treatment than do the females, but no gender × treatment interaction is in the data. *Lower graph*: the data from the example given in the text: there is evidence for gender × treatment interaction because the males respond better to the new medicine, while the females respond better to the control treatment

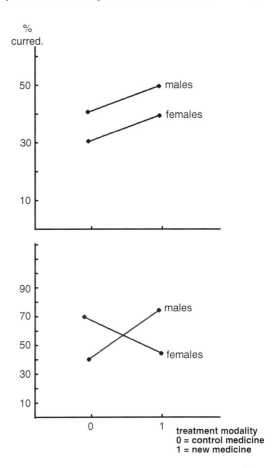

3   How to Test Interaction Statistically, a Real Data Example with a Concomitant Medication as Interacting Factor: Incorrect Method

In the above example the presence of interaction is suggested. We can statistically test whether the difference between new medicine and control is significantly different using e.g. a chi-square or an odds ratio test. The tests produce p-values of >0.10 for the females and <0.001 for the males. It is tempting to state that the difference in p-values establishes a difference between the females and the males. P-values are composite estimators of not only effect size, but also spread in the data. Differences in p-values can arise because of differences in effect sizes or standard errors.

The correct approach is to compare directly the effect sizes relative to the standard errors, e.g. by using the odds ratios of treatment success in either subgroup (Table 30.1). This procedure produces a p-value between 0.05 and 0.10. Obviously, there is a tendency to interaction. However, definitive evidence is lacking.

Table 30.1 Difference between females and males in odds ratios of treatment success

	Standard error	p-value
Odds ratio treatment success females		
0.658	1.336	>0.10
Odds ratio treatment success males		
3.667	1.357	<0.001
Difference in odds ratios[a]		
5.573	2.563	0.05<p<0.10

[a]The difference in odds ratios is calculated by subtracting their logarithmic transformations and turning this subtraction sum into its antilogarithmic term

4   Three Analysis Methods

Verapamil	Metoprolol	
Males		
52	28	
48	35	
43	34	
50	32	
43	34	
44	27	
46	31	
46	27	
43	29	
49	25	
464	302	766
Females		
38	43	
42	34	
42	33	
35	42	
33	41	
38	37	
39	37	
34	40	
33	36	
34	35	
368	378	746
832	680	

As an example we give a study of treatments for paroxysmal atrial fibrillation, the number of episodes per patient is the outcome variable.

Overall metoprolol seems to perform better. However, this is only true only for one subgroup (males).

4.1   First Method, t-Test

	Males	Females
Mean$_{verapamil}$ (SD)	46.4 (3.23866)	36.8 (3.489667)
Mean$_{metoprolol}$ (SD)	30.2 (3.48966) –	37.8 (3.489667) –
Difference means (SE)	16.2 (1.50554)	−1.0 (1.5606)
Difference of males and females 17.2 (2.166)		
t-value = 17.2/2.166 = 8		
p < 0.0001		

There is a significant difference between the males and females, and, thus, a significant interaction between gender and treat-efficacy.

4.2   Second Method, Analysis of Variance (ANOVA)

ANOVA Assesses whether the variance due to interaction is large compared to the variance due to chance (residual variance), (SS = sum of squares).

	Verapamil	Metoprolol	
Males	52	48	
	48	35	
	43		
	50	.	
	_____ +	_____ +	
	464	302	766
Females	38	.	
	42	.	
	.	.	
	.	.	
	.	35	
	_____ +	_____ +	
	368+	378+	746+
	832	680	1,512

$$SS_{total} = \frac{52^2 + 48^2 + ...35^2 - (52 + 48 + +...35)^2}{40} = 1,750.4$$

$$SS_{treatment\,by\,gender} = \frac{464^2 + ...378^2}{10} - \frac{(52 + 48 + +...35)^2}{40} = 1,327.2$$

$$SS_{residual} = SS_{total} - SS_{treatment\,by\,gender} = 423.2$$

$$SS_{rows} = \frac{766^2 + 746^2}{20} - \frac{(52 + 48 + +...35)^2}{40} = 10.0\left(= SS_{gender}\right)$$

$$SS_{columns} = \frac{832^2 + 680^2}{20} - \frac{(52 + 48 + +...35)^2}{40} = 577.6\left(= SS_{treatment}\right)$$

$$SS_{interaction} = SS_{treatment\,by\,gender} - SS_{rows} - SS_{columns} = 1,327.2 - 10.0 - 577.6 = 739.6$$

ANOVA-table (dfs = degrees of freedom, MS = mean square, F = F-statistic)

	SS	dfs	MS	F	P
Rows	10.0	1	10	0.851	ns
Columns (treatment)	577.6	1	577.6	49.1	<0.0001
Interaction	739.6	1	739.6	62.9	<0.0001
Residual	423.2	36	11.76		
Total					

In the above analysis both $SS_{treatment}$ and $SS_{interaction}$ are compared to the $SS_{residual}$. Often it is a better approach to use a "random-effects-model". The $SS_{treatment}$ is then compared to the $SS_{interaction}$. A p-value > 0.05 indicates no interaction. Random effects models will be discussed in the Chap. 56.

4.3   Third Method, Regression Analysis

The y-variable is dependent, the x-variables are independent.
y = number of episodes of paroxysmal atrial fibrillation
x_1 = treat-modality (0 of 1)
x_2 = gender (0 of 1)
Add an additional interaction variable $x_3 = x_1 * x_2$ (* = sign of multiplication).
Perform a multiple linear regression analysis including x_3.
Regression-coefficients-table (b = regression coefficient)

	b	SE	t	sig
Constant	46.40	1.084	42.79	0.00
x_1	-16.20	1.533	-10.565	0.00
x_2	-9.60	1.533	-6.261	0.00
x_3 (interactie)	17.20	2.168	7.932	0.00

The t-value for $x_3 = 7.932$. The F-value for interaction in the above ANOVA-model = 62.916. It is interesting to observe that this F-value equals t^2 of the regression model. The two approaches are obviously very similar. We should note that for random-effects-modeling the SPSS software for linear-regression analyses has limited possibilities.

5   Using a Regression Model for Testing Interaction, Another Real Data Example

How do we statistically test for the presence of interaction. Univariate analyses comparing subgroups can be used for that purpose. However, the linear regression model provides better sensitivity because it suffers less from missing data, and enables to analyze all of the data simultaneously. An example is provided by the Regress trial, a randomized parallel group trial of 884 patients treated with pravastatin or placebo for 2 years. The data of this study have already been briefly addressed in the Chaps. 12 and 14 (Hays 1998). One of the primary efficacy variables was the decrease of the diameter of the coronary arteries after 2 years of treatment. The average decrease was 0.057 mm (standard error (SE) 0.013) in the pravastatin group, and it was 0.117 mm (SE 0.015) in the placebo group (t-test: significance of difference at $p < 0.001$) (Fig. 30.2, upper graph); thus the efficacy estimate b_1 was 0.060 (standard error SE = 0.016). Calcium antagonists had been given to 60% of the placebo patients, and to 59% of the pravastatin patients (chi-square: $p = 0.84$): thus, calcium antagonist treatment was not a confounder variable. Also, calcium antagonist medication was not associated with a diameter decrease ($p = 0.62$). In the patients who did not receive concomitant calcium antagonist medication, the diameter decreases were 0.097 (SE 0.014) and 0.088 (SE 0.014) in patients receiving placebo and pravastatin, respectively ($p = 0.71$). In patients who did receive calcium antagonist medication, the diameter decreases were 0.130 (SE 0.014) and 0.035 (SE 0.014), respectively ($p < 0.001$). Thus, pravastatin-efficacy was, on average, 0.097–0.088 = 0.009 mm in the patients without calcium antagonist medication, and 0.130–0.035 = 0.095 in the patients with calcium antagonist medication (Fig. 30.2, lower graph). The two lines cross, suggesting the presence of interaction between pravastatin and calcium antagonists.

Before statistically testing this suggested interaction, we have to assess whether it makes clinically sense. Atherosclerosis is characterized not only by depots of cholesterol but also of calcium in the fatty streaks that consist of foam cells. It does make sense to argue that calcium antagonists, although they do not reduce plasma calcium, reduce calcium levels in the foam cells, and, thus, beneficially influence the process of atherosclerosis, and that interaction with cholesterol lowering treatment is a possibility.

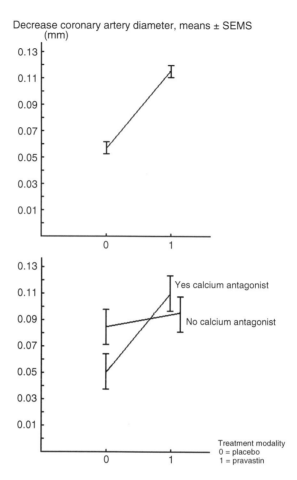

Fig. 30.2 The effect of concomitant calcium antagonists on treatment efficacy of pravastatin estimated by the decrease of coronary artery diameter (ca-diameter) after 2 years' treatment (REGRESS data (Jukema et al. 1995)). *Upper graph*: pravastatin significantly decreased ca-diameter compared to placebo. *Lower graph*: there is evidence for interaction between calcium antagonists and pravastatin, because in the patients receiving no calcium antagonist the benefit of pravastatin was insignificant, while it was highly significant in the patients receiving a concomitant calcium antagonist

We used the following linear regression model for this test:

$$y_i = a + b_1 x_{1i} + b_2 x_{2i} + b_3 x_{3i} + e_i$$

where
y_i = dependent variable = decrease in coronary artery diameter in the ith patient
a = intercept
b_1, b_2, and b_3 = partial regression coefficients for the variables (1) treatment modality, (2) calcium antagonist treatment, (3) interaction between (1) and (2)
e_i = systematic error in the ith patient

Let $x_{1i} = 1$ denote that patient i received pravastatin ($x_{1i} = 0$, if not), let $x_{2i} = 1$ denote that patient i received calcium antagonist medication ($x_{2i} = 0$, if not), and let $x_{3i} = x_{1i}$ times x_{2i}. The estimates were: $b_3 = 0.085$ (SE 0.033), $b_2 = -0.033$ (SE 0.023), and $b_1 = 0.009$ (SE 0.026). Notice that b_1 changed dramatically by including the interaction term x_3 in the linear model; this is a general feature of regression models with interaction terms: the corresponding main-effects (b_1 and b_2) cannot be interpreted independently of the interaction term. Another consequence is that the efficacy estimate no longer exists, but several estimates do exist: in our case there are different efficacy-estimates for patients with ($b_1 + b_3 = 0.009 + 0.085 = 0.094$) and without calcium antagonist medication ($b_1 = 0.009$). This difference was statistically significant (interaction test: $p = 0.011$).

6   Analysis of Variance for Testing Interaction, Other Real Data Examples

6.1   Parallel-Group Study with Treatment × Health Center Interaction

Current clinical trials of new treatments often include patients from multiple health centers, national and international. Differences between centers may affect results. We might say these data are at risk of interaction between centers and treatment efficacy. Hays (1998) described an example: 36 patients were assessed for performance after treatment with either placebo, vitamin supply low dose, and high dose. Patients were randomly selected in six health centers, six patients per center, and every patients was given one treatment at random, and so in each center two patients were given one of the three treatments. The Table 30.2 gives an overview of the results.

The model is $y = \mu + a + b + ab + e$
where y = dependent variable, estimate for performance of patients
   μ = mean result
   a = fixed effect of the three treatments
   b = random effect of health center
   ab = between treatment and health center effect
   e = systematic error
The computations are (SS = sum of squares)

$$SS_{total} = (7.8)^2 + \cdots + (10.5)^2 - \frac{(358.5)^2}{36} = 123.56$$

$$SS_{ab} = \frac{(16.5)^2 + \cdots + (19.1)^2}{2} - \frac{(358.5)^2}{36} = 109.03$$

$$SS_{error} = SS_{total} - SS_{ab} = 123.57 - 109.03 = 14.54$$

Table 30.2 Results of three treatments for assessment of performance in 36 patients in six health centers, results are given as scores)

		Vitamin supply		
Treatment	Placebo	low dose	High dose	Total
Health center				
1	7.8	11.7	11.1	
	8.7	10.0	12.0	
	16.5	21.7	23.1	61.3
2	8.0	9.8	11.3	
	9.2	11.9	10.6	
	17.2	21.7	21.9	60.8
3	4.0	11.7	9.8	
	6.9	12.6	10.1	
	10.9	24.3	19.9	55.1
4	10.3	7.9	11.4	
	9.4	8.1	10.5	
	19.7	16.0	21.9	57.6
5	9.3	8.3	13.0	
	10.6	7.9	11.7	
	19.9	16.2	24.7	60.8
6	9.5	8.6	12.2	
	9.8	10.5	12.3	
	19.3	19.1	24.5	62.9
Total	103.5	119.0	136.0	358.5

Data modified from Hays (1998) with permission from the editor

$$SS_{columns} = \frac{(103.5)^2 + (136.0)^2 + (119.0)^2}{12} - \frac{(358.5)^2}{36} = 44.04$$

$$SS_{rows} = \frac{(61.3) + \cdots + (62.9)^2}{6} - \frac{(358.5)^2}{36} = 6.80$$

$$SS_{interaction} = SS_{ab} - SS_{rows} - SS_{columns} = 109.03 - 6.80 - 44.04 = 58.19$$

Table 30.3 gives the ANOVA (analysis of variance) table. The F test for interaction produces an F-value of 7.19 corresponding with a p-value <0.01 which means that the hypothesis of no interaction is rejected. Although there is insufficient evidence to permit to conclude that there are treatment effects or health center effects, there is pretty strong evidence for the presence of interaction effects. There is something about the combination of a particular health center with a particular treatment that accounts for a significant part of the variability in the data. Thus, between the health centers, treatment differences apparently exist. Perhaps the capacity of a treatment to produce a certain result in a given patient depends on his/her health center background.

6.2 *Crossover Study with Treatment × Subjects Interaction*

In a crossover study different treatments are assessed in one and the same subject. Suppose, we have prior arguments to believe that subjects who better respond to one treatment, will also do so to another treatment. For example, in trials involving a similar class of drugs subjects who respond better to one drug, tend to respond better to all of the other drugs from the same class, and those who respond less, will respond less to the entire class. For example, patients with angina pectoris, hypertension, arrhythmias, chronic obstructive pulmonary disease, responsive to one class of drugs may equally well respond to a different compound from the same class. In this situation our interest may focus on the question is there a difference in response between different patients, instead or in addition to the question is there an overall difference between treatments. If the emphasis is on the differences between the subjects, the design is often called a treatments-by-subjects design. An example is in Table 30.4.

Twelve patients are given in random order four different antihypertensive drugs from the same class. Diastolic blood pressures were used as variable. The statistical model with computations are (sd = standard deviation):

$$SS_{subjects} = sd_1^2 + sd_2^2 + \ldots \ldots sd_{12}^2 = 906$$

$$SS_{treatments} = (\text{treatment mean } 1 - \text{grand mean})^2 + (\text{treatment mean } 2 - \text{grand mean})^2$$
$$+ \ldots = 96.0$$

$$SS_{total} = \sum (y - \bar{y})^2 = \sum y^2 - \frac{(\sum y)^2}{n} = (49^2 + \ldots \ldots 40^2) - (2,160)^2 / 48 = 1,232$$

$$SS_{subjects \times treatments} = SS_{total} - SS_{subjects} - SS_{treatments} = 230$$

The layout for this repeated measures situation is given in Table 30.5. The MS (mean square) for treatments divided by the MS for subjects-by-treatments interaction gives an F-ratio of 4.60. If we are using an alpha level of 0.05 for this test, this results will be significant. The four treatments appear to be having different effects

Table 30.3 ANOVA table of analysis for data of Table 30.2

Source	SS	dfs	MS	F
Columns	44.04	3 − 1 = 2	22.02	22.02/5.82 = 3.78
Rows (centers)	6.80	6 − 1 = 5	1.36	1.68
Interaction (treatment × center)	58.19	10	5.82	5.82/0.81 = 7.19
Error	14.54	18 × (2 − 1) = 18	0.81	
Total	123.57	35		

SS sum of squares, *dfs* degrees of freedom, *MS* mean square, *F* test statistic for F test

Table 30.4 Diastolic blood pressures (mmHg) after 4 week treatment with four different treatments in a crossover study of 12 patients

Patient	Treatment 1	Treatment 2	Treatment 3	Treatment 4	sd²
1	98	96	98	90	…
2	94	92	92	86	…
3	92	94	94	88	
4	94	90	90	90	
5	96	98	98	96	
6	94	88	90	92	
7	82	88	82	80	
8	92	90	86	90	
9	86	84	88	80	
10	94	90	92	90	
11	92	90	90	94	
12	90	80	80	80	
	1,104	1,080	1,080	1,056	Add-up sum = 4,320

Table 30.5 ANOVA table for the data of Table 30.4

Source	SS	dfs	MS	F	
Subjects	906	12 − 1 = 1			
Treatments	96	4 − 1 = 3	32	32/7 = 4.60	<0.05
Subjects × treatments	230	3 × 11 = 33	7		
Total	1,232	47			

SS sum of squares, *dfs* degrees of freedom, *MS* mean square, *F* test statistic for F test

to different subsets in this sample. Note that an overall F test on these data requires the SS residual term which is equal to SS subjects – SS treatments. The F-ratio used for an overall F test equals MS treatments/MS residual, and would produce an entirely different result (see also Chap. 2).

From the above analysis it can be concluded that an interaction effect exists between treatments and patients. Some patients, obviously, respond better or worse to the treatments than others. This is probably due to personal factors like genetic polymorphisms, societal and/or developmental factors. This repeated measures model is particularly convenient in drug development that has to account such factors when assessing the elimination rate and other pharmacokinetic properties of new drugs. Statistical models like these are often called mixed effects models, because they are considered to include a fixed effect (the treatment effect), and a random effect (the effect of being in a subset). Mixed effects models will be further discussed in Chap. 56.

7   Discussion

Interaction effects in a clinical trial should be distinguished from confounding effects. In a trial with interaction effects the treatment groups are generally nicely symmetric. However, there are subsets in each treatment group that have an unusually high or low response. With confounding, things are different. For whatever reason the randomization failed, and the treatment groups are different for a clinically relevant factor. For example, in a placebo-controlled trial the two parallel-groups were asymmetric for age. The control group was significantly older than the treatment group, and this could easily explain the treatment difference. More examples of confounding are given in the Chaps. 12 and 17.

Also interaction effects should be distinguished from carryover effects as commonly observed in crossover studies, and sometimes wrongly called treatment by period interaction. If in a crossover study the effect of the first period of treatment carries on into the second period of treatment, then it may influence the response to the latter period. More examples of this phenomenon will be given in the Chaps. 28 and 30.

Clinical trials usually do not include interaction assessments in the protocol. Results of such assessments are, therefore, post-hoc, and of an exploratory and unconfirmed nature. Why should they be performed even so? In cardiovascular research drug-drug interactions, and effects of comorbidities on drug efficacies are numerous. It is valuable to account at least post-hoc for such mechanisms. Second, current clinical trials involve heterogeneous health centers, investigators, and patient groups. Accounting these heterogeneities can be helpful to predict individual responses in future patients, and to develop prediction rules based on the trial data of individuals. Prediction rules like the Framingham risk score may be developed using trial data to further identify subjects at risk of having a good or bad drug response.

Other reasons for interaction assessments include the following. It may be useful and reassuring to know that in a positive study the benefit in subgroups parallels the benefit in the study overall. For example, in a subgroup analysis of the Dietary Approach to Stop-Hypertension (DASH) randomized clinical trial the results were equivalent in different age, gender, and ethnic groups (Svetkey et al. 1999). Also, it may be useful to know if there are in an unexpectedly negative study certain subgroups that might be benefited or harmed by the treatment. For example, estrogen/progestin replacement caused cardiovascular benefit in women with high lipoprotein, harm in those with low lipoprotein (Shlipak et al. 2000).

We should add that the assessment of interaction, otherwise called heterogeneity, is not always wise. In controlled clinical trials a myriad of subgroups can be identified that would qualify for an exploratory examination, and this approach will almost certainly produce one or more spuriously significant interactions. Interaction terms to be assessed should, therefore, make clinically sense. Demonstrating a statistically significant interaction between the treatment effect and the first letters the patients' Christian names makes no sense, and pursuing such a finding is merely data dredging. We should caution that a "scientific" explanation can be found for every subgroup results in one afternoon Pubmed search. As stated by Dr. Barrett-Connor in a commentary on the nine positive interactions demonstrated in a sub-group analysis of the otherwise negative Heart and Estrogen/progestin Replacement Study (HERS) trial, biological plausibility is quite easy to theorize, anyone with 2 h and a little imagination can do it (Barrett-Connor 2002).

Statistical methods for identifying and integrating interaction terms into the data are limited, and have a limited statistical power. Moreover, if we introduce a large number of interaction terms in a regression analysis, the statistical power to demonstrate statistical significance for the primary endpoint will be reduced. Nonetheless, the assessment of a small number of interaction terms in clinical research can be an important part of the evaluation of new drugs.

The issue of testing interaction is different with meta-analyses of clinical trials (Chalmers and Altman 1996). The aim of a meta-analysis is to obtain a pooled estimate of a treatment effect rather the study of subgroups. The studies to be included in a meta-analysis are often heterogeneous, and protocols, therefore, routinely apply a heterogeneity test prior to data pooling. In the presence of a statistically significant heterogeneity, an data pooling may be difficult to accept, and has as an additional problem that confidence intervals are underestimated, because the extra variability between the different trials is ignored.

If a statistically significant interaction is demonstrated post hoc, its existence should be confirmed in a novel prospective clinical trial. If a relevant interaction is expected prior to the trial, its assessment should be properly included in the trial protocol at the planning stage of the trial. Instead of a regression model a factorial trial design is suitable for such purposes.

Linear regression analyses may provide better precision to test interaction than comparison of subgroups (Hays 1998). It is also often more convenient, because it enables to analyze all of the data simultaneously. Different regression models may be adequate for different types of data, e.g., exponential models are more adequate than linear models for risk ratios and mortality data.

8   Conclusions

In pharmaceutical research and development, multiple factors co-determine the efficacy of the new treatment. In statistical terms we say they interact with the new treatment efficacy. Interaction effects, are not routinely assessed in clinical trials. The current paper reviews some important factors that may interact with the treatment efficacy, and comes to the following recommendations:

1. The assessment of a small number of interaction terms is an important part of the evaluation of new medicines. Important factors that may interact with the treatment efficacy are: (a) concomitant drugs and/or comorbidities, (b) health center

factors in multicenter trials, (c) subject factors like genetic polymorphisms relating to the speed of drug metabolism.
2. Interaction terms to be assessed should make clinically sense.
3. Linear regression analyses provide better sensitivity to test interaction than do subgroup analyses, because they suffer less from missing data and enable to analyze all of the data simultaneously. Exponential regression models are more adequate for risk ratios and mortality data.
4. If a relevant interaction is clinically expected, its assessment should be properly included in the trial protocol at the planning stage of the trial.
5. If a statistically significant interaction is demonstrated post hoc, its existence should be confirmed in a novel prospective clinical trial.

We hope that the examples and recommendations in this chapter be guidelines for the analysis of interaction effects in clinical drug trials, in order to better predict the efficacy/safety of new medicines in future clinical treatment of individual patients.

References

Barrett-Connor E (2002) Looking for the pony in the heart and estrogen/progestin replacement study (HERS) data. Circulation 105:902–903

Chalmers I, Altman DG (eds) (1996) Systematic reviews. Br Med J Books, Bristol

De Craen AJM, Westendorp RGJ (2005) The use of age as a variable in clinical research. Ned Tijdschr Geneeskd 149:2958–2963

Hays WL (1998) Random effects and mixed models. In: Statistics, 4th edn. Holt, Rhinehart and Winnston Inc, Chicago, pp 479–543

Jukema AJ, Zwinderman AH, et al. for the REGRESS Study Group (1995) Effects of lipid lowering by pravastatin on progression and regression of coronary artery disease in symptomatic men with normal to moderately elevated serum cholesterol levels. The Regression Growth Evaluation Statin Study (REGRESS). Circulation 91:2528–2540

Riegelman RK (2005) Studying a study and testing a test. Lippincott Williams & Wilkins, Philadelphia

Shlipak MG, Simon JA, Vittinghoff E et al (2000) Estrogen and progestin, lipoprotein (a), and the risk of recurrent coronary heart disease events after menopause. JAMA 283:1845–1852

Svetkey LP, Simons-Morton D, Vollmer WM et al (1999) Effects of dietary patterns on blood pressure: subgroup analysis of the dietary approaches to stop-hypertension (DASH) randomized clinical trial. Arch Intern Med 159:258–293

Chapter 31
Time-Dependent Factor Analysis

1 Introduction

Assessing the effects of health predictors on morbidity/mortality is an important objective in clinical research. Usually, the individual patients' values of a health predictor are evaluated at the time of entry in a study, and the final effects on morbidity/mortality are collected years later. Logistic and Cox regression models are commonly applied to determine, whether the health predictors significantly contributed to the risk of events/hazard of deaths etc. The problem with this approach is the assumption, that the individual patients' values of the health predictors do not change across time. This may be true for short time observations in simple creatures like mosquitoes. However, humans are more complex and creative, and tend to change their lifestyles in the course of time. It would mean, for example, that the risk of smoking on death cannot be estimated from the numbers of cigarettes at the time of entry, if people tend to give up smoking while on trial. Therefore, an ongoing adjustment of the values of risk factors during the time of observation would be a more adequate assessment. However, standard statistical methods do not allow for such adjustments. In 1996 the group of Abrahamowicz (Cox 1972) was the first to present a model for time-dependent factor analysis based on the traditional Cox regression model (Abrahamowicz et al. 1996). It is now available in SPSS (www.SPSS.com) statistical software and other major software programs, but, unfortunately, still rarely applied. The current chapter explains the novel model using examples from survival studies, and was written to assess the performance of the novel method, and to familiarize the clinical research community with this important approach for improved survival analysis.

2   Cox Regression Without Time-Dependent Predictors

Cox regression is immensely popular. It uses exponential models: per time unit the same percentage of patients has an event. This exponential model may be adequate for survival of mosquitoes, they usually die whenever they collide: in a room full of mosquitoes after the 1st day 50% may be alive, after the 2nd day 25%, etc. (Fig. 31.1). However, human beings are much more complex and creative, and do not usually die from collisions. Yet, this exponential model is widely applied for the comparison of Kaplan-Meier curves in humans.

Cox regression uses an exponential model according to the following equation (t = time):

$$\text{proportion survivors} = 1/2\,t = 2^{-t}$$

In true biology: e (= 2.71828) better fits data than 2, and k is used as a constant for the species:

$$\text{proportion survivors} = e^{-kt}$$

Kaplan-Meier curves are analyzed using this exponential model. Examples of such equations are underneath:

$$\text{proportion survivors} = e^{-kt-bx}$$

x = binary variable (only 0 or 1, 0 means treatment-1, 1 means treatment-2), b = the regression coefficient,

$$\text{if } x = 0, \text{ then the equation turns into proportion survivors} = e^{-kt}$$

$$\text{if } x = 1, \text{ then the equation turns into proportion survivors} = e^{-kt-b}$$

Figure 31.2 gives an example of two Kaplan Meier curves of groups of patients surviving cancer after the start of either treatment-1 or -2. The continuous lines give the real data, the dotted lines the curves modeled by the Cox regression program.

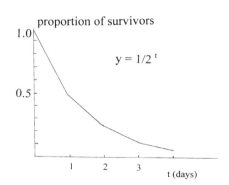

Fig. 31.1 Exponential curve of survival of mosquitoes

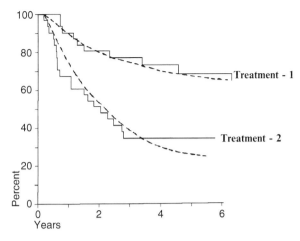

Fig. 31.2 Example of two Kaplan Meier curves of groups of patients surviving cancer after the start of either treatment-1 or -2. The *continuous lines* give the real data, the *dotted lines* the curves modeled by the Cox regression program

We are not so much interested in precise pattern of the separate dotted curves, but rather in the ratio of the two curves (the relative chance of surviving), which is given by: $e^{-kt-b}/e^{-kt} = e^{-b}$.

Consequently, the relative risk death (the hazard ratio) is given by e^b.

$$\text{The hazard ratio}\,(HR) = \text{risk death}_{treatment-2} \,/\, \text{risk death}_{treatment-1} = e^b.$$

$$\text{eLog HR}\,(\text{natural log}) = b.$$

The software calculates the best fit b for the given data, if b is significantly >0, then the HR (= antilog b) is significantly >1, which indicates a significant difference in risk-death between treatment-2 and treatment-1. We use SPSS statistical software for analysis.

Command: Analyze – survival – Cox regression – time: follow months – status: var 2 – define event (1) – Covariates – categorical: treatment – continue – plots – survival => – hazard – continue – ok

The analysis produces a b-value (regression coefficient) of 1.10 with a p-value of 0.01, which means that treatment modality is a significant predictor of survival: treatment-1 is much better than treatment-2 with a hazard ratio of $e^b = e^{1.10} = 3.00$. A nice thing with Cox regression is that like with linear and logistic regression additional x-variables can be added to the model, for example patient characteristics like age, gender, comorbidities etc.

A problem with Cox regression is that it is a major simplification of real life. It assumes that the ratio of risks of dying in the two groups is constant over time, and that this is also true for various subgroups like different age and sex groups. It is inadequate if, for example,

1. treatment effect only starts after 1–2 years,
2. treatment effect starts immediately(coronary intervention),
3. unexpected effect starts to interfere (grapht-versus-host).

Why are these situations inadequate? This is, because the value of the treatment effect changes over time, and this does not happen in a fashion that is a direct function of time. Such situations thus call for an approach that adjusts for the time-dependency. Covariates other than treatment modalities, like elevated LDL cholesterol, and hypertension in cardiovascular research or patients' frailty in oncology research are similarly at risk of changing across time, and do, likewise, qualify for the underneath alternative approach. In the underneath sections the alternative analysis is explained.

3   Cox Regression with a Time-Dependent Predictor

The level of LDL cholesterol is a strong predictor of cardiovascular survival. However, in a survival study virtually no one will die from elevated values in the first decade of observation. LDL cholesterol may be, particularly, a killer in the second decade of observation. Then, in the third decade those with high levels may all have died, and other reasons for dying may occur. In other words the deleterious effect of 10 years elevated LDL-cholesterol may be different from that of 20 years. The Cox regression model is not appropriate for analyzing the effect of LDL cholesterol on survival, because it assumes that the relative hazard of dying is the same in the first, second and third decade. Thus, there seems to be a time-dependent disproportional hazard, and if you want to analyze such data, an extended Cox regression model allowing for non-proportional hazards can be applied, and is available in SPSS (www.SPSS.com) statistical software. In the underneath example 60 patients are followed for 30 years for the occurrence of a cardiovascular event. Each row represents a patient, the columns are the patient characteristics, otherwise called the variables.

Variable					
1	2	3	4	5	6
1,00	1	0	65,00	0,00	2,00
1,00	1	0	66,00	0,00	2,00
2,00	1	0	73,00	0,00	2,00
2,00	1	0	54,00	0,00	2,00
2,00	1	0	46,00	0,00	2,00
2,00	1	0	37,00	0,00	2,00
2,00	1	0	54,00	0,00	2,00
2,00	1	0	66,00	0,00	2,00
2,00	1	0	44,00	0,00	2,00

(continued)

(continued)

Variable					
1	2	3	4	5	6
3,00	0	0	62,00	0,00	2,00
4,00	1	0	57,00	0,00	2,00
5,00	1	0	43,00	0,00	2,00
6,00	1	0	85,00	0,00	2,00
6,00	1	0	46,00	0,00	2,00
7,00	1	0	76,00	0,00	2,00
9,00	1	0	76,00	0,00	2,00
9,00	1	0	65,00	0,00	2,00
11,00	1	0	54,00	0,00	1,00
12,00	1	0	34,00	0,00	1,00
14,00	1	0	45,00	0,00	1,00
16,00	1	0	56,00	1,00	1,00
17,00	1	0	67,00	1,00	1,00
18,00	1	0	86,00	1,00	1,00
30,00	1	0	75,00	1,00	2,00
30,00	1	0	65,00	1,00	2,00
30,00	1	0	54,00	1,00	2,00
30,00	1	0	46,00	1,00	2,00
30,00	1	0	54,00	1,00	2,00
30,00	1	0	75,00	1,00	2,00
30,00	1	0	56,00	1,00	2,00
30,00	1	1	56,00	1,00	2,00
30,00	1	1	53,00	1,00	2,00
30,00	1	1	34,00	1,00	2,00
30,00	1	1	35,00	1,00	2,00
30,00	1	1	37,00	1,00	2,00
30,00	1	1	65,00	1,00	2,00
30,00	1	1	45,00	1,00	2,00
30,00	1	1	66,00	1,00	2,00
30,00	1	1	55,00	1,00	2,00
30,00	1	1	88,00	1,00	2,00
29,00	1	1	67,00	1,00	1,00
29,00	1	1	56,00	1,00	1,00
29,00	1	1	54,00	1,00	1,00
28,00	0	1	57,00	1,00	1,00
28,00	1	1	57,00	1,00	1,00
28,00	1	1	76,00	1,00	1,00
27,00	1	1	67,00	1,00	1,00
26,00	1	1	66,00	1,00	1,00
24,00	1	1	56,00	1,00	1,00
23,00	1	1	66,00	1,00	1,00
22,00	1	1	84,00	1,00	1,00
22,00	0	1	56,00	1,00	1,00
21,00	1	1	46,00	1,00	1,00
20,00	1	1	45,00	1,00	1,00

(continued)

(continued)

Variable					
1	2	3	4	5	6
19,00	1	1	76,00	1,00	1,00
19,00	1	1	65,00	1,00	1,00
18,00	1	1	45,00	1,00	1,00
17,00	1	1	76,00	1,00	1,00
16,00	1	1	56,00	1,00	1,00
16,00	1	1	45,00	1,00	1,00

Var 00001 = follow-up period (years) (Var = variable)

Var 00002 = event (0 or 1, event or lost for follow-up = censored)

Var 00003 = treatment modality (0 = treatment-1, 1 = treatment-2)

Var 00004 = age (years)

Var 00005 = gender (0 or 1, male or female)

Var 00006 = LDL-cholesterol (0 or 1, <3.9 or >= 3.9 mmol/l)

First, a usual Cox regression is performed with LDL-cholesterol as predictor of survival.

Command: Analyze – survival – Cox regression – time: follow months – status: var 2 – define event (1) – Covariates – categorical: elevated LDL-cholesterol (Var 00006) => categorical variables – continue – plots – survival => – hazard – continue – ok

The Table 31.1 shows that elevated LDL-cholesterol is not a significant predictor of survival with a p-value as large as 0.117 and a hazard ratio of 0.618. In order to assess, whether elevated LDL-cholesterol adjusted for time has an effect on survival, a time-dependent Cox regression will be performed. For that purpose the time-dependent covariate is defined as a function of both the variable time (called "T_" in SPSS) and the LDL-cholesterol-variable, while using the product of the two. This product is applied as the "time-dependent" predictor of survival, and a usual Cox model is, subsequently, performed (Cov = covariate).

Command: Analyze – survival – Cox w/Time–Dep Cov – Compute Time–Dep Cov – Time (T_) => in box Expression for T_Cov – add the sign * – add the LDL-cholesterol variable – model – time: follow months – status: var 00002 – ?: define event:1 – continue – T_Cov => in box covariates – ok

The Table 31.2 shows that elevated LDL-cholesterol after adjustment for differences in time is a highly significant predictor of survival. If we look at the actual data of the file, we will observe that, overall, the LDL-cholesterol variable is not an important factor. But, if we look at the blood pressures of the three decades separately, then it is observed that something very special is going on: in the first decade virtually no one with elevated LDL-cholesterol dies. In the second decade virtually everyone with an elevated LDL-cholesterol does: LDL cholesterol seems to be particularly a killer in the second decade. Then, in the third decade other reasons for dying seem to have occurred.

Table 31.1 Result of usual Cox regression using the variable VAR0006 (elevated LDL-cholesterol or not) as predictor and survival as outcome

Variables in the equation						
	B	SE	Wald	df	Sig.	Exp(B)
VAR00006	−,482	,307	2,462	1	,117	,618

Table 31.2 Result of the time-dependent Cox regression using the variable VAR0006 (elevated LDL-cholesterol or not) as a time-dependent predictor and survival as outcome

Variables in the equation						
	B	SE	Wald	df	Sig.	Exp(B)
T_COV_	−,131	,033	15,904	1	,000	,877

4 Cox Regression with a Segmented Time-Dependent Predictor

Some variables may have different values at different time periods. For example, elevated blood pressure may be, particularly, harmful not after decades but at the very time-point it is highest. The blood pressure is highest in the first and third decade of the study. However, in the second decade it is mostly low, because the patients were adequately treated at that time. For the analysis we have to use the socalled logical expressions. They take the value 1, if the time is true, and 0, if false. Using a series of logical expressions, we can create our time-dependent predictor, that can, then, be analyzed by the usual Cox model. In the underneath example 60 patients are followed for 30 years for the occurrence of a cardiovascular event. Each row represents again a patient, the columns are the patient characteristics.

Var 1	2	3	4	5	6	7
1,00	1	65	,00	135,00	–	–
1,00	1	66	,00	130,00	–	–
2,00	1	73	,00	132,00	–	–
2,00	1	54	,00	134,00	–	–
2,00	1	46	,00	132,00	–	–
2,00	1	37	,00	129,00	–	–
2,00	1	54	,00	130,00	–	–
2,00	1	66	,00	132,00	–	–
2,00	1	44	,00	134,00	–	–
3,00	0	62	,00	129,00	–	–
4,00	1	57	,00	130,00	–	–
5,00	1	43	,00	134,00	–	–
6,00	1	85	,00	140,00	–	–
6,00	1	46	,00	143,00	–	–
7,00	1	76	,00	133,00	–	–
9,00	1	76	,00	134,00	–	–

(continued)

(continued)

Var 1	2	3	4	5	6	7
9,00	1	65	,00	143,00	–	–
11,00	1	54	,00	134,00	110,00	–
12,00	1	34	,00	143,00	111,00	–
14,00	1	45	,00	135,00	110,00	–
16,00	1	56	1,00	123,00	103,00	–
17,00	1	67	1,00	133,00	107,00	–
18,00	1	86	1,00	134,00	108,00	–
30,00	1	75	1,00	134,00	102,00	134,00
30,00	1	65	1,00	132,00	121,00	126,00
30,00	1	54	1,00	154,00	119,00	130,00
30,00	1	46	1,00	132,00	110,00	131,00
30,00	1	54	1,00	143,00	120,00	132,00
30,00	1	75	1,00	123,00	123,00	133,00
30,00	1	56	1,00	130,00	124,00	130,00
30,00	1	56	1,00	130,00	116,00	129,00
30,00	1	53	1,00	134,00	130,00	128,00
30,00	1	34	1,00	126,00	110,00	127,00
30,00	1	35	1,00	130,00	115,00	133,00
30,00	1	37	1,00	132,00	125,00	134,00
30,00	1	65	1,00	134,00	124,00	133,00
30,00	1	45	1,00	126,00	116,00	132,00
30,00	1	66	1,00	132,00	129,00	131,00
30,00	1	55	1,00	128,00	111,00	130,00
30,00	1	88	1,00	134,00	120,00	132,00
29,00	1	67	1,00	126,00	121,00	131,00
29,00	1	56	1,00	133,00	122,00	129,00
29,00	1	54	1,00	127,00	120,00	128,00
28,00	0	57	1,00	132,00	119,00	130,00
28,00	1	57	1,00	128,00	118,00	131,00
28,00	1	76	1,00	134,00	120,00	132,00
27,00	1	67	1,00	132,00	121,00	130,00
26,00	1	66	1,00	128,00	119,00	129,00
24,00	1	56	1,00	126,00	113,00	128,00
23,00	1	66	1,00	130,00	117,00	131,00
22,00	1	84	1,00	131,00	117,00	133,00
22,00	0	56	1,00	129,00	118,00	132,00
21,00	1	46	1,00	129,00	119,00	131,00
20,00	1	45	1,00	131,00	110,00	–
19,00	1	76	1,00	130,00	111,00	–
19,00	1	65	1,00	134,00	112,00	–
18,00	1	45	1,00	126,00	113,00	–
17,00	1	76	1,00	129,00	114,00	–
16,00	1	56	1,00	131,00	106,00	–
16,00	1	45	1,00	130,00	110,00	–

Var 00001 = follow-up period years (Var = variable)

Table 31.3 Result of Cox regression with a segmented time-dependent predictor constructed with the relevant blood pressures from three decades of the study and survival as outcome

Variables in the equation						
	B	SE	Wald	df	Sig.	Exp(B)
T_COV_	−,066	,032	4,238	1	,040	,936

Var 00002 = event (0 or 1, event or lst for follow-up = censored)
Var 00003 = age (years)
Var 00004 = gender
Var 00005 = mean blood pressure in the first decade
Var 00006 = mean blood pressure in the second decade
Var 00007 = mean blood pressure in the third decade

The above data file shows that in the second and third decade an increasing number of patients have been lost. The following time-dependent covariate has been constructed for the analysis of these data (* = sign of multiplication):

$$(T\_ >= 1 \& T\_ < 11) * Var\ 5 + (T\_ >= 11 \& T\_ < 21) * Var\ 6 + (T\_ >= 21 \& T\_ < 31) * Var\ 7$$

This predictor is entered in the usual way with the commands (Cov = covariate):

model – time: follow months – status: var 00002 – ?: define event:1 – continue – T_Cov => in box covariates – ok

The Table 31.3 shows that, indeed, a mean blood pressure after adjustment for difference in decades is a significant predictor of survival at p = 0.040, and with a hazard ratio of 0.936 per mmHg. In spite of the better blood pressures in the second decade, blood pressure is a significant killer in the overall analysis.

5   Multiple Cox Regression with a Time-Dependent Predictor

Time-dependent predictors can be included in multiple Cox regression analyses together with time-independent predictors. The example of Sect. 2 is used once more. The data of the effects of two treatments on mortality/morbidity are evaluated using a Cox regression model with treatment modality, Var 00003, as predictor. Table 31.4 shows that treatment modality is a significant predictor of survival: the patients with treatment-2 live significantly shorter than those with treatment-1 with a hazard ratio of 0.524 and a p-value of 0.017. Based on the analysis in the above Sect. 3, we can not exclude that this result is confounded with the time-dependent predictor LDL-cholesterol. For the assessment of this question a multiple Cox model is used with both treatment modality (Var 00003) and the time-dependent LDL-cholesterol (T_Cov) as predictors of survival. Table 31.5 shows that both variables are highly significant predictors independent of one another. A hazard ratio of only 0.226 of one treatment versus the other is observed.

Table 31.4 Simple Cox regression with treatment modality as predictor and survival as outcome

Variables in the equation

	B	SE	Wald	df	Sig.	Exp(B)
VAR00003	−,645	,270	5,713	1	,017	,524

Table 31.5 Multiple Cox regression with treatment modalities and the time-dependent LDL-cholesterol predictor as predictor variables and survival as outcome

Variables in the equation

	B	SE	Wald	df	Sig.	Exp(B)
VAR00003	−1,488	,365	16,647	1	,000	,226
T_COV_	−,092	,017	29,017	1	,000	,912

This result is not only more spectacular but also more precise given the better p-value, than that of the unadjusted assessment of the effect of treatment modality. Obviously, the time-dependent predictor was a major confounder which has now been adjusted.

6   Discussion

Transient frailty and changes in lifestyle may be time-dependent predictors in log-term research. Some readers may find it hard to understand how to code a time-dependent predictor for Cox regression. Particularly in the SPSS program the term T_ is not always well understood. T_ is actually the current time, which is only relevant for a case that is of this time. There are, generally, two types of time-dependent predictors that investigators want to use. One involves multiplying a predictor by time in order to test the proportional hazard function or fit a model with non-proportional hazards. Compute the time-dependent predictor as: T_*covariate (* = sign of multiplication). This produces a new variable which is analyzed like with the usual Cox proportional hazard method.

The other kind of time-dependent predictor is called the segmented time-dependent predictor. It is a predictor where the value may change over time, but not in a fashion that is a direct function of time. For example, in the data file from Sect. 4 the blood pressures change over time, going up and down in a way that is not a consistent function of the time. The new predictor is set up so that for each possible time interval one of the three period variables will operate.

Currently, clinical investigators increasingly perform their own data-analysis without the help of a professional statistician. User-friendly software like SPSS is available for the purpose. Also, more advanced statistical methods are possible. The time-dependent Cox regression is more complicated than the fixed time-independent Cox regression. However, as demonstrated above, it can be readily performed by non-mathematicians along the procedures as described above.

We recommend that researchers, particularly those, whose results do not confirm their prior expectations, perform more often the extended Cox regression models, as explained in this chapter.

We conclude.

1. Many predictors of survival change across time, e.g., the effect of smoking, cholesterol, and increased blood pressure in cardiovascular research, and patients' frailty in oncology research.
2. Analytical models for survival analysis adjusting such changes are welcome.
3. The time-dependent and segmented time-dependent predictors are adequate for the purpose.
4. The usual multiple Cox regression model can include both time-dependent and time-independent predictors.

7 Conclusions

Individual patients' predictors of survival may change across time, because people may change their lifestyles. Standard statistical methods do not allow adjustments for time-dependent predictors. In the past decade time-dependent factor analysis has been introduced as a novel approach adequate for the purpose.

Using examples from survival studies we assess the performance of the novel method. SPSS statistical software is used.

1. Cox regression is a major simplification of real life: it assumes that the ratio of the risks of dying in parallel groups is constant over time. It is, therefore, inadequate to analyze, for example, the effect of elevated LDL cholesterol on survival, because the relative hazard of dying is different in the first, second and third decade. The time-dependent Cox regression model allowing for non-proportional hazards is applied, and provides a better precision than the usual Cox regression (p-value 0.117 versus 0.0001).
2. Elevated blood pressure produces the highest risk at the time it is highest. An overall analysis of the effect of blood pressure on survival is not significant, but, after adjustment for the periods with highest blood pressures using the segmented time-dependent Cox regression method, blood pressures is a significant predictor of survival (p=0.04).
3. In a long term therapeutic study treatment modality is a significant predictor of survival, but after the inclusion of the time-dependent LDL-cholesterol variable, the precision of the estimate improves from a p-value of 0.02 to 0.0001.

We conclude:

1. Predictors of survival may change across time, e.g., the effect of smoking, cholesterol, and increased blood pressure in cardiovascular research, and patients' frailty in oncology research.
2. Analytical models for survival analysis adjusting such changes are welcome.

3. The time-dependent and segmented time-dependent predictors are adequate for the purpose.
4. The usual *multiple* Cox regression model can include both time-dependent and time-independent predictors.

References

Abrahamowicz M, Mackenzie T, Esdaille JM (1996) Time-dependent hazard ratio modeling and hypothesis testing with application in lupus nephritis. J Am Stat Assoc 91:1432–1439
Cox DR (1972) Regression models and life tables. J Royal Stat Soc 34:187–220

Chapter 32
Meta-analysis, Basic Approach

1 Introduction

Problems with meta-analyses are frequent: regressions are often nonlinear; effects are often multivariate rather than univariate; continuous data frequently have to be transformed into binary data for the purpose of comparability; bad studies may be included; coverage may be limited; data may not be homogeneous; failure to relate data to hypotheses may obscure discrepancies. In spite of these well-recognized flaws, the method of meta-analysis is an invaluable scientific activity: Meta-analyses establish whether scientific findings are consistent and can be generalized across populations and treatment variations, or whether findings vary significantly between particular subsets. Explicit methods used limit bias and improve reliability and accuracy of conclusions, and increase the power and precision of estimates of treatment effects and risk exposures. In the past decade, despite reservations on the part of regulatory bodies, the method of meta-analysis has increasingly been employed in drug development programs for the purpose of exploration of changes in treatment effect over time, integrated summaries of safety and efficacy of new treatments, integrating existing information, providing data for rational decision making, and even prospective planning in drug development.

Meta-analyses are increasingly considered an integral part of phase III drug research programs for two reasons. First, meta-analysis of existing data instead of an unsystematic literature search before starting a phase III drug trial has been documentedly helpful in defining the hypothesis to be tested. Second, although meta-analyses are traditionally considered post-hoc analyses that do not test the primary hypotheses of the data, they do test hypotheses that are extremely close to the primary ones. It may be argued, therefore, that with the established uniform guidelines as proposed by Oxman and Guyatt and implemented by the Cochrane Collaborators, probability statements are almost as valid as they are in completely randomized controlled trials.

Meta-analyses should be conducted under the collective responsibility of experienced clinicians and biostatisticians familiar with relevant mathematical approaches. They may still be improved, by a combination of experience and theory, to the point

T.J. Cleophas and A.H. Zwinderman, *Statistics Applied to Clinical Studies*,   365
DOI 10.1007/978-94-007-2863-9_32, © Springer Science+Business Media B.V. 2012

at which findings can be taken as sufficiently reliable where there is no other analysis or confirmation is available.

Meta-analyses depend upon quantity and quality of original research studies as reported. Helpful initiatives to both ends include the Unpublished Paper Amnesty Movement endorsed by the editors of nearly 100 international journals in September 1997 which will help to reduce the quantity of unpublished papers, and the Consolidated Standards of Reporting Trials (CONSORT) Statement (1997) developed by high impact journals which is concerned with quality and standardization of submitted papers.

Meta-analysis can help reduce uncertainty, prevent unnecessary repetition of costly research, and shorten the time between research discoveries and clinical implementation of effective diagnostic and therapeutic treatments, but it can only do so when its results are made available. The continuously updated Cochrane Database of Systematic Reviews on the Internet is an excellent example for that purpose. Medical journals including specialist journals have a responsibility of their own. So much so that they may be able to lead the way for biased experts, who are so convinced of their own biased experience and so little familiar with meta-analysis.

2 Examples

We have come a long way since psychologists in the early 1970s drew attention to the systematic steps needed to minimize biases and random errors in reviews of research. For example, we currently have wonderful meta-analyses of pharmacological treatments for cardiovascular diseases which helped us very much to make proper listings of effective treatments (as well as less effective ones). So, now we are able to answer (1) what is best for our patients, (2) how we should distribute our resources. For example, for acute myocardial infarction, thrombolytic therapy as well as aspirin are highly effective, while lidocaine and calcium channel blockers are not so. For secondary prevention myocardial infarction cholesterol-reducing therapy were highly effective while other therapies were less so or was even counterproductive, e.g., class I antiarrhythmic agents as demonstrated in Fig. 32.1.

On the x-axis we have odds ratios. Many physicians have difficulties to understand the meaning of odds ratios. Odds = likelihood = chance = probability = risk that an event will occur divided by the chance that it won't. It can be best explained by considering a four cell contingency table.

Contingency table	Numbers of subjects who died	Numbers of subjects who did not die
Test treatment (group$_1$)	a	b
Control treatment (group$_2$)	c	d

The proportion of subjects who died in group$_1$ (or the risk (R) or probability of having an effect)

$$= p = a / (a + b), \text{ in group 2 } p = c / (c + d),$$

the ratio of $a/(a+b)$ and $c/(c+d)$ is called risk ratio (RR)

Fig. 32.1 Pooled results (odds ratios = odds of infarction in treated subjects/ odds of infarction in controls) of secondary prevention trials heart infarction

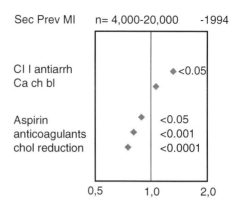

Another approach is the odds approach, where a/b and c/d are odds, and their ratio is the odds ratio(OR). In meta-analyses of clinical trials we use ORs as surrogate RRs, because, here, a/(a+b) is simply nonsense.

For example:

	Treatment group (n)		Control group (n)		Whole population (n)
Sleepiness (n)	32	a	4	b	4,000
No sleepiness (n)	24	c	52	d	52,000

n = numbers of patients

We assume that the control group is just a sample from the population, but its ratio, b/d, is that of the population. So, suppose 4=4,000, and 52=52,000, then the term $\dfrac{a/(a+b)}{c/(c+d)}$ suddenly becomes close to the term $\dfrac{a/b}{c/d} = RR$ of the population.

Currently, even epidemiologists are borrowing from clinical pharmacologists and clinical investigators, and they are quite successful in showing the likeliness of various epidemiological issues such as the epidemiology of various cardiovascular conditions. It should be emphasized that the logic behind meta-analysis is simple and straightforward. All it requires, is to stick to the scientific methods, that is (1) a clearly defined prior hypothesis, (2) thorough search of trials, (3) strict inclusion criteria for trials, and (4) uniform guidelines for data analysis.

3 Clearly Defined Hypotheses

In Chap. 1 we discussed that drug trials principally address efficacy and safety of new drugs. It is specified in advance – in the statistical analysis plan – what are the main outcome variables, and how they should be tested.

A meta-analysis is very much similar to a single trial, and similarly to a single trial it tests a very small number of primary hypotheses, mostly the hypotheses that the new compound is more efficacious and safe than the reference compound. This implies that data dredging is as unacceptable for meta-analyses as it is for separate clinical trials.

4   Thorough Search of Trials

The activity of thoroughly searching-published-research requires a systematic procedure. For example, searching medline requires a whole lot of tricks, and has to be learned. Unless you already know, you may pick up a checklist for this purpose, similarly to the checklist used by aircraft staff before take off, a nice simile used by Dr Oxman from McMasters University, one of the enlightened specialists of meta-analyses. A faulty review of trials is as perilous as a faulty aircraft and both of them are equally deadly, the former particularly so if we are going to use it for making decisions about health care. Search terms will soon put you on the right track when searching Medline. SH, e.g., means "subject-heading" which is controlled vocabulary; TW means "free-text-word" (searching with a lot of TWs increases sensitivity but reduces specificity of the search). There are sensitive ways to look for RCTs. ADJ is another TW and is more precise than AND. NOT means that first and third step are combined and second step is excluded. Use of checklists consistent of search terms of controlled vocabulary and frequent use of free text words makes things so much easier and overcomes the risk of being unsuccessful.

5   Strict Inclusion Criteria

The third scientific rule is strict inclusion criteria. Inclusion criteria are concerned with validity of the trials to be included, which means their likeliness of being unbiased. Strict inclusion criteria means that we subsequently only include the valid studies. A valid study is an unbiased study, a study that is unlikely to include systematic errors. The most dangerous errors in reviews are systematic errors otherwise called biases. Checking validity is thus the most important thing both for doers and for users of systematic reviews. Some factors have empirically been shown to beneficially influence validity. These factors include: blinding the study; random assignment of patients; explicit description of methods; accurate statistics; accurate ethics including written informed consent.

6   Uniform Data Analysis

Statistical analysis is a tool which, when used appropriately, can help us to derive meaningful conclusions from the data. And it can help us to avoid analytic errors. Statistics should be simple and should test primary hypotheses in the first place. Before any analysis or plotting of data can be performed we have to decide what kind of data we have.

6.1   *Individual Data*

Primary data of previously published studies are generally not available for use. Usually, we have to accept the summary statistics from studies instead. This is of course less informative and less precise than a synthesis of primary data but can still provide useful information.

6.2   *Continuous Data, Means and Standard Errors of the Mean (SEMs)*

We just take the mean result of the mean difference of the outcome variable we want to meta-analyze and add up. The data can be statistically tested according to unpaired t-test of the sum of multiple means:

$$t = \frac{mean_1 + mean_2 + mean_3 \dots}{\sqrt{SEM_1^2 + SEM_2^2 + SEM_3^2 + \dots}} \text{ with degrees of freedom} = n_1 + n_2 + n_3 + \dots n_k - k$$

n_i = sample size ith sample, k = number of samples, SEM = standard error of the mean

If the standard deviations are very different in size, e.g., if one is twice the other, then a more adequate calculation of the pooled standard error is as follows. This formula gives greater weight to the pooled SEM the greater the samples.

$$\text{Pooled SEM} = \sqrt{\frac{(n_1 - 1)SD_1^2 + (n_2 - 1)SD_2^2 + \dots}{n_1 + n_2 + \dots - k} \times (\frac{1}{n_1} + \frac{1}{n_2} + \dots)}$$

Similarly, if the samples are very different in size, then a more adequate calculation of the nominator of t is as follows.

$$k \left(\frac{mean_1 n_1 + mean_2 n_2 + \dots}{n_1 + n_2 + \dots} \right)$$

6.3   *Proportions: Relative Risks (RRs), Odds Ratios (ORs), Differences Between Relative Risks (RDs)*

Probably, 99% of meta-analyses make use of proportions rather than continuous data, even if original studies provided predominantly the latter particularly for efficacy data (mean fall in blood pressure etc.). This is so both for efficacy and safety meta-analyses. Sometimes data have to be remodeled from quantitative into binary ones for that purpose.

Calculation of point estimates and their variances

Contingency table	Numbers of patients with disease improvement	Numbers of patients with no improvement	Total
Test treatment	a	b	a+b
Reference treatment	c	d	c+d
Total	a+c	b+d	n

Point estimators RR, OR, or RD:

$$RR = \frac{a/(a+b)}{c/(c+d)}$$

$$OR = \frac{a/b}{c/d}$$

$$RD = \frac{a}{(a+b)} - \frac{c}{(c+d)}$$

The data can be statistically tested by use of a chi-square test of the added point estimators.

Instead of RR and OR we take lnRR and lnOR in order to approximate normality

$$Chi\text{-}square = \frac{\left(\dfrac{lnRR_1}{s_1^2} + \dfrac{lnRR_2}{s_2^2} + \dfrac{lnRR_3}{s_3^2} \ldots\right)^2}{\dfrac{1}{s_1^2} + \dfrac{1}{s_2^2} + \dfrac{1}{s_3^2} + \ldots} \quad degrees\ of\ freedom\ 1(one).$$

s^2 = variance of point estimate:

$$s_{lnRR}^2 = 1/a - 1/(a+b) + 1/c - 1/(c+d)$$
$$s_{lnOR}^2 = 1/a + 1/b + 1/c + 1/d$$
$$s_{RD}^2 = ab/(a+b)^3 + cd/(c+d)^3$$

for RD, which does not have so much skewed a distribution, ln-transformation is not needed.

$$Chi\text{-}square = \frac{\left(\dfrac{RD_1}{s_1^2} + \dfrac{RD_2}{s_2^2} + \dfrac{RD_3}{s_3^2} \ldots\right)^2}{\dfrac{1}{s_1^2} + \dfrac{1}{s_2^2} + \dfrac{1}{s_3^2} + \ldots}$$

As alternative approach Mantel-Haenszl-summary chi-square can be used: Mantel-Haenszl summary chi-square test:

$$\chi_{M\text{-}H}^2 = \frac{\left(\sum a_i - \sum\left[(a_i + b_i)(a_i + c_i)/(a_i + b_i + c_i + d_i)\right]\right)^2}{\sum\left[(a_i + b_i)(c_i + d_i)(a_i + c_i)(b_i + d_i)/(a_i + b_i + c_i + d_i)^3\right]}$$

a_i, b_i, c_i, and d_i are the a-value, b-value, c-value, and d-value of the ith sample

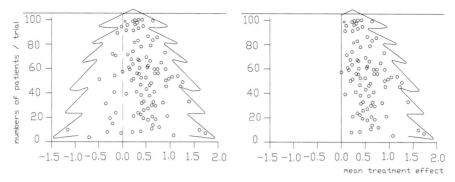

Fig. 32.2 This Christmas tree otherwise called funnel plot of 100 published trials shows on the x-axis the mean result of each trial; on the y-axis it shows the numbers of pts involved in each trial. As you can see on the *left*, there is a Christmas-tree or upside- down-funnel-pattern of distribution of the results. The smaller the trial, the larger the distribution of results. *Right graph* gives a simulated pattern, suggestive for **publication bias**: the negative trials are not published and thus missing. This cut Christmas-tree can help us suspect that there is a considerable publication bias in the meta- analysis

This approach has been explained in Chap. 3. Results of the two approaches yield similar results. However, with Mantel-Haenszl the calculation of pooled variances is rather complex, and a computer program is required.

A good starting point with any statistical analysis is plotting the data (Fig. 32.2).

6.4 Publication Bias

This socalled funnel plot of 100 published trials shows on the x-axis the mean result of each trial; on the y-axis it shows the numbers of pts involved in each trial. As you can see on the left, there is a Christmas-tree or upside-down-funnel-pattern of distribution of the results. The smaller the trial, the larger the distribution of results. Right graph gives a simulated pattern, suggestive for publication bias: the negative trials are not published and thus missing. This cut Christmas-tree can help us suspect that there is a considerable publication bias in the meta-analysis. **Publication bias** can also be statistically tested by rank correlation between variances and odds ratios. If small studies with negative results are less likely to be published, rank correlation would be high, if not it would be low. This can be assessed by the **Kendall tau test**:

Normally, the correlation coefficient r measures actual results. The Kendall tau-test basically does the same, but uses ranked data instead of actual data.

Trial	A	B	C	D	E	F	G	H	I	
Ranknumber of size of trial	1	2	3	4	5	6	7	8	9	10
Ranknumber of size of mean result	5	3	1	4	2	7	9	6	10	8

Lower row add up rank numbers higher than 5, respectively 3, respectively 1, respectively 4: we find $5+6+7+5+5+3+1+2+0+0=34$.

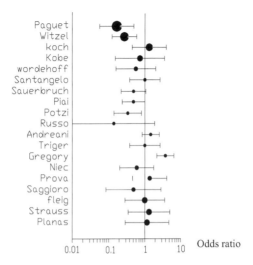

Fig. 32.3 Heterogeneous trials, 19 trials of endoscopic intervention vs no intervention for upper intestinal bleeding. On the y-axis the individual studies, on the x-axis the results, the sizes of the *bullets* correspond to the sizes of the studies (Thompson 1995, with permission from the editor)

Then lower row add up rank numbers lower than 5, 3, 1, etc.: we find $4+2+0+1+0+1+2+0+1+0=11$.

The standard error of this result is $\sqrt{\dfrac{n(n-1)(2n+5)}{18}}$, and we assume a normal distribution. We can now test this correlation and find

$$\frac{(34-11)}{\sqrt{\dfrac{n(n-1)(2n+5)}{18}}} = 1.968$$

which is approximately $1.96 = 2 =$ the number of SEMs distant from which is $\leq 5\%$ of the data. And so, the null-hypothesis of no publication bias has to be rejected. **Publication bias** can also be tested by calculating the shift of odds ratios caused by the addition of unpublished trials e.g. from abstract-reports or proceedings.

6.5   *Heterogeneity*

Figure 32.3 gives an example of a meta-analysis with means and 95% confidence intervals (CIs), telling us something about heterogeneity.

On the x-axis is the result, on the y-axis are the trials. This example has been previously used by Dr Thompson from London School of Hygiene and Tropical Medicine. We see the results of 19 trials of endoscopic sclerotherapy for esophageal varices bleeding: odds ratios less than one represent a beneficial effect. These trials were considerably different in patient-selection, baseline-severity-of-condition, sclerotechniques, management-of –bleeding-otherwise, and duration-of-follow-up. And so, this is a meta-analysis which is clinically very heterogeneous. Is it also statistically heterogeneous? For that purpose we test whether there is a greater variation between the results of the trials than is compatible with the play of chance, simply using a chi-square test. In so doing, we find $\chi^2 = 43$ for $19 - 1 = 18$ degrees of freedom (dfs). The p value is <001 giving substantial evidence for statistical heterogeneity. For the interpretation of such tests it is useful to know that a χ^2 statistic has on average a value equal to the degrees of freedom, so a result of $\chi^2 = 18$ with 18 dfs would give no evidence for heterogeneity, values much larger such as here observed do so for the opposite.

With very few studies in the meta-analysis, or with small studies, the fixed model approach has little power, and is susceptible to type II errors of not finding heterogeneity which may actually be in the data. A little bit better power is then provided by the random effect model of Dersimonian and Laird, which assumes an additional variable. The variable $s_{between trials}$ is added to the model, meaning the size of variance between the trials. The fixed model for testing the presence of heterogeneity of ordinal data is demonstrated underneath. For continuous data multiple group analysis of variance (ANOVA) may be used.

Fixed effect model (Cochran-Q test)
This test for homogeneity (k-1 degrees of freedom) is based on the Cochran-Q test (see Chap. 3 Sect. 5, for further explanation of this test).

$$\chi^2 = \frac{RD_1^2}{s_1^2} + \frac{RD_2^2}{s_2^2} + \frac{RD_3^2}{s_3^2} \ldots - \frac{\left[\frac{RD_1}{s_1^2} + \frac{RD_2}{s_2^2} + \frac{RD_3}{s_3^2}\right]^2}{\frac{1}{s_1^2} + \frac{1}{s_2^2} + \frac{1}{s_3^2} + \ldots}$$

Random effect model (DerSimonian and Laird)
This test for heterogeneity is identical, except for variances s^2 which are replaced with

$$\left(s^2 + s_{between trials}^2\right).$$

Example of random effect model analysis					
	Test treatment			Reference treatment	
Trial	Death	Survivors		Death	Survivors
1	1	24		5	20
2	5	95		15	85
3	25	475		50	450

In the above example, the test for heterogeneity fixed effect model provides $\chi^2 = 1.15$ with dfs $3-1 = 2$, while the test with the random effect model provides a

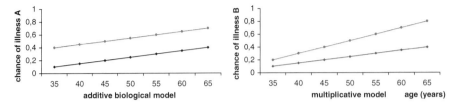

Fig. 32.4 Age is a determinant of illness, but in the *right graph* the risk difference is heterogeneous because it increases with age

$\chi^2 = 1.29$ with dfs equally 2, both lower than 2. The between-trial variance $s_{between\ trials}^2$ is thus accepted to be not significantly different from zero and so are the weights of the two models. Heterogeneity can be neglected. With the simple example given, the two approaches to test homogeneity raise similar results (the null hypothesis is tested that studies are equal). And so, between-trial variance $s_{between\ trials}^2$ is accepted to be zero and the results of the two models are equal.

Heterogeneity can be neglected in this example.

6.5.1   Heterogeneity and Sub-group Analysis

When there is heterogeneity, to analists of systematic reviews, that's when things first get really exciting. A careful investigation of the potential cause of heterogeneity has to be accomplished. The main focus then should be on trying to understand any sources of heterogeneity in the data. In practice, this may be less hard to assess since the doers have frequently noticed clinical differences already, and it thus becomes relatively easy to test the data accordingly. Figure 32.4 below shows how age e.g. is a determinant of illness, but in the right graph the risk difference is heterogeneous because it increases with age.

Except age, outliers may give an important clue about the cause of heterogeneity.

Figure 32.5 shows the relation between cholesterol and coronary heart disease. The two outliers on top were the main cause for heterogeneity in the data: one study was different because it achieved a very small reduction of cholesterol; the other was a very short-term study.

Still other causes of heterogeneity may be involved. 33 Studies of cholesterol and risk of carcinomas showed that heterogeneity was huge. When the trials were divided according to social class, the effect in the lowest class was 4–5 times those of the middle and upper class, explaining everything about this heterogeneous result.

We should, of course, warn of the danger of overinterpretation of heterogeneity. Heterogeneity may occur by chance. This is particularly an important possibility to consider when no clinical explanation is found. Also, we should warn that a great deal of uniformity among the results of independently performed studies is not necessarily good; it can suggest consistency-in-bias rather than consistency-in-real-effects.

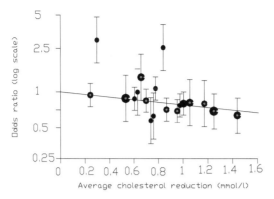

Fig. 32.5 The relation between cholesterol and coronary heart disease. The two outliers on top were the main cause for heterogeneity in the data, the sizes of the *bullets* correspond to the sizes of the studies (Shipley et al. 1991, with permission from the editor)

6.6   *Robustness*

Sensitivity or robustness of a meta-analysis is one last important aspect to be addressed in the analysis of the data. When talking of strict inclusion criteria, we discussed studies with lower levels of validity, as assessed by factors such as blinding, random assignments, accurate and explicit description of results and statistics. It may be worthwhile not to completely reject the studies with lower methodology. They can be used for assessing another characteristic of meta-analyses, namely its sensitivity.

This left upper graph (Fig. 32.6) gives an example of how the pooled data of three high-quality-studies provide a smaller result, than do four studies-of-borderline-quality. The summary result is mainly determined by the borderline-quality-studies, as is also shown in the cumulative-right-upper -graph. When studies are ordered according to their being blinded or not as shown in the lower graph, differences may be large or may be not so. In studies using objective variables, e.g., blood pressures, heart rates, blinding is not so important than in studies using subjective variables (pain scores etc.). In this particular example differences were negligible. So, in conclusion, when examining the influence of various inclusion criteria on the overall odds ratios, we may come to conclude that the criteria themselves are an important factor in determining the summary result. We say in that case that the meta-analysis lacks robustness (otherwise called sensitivity or precision of point estimates). Interpretation then has to be cautious, pooling may have to be left out altogether. Just leaving out trials at this stage of the meta-analysis is inappropriate either, because it would introduce bias similar to publication-bias or bias-introduced-by-not-complying-with-the-intention-to-treat-principle.

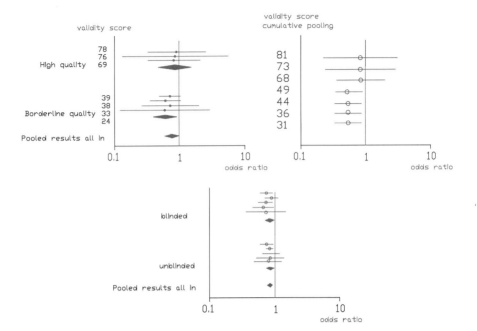

Fig. 32.6 The *left upper graph* gives an example of how the pooled data of three high-quality-studies provide a smaller result, than do four studies-of-borderline-quality. The summary result is mainly determined by the borderline-quality-studies, as is also shown in the cumulative-*right-upper -graph*. When studies are ordered according to their being blinded or not as shown in the *lower graph*, differences may be large or may be not so. In studies using objective variables, e.g., blood pressures, heart rates, blinding is not so important than in studies using subjective variables (pain scores etc.). In this particular example differences were negligible

7   Discussion, Where Are We Now?

Several recent publications were critical of the method of meta-analysis: e.g., Chalmers and Lau in JAMA 1996 and Lelorier in NEJM 1997 concluded that meta-analyses did not accurately predict the outcomes of subsequent large trials. Colditz and Berlin JAMA 1999 concluded that meta-analyses were not or at least not-yet good enough to identify adverse drug reactions. Why so? Probably, the answer is (1) trials must get better, and (2) publication bias must disappear altogether. There are several important initiatives being taken at this very moment that may be helpful to this aim. In May 1998 editors of 70 journals have endorsed the Consolidated-Standards-of-Reporting-Trials-Statement (the CONSORT-Statement) developed by JAMA, BMJ, Lancet, and Annals-of-Intern-Med in an effort to standardize the way trials are reported, with special-emphasis on the-intention-to-treat-principle in order to reduce treatment-related selection-bias. For investigators, <reporting> according to such standards will become much easier, and will even become a non-issue if requirements as requested by CONSORT are met. This initiative may have important potential to improve the level of validity of trials and thus facilitate their suitability for meta-analyses. Another important milestone is the initiative of the Unpublished-Paper-Amnesty-Movement. In September 1997 the editors of nearly 100 international journals invited investigators to submit unpublished study data in the form of unreported-trial-registration-forms. Submitted materials are routinely made available to the world through listing the trial-details on the journals' web sites, in addition to other ways. The International-Committee-of-Medical-Editors and the World-Association-of-Medical-Editors are currently helping these initiatives by standardizing the peer review system and training referees.

Where do we go? We go for the aim of meta-analyses being accepted as gold standard for:

1. Reporting randomized experimental research.
2. Setting the stage for the development of new drugs.
3. Determination of individual therapies.
4. Leading the way for regulatory organs.
5. Maybe soon even epidemiological research.

We will only accomplish these efforts if we stick to the scientific method, which we summed up for you earlier. However, today many meta-analyses are presented or published, that do not follow these simple scientific principles, and that just leave out validity assessment of trials included, or tests for heterogeneity and publication bias. Both journal editors and readers of meta-analyses must be critical and alert since a flawed meta-analysis of unreliable and biased material is deadly, not only to research but also to health care. The above guidelines enable not only to perform meta-analyses but also to identify flawed meta-analyses, and, more importantly, to identify and appreciate well-performed meta-analyses.

8 Conclusions

The scientific methods governing the practice of meta-analysis include (1) a clearly defined prior hypothesis, (2) a thorough search of trials, (3) strict inclusion criteria, and (4) a uniform data analysis. In the statistical analysis of the meta-data three pitfalls have to be accounted: (1) publication bias, (2) heterogeneity, (3) lack of robustness.

References

Shipley MJ, Pocock SJ, Marmot MG (1991) Does plasma cholesterol concentration predict mortality from coronary heart disease in elderly people? 18 year follow-up in Whitehall study. BMJ 303:89–92

Thompson SG (1995) Why sources of heterogeneity should be investigated. In: Chalmers I, Altman DG (eds) Systematic reviews. BMJ Publishing Group, London, pp 48–63

Chapter 33
Meta-analysis, Review and Update of Methodologies

1 Introduction

In 1982 thrombolytic therapy for acute coronary syndromes was controversial. In a meta-analysis of seven trials Stampfer et al. found a reduced risk of mortality of 0.80 (95% confidence interval 0.68–0.95). These findings (Stampfer et al. 1982) were not accepted by cardiologists until 1986, when a large clinical trial confirmed the conclusions (Gruppo Italiano per lo Studio della Streptochinasi nell'Infarto Miocardico (GISSI) 1986), and streptokinase became widely applied.

Meta-analyses can be defined as systematic reviews with pooled data. Traditionally, they are post-hoc analyses. However, probability statements may be more valid, than they usually are with post-hoc studies, particularly if performed on outcomes that were primary outcomes in the original trials. Problems with pooling are frequent: correlations are often nonlinear (Glass and Smith 1979); effects are often multifactorial rather than unifactorial (Fleiss and Gross 1991); continuous data frequently have to be transformed into binary data for the purpose of comparability (Stein 1998); poor studies may be included and coverage may be limited (Zhou et al. 2003); data may not be homogeneous and may fail to relate to hypotheses (Turnbul 2003). In spite of these problems, the methods of meta-analysis are an invaluable scientific activity: they establish whether scientific findings are consistent (Cook et al. 1998), and can be generalized across populations and treatment variations (Straus and Sackett 1998), and whether findings vary between subgroups (Bero et al. 1998). The methods also limit bias, improve reliability and accuracy of conclusions (Jones 1995), and increase the power and precision of treatment effects and risk exposures (Zhou et al. 2003).

The objective of this chapter is to review statistical procedures for the meta-analysis of clinical research. The Google data base system provides 659,000 references on the methods of meta-analysis, and refers to hundreds of books of up to 600 pages (Hunter and Schmidt 2004), illustrating the complexity of this subject. The basic statistical analysis of meta-analyses is, however, not complex, if the basic scientific methods are met (Cleophas 2006). We first will review the scientific methods, and, then, introduce the statistical analysis, including the analysis of potential pitfalls. Finally, we will cover some new developments.

2   Four Scientific Rules

The logic behind meta-analyses is simple and straightforward. What it requires, is to stick to scientific methods, largely similar to those required for clinical trials. They can be summarized: (1) a clearly defined prior hypothesis, (2) thorough search of trials, (3) strict inclusion criteria, and (4) uniform data analysis (Cleophas 2006).

2.1   Clearly Defined Hypothesis

Clinical trials address efficacy and safety of new drugs or interventions. It is specified in advance what are the main outcome variables, and how they should be tested. A meta-analysis is very much similar to a single trial, and, similarly to a single trial, it tests a very small number of primary hypotheses, mostly that the new compound or intervention is more efficacious and safe than the reference compound or intervention.

2.2   Thorough Search of Trials

The activity of thoroughly searching-published-research requires a systematic procedure, and has to be learned. You may pick up a checklist for this purpose, similarly to the checklist used by aircraft staff before take off, a nice simile used by Oxman and Guyatt (1988). A faulty review of trials is as perilous as a faulty aircraft and both of them are equally deadly, particularly so if we are going to use it for making decisions about health care. For a systematic review Medline (Greenhalgh 1997) is not enough, and other data bases have to be searched, e.g., EMBASE-Excerpta Medica (Lefebvre and McDonald 1996) and the Cochrane Library (2011).

2.3   Strict Inclusion Criteria

Inclusion criteria are concerned with the levels of validity, otherwise called quality criteria, of the trials to be included. Strict inclusion criteria means that we will, subsequently, only include the valid studies. Some factors have empirically been shown to beneficially influence validity. These factors include: blinding the study; random assignment of patients; explicit description of methods; accurate statistics; accurate ethics including written informed consent. We should add that the inclusion of unpublished studies may reduce the magnitude of publication bias, an issue which will be discussed in the Sect. 4.

2.4   Uniform Data Analysis

Statistical analysis is a tool which helps to derive meaningful conclusions from the data, and to avoid analytic errors. Statistics should be simple and test primary hypotheses in the first place. Prior to any analysis or data plots, we have to decide what kind of data we have.

3   General Framework of Meta-analysis

In general, meta-analysis refers to statistical analysis of the results of different studies. The simplest analysis is to calculate an average, and in a meta-analysis a weighted average is computed. Consider a meta-analysis of k different clinical trials, and let $x_1, x_2,..., x_k$ be the summary statistics. The weighted average effect is then calculated as

$$\overline{X}_w = \frac{\sum_{i=1}^{k} w_i x_i}{\sum_{i=1}^{k} w_i}, \text{ and its standard error is}$$

$$se(\overline{X}_w) = \left[\frac{\sum_{i=1}^{k} (w_i)^2 Var(x_i)}{[\sum_{i=1}^{k} w_i]^2} \right]^{1/2}.$$

The weights w_i are a function of the standard error of x_i, denoted as $se(x_i)$, and of the variance σ^2 of the true effects of the compound between k different studies:

$$w_i = \frac{1}{(se(x_i)^2 + \sigma^2)}.$$

If all k studies have the same true quantitative effect, $\sigma^2 = 0$ and the weighted average effect is called a *fixed-effect* estimate. If the true effects of the compound vary between studies, $\sigma^2 > 0$ and the weighted average effect is called a *random-effects* estimate. For the fixed-effect estimate (i.e. $\sigma^2 = 0$) the calculations are quite simple, for the random-effects estimate the calculations are more complex, but available in computer packages (SAS 2011; SPSS Statistical Software 2011; Cochrane Revman 2011; Stata statistical software for professionals 2011; Comprehensive Meta-analysis, by Biostat 2011).

Depending on the type of outcome variable, the summary statistics x_1, x_2, …, x_k have different forms.

1. *Continuous data*

   Continuous data are summarized with means and standard deviations; $mean_{1i}$ and SD_{1i} in the placebo-group, and $mean_{2i}$ and SD_{2i} in the active-treatment group of trial i. The summary statistic equals $x_i = mean_{1i} - mean_{2i}$ and

   $$se(x_i) = \sqrt{\frac{SD_{1i}^2}{n_{1i}} + \frac{SD_{2i}^2}{n_{2i}}},$$ where n_{1i} and n_{2i} are the sample sizes of the two treatments.

   If a trial compares two treatments in the same patients, the summary statistic is $x_i = mean_{1i} - mean_{2i}$, where $mean_{1i}$ and $mean_{2i}$ are the means of the two treatments, and

   $$se(x_i) = \sqrt{\frac{SD_{1i}^2}{n_i} + \frac{SD_{2i}^2}{n_i} - \frac{2r\,SD_{1i}\,SD_{2i}}{n_i}},$$ where r is the correlation between the outcomes in the two treatments.

   If the distribution of the outcomes is very skewed, it is more useful to summarize the outcomes with medians than means.

2. *Binary data*

   Binary data are summarized as proportions of patients with a positive outcome in the treatment arms, denoted by p_{i1} and p_{i2}. Three different summary statistics are used:

   (a) Risk-difference.

   The summary statistic of trial i equals $xi = p_{1i} - p_{2i}$, the standard error equals

   $$se(x_i) = \sqrt{\frac{p_{1i}(1-p_{1i})}{n_{1i}} + \frac{p_{2i}(1-p_{2i})}{n_{2i}}},$$ where n_{1i} and n_{2i} are the sample sizes of

   the two treatments of trial i.

   (b) Relative Risk.

   The summary statistic of trial i equals the ratio of the two proportions, but its distribution is often very skewed. Therefore, we prefer to analyze the natural logarithm of the relative risk, ln(RR). The summary statistic thus equals

   $x_i = ln\ (p_{i1}/p_{i2})$, and the standard error equals $se(x_i) = \sqrt{\dfrac{1-p_{1i}}{p_{1i}n_{1i}} + \dfrac{1-p_{2i}}{p_{2i}n_{2i}}}$.

   (c) Odds Ratio.

   The summary statistic of trial i equals the ratio of the odds, but since the odds ratio is strictly positive, we again prefer to analyze the natural logarithm of the odds ratio. Thus the summary statistic equals $x_i = ln\left(\dfrac{p_{1i}/(1-p_{1i})}{p_{2i}/(1-p_{2i})}\right)$, and the standard error equals

   $$se(x_i) = \sqrt{\frac{1}{n_{1i}p_{1i}} + \frac{1}{n_{1i}(1-p_{1i})} + \frac{1}{n_{2i}p_{2i}} + \frac{1}{n_{2i}(1-p_{2i})}}.$$

(d) Other methods.

The Mantel-Haenszel method has been developed for the stratified analysis of odds ratios, and has been extended to the stratified analysis of risk ratios and risk differences (Greenland and Robins 1985). Like the general model a weighted average effect is calculated. For the calculation of combined odds ratios Peto's method is also often used (Yusuf et al. 1985). It applies a way to calculate odds ratios which may cause under- or overestimation of extreme values like odds ratios <0.2 or >5.0.

Sometimes valuable information can be obtained from crossover studies, and, if the paired nature of the data are taken into account, such data can be included in a meta-analysis. The Cochrane Library CD-ROM provides the Generic inverse variance method for that purpose (Cochrane Library 2011).

3. *Survival data*

Survival trials are summarized with Kaplan-Meier curves, and the difference between the survival in two treatment arms is quantified with the log (hazard ratio) calculated from the Cox regression model. To test whether the weighted average is significantly different from 0.0, a chi-square test is used: $\chi^2 = \left(\dfrac{\overline{X}_w}{se(\overline{X}_w)} \right)^2$ with one degree of freedom. A calculated χ^2-value larger than 3.841, indicates that the pooled average is significantly different from 0.0 at $p<0.05$, and, thus, that a significant different exists between the test and reference treatments. The Generic inverse variance method is also possible for the analysis of hazard ratios (Cochrane Library 2011).

4   Pitfalls of Data Analysis

Meta-analyses will suffer from any bias that the individual studies included suffer from, including incorrect and incomplete data. Two publications underline these problems: (1) out of 49 recently published studies, 83% of the unrandomized and 25% of the randomized studies were partly refuted soon after publication (Ioannides 2005); (2) out of 519 recently published trials 20% selectively reported positive results, and reported negative results incompletely (Chan and Altman 2005). Three common pitfalls of meta-analyses are listed underneath.

4.1   Publication Bias

A good starting point with any statistical analysis is plotting the data (Fig. 32.2, Chap. 32). A Christmas tree (Cleophas 2006) or upside-down-funnel-pattern of distribution of the results of 100 published trials shows on the x-axis the mean result of each trial, on the y-axis the sample size of the trials. The smaller the trial, the wider the distribution of results. The right graph gives a simulated pattern, suggestive of publication bias: the negative trials are not published and thus missing. This cut Christmas-tree can help suspect that there is **publication bias** in the meta-analysis. Publication bias can be tested by calculating the shift of odds ratios caused by the addition of unpublished trials from abstract-reports or proceedings (Chalmers and Altman 1995).

4.2   Heterogeneity

In order to visually assess heterogeneity between studies several types of plots are proposed, including forest plots, radial and L' Abbe plots (National Council of Social Studies 2011). The forest plot of Fig. 32.3 in Chap. 32 gives an example used by Thompson (1995) of a meta-analysis with odds ratios and 95% confidence intervals (CIs), telling something about heterogeneity. On the x-axis are the results, on the y-axis the trials. We see the results of 19 trials of endoscopic intervention vs no intervention for upper intestinal bleeding: odds ratios less than one represent a beneficial effect. These trials were considerably different in patient-selection, baseline-severity-of-condition, endoscopic-techniques, management-of-bleeding-otherwise, and duration-of-follow-up. And so, this is a meta-analysis which is, clinically, very heterogeneous. Is it also statistically heterogeneous? For that purpose we may use a fixed-effect model which tests whether there is a greater variation between the results of the trials than is compatible with the play of chance, using a chi-square test. The null-hypothesis is that all studies have the same true odds ratio, and that the observed odds ratios vary only due to sampling variation in each study. The alternative hypothesis is that the variation of the observed odds ratio is also due to systematic differences in true odds ratios between studies. The Cochran Q test with the Q statistic is used to test the above null hypothesis with summary statistics x_i and weights w_i:

$$Q = \sum_{i=1}^{k} w_i (x_i - \overline{X}_w)^2 \quad \text{with } k - 1 \text{ degrees of freedom.}$$

We find $Q = 43$ for $19 - 1 = 18$ degrees of freedom (dfs) for the example of the endoscopic intervention. The p-value is <0.001 giving substantial evidence for statistical heterogeneity. For the interpretation it is useful to know that, when the null-hypothesis is true, a Q statistic has on average a value close to the degrees of freedom, and increases with increasing degrees of freedom. So, a result of $Q = 18$ with 18 dfs would give no evidence for heterogeneity, values much larger such do so for the opposite.

If the above test is positive, it is common to also calculate a random-effects estimate of the weighted average, as suggested by Dersimonian and Laird (1986). We should add that, in most situations, the use of the random-effects model will lead to wider confidence intervals and a lower chance to call a difference statistically significant. A disadvantage of the random-effects analysis is that small and large studies are given almost similar weights (Berlin et al. 1989). Complementary to the Q-statistic, the amount of heterogeneity between studies is often quantified with the I^2-statistic (Higgins and Thompson 2002)

$$I^2 = 100\% * \left[Q - (k-1) \right] / Q$$

which is interpreted as the proportion of total variation in study estimates due to heterogeneity rather than sampling error. Fifty percent is often used as a cut-off for heterogeneity.

4.3   Investigating the Cause for Heterogeneity

When there is heterogeneity, careful investigation of the potential cause has to be accomplished. The main focus should be trying to understand any sources of heterogeneity in the data. In practice, it may be less hard to assess since the do-ers already have noticed clinical differences, and it, thus, becomes easy to test the data accordingly. The general approach is to quantify the association between the outcomes and characteristics of the different trials. Not only patient-characteristics, but also trial-quality-characteristics such the use of blinding, randomization, and placebo-controls have to be considered. Scatterplots are helpful to investigating the association between outcome and a covariate, but these must be inspected carefully because differences in trial sample-sizes may distort the existence of association, and meta-regression techniques may be needed to investigate associations.

Outliers may also give a clue about the cause of heterogeneity. Figure 32.5 in Chap. 32 shows the relation between cholesterol and coronary heart disease (Shipley et al. 1991). The two outliers on top were the main cause for heterogeneity in the data.

Still other causes for heterogeneity may be involved. As an example, 33 studies of cholesterol and the risk of carcinomas showed that heterogeneity was huge (Khan et al. 1996). When the trials were divided according to social class, the effect in the lowest class was 4–5 times those of the middle and upper class, explaining everything about this heterogeneous result.

There is some danger of over-interpretation of heterogeneity. Heterogeneity may occur by chance, and will almost certainly be found with large meta-analyses involving many and large studies. This is particularly an important possibility when no clinical explanation is found, or when the heterogeneity is clinically irrelevant. Also, we should warn that a great deal of uniformity among the results of independently performed studies is not necessarily good; it can indicate consistency-in-bias rather than consistency-in-real-effects as suggested by Riegelman (2005).

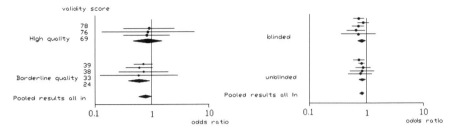

Fig. 33.1 *Left graph*: three high-quality-studies provide a smaller result, than do four studies-of-borderline-quality; the summary result is mainly determined by the borderline-quality-studies. *Right graph*: when studies using objective variables are ordered according to their being blinded, differences may not be large

4.4   Lack of Robustness

Sensitivity or robustness of a meta-analysis is one last aspect to be addressed. When talking of strict inclusion criteria, we discussed studies with lower levels of validity. It may be worthwhile not to completely reject the studies with lower methodology (Khan et al. 1996). They can be used for assessing sensitivity.

The left graph of Fig. 33.1 gives an example of how the pooled data of three high-quality-studies provide a smaller result, than do four studies-of-borderline-quality. The summary result is mainly determined by the borderline-quality-studies. When studies are ordered according to their being blinded as shown in the right graph, differences may be large or not. In studies using objective variables, for example blood pressures or heart rates, blinding is not as important as it is in studies using subjective variables (pain scores etc.). In this particular example differences were negligible. When examining the influence of various inclusion criteria on the overall odds ratios, we have to conclude that the criteria themselves are an important factor in determining the summary result. In that case the meta-analysis lacks robustness. Interpretation has to be cautious, and pooling may have to be left out altogether. Just leaving out trials at this stage of the meta-analysis is inappropriate either, because it would introduce bias similar to publication-bias or bias-introduced-by-not-complying-with-the-intention-to-treat-principle.

5   New Developments

Software programs for the analysis of meta-data are provided by SAS (2011), the Cochrane Revman (2011), S-plus (2011), StatsDirect (2011), StatXact (2011), True Epistat (2011). Most of these programs are expensive, but common procedures are available through Microsoft's Excel and in Excel-add-ins (2011), while many websites offer online statistical analyses for free, including BUGS (2011) and R (2011).

Leandro's software program (Leandro 2005) visualizes heterogeneity directly from a computer graph based on Galbraith (1988) plots.

New statistical methods are being developed. Boekholdt et al. (2005). showed that observational studies and clinical trials can be simultaneously included in a meta-analysis. Van Houwelingen et al. (2002). assessed heterogeneity with multivariate methods for bivariate and multivariate outcome parameters. If trials directly comparing the treatments under study are not available, indirect comparisons with a common comparator may be used (Glenny et al. 2005). A method like leave-one-out cross-validation is a standard sensitivity technique for such purpose. Lumley (2002) developed network meta-analysis to compare competing treatments not directly compared in trials. Terrin et al. (2003) and Tang and Liu (2000) recently demonstrated that an asymmetric Christmas tree is only related to publication bias if the trials included are homogeneous, and that registries are a good alternative approach. In recent years the method of meta-regression brought new insights (Schmid et al. 2004; Higgins and Thompson 2004). For example, it showed that group-level instead of patient-level analyses easily fails to detect heterogeneities between individual patients, otherwise called ecological biases. Robustness is hard to assess if low quality studies are lacking. Casas et al. (2004) showed that it can be assessed by evaluating the extent to which different variables contribute to the variability between the studies. It can also be assessed using cumulative meta-analysis (Lau et al. 1995), while quality measures can be adjusted for in meta-regression.

Meta-analyses including few studies, e.g., 3 or 4, have little power to test the pitfalls. In contrast, meta-analyses including many studies may have so much power that they demonstrate small pitfalls, that are not clinically relevant. For example, a meta-analysis of 43 angiotensin blocker studies (Conlin et al. 2000) found 95% confidence intervals of the heterogeneity and publication bias effects were not wider than 5% of the treatment effects. Another reason why the pitfalls receive less attention today than 5 years ago is, that an increasing part of the current meta-analyses are performed in the form of working papers of an explorative nature, where the primary question is not a result representative for the entire population, but rather the estimates of the treatment effects in subgroups and interactions. These meta-analyses contain many details, and look a bit like working papers of technological evaluations as produced by physicists. The trend to increasingly publish detailed data, rather than study reports as allowed by journals, is enhanced by the Internet, which enables to register many more data than do medical journals.

Meta-analyses were 'invented' in the early 1970s by psychologists, but pooling study results extends back to the early 1900s by statisticians such as Karl Pearson, and Ronald Fisher. In the first years pooling of the data was often impossible due to heterogeneity of the studies. However, after 1995 trials became more homogeneous. In the late 1990s several publications concluded that meta-analyses did not accurately predict treatment (LeLorier et al. 1997; Temple 1999) and adverse effects (Brewer and Colditz 1999). The pitfalls were held responsible. Initiatives against them include (1) the Consolidated-Standards-of-Reporting-Trials-Movement (CONSORT), (2) the Unpublished-Paper-Amnesty-Movement of the English journals, and (3) the World Association of Medical Editors' initiative to standardize the peer review system. Guidelines/checklists for reporting meta-analyses were published like QUOROM (Quality of Reporting of Meta-analyses) and MOOSE (Meta-analysis Of Observational Studies in Epidemiology).

6 Conclusions

Meta-analysis is important in clinical research, because it establishes whether scientific findings are consistent, and can be generalized across populations. The statistical analysis consists of the computation of weighted averages of study characteristics and their standard errors. Common pitfalls of data-analysis are (1) publication bias, (2) heterogeneity, (3) lack of robustness. New developments in the statistical analysis include (1) new software easy to use, (2) new arithmetical methods that facilitate the assessment of heterogeneity and comparability of studies, (3) a current trend towards more extensive data reporting including multiple subgroup and interaction analyses. Meta-analyses are governed by the traditional rules for scientific research, and the pitfalls are, particularly, relevant to hypothesis-driven meta-analyses, but less so to current working papers with emphasis on entire data coverage.

References

Berlin JA, Laird NM, Sacks HS, Chalmers TC (1989) A comparison of statistical methods for combining event rates from clinical trials. Stat Med 8:141–151

Bero LA, Grilli R, Grimshaw JM, Harvey E, Oxman AD, Thomson MA (1998) Closing the gap between research and practice: an overview of systematic reviews of interventions to promote the implementation of research findings. BMJ 317:465–468

Boekholdt SM, Sacks FM, Jukema JW, Shepherd J, Freeman DJ, McMahon AD, Cambien F, Nicaud V, GJ De grooth, Talmud PJ, Humphries SE, Miller GJ, Eiriksdottir G, Gudnason V, Kauma H, Kakko S, Savolainen MJ, Arca M, Montasli A, Liu S, Lanz HJ, Zwinderman AH, Kuivenhoven JA, Kastelein JJ (2005) Cholesterol ester transfer protein TaqiB variant, high density lipoprotein cholesterol levels, cardiovascular risk, and efficacy of pravastatin treatment. Circulation 111:278–287

Brewer T, Colditz GA (1999) Postmarketing surveillance and adverse drug reactions; current perspectives. JAMA 281:824–829

BUGS y WinBUGS. http://www.mrc-bsu.cam.ac.uk/bugs

Casas JP, Leonelo EB, Humphries SE (2004) Endothelial NO synthase genotype and ischemic heart disease. Circulation 109:1359–1365

Chalmers I, Altman DG (1995) Systematic reviews. BMJ Publishing Group, London

Chan AW, Altman DG (2005) Identifying outcome reporting bias in randomised trials on PubMed: review of publications and survey of authors. BMJ 330:753–756

Cleophas TJ (2006) Meta-analysis. In: Cleophas TJ, Zwinderman AH, Cleophas AF (eds) Statistics applied to clinical trials, 3rd edn. Springer, Dordrecht, pp 205–218

Cochrane Library. http://www.cochrane.org/cochrane/hbook.htm. Accessed 15 Dec 2011

Cochrane Revman. http://www.cochrane.org/cochrane/revman.htm. Accessed 15 Dec 2011

Comprehensive Meta-analysis, by Biostat. http://www.meta-analysis.com. Accessed 15 Dec 2011

Conlin PR, Spence JD, Williams B, Ribeiro AB, Saito I, Benedict C, Bunt AM (2000) Angiotensin II antagonists for hypertension: are there differences in efficacy? Am J Hypertens 13:418–426

Cook DJ, Mulrow CD, Haynes RB (1998) Systematic reviews: synthesis of the best evidence for clinical decisions. Ann Intern Med 317:339–342

Dersimonian R, Laird NM (1986) Meta-analysis in clinical trials. Control Clin Trials 7:177–188

Fleiss JL, Gross AJ (1991) Meta-analysis in epidemiology, with special reference to studies of the association between exposure to environmental tobacco smoke and lung cancer. J Clin Epidemiol 44:127–129

Galbraith RF (1988) A note on graphical presentation of estimated odds ratios from several trials. Stat Med 7:889–894

Glass GV, Smith ML (1979) Meta-analysis of research on class size and achievement. Educ Evol Policy Anal 1:2–16

Glenny AM, Altman DG, Song F, Sakarovitch C, Deeks JJ, D'Amico RD, Bradburn M, Eastwood AJ (2005) Indirect comparisons of competing interventions. Health Technol Assess 9:1–148

Greenhalgh T (1997) How to read a paper. The Medline database. BMJ 315:180–183

Greenland S, Robins JM (1985) Estimation of common effect parameter from sparse follow-up data. Biometrics 41:55–68

Gruppo Italiano per lo Studio della Streptochinasi nell'Infarto Miocardico (GISSI) (1986) Effectiveness of intravenous thrombolytic treatment in acute myocardial infarction. Lancet 1:397–402

Higgins JPT, Thompson SG (2002) Quantifying heterogeneity in a meta-analysis. Stat Med 21:1539–1558

Higgins JPT, Thompson SG (2004) Controlling the risk of spurious findings from meta-regression. Stat Med 23:1662–1682

Hunter JE, Schmidt FL (2004) Methods in meta-analysis, 2nd edn. Sage Public Inc, Thousand Oaks

Ioannides JP (2005) Contradicted and initially stronger effects in highly cited clinical research. JAMA 294:210–228

Jones DR (1995) Meta-analysis: weighing the evidence. Stat Med 14:137–139

Khan KS, Daya S, Jadad AR (1996) The importance of quality of primary studies in producing unbiased systematic reviews. Arch Int Med 156:661–666

Lau J, Schmid CH, Chalmers TC (1995) Cumulative meta-analysis of clinical trials builds evidence for exemplary medical care. J Clin Epidemiol 48:45–57

Leandro G (2005) Meta-analysis in medical research. BMJ books, London

Lefebvre C, McDonald S (1996) Development of a sensitive search strategy for reports of randomized trials in EMBASE. In: Paper presented at the fourth international Cochrane colloquium, Adelaide, Australia, 20–24 Oct 1996

LeLorier J, Gregoire G, Benhaddad A, Lapierre J, Derderien F (1997) Discrepancies between meta-analyses and subsequent large randomized controlled trials. N Engl J Med 337:536–542

Lumley T (2002) Network meta-analysis for indirect treatment comparisons. Stat Med 21:2313–2324

Meta-analysis Mark X. Microsoft's Excel. Accessed 15 Dec 2011

National Council of Social Studies. Statistical and power analysis software. http://www.ncss.com/metaanal.html. Accessed 15 Dec 2011

Oxman AD, Guyatt G (1988) Guidelines for reading reviews. Can Med Assoc J 138:697–703

R. http://cran.r-project.org. Accessed 15 Dec 2011

Riegelman RK (2005) Meta-analysis. In: Riegelman RK (ed) Studying a study & testing a test, 2005th edn. Lippincott Williams & Wilkins, Philadelphia, pp 99–115

S-plus.http://www.mathsoft.com/splus. Accessed 15 Dec 2011

SAS. http://www.prw.le.ac.uk/epidemiol/personal/ajs22/meta/macros.sas. Accessed 15 Dec 2011

Schmid CH, Stark PC, Berlin JA, Landais P, Lau J (2004) Meta-regression detected associations between heterogeneous treatment effects and study-level, but not patient-level, factors. J Clin Epidemiol 57:683–697

Shipley MJ, Pocock SJ, Marmot MG (1991) Does plasma cholesterol concentration predict mortality from coronary heart disease in elderly people? 18 year follow-up in Whitehall study. BMJ 303:89–92

SPSS Statistical Software. http://www.spss.com. Accessed 15 Dec 2011

Stampfer MJ, Goldhaber SZ, Yusuf S (1982) Effects of intravenous streptokinase on acute myocardial infarction: pooled results from randomized trials. N Engl J Med 307:1180–1182

Stata, statistical software for professionals. http://www.stat.com. Accessed 15 Dec 2011

StatsDirect. http://www.camcode.com. Accessed 15 Dec 2011

StatXact. http://www.cytel.com/products/statxact/statact1.html. Accessed 15 Dec 2011

Stein RA (1998) Meta-analysis from one FOA reviewer's perspective. Proceedings of the Biopharmaceutical Section of the American Statistical Association 2:34–38

Straus SE, Sackett DL (1998) Using research findings in clinical practice. BMJ 317:339–342

Tang JL, Liu JL (2000) Misleading funnel plots for detection of bias in meta-analysis. J Clin Epidemiol 53:477–484

Temple R (1999) Meta-analyses and epidemiological studies in drug development and postmarketing studies. JAMA 281:841–844

Terrin N, Schmid CH, Griffith JL, D'Agostino RB, Selker HP (2003) External validation of predictive models: a comparison of logistic regression, classification trees, and neural networks. J Clin Epidemiol 56:721–729

Thompson SG (1995) Why sources of heterogeneity should be investigated. In: Chalmers I, Altman DG (eds) Systematic reviews. BMJ Publishing Group, London, pp 48–63

True Epistat. http://ic.net/~biomware/biohp2te.htm. Accessed 15 Dec 2011

Turnbul F for the Blood Pressure Lowering Trialists' Collaboration (2003) Effects of different blood pressure lowering regimens on major cardiovascular events: results of prospectively designed overviews of randomised controlled trials. Lancet 362:1527–1535

Van Houwelingen HC, Arends LR, Stijnen T (2002) Advanced methods in meta-analysis: multivariate approach and meta-regression. Stat Med 21:589–624

Yusuf S, Peto R, Lewis J, Collins R, Sleight P (1985) Beta blockade during and after myocardial infarction: an overview of the randomized trials. Prog Cardiovasc Dis 27:335–371

Zhou X, Fang J, Yu C, Xu Z, Lu Y (2003) Meta-analysis. In: Lu Y, Fang J (eds) Advanced medical statistics. World Scientific, River Edge, pp 233–316

Chapter 34
Meta-regression

1 Introduction

The previous two chapters showed that pooling a meta-analysis of separate studies is pretty meaningless, if the results are significantly heterogeneous across studies. Instead, a careful investigation of the potential causes of heterogeneity has to be accomplished. Differences in age groups, co-morbidities, co-medications, gender differences and other characteristics are common causes. Subgroup comparisons are commonly applied for the purpose. However, in the past few years multiple regression analysis has been increasingly used as an alternative approach. The main study outcome is the dependent variable and the potential causes of heterogeneity are the independent variables. Advantages of this method include that the effects of multiple factors can be studied simultaneously, and that confounders and interacting-factors can be adjusted (see also the Chaps. 28 and 30). In the present chapter an example was used of a recently published meta-analysis from our group (Atiqi et al. 2009).

2 An Example of a Heterogeneous Meta-analysis

Table 34.1 shows the individual studies included in a meta-analysis of 20 studies on adverse drug admissions (ADEs) (Atiqi et al. 2009). The pooled result of the 20 studies as included in the meta-analysis provided an overall percentage of ADEs of 5.4% (5.0–5.8). However, the meaning of this pooled result was limited due to a significant heterogeneity between the individual studies: both the fixed effects and random effects tests for heterogeneity were highly significant (both $p < 0.001$, $I^2 > 90\%$, see also previous two chapters for explanation of the terms).

In order to explore the cause for this heterogeneity the studies of elderly were analyzed separately. The pooled percentages for the elderly (Table 34.2: studies 1–3, 6, 16, 17) was 4.8% (3.4–5.2) and for the studies on younger patients

T.J. Cleophas and A.H. Zwinderman, *Statistics Applied to Clinical Studies*,
DOI 10.1007/978-94-007-2863-9_34, © Springer Science+Business Media B.V. 2012

Table 34.1 Recent studies on patients admitted to hospital due to adverse drug effect

Study	Study size	Percentage of all admissions	95% confidence intervals
1. Mannesse et al. (2000)	106	21.0%	13.0–29.0%
2. Malhotra et al. (2001)	578	14.4%	11.5–17.3%
3. Chan et al. (2001)	240	30.4%	24.5–36.3%
4. Olivier et al. (2002)	671	6.1%	4.3–7.9%
5. Mjorndal et al. (2002)	681	12.0%	9.5–14.5%
6. Onder et al. (2002)	28,411	3.4%	3.2–3.6%
7. Koh et al. (2003)	347	6.6%	4.0–9.2%
8. Easton–Carter et al. (2003)	8,601	3.3%	2.9–3.7%
9. Dormann et al. (2003)	915	4.9%	4.9–14.3%
10. Peyriere et al. (2003)	156	9.6%	4.9–14.3%
11. Howard et al. (2004)	4,093	6.5%	5.7–7.3%
12. Pirmohamed et al. (2004)	18,820	6.5%	6.2–6.8%
13. Hardmeier et al. (2004)	6,383	4.1%	3.6–4.6%
14. Easton et al. (2004)	2,933	4.3%	3.6–5.0%
15. Capuano et al. (2004)	480	3.5%	1.9–5.1%
16. Caamano et al. (2005)	19,070	4.3%	3.7–4.6%
17. Yee et al. (2005)	2,169	12.6%	11.2–14.0%
18. Baena et al. (2006)	2,261	33.2%	31.2–35.2%
19. Leendertse et al. (2006)	12,793	5.6%	5.2–6.0%
20. Van der Hooft et al. (2008)	355	5.1%	2.8–7.4%
Pooled	113,203	5.4%	5.0–5.8%

Table 34.2 Data file for a meta-regression

Study no	% ADEs	Study magnitude	Clinicians' study yes = 1	Elderly study yes = 1
1	21.00	106.00	1.00	1.00
2	14.40	578.00	1.00	1.00
3	30.40	240.00	1.00	1.00
4	6.10	671.00	0.00	0.00
5	12.00	681.00	0.00	0.00
6	3.40	28,411.00	1.00	0.00
7	6.60	347.00	0.00	0.00
8	3.30	8,601.00	0.00	0.00
9	4.90	915.00	0.00	0.00
10	9.60	156.00	0.00	0.00
11	6.50	4,093.00	0.00	0.00
12	6.50	18,820.00	0.00	0.00
13	4.10	6,383.00	0.00	0.00
14	4.30	2,933.00	0.00	0.00
15	3.50	480.00	0.00	0.00
16	4.30	19,070.00	1.00	0.00
17	12.60	2,169.00	1.00	0.00
18	33.20	2,261.00	0.00	1.00
19	5.60	12,793.00	0.00	0.00
20	5.10	355.00	0.00	0.00

ADEs admissions due to adverse drug effects

Table 34.3 Assessment of studies for type of department

Study number
1. Dept Geriatrics, Erasmus University Hospital Rotterdam, Netherlands
2. Dept Internal Medicine, Chandigarh, India
3. Dept Medicine, Hobart General Hospital, Hobart, Australia
4. Dept Clinical Pharmacology, Umea University Hospital, Sweden,
5. Center Gerontology and health Care Research Brown University Providence, USA
6. Non-communicable Disease Epidemiology Unit London School of Hygiene
7. Department of Pharmacy National University of Singapore, Singapore
8. Faculty of Pharmacy University of Sydney, Australia
9. Dept Experimental and Clinical Pharmacology and Toxicology, University Erlangen
10. Lab Clinical Pharmacy University Montpellier France
11. School of Community Health Sciences, University Nottingham, UK
12. Dept Pharmacology University of Liverpool UK
13. Dept Clinical Pharmacy University Zurich Switzerland
14. Faculty of Pharmacy University of Sydney, Australia
15. Centre for Pharmacoepidemics and Pharmacosurveillance, Second University of Naples
16. Dept Epidemiology and Public Health Santiago de Compostella University, Spain
17. Clinical Pharmacist, Drug Information, Blue Shield of California, San Francisco
18. Emergency department, University Hospital, Granada, Spain
19. Department of Pharmacoepidemiology University Utrecht, Netherlands
20. Pharmacoepidemiology Unit Erasmus University Rotterdam, Netherlands

(remainder of studies) 3.5% (95% confidence interval 3.1–3.9). Although the percentage ADEs in elderly patients tended to be larger than that in the younger ($0.05 < p < 0.1$), the overall percentage of 5.4% was not significantly smaller than the percentage of ADEs in the elderly, which suggests that age was not an important cause for heterogeneity in these studies.

We also assessed the studies for type-of-research-group. Because medical articles are often co-authored by specialists from different disciplines and/or guest-authors, we decided to name the type-of-research-group after the type of department of the first two authors. Table 34.3 shows that in the studies performed by clinicians (studies 1, 2, 3, and 18) the percentages ADEs were much higher (pooled data 29.2%, 26.4–32.0) than those of the other studies (pooled data 4.8%, 4.1–5.5). A careful further examination of these data revealed that the difference between the type of research groups was associated with a significant difference in magnitude of the studies: the four clinicians' studies had a mean sample size of 796 (740–852), while the remainder of the studies averaged at 6,680 (6,516–6,844) patients per study, different at $p < 0.001$. This effect was ascribed to the presence of publication bias in this meta-analysis (small studies with small results were under-published).

In order to simultaneously assess the effects of study-magnitude, patients' age, and type-of- research-group a multiple linear regression was, subsequently, performed (Table 34.4). After adjustment for patients' age and type-of-research-group the study-magnitude was no significant predictor of study effect anymore. In contrast, the type-of-research-group was the single and highly significant predictor of study result.

Table 34.4 SPSS (www.spss.com) multiple linear meta-regression table with study result (percentage ADEs) as dependent variable and study-magnitude, patients' age, and type-of-research-group as independent variables

Covariate	Unstandardized coefficients		Standardized coefficients		
	B	Std error	Beta	t	sig.
Constant	6.92	1.45		4.76	0.000
Study magnitude	−7.7.e-0.05	0.00	−0.071	−0.50	0.62
Patients' age	−1.39	2.89	−0.075	−0.48	0.64
Type research group	18.93	3.36	0.89	5.64	0.000

After adjustment for patients' age and type-of-research-group the study-magnitude is no significant predictor of study effect anymore. In contrast, the type-of-research-group is the single highly-significant predictor of the study result
Dependent variable: study result
std error standard error, *t* t-value, *sig.* level of significance

3   Discussion

An important hypothesis of the above example study was, that the real burden of ADEs in present health care may be best assessed by clinicians who have to make a diagnosis and are, subsequently, in charge for starting a treatment. Indeed, the studies performed by clinicians produced much larger percentages of ADE admissions. This effect was accompanied by the finding that the clinicians' studies were significantly smaller than the remainder of the studies. According to the meta-regression the larger percentages ADEs in the clinicians' studies could not be explained by the magnitude of the studies: the type-of-research-group remained the single highly significant predictor of study results after adjustment for difference in study-magnitudes. And, so, the type of study group could be held largely responsible for the clinical heterogeneity observed. Meta-regression can be considered as an extension to subgroup analyses, and in principle allows the effects of multiple factors to be investigated simultaneously. We should add that mostly the numbers of studies are small and, therefore, do not allow for inclusion of more than 2 or 3 variables. Like with usual testing meta-analysis for heterogeneity, both a fixed effects and a random effects meta-regression is possible. The Stata software program offers it in "metareg macro" (Meta-regression 2011). Limitations of meta-regressions have to be mentioned. They include problems associated with looking at irrelevant characteristics of participants, power loss associated with the inclusion of multiple variables, increased risks of type I errors due to multiple testing, little availability of software to date (Stanley and Jarrell 1989; Higgins and Beyene 2011).

Due to the omnipresent computer the use of arithmetically increasingly complex methods has expanded tremendously. The field of statistics has now great difficulty with finding adequate names for its novel methods. Often a name represents various methods like, e.g. the term "mixed model" is used both for mixed effects models (Chap. 56) and mixed linear models (Chap. 55), although the two methods are entirely different. A similar phenomenon is observed with the term "meta-regression".

Table 34.5 Meta-analysis of regression analyses is different from regression analysis of a meta-analysis: an example of the former

Study no.	B	SE	n	dfs	t	p
1	1.5	0.8	20	19	1.875	0.076
2	1.7	0.9	20	19	1.888	0.074
3	1.9	1.0	20	19	1.900	0.073
Pooled result	5.1	1.6	60	57	3.259	0.002

Pooled t-value is calculated according to $(B_1 + B_2 + B_3)/\sqrt{(SE_1^2 + SE_2^2 + SE_3^2)}$

B regression coefficient, SE standard error, n sample size, t t-value, p p-value

Although usually applied to name the regression of a meta-analysis, it is currently also sometimes used to name the meta-analysis of regression analyses. Like with meta-analysis of means of studies, the main results of regression analyses may be pooled in order to improve the power of testing. In Table 34.5 an example is given. The B-value behaves like a mean value and can be considered to follow a t-distribution. Pooling can be performed as explained in Chap. 32, Sect. 6. If the magnitudes of the standard deviations or the B-values are very different across studies a more adequate calculation of the t-values should be performed (Chap. 32, Sect. 6). It can be observed in the Table 34.5 that, indeed, the pooled result of the three regression studies produced a much better t- and p-value than did the separate studies.

4 Conclusions

In the past few years multiple regression analysis has been increasingly used as an approach alternative to subgroup analysis to assess heterogeneity in meta-analyses. This chapter was written to explain how it works. In a real data example of a published heterogenous meta-analysis of 20 studies on adverse drug effect admissions (ADEs) the main study outcome was the dependent variable and the potential causes of heterogeneity were the independent variables.

The following observations were made.

1. A difference in age and difference in type of research group was largely held responsible for the heterogeneity observed, $0.05 < p < 0.10$ and $p < 0.0001$.
2. It was also observed that the magnitudes of the clinicians' studies were much smaller than those of the rest, $p < 0.001$, and it could, therefore, not be excluded that the type of study group rather than the study magnitude was responsible for the heterogeneity.
3. Multiple linear regression with numbers of ADEs as outcome and age, type of study group, and magnitude of study as exposure variable showed, indeed, that the larger percentages ADEs in the clinicians' studies could not be explained by the magnitude of the studies: the type-of-research-group remained the single highly significant predictor of study results after adjustment for difference in study-magnitudes, $p < 0.0001$.

We conclude that the advantages of meta-regression compared to simple subgroups comparisons for the assessment of heterogeneity include that (1) the effects of multiple factors can be studied simultaneously, and that (2) confounders and interacting-factors can be adjusted. The most important variable responsible for the heterogeneity can be readily identified. Problems, of course, include the increased risks of type I errors and power loss with small meta-analyses.

References

Atiqi R, Cleophas TJ, Van Bommel E, Zwinderman AH (2009) Meta-analysis of recent studies on patients admitted to hospital due to adverse drug effects. Int J Clin Pharmacol Ther 47:549–556

Higgins J, Beyene J. An introduction to meta-regression. www.cochrane.org/colloquia. Accessed 15 Dec 2011

Meta-regression. www.mrc.bsu.cam.ac.uk/cochrane/handbook/chapter_9/9_6_4_meta_regression. Accessed 15 Dec 2011

Stanley TD, Jarrell SB (1989) Meta-regression analysis: a quantitative method of literature surveys. J Econ Surv 3:161–170

Chapter 35
Crossover Studies with Continuous Variables

1 Introduction

Crossover studies with continuous variables are routinely used in clinical drug research: for example, no less than 22% of the double-blind placebo-controlled hypertension trials in 1993 were accordingly designed (Niemeyer et al. 1998). A major advantage of the crossover design is that it eliminates between-subject variability of symptoms. However, problems include the occurrence of carryover effect, sometimes called treatment-by-period interaction (see also Chap. 30): if the effect of the first period carries on into the next one, then it may influence the response to the latter period. Second, the possibility of time effects due to external factors such as the change of the seasons has to be taken into account in lengthy crossover studies. Third, negative correlations between drug responses, although recently recognized in clinical pharmacology, is an important possibility not considered in the design and analysis of clinical trials so far. Many crossover studies may have a positive correlation-between-drug-response, not only because treatments in a given comparison are frequently from the same class of drugs, but also because one subject is used for comparisons of two treatments. Still, in treatment comparisons of completely different treatments patients may fall into different populations, those who respond better to the test-treatment and those who do so to the reference-treatment. This phenomenon has already lead to treatment protocols based on individualized rather than stepped care (Scheffé 1959). Power analyses for crossover studies with continuous variables so far only accounted for the possibility of approximately zero levels of correlations (Cleophas 1993; Willan and Pater 1986; Freeman 1989; Fleiss 1989; Senn 1994; Grieve 1994). While considering different levels of correlation, we recently demonstrated (Cleophas and Van Lier 1996) that the crossover design with binary variables is a powerful means of determining the efficacy of new drugs in spite of such factors as carryover effects. Crossover trials with continuous variables, however, have not yet been similarly studied.

T.J. Cleophas and A.H. Zwinderman, *Statistics Applied to Clinical Studies*,
DOI 10.1007/978-94-007-2863-9_35, © Springer Science+Business Media B.V. 2012

In the current chapter while taking both positive and negative correlations into account we drew power curves of hypothesized crossover studies with different amounts of treatment effect, carryover effect and time effect.

2   Mathematical Model

According to Scheffé (Nies and Spielberg 1996) the notion for a simple two-period two-group crossover study is

	Period 1		Period 2	
Group	Treatment	Mean effect	Treatment	Mean effect
1 (n_1)	1	$y_{1.1}$	2	$y_{1.2}$
2 (n_2)	2	$y_{2.1}$	1	$y_{2.2}$

where y_{ijk} = the response in the jth patient in the ith group in the kth period. We assume that $n_1 = n_2 = n$ and that we have normal distributions or t-distributions. $y_{i.k} = \sum y_{ijk}/n$.

Treatment, carryover and time effects are assessed according to Grizzle (1965). To test treatment effect φ the sum of the results of treatment 1 is compared with the treatment 2 results ($y_{1.1} + y_{2.2}$ versus $y_{1.2} + y_{2.1}$). To trace carryover effect (λ) the sum of the results in group 1 is compared with the group 2 results ($y_{1.1} + y_{1.2}$ versus $y_{2.1} + y_{2.2}$). To trace time effect (π) the sum of the results in period 1 is compared with the period 2 results ($y_{1.1} + y_{2.1}$ versus $y_{1.2} + y_{2.2}$).

The null-hypotheses that φ, λ, and π are zero

$$\varphi\left[\left(y_{1.1} + y_{2.2}\right) - \left(y_{1.2} + y_{2.1}\right)\right] = 0$$

$$\lambda\left[\left(y_{2.1} + y_{2.2}\right) - \left(y_{1.1} + y_{1.2}\right)\right] = 0$$

$$\pi\left[\left(y_{1.1} + y_{2.1}\right) - \left(y_{1.2} + y_{2.2}\right)\right] = 0$$

should be slightly remodeled into paired comparisons, because otherwise calculations cannot be appropriately accomplished.

$$\varphi\left[\left(y_{1.1} - y_{1.2}\right) - \left(y_{2.1} - y_{2.2}\right)\right] = 0$$

$$\lambda\left[\left(y_{2.1} + y_{2.2}\right) - \left(y_{1.1} + y_{1.2}\right)\right] = 0$$

$$\pi\left[\left(y_{1.1} - y_{1.2}\right) + \left(y_{2.1} - y_{2.2}\right)\right] = 0$$

In this way 2×2 paired cells can be adequately added or subtracted in a cell by cell manner.

3 Hypothesis Testing

These null hypotheses can be tested, for example, by paired t-statistic or repeated measures analysis of variance (ANOVA). The larger the extent to which the t or F value of our distribution differs from zero, the more sensitivity the statistical approach does provide.

$$t = \frac{d}{SE}\left(\text{or repeated measures ANOVA, F value}\right)$$

where d is φ, λ, or π, and SE is their standard error.

SE is calculated by use of the standard formulas for the variance ($\sqrt{\sigma^2/n}$) of paired and unpaired sums and differences.

$$\sigma^2_{\text{paired sums}} = \sigma_1^2 + \sigma_2^2 + 2\rho\sigma_1\sigma_2$$

$$\sigma^2_{\text{paired differences}} = \sigma_1^2 + \sigma_2^2 - 2\rho\sigma_1\sigma_2$$

$$\sigma^2_{\text{unpaired sums}} = \sigma_1^2 + \sigma_2^2$$

$$\sigma^2_{\text{unpaired differences}} = \sigma_1^2 + \sigma_2^2$$

If we assume that $\sigma = \sigma_{Y1.1} = \sigma_{Y1.2} = \sigma_{Y2.1} = \sigma_{Y2.2} =$ standard deviation of the samples in each of the cells, and that $\rho = \rho_{Y1.1 \text{ vs } Y1.2} = \rho_{Y2.1 \text{ vs } Y2.2} =$ correlation coefficient between the samples of each of the two paired cells, then

$$\sigma_\varphi^2 = 2\left(2\sigma^2\right)\left(1 - \rho\right)$$

$$\sigma_\lambda^2 = 2\left(2\sigma^2\right)\left(1 + \rho\right)$$

$$\sigma_\pi^2 = 2\left(2\sigma^2\right)\left(1 - \rho\right)$$

Because $n_1 = n_2 = n$, we now can calculate the SEs as follows:

$$SE_\varphi = \sqrt{4\sigma^2(1-p)\left(\frac{1}{2n} + \frac{1}{2n}\right)} = \sqrt{\frac{4\sigma^2(1-p)}{n}}$$

and accordingly

$$SE_\lambda = \sqrt{\frac{4\sigma^2(1+p)}{n}}$$

$$SE_\pi = \sqrt{\frac{4\sigma^2(1-p)}{n}}$$

Suppose $\lambda = \varphi$ and $\rho = 0$, then $t_\lambda = t_\varphi$. In this situation the sensitivity to test carry-over and treatment effect are equal.

$$\text{If } \lambda = \varphi \text{ and } \rho > 0 \quad \text{then } t_\lambda < t_\varphi$$
$$\text{If } \lambda = \varphi \text{ and } \rho < 0 \quad \text{then } t_\lambda > t_\varphi$$

So, the sensitivity of testing is largely dependent on the correlation between treatment modalities ρ. Whenever $\rho > 0$ we soon will have a much larger t-value, and, thus, better sensitivity to test treatment effect than carryover effect of similar size. We should add that in practice $\sigma_{Y1.2}$ may be somewhat larger than $\sigma_{Y1.1}$, because the larger the data the larger the variances. If, e.g., $\sigma_{Y1.2}$ is 10% larger than $\sigma_{Y1.1}$, ρ will change from 0.00 to 0.05. So, in this situation the level of positive correlation required tends to rise.

Time effect (π) is generally considered to influence one treatment similarly to the other, and its influence on the size of the treatment difference is, thus, negligible.

	Period 1		Period 2	
Group	Treatment	Mean response	Treatment	Mean response
1	1	$y_{1.1}$	2	$y_{1.2} + \tfrac{1}{2}\pi$
2	2	$y_{2.1}$	1	$y_{2.2} + \tfrac{1}{2}\pi$

Under the assumption $\varphi = 0$ we have

$$\varphi = (y_{1.1} - y_{1.2} - \tfrac{1}{2}\pi) - (y_{2.1} - y_{2.2} - \tfrac{1}{2}\pi)$$
$$= y_{1.1} - y_{1.2} - y_{2.1} + y_{2.2}$$

Although time or period effects may introduce extra variance in the study, the crossover design in a way adjusts for time effects, and some even believe that time effects do not have to be taken into account in the routine analysis of crossover studies, unless there is a clinical interest to know (Senn 1994).

4   Statistical Power of Testing

Figure 35.1 gives an example of a t-distribution (H_1) and its null hypothesis of no effect (H_0). $\alpha = \%$ chance of erroneously rejecting this null hypothesis (usually taken as 5%), and $\beta = \%$ chance of erroneously accepting this null hypothesis. Statistical power is defined as $(1 - \beta) \times 100\%$. Statistical power can be approximated from the equation (prob = probability):

$$\text{POWER} = 1 - \beta = 1 - \text{prob}\left[Z \leq \left(t - t^1 \right) \right]$$

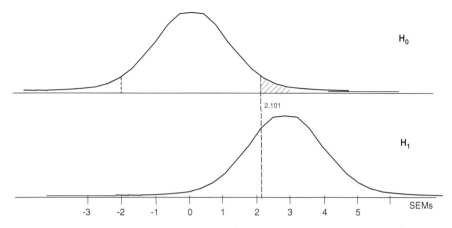

Fig. 35.1 Example of a t-distribution (H_1) and its null hypothesis (H_0) α % chance of erroneously rejecting this null hypothesis (usually taken as 5%), β % chance of erroneously accepting this null hypothesis. Statistical power is defined as $(1-\beta) \times 100\%$

where Z represents the standardized value for the differences between mean and zero and t^1 represents the upper critical value of t for the given degrees of freedom and α has been specified ($\alpha = 0.05$).

Suppose we have a crossover study with $n = 10$ per group, because this is a size frequently used in such studies, and with $\varphi = \sigma =$ standard deviation of the samples in each cell, because this is frequently approximately so. Then increasing amounts of λ are added with $\sigma_\lambda = \lambda$. The influence of this procedure on the statistical power of testing λ and φ are then assessed. The amounts of λ are expressed as λ/φ ratios. Power graphs are calculated for three different levels of correlation-between-drug-response ($\rho \cong -1$; $\rho \cong 0$; $\rho \cong +1$).

Figure 35.2 shows the results. First, there are three power curves of treatment effect for the three levels of correlation. As λ/φ increases, all three gradually come down. The negative correlation curve is the first to do so. Consequently, this situation has generally little power of rightly coming to the right conclusion. At $\lambda/\varphi = 1.0$, when treatment effect is equal to carryover effect, there is less than 30% power left. It means we have a more than 70% chance that treatment effect is erroneously unobserved in this study. Considering that a power of approximately 80% is required for reliable testing, we cannot test carryover here in a sensitive manner. The zero and positive correlation situations provide essentially better power.

There are also three power curves of carryover effect for three correlation levels. The negative correlation curve provides essentially better power than the zero and positive correlation curves do. This example shows that strong positive correlations leave little power to test carryover effect. It also shows that strong negative correlations produce excessive power to test carryover effect.

Fig. 35.2 Statistical power
of testing carryover effect
(*slope upwards*) and
treatment effect (*slope
downwards*); λ carryover
effect, φ treatment effect, ρ
correlation coefficient
(_____ ρ≅−1;
_ _ _ _ _ _ _ _   ρ≅0;
------------------------- ρ≅+1)

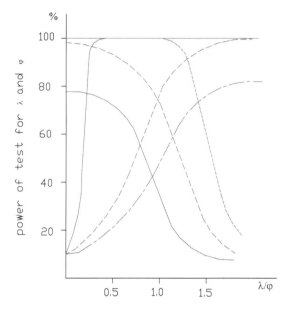

Fig. 35.3 Statistical power
of testing time effect (*slope
upwards*) and treatment effect
(*slope downwards*) π time
effect, φ treatment effect, ρ
correlation coefficient
(_____ ρ≅−1;
_ _ _ _ _ _ _ _   ρ≅0;
------------------------- ρ≅+1)

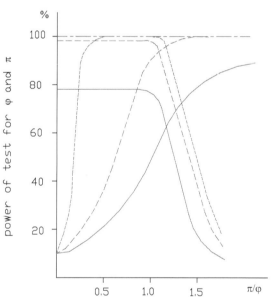

The amounts of time effect are generally assumed to influence the two treatment
groups similarly, and it, therefore, may hardly influence the treat comparison.
Suppose in the above example time effect (π) instead of carryover effect (λ) is added
in increasing amounts with $\sigma_\pi = \pi$.

Figure 35.3 shows the influence of increasing ratios π/φ on the statistical power
of testing π and φ. First, small time effects unlike carryover effects hardly influence

nor the amount nor the statistical power of testing treatment effect. Also the power of demonstrating time effect is largely dependent on the level of correlation-between-drug-response: with a negative correlation we have little power to demonstrate time-effect. In contrast, with a positive correlation we have a lot of power to do so.

We conclude that the level of correlation-between-drug-response is a major determinant of not only the power of demonstrating treatment effect but also that of time effect in the current approach.

5 Discussion

The crossover design for treatment comparisons with continuous variables provides approximately equal statistical power to test carryover, time, and treatment effects when between-treatment correlation is not strong positive/negative. For example, in the hypothesized crossover situation from our example the statistical power to demonstrate similarly-sized treatment and carryover, or treatment and time effects is approximately 80% (as demonstrated in the above figures), which is generally considered to be an acceptable level for reliable testing. However, whenever the correlation coefficient is >0, we will soon have better sensitivity to test treatment than carryover or time effect of similar size. Inversely, whenever it is <0, we will soon have better sensitivity to demonstrate the latter two rather than the former.

We should add that calculations are made under the assumption that either carryover or time effect are in the study. If both effects are simultaneously in the study, variances have to be added up and powers will be somewhat smaller. The assumption does not invalidate the overall conclusion of the procedure as it produces the largest powers for the given data.

5.1 Analysis of Covariance (ANCOVA)

Analysis of covariance is used if two x-variables are dependent on one another.

When F-tests are used instead of t-tests, the sensitivity of testing can be somewhat improved by analysis of covariance (ANCOVA) according to

adjusted $SS_{treatment}$ between groups =
unadjusted $SS_{treatment}$ between groups +
$(SP$ within groups$)^2/SS_{carryover}$ within groups −
$(SP$ total$)^2/SS_{carryover}$ total

adjusted SS within groups = unadjusted SS within groups −
$(SP$ within groups$)^2/SS_{carryover}$ within groups

where SS = sum of squares, and SP = sum of products of
treatment by carryover effects
(treatment effect × carryover effect).

Computation can be found, e.g., in Hays' textbook Statistics (SPSS for Windows 2011), and can be readily made by statistical packages, e.g., SPSS (Hays 1988) under the subprogram "ANOVA".

In this way, power of testing may improve by a few percentages. However, this method of adjustment can be used only when correlations are not strong + or −, and when n is at least 20 or more, which is not so in many crossover studies. Also the method only adjusts statistical sensitivity, but not amounts of treatment, carryover or time effects, and so its usefulness is limited.

Although the analysis uses multiple comparisons testing, the p-values do not have to be multiplied by the number of tests, because although the chance of a positive test increases, the chance of e.g., a positive test for carryover does not as it is only tested once.

The current chapter stresses the major impact of correlation level between treatment comparison, and particularly the phenomenon of negative correlations. This phenomenon is only shortly being recognized and may have flawed many trials so far. In a trial the test treatment is frequently a slight modification of the reference treatment or is equivalent to it with addition of just a new component. In this situation there is obviously a positive correlation between responses to test and reference treatments. However, completely new classes of drugs are continually being developed and are tested against established classes of drugs. With the comparison of drugs from completely different classes patients may fall into different populations: those who respond better to one class and those who do so to the other class. For example, patients with angina pectoris unresponsive to calcium channel blockers or nitrates may respond very well to beta blockers. Also hypertension, cardiac arrhythmias, chronic obstructive pulmonary disease are conditions where a non-response is frequently associated with an excellent response to a completely different compound. These are situations where a crossover study may give rise to a strong negative correlation. It would mean that a crossover design for the comparisons of treatment from completely different classes of drugs is endangered of being flawed and that such comparisons had better be assessed in the form of a parallel group comparison which evens out within subject variability.

6   Conclusion

Background: The crossover design is a sensitive means of determining the efficacy of new drugs because it eliminates between subject-variability. However, when the response in the first period carries on into the second (carryover effects) or when time factors can not be kept constant in a lengthy crossover (time effects), the statistical power of testing may be jeopardized. We recently demonstrated that the crossover design with binary variables is a powerful method in spite of such factors as carryover effects (Cleophas and Van Lier 1996). Power analysis of crossover trials with continuous variables has not been widely published.

Objective: Using the Grizzle model for the assessment of treatment effect, carryover effect and time effect, we drew power curves of hypothesized crossover studies with different levels of correlation between drug responses.

Results: We demonstrate that the sensitivity of testing is largely dependent on the levels of correlation between drug response. Whenever the correlation coefficient is >0, we soon will have better sensitivity to test treatment effect than carryover effect or time effect of similar size. Whenever levels of correlation are not strong positive or negative the statistical power to demonstrate similarly-sized treatment and carryover effect, or treatment and time effect is approximately 80%, which is an acceptable level for reliable testing.

Conclusions: The crossover design is a powerful method for assessing positively correlated treatment comparisons, despite the risk of carryover and time effects.

References

Cleophas TJ (1993) Crossover studies: a modified analysis with more power. Clin Pharmacol Ther 53:515–520

Cleophas TJ, Van Lier HH (1996) Clinical trials with binary responses: power analyses. J Clin Pharmacol 36:198–204

Fleiss JA (1989) A critique of recent research on the two-treatment crossover design. Control Clin Trials 10:237–241

Freeman PR (1989) The performance of the two-stage analysis of two-treatment, two-period cross-over trials. Stat Med 8:1421–1432

Grieve AP (1994) Bayesian analyses of two-treatment crossover studies. Stat Methods Med Res 3:407–429

Grizzle JE (1965) The two-period change-over design and its use in clinical trials. Biometrics 22:469–480

Hays WL (1988) Statistics, 4th edn. Holt, Rinehart and Winston, Inc, Fort Worth

Niemeyer MG, Zwinderman AH, Cleophas TJ, De Vogel EM (1998) Crossover studies are a better format for comparing equivalent treatments than parallel-group studies. In: Kuhlmann J, Mrozikiewicz A (eds) What should a clinical pharmacologist know to start a clinical trial (phase I and II). Zuckschwerdt Verlag, Munich, pp 40–48

Nies AS, Spielberg SP (1996) Individualization of drug therapy. In: Hardman JL et al (eds) Goodman and Gilman's pharmacological basis of therapeutics. McGraw-Hill, New York, pp 43–63

Scheffé H (1959) Mixed models. In: Scheffé H (ed) The analysis of variance. Wiley, New York, pp 261–291

Senn S (1994) The AB/BA crossover: past, present and future. Stat Methods Med Res 3:303–324

SPSS for Windows. www.SPSS.com. Accessed 15 Dec 2011

Willan AR, Pater JL (1986) Carryover and the two-period crossover clinical trial. Biometrics 42:593–599

Chapter 36
Crossover Studies with Binary Responses

1 Introduction

The crossover design is widely used in clinical research especially in the case of a limited number of patients. The main advantage of within-patient over between-patient comparisons is that between-subject variability is not used in the comparisons. However, a prerequisite is that the order of the treatments does not influence the outcome of the treatment. If the effect of the treatment administered in the first period carries on into the second period, then it may influence the measured response in the second period. This essentially means that only symptomatic treatments qualify for crossover comparisons and curative treatments do not. However, symptomatic treatments frequently have small curative effects, e.g., wound healing by vasodilators or, more recently, cardiac remodelling by after load reduction. The treatment group that is treated with the effective compound first and with the less effective compound or placebo second is frequently biased by carryover effect from the first period into the second, whereas the alternative group that is treated in the reverse order is not so (Cleophas 1995). For example, of 73 recently published crossovers only six reported the data of the separate periods. In five of them (83%) this very type of carryover effect was demonstrable. Such a mechanism may cause a severe underestimation of the treatment results (Cleophas 1990) and this possibility should, therefore, be assessed in the analysis. Most of the reports on the subject of order effects so far have addressed crossover studies with a quantitative rather than binary response (Brown 1980; Barker et al. 1982; Louis et al. 1984; Willan and Pater 1986; Packer 1989; Fleiss 1989; Freeman 1989; Senn 1993). Although Hills and Armitage (and 1979) in an overview of methods in crossover clinical trials mentioned the tests of Gart (1969) and Prescott (1981) for crossover trials with a binary response and Fidler (1984) presented a model, little attention has been paid to this kind of trials. A binary response is different from a quantitative in that it generally does not answer what exactly can be expected in an individual. Rather it addresses whether or not a particular result has a predictive value, which one of two treatments is better, or whether there is a treatment effect in the data. One might contend, therefore, that some undervaluation of a difference in binary data is not that important as long as it does not cause a type II error of finding no difference were there is one. The main issue of the present chapter is the question whether in a crossover trial with a binary response a significant carryover effect does leave enough power in the data to demonstrate a treatment effect.

2   Assessment of Carryover and Treatment Effect

In a crossover trial with two treatments and two periods the patients are randomized into two symmetric groups that are treated with treatments A and B in a different order (Table 36.1). If groups are symmetric and the results are not influenced by the order of the treatments, the probabilities of treatment success in group I and II should be virtually the same in each period for each treatment: p_A being the probability of treatment success from treatment A, p_B from treatment B (Table 36.1).

The group that is treated with the less effective treatment or placebo after the more effective is endangered of being biased by carryover effect from the first period into the second.

Suppose treatment A is far less effective than B (Table 36.1). Then, if in Group II treatment B has a carryover effect on the outcome of treatment A, the probability of treatment success changes from p_B into p_C. To detect a carryover effect we compare the outcomes of treatment A in Group I to those in group II: p_A versus p_C, an unpaired comparison. The amount of carryover effect in group II is considered to be the difference between p_C and p_A. Carryover effect in Group I (ineffective treatment period prior to effective) is assumed to be negligible. Time effect is assumed to be negligible as well, because we study stable disease only. It thus seems that neither a test for carryover effect in Group I, nor a test for time effects needs to be included in our assessment. Treatment effect is assessed by taking the two groups together after which all of the outcomes of the treatments A are compared with those of the treatments B in a paired comparison. The assumption that carryover effect is negligible implies that the test for carryover effect uses only half of the available data and might therefore be expected to be less sensitive. However, sensitivity not only depends on sample size but also on the size of differences and their variances.

Table 36.1 Example of a crossover design with a binary response

	Period I		Period II	
		Probability of		Probability of
Group	Treatment	treatment success	Treatment	treatment success
I	p_A		B	p_B
II	p_B		A	$p_A{}^a$

[a]If in Group II treatment B has a carryover effect on the outcome of treatment A, p_A changes to p_C. If $P_B = p_C$, carryover effect is maximal

3 Statistical Model for Testing Treatment and Carryover Effects

We assume an unidirectional assessment where p is between 0.0 (no symptoms anymore) and 1.0 (=100% remains symptomatic in spite of treatment). When carryover effect is in the data, p_A in Group II turns into p_C (Table 36.1). The difference between p_C and p_A is considered to be the amount of carryover effect in the data. Fisher exact test, as explained in Chap. 3, is used for testing whether p_C is significantly different from p_A. With the program of Bavry (1988) those values of p_C are determined that should yield a significant carryover effect in 80% of the trials (i.e. the power equals 80%). The number of patients in both groups is chosen between 10 and 25, because many crossover trials have 20–50 patients. These values of p_C are then used for determining whether in crossover trials with significant carryover effect and a binary response enough power is left in the data for demonstrating a significant treatment effect.

For testing the treatment effect all of the data of the treatment A are taken together and compared with those of the treatments B. The power of this test depends not only on the probabilities p_A and p_B, but also on the correlation between the treatment responses. This correlation is expressed as $\rho = p_{A/B} - p_A$, where $p_{A/B}$ is the probability of a treatment success with A, given that treatment B was successful. When $\rho = 0$, treatments A and B act independently. When p_B equals p_C, this would mean that carryover effect in group II is not only significant but also maximal given the amount of treatment effect. Considering this situation of maximal carryover effect, we calculate the power of detecting treatment effects. The power of McNemar's test with p_B being equal to p_C and with various values of p_A was calculated according to Bavry (1988) .

4 Results

4.1 Calculation of p_C Values Just Yielding a Significant Test for Carryover Effect

For various numbers of patients and various values of p_{Ac} (the probability of success with treatment A in period I, Table 36.1), the p_C values (the probability of success with treatment A in period II) are calculated that with a power of 80% will give a significant test for carryover effect (p_A versus p_C, $\alpha = 0.05$).

Table 36.2 shows that carryover effects (difference between p_A and p_C) as large as 0.60, 0.50, 0.40 and 0.35 are required for a significant test. For $\alpha = 0.01$, these values are about 0.70, 0.60, 0.50 and 0.45. Using these p_C values, we then calculated the probability of detecting a treatment effect (i.e. power of testing treatment effect). We report minimal values of power only, i.e., the situation where $p_B = p_C$. Whenever $p_B < p_C$, we would have even better power of testing treatment effect.

Table 36.2 Power to demonstrate a treatment effect in spite of the presence of a significant carryover effect

| p_A | Total number of patients | | | |
	2×10	2×15	2×20	2×25
0.10				
0.20				
0.30				98 (0.02)
0.40		96 (0.02)	97 (0.05)	96 (0.08)
0.50		97 (0.06)	96 (0.11)	96 (0.14)
0.60	97[a] (0.04)[b]	98 (0.11)	96 (0.18)	95 (0.23)
0.70	96 (0.11)	97 (0.20)	97 (0.26)	94 (0.33)
0.80	96 (0.20)	97 (0.30)	97 (0.37)	96 (0.43)
0.90	96 (0.31)	97 (0.43)	96 (0.47)	96 (0.52)

[a] Power (%) of McNemar's test for treatment effect ($\alpha=0.05$, $\rho=0$)
[b] p_C value just yielding a significant test for carryover effect ($\alpha=0.05$, power$=80\%$)

4.2   Power of Paired Comparison for Treatment Effect

When the result of treatment B (p_B) is taken equal to the maximal values of p_C and treatments A and B act independently ($\rho=0$), the probability of detecting a treatment effect (i.e. the power) in the crossover situation with n between 20 and 50 is always more than 94% (Table 36.2). Usually, however, treatments A and B do not act independently. With a negative correlation between the two treatments modalities power is lost, with a positive correlation it is augmented. Table 36.3 shows power values adjusted for different levels of ρ. With negative levels of ρ and 20 patients the power for detecting a treatment difference is not less than 74% which is about as large as that chosen for the test on carryover effect (80%). When more patients are admitted to the trial this value will be about 90%.

5   Examples

Suppose we have a negative crossover where probability of treatment success group II p_C (Table 36.4) may have changed from 0.8 into 0.2 due to carryover effect from the effective treatment B into the second period. Fisher exact test for demonstrating a carryover effect (p_A versus p_C) is calculated according to

$$\text{Point probability for carryover effect} = \frac{10!\,10!\,10!\,10!}{20!\,2!\,8!\,2!\,8!} = 0.011$$

Cumulative tail probability $= 0.011 + 0.003 + 0.007 = 0.021$ and is thus significant at an $\alpha=0.021$ level.

Table 36.3 Power (%) to demonstrate a treatment effect in spite of the presence of a significant carryover effect

	ρ	Total number of patients			
		2×10	2×15	2×20	2×25
$\alpha_1{}^a=0.05$	−0.20	89	94	96	95
$\alpha_2=0.05$	−0.10	92	96	97	97
	0	96	96	96	94
	0.10	98	97	98	99
	0.20	98	98	99	99
$\alpha_1=0.01$	−0.20	95	99	94	99
$\alpha_2=0.01$	−0.10	97	100	99	99
	0	99	99	99	99
	0.10	100	100	100	100
	0.20	100	100	100	100
$\alpha_1=0.10$	−0.20	74	84	89	88
$\alpha_2=0.05$	−0.10	79	91	92	90
	0	85	90	89	88
	0.10	89	95	95	94
	0.20	95	94	97	97
$\alpha_1=0.05$	−0.20	75	87	90	90
$\alpha_2=0.01$	−0.10	81	92	92	93
	0	88	90	90	89
	0.10	92	93	95	96
	0.20	96	96	98	98

[a] α_1 level of significance of test for carryover effect
α_2 level of significance of test for treatment effect
ρ level of correlation between treatments A and B

Table 36.4 Example

	Period I		Period II	
Group	Treatment	Probability of treatment success	Treatment	Probability of treatment success
I (n=10)	A	$p_A=0.8$	B	$p_B=0.2$
II (n=10)	B	$p_B=0.2$	A	$p_C=0.2$

If we perform a similar unpaired analysis of the first period for demonstrating a treatment effect we likewise obtain a significant test at $\alpha=0.021$ level. Suppose carryover effect would be smaller, e.g., $p_A=0.8$, $p_B=0.0$, $p_C=0.2$. Then the test for treatment effect would yield an even better result:

$$\text{Point probability for carryover effect} = \frac{29!\,8!\,10!\,10!}{20!\,2!\,8!\,10!\,0!} = 0.004$$

Cumulative tail probability $= 0.004 + 0.001 + 0.003 = 0.008$.

So, in crossovers with a binary response and a negative result, it does make sense to test for carryover effect by comparing the two periods with the less effective treatment modalities. If a significant test is demonstrated, we obviously will find a significant difference at a similar or even lower level of significance when taking the first period for estimating the difference between treatment A and B. Thus, it would seem appropriate for our purpose to disregard the data of the second period in this particular situation (although the second period might still provide interesting information).

6   Discussion

The power of crossover studies is frequently reduced by carryover effect. This is particularly so when a group that is treated with an effective treatment first, is then treated with an ineffective treatment or placebo second. In studies with a quantitative response this very effect may cause severe underestimation of the treatment effect (Cleophas 1995). Studies with a binary response are, however, different from studies with a quantitative response in that they are mostly designed to answer whether a treatment has any effect rather than what size such effect does have. One might contend, therefore, that underestimation in such studies is not that important as long as the null hypothesis of no treatment effect doesn't have to be erroneously accepted. We demonstrate that in crossovers with a binary response and significant carryover effect the power of testing the treatment effect remains substantial even so. This would imply that routinely testing for carryover effects in such studies is not necessary as long as the result of the treatment comparison is positive. When a study is negative it does make sense, however, to test for carryover effect by comparing p_A versus p_C (Table 36.1).

When p_A is significantly different from p_C, we assume that there is carryover effect in group II. In this situation a parallel-group analysis of period I (p_A versus p_B) can effectively be used for the purpose of demonstrating a treatment effect. It will provide a significant difference at the same or even a lower level of significance than the test for carryover effect. This is so, because when carryover effect is maximal, p_B equals p_C. The difference between p_B and p_A will, therefore, be at least as large as the difference between p_C and p_A but probably larger. Therefore, no further test for treatment effect seems to be required for our purpose and it seems appropriate that the results of the second period be disregarded.

Considering that the problem of carryover effects influence in crossover trials with a binary response may not be too hard to handle, we may as well shift our standard of choosing this particular trial design somewhat, and make use of its additional advantages more frequently. The design is, e.g., particularly powerful for the study of rapid relief of symptoms in chronic disease where the long-term condition of the patient remains fairly stable (Cleophas and Tavenier 1995). This is so, because between-subject variability is not used in a within-subject comparison. Also, we can make use of positive correlations between the treatment modalities tested, because the statistical power of testing treatment comparisons with a positive correlation can be largely enhanced by within-subject comparisons (Cleophas and Tavenier 1994). Furthermore, none of the patients in the trial has to be treated throughout the trial with a less adequate dose or placebo, which is why a crossover raises usually less ethical problems than does a parallel-group study where one group is treated with a placebo or less adequate dosage throughout the trial. Also, we have the advantage that patients can express their own opinions about which of the treatments they personally prefer. This is especially important with subjective variables, such as pain scores.

Furthermore, not so large a group is required because of within-subject comparisons, which facilitates the recruitment procedure and reduces costs. Finally, double-blinding cannot be effectively executed in self-controlled studies without some kind of crossover design.

In summary:

1. Crossover studies with a binary response and positive results do not have to be tested for carryover effects.
2. If such studies have a negative result, testing for carryover effect does make sense.
3. If a carryover effect is demonstrated, the treatment results should be analyzed in the form of a parallel-group study of the first period.

7 Conclusions

The two-period crossover trial has the evident advantage that by the use of within-patients comparisons, the usually larger between-patient variability is not used as a measuring stick to compare treatments. However, a prerequisite is that the order of the treatments does not substantially influence the outcome of the treatment. Crossover studies with a binary response (such as yes/no or present/absent), although widely used for initial screening of new compounds, have not previously been studied for such order effects. In the present chapter we use a mathematical model based on standard statistical tests to study to what extent such order effects, otherwise called carryover effects, may reduce the power of detecting a treatment effect. We come to the conclusion that in spite of large carryover effects the crossover study with a binary response remains a powerful method and that testing for carryover effects makes sense only if the null-hypothesis of no treatment effect cannot be rejected.

References

Barker M, Hew RJ, Huitson A, Poloniecki J (1982) The two-period crossover trial. Bias 9:67–112
Bavry JH (1988) Design power (TM). Scientific software Inc, Hillsdale

Brown BW (1980) The crossover experiment for clinical trials. Biometrics 36:69–79

Cleophas TJ (1990) Underestimation of treatment effect in crossover trials. Angiology 41:855–864

Cleophas TJM (1995) A simple analysis of carryover studies with one-group interaction. Int J Clin Pharmacol Ther 32:322–328

Cleophas TJM, Tavenier P (1994) Fundamental issues of choosing the right type of trial. Am J Ther 1:327–332

Cleophas TJM, Tavenier P (1995) Clinical trials of chronic diseases. J Clin Pharmacol 35:594–598

Fidler V (1984) Change-over clinical trials with binary data: mixed model-based comparisons of tests. Biometrics 40:1063–1079

Fleiss JL (1989) A critique of recent research on the two-treatment crossover design. Control Clin Trials 10:237–243

Freeman PR (1989) The performance of the two-stage analysis of two-treatment, two-period crossover trials. Stat Med 8:1421–1432

Gart JJ (1969) An exact test for comparing matched proportions in crossover designs. Biometrika 56:57–80

Hills M, Armitage P (1979) The two-period crossover trial. Br J Clin Pharmacol 8:7–20

Louis TA, Lavori PW, Bailar JC, Polansky M (1984) Crossover and self-controlled design in clinical research. N Engl J Med 310:24–31

Packer M (1989) Combined beta-adrenergic and calcium entry blockade in angina pectoris. N Engl J Med 320:709–718

Prescott RJ (1981) The comparison of success rates in crossover trials in the presence of an order effect. Appl Stat 30:9–15

Senn S (1993) Crossover trials in clinical research. Wiley, Chicester

Willan AR, Pater JL (1986) Carryover and the two-period clinical trial. Biometrics 42:593–599

Chapter 37
Cross-Over Trials Should Not Be Used to Test Treatments with Different Chemical Class

1 Introduction

So many unpredictable variables often play a role in clinical trials of new medical treatments that a trial without controls has become almost unconceivable. Usually, a parallel-group design is used: with every patient given a new therapy, a control patient is given standard therapy or a placebo. For the study of reversible treatments of chronic stable conditions with responses that can be measured on relatively short notice a cross-over design can be chosen: a single patient receives both new therapy and a standard therapy or placebo. Of course, we have to be fairly sure that carry-over effects of one treatment period carrying on into the other or time effects are negligible. But then the cross-over design has the advantage that it eliminates between-subject variability of symptoms in a treatment comparison. And this makes the design sensitive, particularly with conditions where between-subject variability is notoriously large, e.g., angina pectoris and many other pain syndromes.

In 1965 the biostatistician James Grizzle (1965) gave uniform guidelines for the cross-over design, and it was he who first recognized the problem of negative correlations between treatment responses that may endanger the validity of the cross-over design. In his example two completely different treatments (A = ferrous sulphate and B = folic acid) were tested for their abilities to increase hemoglobin (Fig. 37.1). Obviously, there was an inverse correlation between the two treatments: ferrous sulphate was only beneficial when folic acid was not, and so was folic acid when ferrous sulphate was not. Although the mean result of ferrous sulphate treatment was 1.7 mmol different from that of folic acid which is quite a difference, it did not reach statistical significance ($p = 0.12$). This was probably due to the significant negative correlation in the treatment comparison. How a negative correlation reduces the sensitivity of a paired comparison can be explained as follows:

t = mean result/pooled SEM.
where pooled SEM = pooled standard error of the mean

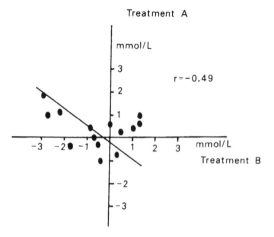

Fig. 37.1 Two completely different treatments (A=ferrous sulphate and B=folic acid) were tested for their abilities to increase hemoglobin. There was an inverse correlation between the two treatments: ferrous sulphate was only beneficial when folic acid was not, and so was folic acid when ferrous sulphate was not. Although the mean result of ferrous sulphate treatment was 1.7 mmol different from that of folic acid, the difference did not reach statistical significance (p=0.12). This was probably due to the negative correlation in the treatment comparison (Grizzle 1965)

the formula for pooled SEM is:

$$(\text{pooled SEM})^2 = \text{SEM}_1{}^2 + \text{SEM}_2{}^2 - 2 \text{ r SEM}_1.\text{SEM}_2$$

where SEM_1 and SEM_2 are standard errors of the mean of separate treatments and r=correlation coefficient.

When we assume $\text{SEM}_1 = \text{SEM}_2 = \text{SEM}$, then

$$(\text{pooled SEM})^2 = (1-r) \, 2 \, \text{SEM}^2$$

If r would have been 0 instead of −0.49 (Fig. 37.1) the t-value of this comparison would have been $\sqrt{(1-r)} = \sqrt{1.49} = 1.225$ larger than the present t-value and the treatment comparison would have reached statistical significance.

We currently are aware that ferrous sulphate and folic acid are treatments with a totally different chemical class/mode of action. And so, although both of the compounds improve hemoglobin, certainly nobody nowadays would use the compounds in a treatment comparison anymore. However, we continue to compare many other treatments from different classes of drugs all the time, even if we know that their mode of action is totally different, e.g., beta-blockers are compared with calcium channel blockers or nitrates for the treatment of angina pectoris. Compounds from different chemical classes are compared for the treatment of hypertension, Raynaud's phenomenon, cardiac arrhythmias, chronic obstructive pulmonary disease and many more conditions.

The current chapter shows that it is not correct to use a cross-over design for testing such kind of treatment comparisons because of the risk of negative correlations between treatment responses, and thus of a flawed study. We will test this hypothesis in a non-mathematical way by giving examples in which a cross-over design should NOT have been used. Also, we will estimate the size of the problem by reviewing hypertension trials published for their design in relation to the type of treatment comparison. A more mathematical approach of the problems of negative correlations can be found elsewhere (Cleophas 1999).

2 Examples from the Literature in Which Cross-Over Trials Are Correctly Used

Cross-over trials generally have a strong positive correlation between treatment responses for two reasons. First, this is so, because one subject is used to the comparison of two treatments. Second, in controlled clinical trials the new treatment may be a slight modification of the standard or be equivalent to it with the addition of a new component. In this situation there is a positive correlation between the response to the new treatment and the standard treatment: treatment 1 performs highly when treatment 2 does so.

Table 37.1 gives seven examples of cross-over studies where compounds from the same chemical class/mode of action are compared. For example, two beta-adrenergic agonists, two calcium channel blockers, two beta-blockers, two different dosages of the same compound are compared. Such comparisons should have a strong positive correlation, and the table shows that this is so. Correlation coefficients calculated from the data were consistently positive. These studies were appropriately performed in the form of a cross-over study. The cross-over design provided extra sensitivity by accounting for the positive correlation. A parallel-group study would have lacked the extra sensitivity.

3 Examples from the Literature in Which Cross-Over Trials Should Not Have Been Used

In trials with completely different treatments patients tend to fall apart into different populations: those who respond better to treatment 1 and those who do so to treatment 2. For example, patients with angina pectoris irresponsive to beta-blockers may respond either to calcium channel blockers or nitrates. Also, hypertension, Raynaud's phenomenon, different types of cardiac arrhythmias and chronic obstructive pulmonary disease are known to be conditions where a non-response to a particular compound is frequently associated with an excellent response to a completely different compound. These are examples of situations in which a strong negative

Table 37.1 Examples from the literature in which cross-over trials are correctly used

	Treatment	Efficacy[a] (mean ± SEM)	p-value	Correlation coefficient[b]
1. Angiology 1985; 36:219–226	Beta-adrenergic agonist	22.7 ± 0.5	<0.01	r=+0.56
n = 12	Alpha-adrenergic antagonist with beta- agonistic property	27.7 ± 1.0		
2. Lancet 1986; ii: 189–192	Platelet activating factor	−1.5 ± 1.0	<0.001	r=+0.66
n = 6	Its precursor	+0.2 ± 1.0		
3. Lancet 1986; ii: 740–741	Cholesterol lowering drug A	42 ± 12	<0.05	r=+0.20
n = 7	Cholesterol lowering drug B	50 ± 12		
4. Lancet 1987; i: 647–652	High alcohol intake	143 ± 5	<0.01	r=+0.41
n = 40	Low alcohol intake	137 ± 5		
5. Lancet 1987; ii: 650–653	Atenolol	74.3 ± 4.5[c]	<0.01	r=+0.39
n = 20	Labetalol	79.9 ± 7.2		
6. Br Heart J 1993; 70:252–258	Gallopamil	29.9 ± 11.0	<0.0001	r=+0.56
n = 18	Nifedipine	49.7 ± 26.8		
7. Int J Clin Pharmacol Ther 1997; 35:514–518	Amlodipine	1.58 ± 0.32	<0.001	r=+0.65
n = 8	Felodipine	4.43 ± 1.86		

[a]Denotes in study 1 finger temperature after finger cooling (°C), study 2 bronchial responsiveness to methacholine (doubling dilutions), in study 3 plasma level of HDL-cholesterol (mg/dl), in study 4 systolic blood pressure (mmHg), in study 5 heart rate (beats/min), in study 6 QRS voltage (% of standardized maximum), in study 7 peak-trough ratio

[b]Correlation coefficient (r) was calculated using t-statistic: p-values were turned into t-values after adjustment for the degrees of freedom, and r was calculated using the formula for the pooled standard error of the mean (SEM): (pooled SEM)^2 = SEM$_1^2$ + SEM$_2^2$ − 2 r SEM$_1$.SEM$_2$

[c]For the paired analysis two-sided ANOVA was used which for two groups of paired data yields the same results as a paired t - test, however

correlation may exist. This may be even so with self-controlled studies that otherwise are more likely to have a positive correlation because one subject is used to the comparison of two treatments. As demonstrated above the problem with negative correlations in a cross-over study is lack of sensitivity: the pooled SEM is approximately $\sqrt{(1-r)}$ times larger with a negative correlation than it would have been with a zero correlation (parallel-group study), and this reduces the probability level of testing, and, thus, produces erroneously negative studies. The examples in Table 37.2 show that the problem can be readily detected in the literature. All of these studies were negative, and this was presumably so because of the negative correlation coefficient between treatment responses. Had they been performed in the form of a parallel-group study, most of them probably would have had a statistically significant effect. At least, when we tested the studies as though they were unpaired, in most of them p-values of 0.05 or less were obtained.

Table 37.2 Examples from the literature in which cross-over trials should NOT have been used

	Treatment	Efficacy[a] (mean ± SEM)	p-value	Correlation coefficient[b]
1. Lancet 1986; i:997–1001	NSAID with renal	127 ± 3	n.s.	r = −0.29
n = 20	NSAID without renal prostaglandin synthesis	131 ± 3		
2. N Engl J Med 1986; 314:1280–1286	Tolazolin	140 ± 34	n.s.	r = −0.30
n = 12	Insulin	112 ± 15		
3. N Engl J Med 1986; 315:735–739	Beta-adrenergic agonist	42 ± 18	n.s.	r = −0.30
n = 11	Anticholinergic agent	25 ± 14		
4. Br J Clin Pharmacol 1991; 31:305–312	Xamoterol	80.1 ± 2.6	n.s.	r = −0.25
n = 38	Enalapril	75.1 ± 1.6		
5. Br J Clin Pharmacol 1991; 32:758–760	Nitroprusside	13 ± 5	n.s.	r = −0.42
n = 6	Bradykinine	91 ± 2		
6. Curr Ther Res 1991; 49:340–350	Nifedipine	14.0 ± 3.6	n.s.	r = −0.46
n = 42	Captopril	6.7 ± 2.1		
7. Eur J Gastroenterol Hepat 1993; 5:627–629	Atenolol	3.9 ± 0.2	n.s.	r = −0.70
n = 18	Nifedipine	2.9 ± 0.3		

SEM standard error of the mean, *n.s.* not significant

[a]Denotes in study 1 systolic blood pressure (mmHg), in study 2 plasma glucose level (mg/dl), in study 3 forced expiratory volume in one second (% change from baseline), in study 4 diastolic blood pressure (mmHg), in study 5 plasma ureum (mmol/l), in study 6 fall in mean blood pressure (mmHg), in study 7 oesophageal sphincter pressure (mmHg)

[b]Correlation coefficient (r) was calculated using t-statistic: p-values were turned into t-values for the degrees of freedom, and r was calculated using the formula for the pooled standard error of the mean (SEM): (pooled SEM)^2 = SEM$_1^2$ + SEM$_2^2$ − 2 r SEM$_1$·SEM$_2$

4 Estimate of the Size of the Problem by Review of Hypertension Trials Published

The above examples indicate the existence of a potential problem with negative correlations in cross-over trials. However, they do not answer how prevalent the problem is. In order to address this question we assessed the double blind randomized hypertension trials listed in Cardiology Dialogue (Rapid Literature Service 1994). Hypertension treatments frequently have pharmacologically completely different modes of action: diuretics reduce blood pressure by volume depletion, beta-blockers and calcium channel blockers/angiotensin converting enzyme inhibitors do so by reducing cardiac output and peripheral resistance respectively. Of 73 randomized controlled trials (Table 37.3) a significantly smaller percentage of cross-over

Table 37.3 Double blind randomized hypertension trials listed in the 1994 volume of Cardiology Dialogue (Nies and Spielberg 1996)

	Parallel-group studies		Cross-over studies	
	N	Different treatments (%)	N	Different treatments (%)
Am J Cardiol	3	2	2	1
J Am Coll Cardiol	1	0		
Am J Hypertens	7	5	1	0
Curr Ther Res	5	2	1	0
Clin Med			1	0
NEJM	2	0		
Clin Exp Hypertens	1	0	2	0
J Human Hypertens	7	6	2	0
Br J Clin Pharmacol	3	3	1	1
Cardiovasc Drug Ther			1	1
Clin Lab Invest	1	1		
Herz Kreislauf	2	1		
Zeitschr Kardiol	1	1		
J Cardiovasc Pharmacol	4	3		
J Clin Pharmacol	3	2	1	0
Clin Ther			1	0
Clin Pharmacol Ther	2	2		
Cardiol	4	3		
J Int Med	1	1		
Eur J Clin Pharmacol	1	1		
Hypertens	1	1		
Arch Int Med	1	1		
B J Clin Pract			1	1
Clin Pharmacol Res	1	1		
JAMA	1	1		
Postgrad Med	1	1		
Drug Invest			1	0
Total numbers	53	38 (72%)	15	4 (27%)

than of parallel-group studies compared treatments with a totally different chemical class/mode of action (for example, diuretic versus vasodilator, or beta-blocker versus vasodilator etc., 27 versus 72%, P<0.001). Apparently, the scientific community has some intuition of doing the right thing at the right time: in 73% of the cases the cross-over design was correctly used. Nonetheless, in 4 (27%) of the cases this was not so. Two of these studies were not able to reject the null-hypothesis of no effect and the other two would probably have been more sensitive, had they been performed in the form of a parallel-group study.

5 Discussion

The current chapter shows that clinical trials comparing treatments with a totally different chemical class/mode of action are at risk of negative correlation between treatment responses. Such negative correlations have to be added to the standard errors in a cross-over trial, thus reducing the sensitivity of testing differences, making the design a flawed method for evaluating new treatments. The examples suggest that the phenomenon of negative correlations is not uncommon in practice, and that it should be taken into account when planning drug research.

The mechanism of between-group disparities in drug response is currently being recognized in clinical pharmacology, and is, in fact, the main reason that in treatment protocols the principle of stepped care is being replaced by individualized care (Nies and Spielberg 1996). However, when it comes to research, clinicians and clinical pharmacologists are still unfamiliar with the problems this issue raises and virtually never take account of it. The recognition of between-group disparities in drug response also implies that negative correlations in a treatment comparison are routinely tested, and that a cross-over design is not always appropriate.

So far, statisticians have assumed that a negative correlation in cross-over studies was virtually non-existent, because one subject is used for comparison of two treatments. For example, Grieve recently stated one should not contemplate a cross-over design if there is any likelihood of correlation not being positive (Grieve 1994). The examples in the current paper show, however, that with completely different treatments, the risk of a negative correlation is a real possibility, and that it does give rise to erroneously negative studies. It makes sense, therefore, to restate Grieve's statement as follows: one should not contemplate a cross-over design if treatments with a totally different chemical class/mode of action are to be compared.

At the same time, however, we should admit that the cross-over design is very sensitive for comparing treatments of one class and presumably one mode of action. The positive correlation in such treatment comparisons adds sensitivity, similarly to the way it reduces sensitivity with negative correlations: the pooled SEM is approximately $\sqrt{(1-r)}$ times smaller with positive correlation than it would have been with a zero correlation (parallel-group study), and this increases the probability level of testing accordingly. This means that the cross-over is a very sensitive method for evaluating studies with presumable positive correlation between treatment responses, and that there is, thus, room left for this study design in drug research.

6 Conclusions

Comparisons of treatments with totally different chemical class/mode of action are at risk of a negative correlation between treatment responses: patients tend to fall apart into different populations, those who respond better to treatment 1 and those who do so to treatment 2. The cross-over design is flawed when this phenomenon takes place. The objective of this chapter was to assess whether this flaw is prevalent in the literature.

Fourteen randomized controlled cross-over studies were assessed for correlation levels in relation to their type of treatment comparison. Correlation coefficient (r) was calculated using T-statistic: P-values were turned into T-values for the degrees of freedom, and r was calculated using the formula for the pooled standard error of the mean (SEM): (pooled $SEM)^2 = SEM_1^2 + SEM_2^2 - 2$ r $SEM_1.SEM_2$. Randomized controlled hypertension trials of 1994 were listed for study design in relation to type of treatment comparison.

Cross-over studies comparing treatments with a totally different chemical class/mode of action were frequently negative, and this was, obviously, due to their negative correlation between treatment responses. Cross-over studies comparing similar treatments had frequently a positive correlation, and this added extra sensitivity to the treatment comparison. Twenty-seven percent of the cross-over hypertension studies compared completely different treatments, and these studies should, therefore, not have been performed in the form of a cross-over study.

Cross-over trials lack sensitivity to test one treatment against another treatment with a totally different chemical class/mode of action, and should, therefore, not be used for that purpose. In contrast, they are, particularly, sensitive to compare treatments from one chemical class/with one mode of action. It is hoped that this chapter affects the design of future crossover trials.

References

Cleophas TJ (1999) Between-group disparities in drug response. In: Human experimentation. Kluwer Academic Publishers, Boston, pp 48–56

Grieve AP (1994) Bayesian analysis of two-treatment crossover studies. Stat Meth Med Res 3:407–429

Grizzle JE (1965) The two-period change-over design and its use in clinical trials. Biometrics 22:467–480

Nies AS, Spielberg SP (1996) Individualization of drug therapy. In: Hardman JL, Limbird LE (eds) Goodman and Gilman's pharmacological basis of therapeutics. McGraw-Hill, New York, pp 43–63

Rapid Literature Service (ed) (1994) Cardiology dialogue. Limbach GMBH, Cologne

Chapter 38
Quality-Of-Life Assessments in Clinical Trials

1 Introduction

Less than 10 years ago the scientific community believed that quality of life (QOL) was part of the art of medicine rather than the science of medicine. In the past few years index methods have been developed and have proven to be sensitive and specific to assess patients' health status not only on a physical, but also on a psychological and social base. We increasingly witness that QOL is implemented in the scientific evaluation of medicine. However, major problems with QOL assessments so far, include the contributing factor patients' opinion, which is very subjective and, therefore, scientifically difficult to handle, and, second, the low sensitivity of QOL-questionnaires to reflect true changes in QOL. The Dutch Mononitrate Quality Of Life (DUMQOL) Study Group has recently addressed both problems. In their hands, the patients' opinion was a consistent and statistically independent determinant of QOL in patients with angina pectoris. The problem of low sensitivity of QOL-assessments could be improved by replacing the absolute score-scales with relative ones, using for that purpose odds ratios of scores. The current chapter reviews the main results of this so far only partly published research (Frieswijk et al. 2000; Zwinderman et al. 1999) from the Netherlands.

2 Some Terminology

QOL battery	A questionnaire large enough to adequately address important domains of QOL.
Domains of QOL	Physical, psychological, and social areas of health seen distinct and important to a person's perception of QOL.

(continued)

(continued)

Items	Items, otherwise called questions, constitute a domain, e.g., the DUMQOL-questionnaire for angina pectoris, consists of respectively 8, 7, and 4 questions to assess the domains (1) mobility, (2) somatic symptoms, and (3) psychological distress.
Absolute score scales	For every item the individual response is scored on a (linear) scale. Mean of scores a group of patients are calculated. Mean domain scores are calculated as overall means of the latter mean scores.
Relative score scales	The same procedure. However, results are reported in the form of odds ratios.
Odds ratios	Mean of the domain scores in patients with a particular characteristic/mean of the domain scores in patients without this particular characteristic.
Validated QOL batteries	This is controversial. QOL batteries are diagnostic tests, and validation of any diagnostic test is hard to accomplish without a gold standard for comparison. Surrogate validation is sometimes used: actual QOL scores are compared with scores expected based on levels of morbidity.
Internal consistency of domain items	There should be a strong correlation between the answers given to questions within one domain: all of questions should approximately predict one and the same thing. The level of correlation is expressed as Cronbach's alpha: 0 means poor, 1 perfect relationship.
Cronbach's alpha	$$alpha = \frac{k}{(k-1)} \left(1 - \sum \frac{s_i^2}{s_T^2} \right)$$ k = number of items s_i^2 = variance of ith item s_T^2 = variance of total score obtained by summing up all of the items
Multicollinearity	There should not be a too strong correlation between different domain scores because different domains different areas of QOL. A Pearson's correlation >0.90 means the presence of multicollinearity and, thus, of a flawed multiple regression analysis.
Pearson's correlation coefficient (r)	$$r = \frac{\sum (x - \bar{x})(y - \bar{y})}{\sqrt{\sum (x - \bar{x})^2 \sum (y - \bar{y})^2}}$$
Sensitivity of QOL assessment	Sensitivity or precision means ability of the measurement to reflect true changes in QOL.
QOL estimator	Mean (or pooled) result of the data from a single domain.
Index methods	Index methods combine the results of various domains of a QOL battery to provide an index for overall QOL.

3   Defining QOL in a Subjective or Objective Way?

In 1992 Brazier et al (1992) validated the Short Form (SF)-36 health survey questionnaire of Stewart et al. (1988), a self-administered questionnaire, addressing any aspects that, according to the designer, might be important to the patients' QOL. However, at each item in the questionnaire, the question "is it important to you?" was missing. In 1994 Gill and Feinstein (1994) in their "Critical appraisal of quality of life assessments" emphasized that, from their personal experience in patient care, they believed that QOL, rather than a description of health status, should describe the way patients perceive their health status. One year later Marquis et al (1995) designed a questionnaire for patients with angina pectoris based on psychological factors, in addition to clinical symptoms, and concluded that the former is probably a better predictor of QOL than the latter. In subsequent years QOL assessments increasingly allowed for patients giving their own opinion, in addition to patients answering questions about health status. However, the latter was consistently given more weight than the former. For example, Testa and Simonson (1996) allowed for one such question out of six questions in each QOL-domain giving the question just about 1/6 of the total weight in various domains. The problem with the subjective approach to QOL, as recently pointed out by Thompson et al (1998), is that it is difficult to match with the accepted rule that scientific data should be objective. In addition, the patients' opinion may be a variable so unpredictable, that it cannot be applied as a reliable measure for clinical assessment of groups of patients. So far, the concept that the patients' opinion is a relevant variable in the assessment of QOL has never been proven to be true. In order to test this issue the DUMQOL Study Group has recently completed some relevant research.

4   The Patients' Opinion Is an Important
Independent-Contributor to QOL

The DUMQOL Study Group used the validated form of Stewart's SF-36 Questionnaire for the purpose of scoring QOL (Stewart et al. 1988), and the DUMQOL-50 questionnaire for scoring psychological distress and health status according to the patients' judgment (Niemeyer et al. 1997). The patients' opinion (patients were requested to estimate the overall amount of his/her QOL as compared to patients they knew with a similar condition) and health status according to the physicians' judgement (the physician was requested to estimate the patients' health status) were scored like the others on 5 point-scales. Internal consistency and retreatment reliability of the test-battery was adequate with Cronbach's alpha 0.66. Table 38.1 shows the results from a cohort of 82 outpatient-clinic patients with stable angina pectoris. Obviously, QOL was strongly associated with the patients' opinion. In none of the comparisons were adjustment for multicollinearity required (Pearson's correlation coefficient >0.9). Table 38.2 shows that psychological distress was the most important contributor to QOL. Also, the patients' opinion

Table 38.1 Correlation matrix to assess multicollinearity in the data, Pearson's correlation coefficient are given (r)

	Patients' opinion	Psychological distress	Health status patients' judgment	Health status physicians' judgment
Psychological distress	0.35			
Health status patients' judgment	0.36	0.30		
Health status physicians' judgment	0.42	0.41	0.48	
Quality of life	0.42	0.58	0.43	0.27

R < 0.20 weak correlation; 0.20 < r < 0.40 moderate correlation; r > 0.40 strong correlation

Table 38.2 Stepwise multiple regression analysis of the associations of various (dependent) predictors on QOL in patients with angina pectoris

	Beta	t	p-value
Psychological distress	0.43	4.22	0.000
Patients' opinion	0.22	2.19	0.032
Health status (patients' judgment)	0.19	1.88	0.071
Health status (physicians' judgment)	0.11	0.16	0.872

beta standardized partial correlation coefficient

significantly contributed to QOL. Physical health status according to the patients' judgment only made a borderline contribution, while the physicians' judgment was not associated with QOL at all. These data strongly support the relevance of the patients' opinion as an important independent-contributor to QOL.

5   Lack of Sensitivity of QOL-Assessments

Sensitivity defined as ability of the measurement to reflect true changes in QOL is frequently poor in QOL assessments (Ware et al. 1993). A well-established problem with QOL scales is their inconsistent relationship between ranges of response and true changes in QOL (Testa and Simonson 1996). A good example of this problem is the physical scale of the SF-36 questionnaire. It ranges from 0 to 100 points. However, while healthy youngsters may score as high as 95 and topsporters even 100, 60 year-old subjects usually score no better than 20. A patient with angina pectoris may score 5 points. If he would score 10, instead of 5, after the allowance for sublingual nitrates ad libitum, this improvement would equal 5% on the absolute scale of 100 points, which does not seem to be very much. However, on a relative scale this score of 10 points is 100% better than a score of 5 points, and, in terms of improvement of QOL, this difference on the SF-36-scale between 5 and 10 points does mean a world of difference. It, for example, means the difference between a largely dependent and independent way of life. In this example the low score on the absolute-scale masks important and meaningful changes in QOL. The DUMQOL Study Group took issue with this well-recognized but unsolved phenomenon and performed an odds ratio analysis of patient characteristics in a cohort of 1,350 patients with stable angina pectoris. They showed that this approach provided increased precision to estimate effects on QOL estimators.

6   Odds Ratio Analysis of Effects of Patient Characteristics on QOL Data Provides Increased Precision

Table 38.3 gives an overview of effects of patient characteristics on QOL estimators in 1,350 patients with stable angina pectoris. Results are presented as odds ratios. The odds ratio presents the relative risk of QOL difficulties and is defined as the ratio between mean domain score of patients with a particular characteristic and that of patients without this particular characteristic.

The procedure readily identifies categories of patients that, obviously, have poor QOL scores. For example,

1. Increased QOL-difficulties were observed in patients with advanced New York Heart Association (NYHA) anginal class: the higher the anginal class the larger the risk of mobility difficulties, pain, chest pain, anginal pain, and distress.
2. The risk of mobility difficulties was increased in patients with diabetes mellitus, arrhythmias, and peripheral vascular diseases.
3. Patients using sublingual nitrates (and thus presumably very symptomatic) reported more (severe) mobility difficulties, pain, chest pain, and psychological distress.
4. Female patients reported more (severe) mobility difficulties, pain, anginal pain, and distress than their male counterparts.
5. The risk of mobility difficulties increased with age, but, in contrast, elderly patients reported less pain, anginal pain, and distress.

The above categories of patients are, obviously, very symptomatic and should, therefore, particularly benefit from treatments. The beneficial effects of treatments in patients with particular characteristics can be predicted according to the following procedure:

1. Odds Ratio$_{\text{active treatment/placebo}}$ = mean domain score in patients on active treatment/ mean domain score in patients on placebo.
2. Odds Ratio$_{\text{characteristic/no characteristic}}$ = mean domain score in patients with particular characteristic/mean domain score in patients without this particular characteristic.

The relative risk of scoring in patients with a particular characteristic if they used active treatment can be estimated and calculated according to:

3. Odds Ratio$_{\text{characteristic/no characteristic}}$ × Odds Ratio$_{\text{active treatment/placebo}}$.

Table 38.3 Stable angina pectoris: effects of patient characteristics on quality of life estimators. Odds ratios and 95% confidence intervals are given

	Mobility difficulties	Pain in general	Early morning pain	Psychological distress	Chest pain	Patient satisfaction
Gender (females/males)	2.5 (1.8–3.3)***	2.0 (1.3–3.0)***	1.7 (0.6–4.7)	1.3 (0.9–2.0)	2.1 (1.1–3.9)**	0.8 (0.3–1.9)
Age (>68/<86 years)	1.4 (1.2–1.5)**	1.0(0.9–1.1)	0.9 (0.9–1.0)	1.0 (0.9–1.0)	1.0 (0.9–1.0)	1.0 (0.9–1.0)
NYHA (III-and-IV/II-and-I)	5.6 (4.8–6.6)***	2.8 (2.1–3.5)***	46.8 (26.3–83.1)***	4.4 (3.5–5.5)***	37.2 (23.4–58.9)***	0.6 (0.4–1.1)
Smoking yes/no	0.8 (0.5–1.1)	1.3 (0.8–2.1)	12.9 (3.0–56.2)***	3.2 (2.0–5.2)*	0.5 (0.2–1.2)	5.8(2.1–15.8)**
Cholesterol yes/no	0.9 (0.7–1.3)	1.4 (0.3–2.0)	1.3 (0.5–3.4)	1.8 (1.2–2.8)*	1.8 (0.9–3.4)	1.1 (0.5–2.6)
Hypertension yes/no	0.3 (0.2–0.4)*	0.5 (0.3–0.7)*	0.7 (0.2–0.9)*	0.3 (0.2–0.4)**	0.5 (0.3–0.9)*	1.7 (0.7–4.1)
Diabetes yes/no	2.2 (1.5–3.1)*	1.1 (0.6–1.9)	9.1 (3.0–28.2)***	2.0 (1.1–3.7)*	1.8 (0.7–4.6)	1.1 (0.3–4.2)
Arrhythmias yes/no	2.9 (2.0–4.1)**	1.3 (0.7–2.1)	3.6 (1.3–10)*	3.2 (1.9–5.4)*	10.2 (4.5–23.4)**	1.2 (0.4–3.7)
PVD yes/no	11.0 (7.9–15.1)***	2.2 (1.4–3.6)*	1.1 (0.7–1.7)	2.6 (1.5–4.5)*	1.0 (0.4–2.2)	8.3 (2.7–25.7)**
Beta-blockers yes/no	0.8 (0.7–0.9)*	0.8 (0.5–1.1)	1.7 (0.7–4.0)	0.9 (0.6–1.2)	1.3 (0.7–2.2)	3.2 (1.5–6.9)**
Calcium channel blockers yes/no	1.5 (1.2–1.9)*	1.3 (0.9–1.8)	3.2 (1.5–6.6)*	2.0 (1.4–2.9)*	6.0 (3.4–10.7)**	6.5 (3.0–13.8)*
Sublingual nitrates yes/no	2.6 (2.1–3.3)***	3.0 (2.2–4.2)***	1.0 (0.7–1.4)	3.1 (2.5–4.3)***	7.1 (4.2–12.0)***	3.4 (1.6–6.9)***

Quality of life domains were estimated using a questionnaire based on the medical outcomes short-form 36 health survey and the angina pectoris quality of life questionnaire

Results are given as odds ratios = mean domain scores in patients with characteristic/mean domain scores in patients without characteristic

PVD peripheral vascular disease, *NYHA* New York Heart Association Angina Class

*P<0.05; **P<0.01; ***P<0.001

Along this line the odds ratio approach to QOL-assessments can be helpful to estimate the effects of cardiovascular drugs on quality of life in different categories of patients with increased precision.

7   Discussion

The medical community is, obviously, attracted to the concept that QOL assessments should pay particular attention to the individual, but, at the same time, it believes in the usefulness of a scientific method to measure QOL (Albert et al. 1998). Usually, the objective of a study is not to find the greatest good for a single person but the greatest good for the entire population, moving from an individual perspective to a societal one. Even for quality-of-life measurements, only large clinical studies designed and conducted with rigorous statistical standards allow for a hypothesis to be tested and to offer useful results. Using the patients' opinion as measurement-instrument raises a major problem within this context. The general concept of medical measurements is that measurement-instruments remain constant irrespective of who is using them: a thermometer remains the same whoever's mouth it is placed in. With the patients' opinion this is not so. Rather than true ability, perceived functional ability and willingness to complain is assessed. An assessment tool to reflect the viewpoint of patients is, obviously, a major challenge. Although the medical community expresses sympathy with the latter concept, it expresses doubt about scientific value and even questions whether the patients' opinion is part of medicine at all (Testa and Simonson 1996; Thompson et al. 1998; Albert et al. 1998). The recent research from the DUMQOL Group shows that the patients' opinion in a standardized way, produces data that are sufficiently homogeneous to enable a sensitive statistical analysis. These data strongly support the relevance of the patients' opinion as an independent contributing factor to QOL. This variable should, therefore, be adequately implemented in future QOL assessments.

A second problem with current QOL-batteries is the inconsistent relationship between ranges of response and true changes in QOL-assessments. This is mainly due to very low (and very high) scores on the absolute-scale, masking important and meaningful changes in QOL. The DUMQOL Study Group showed that this problem can be adequately met by the use of relative rather than absolute scores, and it used for that purpose an odds ratio-approach of QOL scores. This approach provided increased precision to estimate effects on QOL estimators. An additional advantage of the latter approach is that odds ratios are well understood and much in use in the medical community, and that (those) results from QOL research can, therefore, be more easily communicated through odds ratios than through the comparison of absolute scores. For example, "the odds ratio of (severe) mobility difficulties for mononitrate therapy in patients with stable angina is 0.83 ($p < 0.001$)" is better understood than "the mean mobility difficulties score decreased from 1.10 to 1.06 on a scale from 0 to 4 ($p = 0.007$)".

We conclude that recent QOL-research from the DUMQOL Study Group allows for some relevant conclusions, pertinent to both clinical practice and clinical research. QOL should be assessed in a subjective rather than objective way, because the patients' opinion is an important independent contributor to QOL. The comparison of absolute QOL-scores lacks sensitivity to truly estimate QOL. For that purpose the odds ratio approach of QOL scores provides increased precision to estimate QOL.

8   Conclusions

Two major issues in quality of life (QOL) research include the patients' opinion as a contributing factor in QOL-assessments, and the lack of sensitivity of QOL-assessments. The objective of this chapter was to review results from recent research by the Dutch Mononitrate Quality Of Life (DUMQOL) Study Group relevant to these issues.

Using a test-battery including Stewart's Short Form (SF)-36 Questionnaire and the DUMQOL-50 questionnaire, the DUMQOL Study Group tested the hypothesis that the patients' opinion might be an independent determinant of QOL and performed for that purpose a stepwise multiple regression analysis of data from 82 outpatient clinic patients with stable angina pectoris. Psychological distress was the most important contributor to QOL (beta 0.43, P<0.0001). Also, the patients' opinion significantly contributed to QOL (beta 0.22, p=0.032). Physical health status according to the patients' judgment only made a borderline contribution (beta 0.19, P=0.71), while the physicians' judgment was not associated with QOL at all (beta 0.11, P=0.87). Using an Odds ratio approach of QOL scores in 1,350 outpatient clinic patients with stable angina pectoris the DUMQOL Study Group assessed the question that relative scores might provide increased precision to estimate the effects of patient characteristics on QOL data. Increased QOL difficulties were observed in New York Heart Association Angina Class (NYHA) III-IV patients, in patients with comorbidity, as well as in females and elderly patients. Odds ratios can be used in these categories to predict the benefit from treatments. We conclude that recent QOL-research of the DUMQOL Study Group allows for conclusions relevant to clinical practice. QOL should be defined in a subjective rather than objective way. The patients' opinion is an important independent contributor to QOL. The comparison of absolute QOL-scores lacks sensitivity to truly estimate QOL. The odds ratio approach of QOL scores provides increased precision to estimate QOL.

References

Albert SM, Frank L, Mrri R, Hylandt AG, Leplége A (1998) Defining and measuring quality of life in medicine. J Am Med Assoc 279:429–431
Brazier JE, Harper R, Jones NM, O'Cathain A, Thomas KJ, Usherwood T, Westlake L (1992) Validating the SF-36 health survey questionnaire: new outcome measure for primary care. Br Med J 305:160–164

Frieswijk N, Buunk BP, Janssen RM, Niemeyer MG, Cleophas TJ, Zwinderman AH (2000) Social comparison and quality of life: evaluation in patients with angina pectoris. Cardiogram 16:26–31

Gill TM, Feinstein AR (1994) A critical appraisal of the quality of quality-of-life measurements. J Am Med Assoc 272:619–626

Marquis P, Fagol C, Joire JE (1995) Quality of life assessment in patients with angina pectoris. Eur Heart J 16:1554–1559

Niemeyer MG, Kleinjans HA, De Ree R, Zwinderman AH, Cleophas TJ, Van der Wall EE (1997) Comparison of multiple dose and once-daily nitrate therapy in 1350 patients with stable angina pectoris. Angiology 48:855–863

Stewart AL, Hays RD, Ware JE (1988) The MOS short form general health survey. Med Care 26:724–735

Testa MA, Simonson DC (1996) Assessment of quality-of-life outcomes. N Engl J Med 334:835–840

Thompson DR, Meadows KA, Lewin RJ (1998) Measuring quality of life in patients with coronary heart disease. Eur Heart J 19:693–695

Ware JE, Snow KK, Kosinski M, Gandek B (1993) SF-36 health survey: manual and interpretation guide. The Health Institute, New England Medical Center, Boston

Zwinderman AH, Niemeyer MG, Kleinjans HA, Cleophas TJ (1999) Application of item response modeling for quality of life assessments in patients with stable angina pectoris. In: Kuhlman J, Mrozikiewicz A (eds) Clinical pharmacology. Zuckschwerd Verlag, New York, pp 48–56

Chapter 39
Item Response Modeling

1 Introduction

Item response models are applied for analyzing item scores of psychological and intelligence tests, and they are based on exponential relationships between the psychological traits and the item responses (Baker and Kim 2004; De Boeck and Wilson 2004). Items are usually questions with "yes" or "no" answers. Item response models were invented by Georg Rasch, a mathematician from Copenhagen who was unable to find work in his discipline in the 30ths and turned to work as a psychometrician (Rasch 1980). These models are, currently, the basis for modern psychological testing including computer-assisted adaptive testing (Van der Linden and Veldkamp 2004). Advantages compared to classical linear testing include first that item response models do not use reliability as a measure of their applicability, but instead use formal goodness of fit tests (Zwinderman 1991). Second, the scale does not need to be of an interval nature. As a consequence the effects of covariates can be analyzed and reported with odds ratios, independently of the item format and population averages. Ceiling effects are, therefore, much less of a problem than they are with classical linear methods (Fischer 1974).

Our group (Zwinderman et al. 1998) and the group of Dr. Kessler and Mrocek (1995) were the first to apply item response modeling to quality of life assessments. Like psychometric properties quality of life is a multidimensional construct and is often investigated in homogeneous populations. Both aspects are a direct threat to the reliability, because reliability is a direct function of the dimensionality of the item pool and of the variance of the true score in the population. Indeed, item response modeling may be suitable for quality of life analyses, although not widely used so far (Uttaro and Lehman 1999; Douglas 1999; Reeve et al. 2007; Teresi and Fleishman 2007; Cook et al. 2007). But this may be a matter of time. Quality of life (QOL) research is still in its infancy, and modern QOL batteries provide better validity and reliability (Cleophas et al. 2009a), making it better suitable for methods like item response modeling.

T.J. Cleophas and A.H. Zwinderman, *Statistics Applied to Clinical Studies*,
DOI 10.1007/978-94-007-2863-9_39, © Springer Science+Business Media B.V. 2012

Not only quality of life, but also current clinical diagnostic batteries are increasingly multidimensional, particularly, in clinical research like diagnostic test batteries in the vascular laboratory or catheterization laboratory: multiple tests are often used to assess the presence of a single disease or disease severity. To date item response modeling has not yet been applied in this field. The current chapter is the first effort for that purpose, and was also written to explain the principles of item response modeling to the readership of clinical investigators. Data examples are given of both a quality of life assessment and a diagnostic test battery in the vascular laboratory.

2   Item Response Modeling, Principles

With psychometric item response modeling the data of a test sample are exponentially modeled according to:

Probability of responding to an item $(yes/no) = e^{(\text{ability level of patient}) - (\text{difficulty level of item})}$.

This equation can also be described as:

Log odds of responding to an item (yes/no) =

(ability level of patient) − (difficulty level of item).

Multiple items in a single test can be simply added up:

Probability of responding to a set of items (yes/no) =

$\Sigma\ e^{(\text{ability levels of patients}) - (\text{difficulty levels of items})}$.

Log odds of responding to a set of items (yes/no) =

Σ (ability levels of patients) − (difficulty levels of items).

Software is used to calculate the best fit ability parameters, otherwise called latent traits, and the best fit difficulty parameters for the data given. Then, based on these parameters, just like with logistic models for making predictions from risk factor profiles, predictions can be made about individual levels of intellectual and psychological abilities (Baker and Kim 2004; De Boeck and Wilson 2004; Rasch 1980; Van der Linden and Veldkamp 2004; Zwinderman 1991; Fischer 1974). Similarly, predictions about levels of quality of life (Zwinderman et al. 1998; Kessler and Mrocek 1995) and, maybe also, severity of clinical diseases can respectively be made with quality of life data and diagnostic laboratory data.

For analysis the data are fitted within the standard Gaussian distribution. A problem is that item response modeling is not available in standard statistical software. However, for dichotomous items plenty software is commercially and freely available, Egret (Anonymous 1991), RSP (Glas and Ellis 1993), OPLM (Verhelst 1993), and Free Software LTA (Uebersax 2006). For polytomous items such software is rapidly being developed (Conquest Generalized Item Response Modeling Software 2011; Full Lifecycle Unified Modeling Language Modeling Software 2011). For Windows BILOG-MG and MULTILOG are available (Item Response Modeling with BILOG MG and MULTILOG for Windows 2011). All of the above software can handle large data files, the numbers of items to be scored are now only limited by the memory capacities of the hardware.

In the current paper, we choose to use the Free Software LTA (latent trait analysis) -2 (with binary items) of John Uebersax (2006).

The interesting things about item response modeling are

1. that they are more realistic than classical methods: e.g., with a classical model the data would produce a quality of life between 0% and 100% while patients with a quality of life of 0% and 100% in reality do not exist; in contrast, with item response modeling quality of life levels are expressed as distances from an average level;
2. that they are more flexible and precise, and, therefore, more suitable for making predictions about individual patients, for example, a set of five items will give five levels of quality of life or severity of disease in the usual classical model, with item response modeling it will give 32 levels.

The following type of data are suitable for item response modeling. A sub-domain of mental depression after a myocardial event is assessed with five items (answer yes/no): (1) not hopeful, (2) blue feeling, (3) tired in the morning, (4) worrier, (5) not talking. If we review the answers, we may observe that, for example, the items (4) and (5) are less often confirmed by our test sample subjects than the other three items. They may, therefore, be expressions of a more severe level of depression. Item response models, unlike the classical models for psychometric assessments, account for and make use of the different levels of severity of items in a test battery. By doing so they change largely qualitative data into fairly accurate quantitative data. They use for that purpose the (slight) differences between individual patients in response pattern to a set of items.

The results of the item response model are fitted to a standard normal Gaussian curve. Both the chi-square goodness of fit and the Kolmogorov-Smirnov (KS) goodness of fit test can be used to assess how closely the results actually follow the Gaussian curve, respectively using a significant chi-square value (Cleophas et al. 2009b) and using the largest cumulative difference between observed and expected frequencies according to the KS table (Cleophas et al. 2009c), as criteria for adequacy of the model for making predictions.

3 Quality Of Life Assessment

As an example we will now analyze the five-item of a mobility-domain of a quality of life battery for patients with coronary artery disease in a group of 1,000 patients. Instead of five many more items can be included. However, for the purpose of the simplicity we will again use five items: the domain mobility in a quality of life battery was assessed by answering "yes or no" to experienced difficulty (1) while climbing stair, (2) on short distances, (3) on long distances, (4) on light household

Table 39.1 A summary of a 5-item mobility-domain quality of life data of 1,000 anginal patients

No. response pattern	Response pattern (1 = yes, 2 = no) to items 1–5	Observed frequencies
1.	11111	4
2.	11112	7
3.	11121	3
4.	11122	12
5.	11211	2
6.	11212	2
7.	11221	4
8.	11222	5
9.	12111	2
10.	12112	9
11.	12121	1
12.	12122	17
13.	12211	1
14.	12212	4
15.	12221	3
16.	12222	16
17.	21111	11
18.	21112	30
19.	21121	15
20.	21122	21
21.	21211	4
22.	21212	29
23.	21221	16
24.	21222	81
25.	22111	17
26.	22112	57
27.	22121	22
28.	22122	174
29.	22211	12
30.	22212	62
31.	22221	29
32.	22222	263
		1,000

work, (5) on heavy household work. In Table 39.1 the data of 1,000 patients are summarized. These data can be fitted into a standard normal Gaussian frequency distribution curve (Fig. 39.1). From the Fig. 39.1 it can be seen that the items used here are more adequate for demonstrating low quality of life than they are for demonstrating high quality of life, but, nonetheless, an entire Gaussian distribution can be extrapolated from the data given. The lack of histogram bars on the right side of the Gaussian curve suggests that more high quality of life items in the questionnaire would be welcome in order to improve the fit of the histogram into the Gaussian curve. Yet it is interesting to observe that, even with a limited set of items, already a fairly accurate frequency distribution pattern of all quality of life levels of the population is obtained.

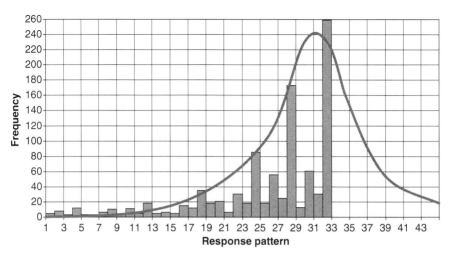

Fig. 39.1 Frequency distribution of response patterns to a 5 item mobility domain of a quality of life battery in 1,000 patients with coronary artery disease. The lack of histogram bars on the *right side* of the Gaussian curve suggests that more high quality of life items in the questionnaire would be welcome in order to improve the fit of the histogram into the Gaussian curve. Yet it is interesting to observe that even with a limited set of items already a fairly accurate frequency distribution pattern of all quality of life levels of the population is obtained

The LTA-2 software program is used (Uebersax 2006). We enter the data file and command: Gaussian error model for IRF shape, chi-square goodness of fit for Fit Statistics, then Frequency table, and, finally, EAP score table. The software program calculates the quality of life scores of the different response patterns as EAP (expected ability a posteriori) scores. These scores can be considered as the z-values of a normal Gaussian curve, meaning that the associated areas under curve of the Gaussian curve is an estimate of the level of quality of life.

There is, approximately,

a 50% quality of life level with an EAP score of 0,
a 35% QOL level with an EAP score of −1 (standard deviations),
a 2.5% QOL level with an EAP score of −2
a 85% QOL level with an EAP score of +1
a 97.5% QOL level with an EAP score of +2

In Table 39.2 the EAP scores per response pattern is given as well as the AUC (= quality of life level) values as calculated by the software program are given. In the fourth column the classical score is given ranging from 0 (no yes answers) to 5 (5 yes answers).

It can be observed, that, unlike the classical scores, running from 0% to 100%, the item scores are more precise and vary from 3.4% to 74.5% with an overall mean score, by definition, of 50%. The item response model produced an adequate fit for the data as demonstrated by chi-square goodness of fit values/degrees of freedom of 0.86. What is even more important, is, that we have 32 different QOL scores instead of no more than five as observed with the classical score method. With six items the

Table 39.2 Results of the item response analysis of the data from Table 39.1

No. response pattern	Response pattern (1 = yes, 2 = no) to items 1–5	EAP scores (SDs)	AUCs (QOL levels) (%)	Classical scores (0–5)
1.	11111	−1.8315	3.4	0
2.	11112	−1.4425	7.5	1
3.	11121	−1.4153	7.8	1
4.	11122	−1.0916	15.4	2
5.	11211	−1.2578	10.4	1
6.	11212	−0.8784	18.9	2
7.	11221	−0.8600	19.4	2
8.	11222	−0.4596	32.3	3
9.	12111	−1.3872	8.2	1
10.	12112	−0.9946	16.1	2
11.	12121	−0.9740	16.6	2
12.	12122	−0.5642	28.8	3
13.	12211	−0.8377	20.1	2
14.	12212	−0.4389	33.0	3
15.	12221	−0.4247	33.4	3
16.	12222	0.0074	50.4	4
17.	21111	−1.3501	8.9	1
18.	21112	−0.9381	17.4	2
19.	21121	−0.9172	17.9	2
20.	21122	−0.4866	31.2	3
21.	21211	−0.7771	21.8	2
22.	21212	−0.3581	35.9	3
23.	21221	−0.3439	36.7	3
24.	21222	0.1120	54.4	4
25.	22111	−0.8925	18.7	2
26.	22112	−0.4641	32.3	3
27.	22121	−0.4484	32.6	3
28.	22122	0.0122	50.4	4
29.	22211	−0.3231	37.5	3
30.	22212	0.1322	55.2	4
31.	22221	0.1433	55.6	4
32.	22222	0.6568	74.5	5

EAP expected ability a posteriori, *QOL* quality of life

numbers of scores would even rise to 64. The interpretation is: the higher the score, the better the quality of life.

4   Clinical and Laboratory Diagnostic-Testing

So far item response modeling has not been used clinical diagnostic procedures. Suppose that instead of five items predicting about quality of life to be answered with a yes or no, we have five vascular-laboratory tests predicting about the presence of peripheral vascular disease, for example (1) an ankle pressure < brachial pressure, (2) a reduction of ankle pressure after 5 min treadmill >25%, (3) a proximal thigh pressure >35 mmHg below brachial, (4) segmental pressures (thigh, calf, ankle) >20 mmHg difference, and (5) a toe pressure <35% different from brachial. Similarly to the above sample, response patterns can be obtained from a data file of patients in analysis for peripheral vascular disease. The classical and item response scores from the response patterns tell us something about the expected magnitude of the vascular disease, but the item response model performs better than the classical score, because the classical score only gives the numbers of positive tests as estimators, while the item response model gives 32 levels injury. The larger the score, the more severe the disease. In 1,350 patients the predictors were measured. The data file was entered in the above LTA-2 analysis program (Uebersax 2006). In Table 39.3 the results of the analysis is given. The areas under the curve present the item response scores. They run from 9.9% to 83.5%. For each response pattern a separate score is produced by the analysis. The item response model produced an adequate fit for the data as demonstrated by chi-square goodness of fit values/degrees of freedom of 0.64.

When using the above item response scores and classical scores in simulated trials, it is observed, as expected, that the item response score method provides a much better sensitivity to demonstrate significant effects than does the classical score method (Table 39.4). This is so both with parallel-group and crossover designs.

5   Discussion

Do we have to assess item response models for reliability/validity? In the above laboratory test example the items were based on add-up sums of previously validated predictors. However, otherwise, they are used here in a somewhat different context, and psychological and quality of life items are generally not based on previously validated predictors. An important advantage of item response models is that they, strictly, do not require parallel tests for such purposes. This is, because the data are internally "sort of" tested for reliability:

1. ability levels of patients are tested against difficulty levels of items,
2. quality of life levels of patients are tested against quality of life levels of the items,
3. health levels of patients are tested against the health predicting levels of the items.

Yet both patient-levels and item-levels are unknown, but they have a meaningful interaction, and this interaction is mainly measured with item response modeling.

A problem is, of course, that the data should fit the Gaussian distribution, but various goodness of fit tests are available for that purpose. The software program applied in the above example makes by default use of chi-square goodness of fit tests, and the analysis does not proceed if an adequate goodness of fit is not obtained.

Table 39.3 Results of item response analysis of 5 laboratory predictors of peripheral vascular disease in 1,350 patients

No. response pattern	Response pattern (1 = yes, 2 = no) to items 1–5	EAP scores (SDs)	AUCs (severity of disease levels) (%)	Classical scores (0–5)
1.	11111	−1.97	12.4	0
2.	11112	−1.61	15.4	1
3.	11121	−2.04	12.1	1
4.	11122	−1.55	16.1	2
5.	11211	−1.73	14.2	1
6.	11212	−1.35	18.9	2
7.	11221	−0.85	19.1	2
8.	11222	−0.46	32.3	3
9.	12111	−1.55	16.1	1
10.	12112	−1.34	9.9	2
11.	12121	−0.80	21.1	2
12.	12122	−0.74	23.0	3
13.	12211	−0.61	27.2	2
14.	12212	−0.44	33.0	3
15.	12221	−0.51	33.4	3
16.	12222	−1.55	16.1	4
17.	21111	−0.56	28.9	1
18.	21112	−0.35	36.2	2
19.	21121	−0.31	37.9	2
20.	21122	0.00	50.2	3
21.	21211	0.00	50.1	2
22.	21212	−0.05	48.1	3
23.	21221	0.23	59.1	3
24.	21222	0.26	60.0	4
25.	22111	0.47	68.2	2
26.	22112	0.06	52.3	3
27.	22121	0.60	72.6	3
28.	22122	0.01	50.4	4
29.	22211	−0.32	37.5	3
30.	22212	0.69	75.3	4
31.	22221	0.73	76.6	4
32.	22222	0.97	83.5	5

EAP expected ability a posteriori, *AUC* area under the curve of Standard Gaussian curve, an estimate of the severity of a disease

Logistic models for predicting risk factors, based on exponential relationships between the predictor and the outcome, have been demonstrated to provide an adequate fit for risk profiling in clinical disease and other fields, and seems to better fit data than does linear modeling. The same may be true with binary quality of life and diagnostic laboratory data. However, more studies are required. Yet, we believe that item response modeling has great potential for improving the accuracy and precision of quality of life and laboratory research.

Table 39.4 When using the item response scores and classical scores from Table 39.3 in simulated trials, it is observed, as expected, that the item response score method provides a much better sensitivity to demonstrate significant effects than does the classical score method. This is so both with parallel-group and crossover designs

Parallel-group study

	Item response scores		Classical scores	
	Group 1	Group 2	Group 1	Group 2
	16.1	33.4	2	3
	18.9	28.9	2	1
	32.3	36.2	3	2
	9.9	50.2	2	3
	23.0	48.1	3	3
	33.0	60.0	4	4
	16.1	52.3	4	3
	36.2	50.4	2	4
	50.2	75.3	3	4
	48.1	83.5	3	5
Mean scores	28.38	51.83	2.7	3.2
Standard deviation	13.843	17.477	0.6749	1.1353
Mean difference	23.45		0.50	
Standard error	7.05		0.42	
	t-value = 3.1		t-value = 1.19	
	p < 0.01		Not significant	

Crossover study

Patient no	Item response	Scores	Differences	Classical	Scores	Differences
1.	16.1	33.4	−17.3	2	3	−1
2.	18.9	28.9	−10.0	2	1	1
3.	32.3	36.2	−3.9	3	2	1
4.	9.9	50.2	−40.3	2	3	−1
5.	23.0	48.1	−25.1	3	3	0
6.	33.0	60.0	−27.0	3	4	−1
7.	16.1	52.3	−36.2	4	3	1
8.	36.2	50.4	−14.2	2	4	−2
9.	50.2	75.3	−25.2	3	4	−1
10.	48.1	83.5	−35.4	3	5	−2
Mean difference			−23.46			−0.7
Standard error			3.79			0.9
			t-value = 6.19			t-value = 0.78
			p < 0.002			Not significant

What is even more important, it does enable to make more exact estimations in individual patients than classical methods do. Also, being more precise and sensitive, it should be more so to estimate patients that have missing data.

We should discuss some limitation of the novel approach. Unlike the classical methods item response modeling is an invariant method, which means that each item is applied as point estimate without variance. This explains part of the sensitivity of the method, but at the same time means that some dispersion in the data is at risk of being underestimated. However, invariant tests are common in physics, and have received increasing attention in clinical research. For example, Fisher exact tests and log likelihood ratio tests are of this kind. In addition, with item response modeling it may be, particularly, justified not to include variance, calculated as (squared) distances from mean scores, because the individual data are scored against a continuum of scores.

We hope that this brief introduction will stimulate clinical investigators to pay more attention to the possibilities item response modeling offers.

6   Conclusions

Item response models using exponential modeling are more sensitive than classical linear methods for making predictions from psychological questionnaires. This chapter is to assess whether they can also be used for making predictions from quality of life questionnaires and clinical and laboratory diagnostic-tests.

Of 1,000 anginal patients assessed for quality of life and 1,350 patients assessed for peripheral vascular disease with diagnostic laboratory tests items response modeling was applied using the Latent Trait Analysis program-2 of Uebersax.

The 32 different response patterns obtained from test batteries of 5 items produced 32 different quality of life scores ranging from 3.4% to 74.5% and 32 different levels peripheral vascular disease ranging from 9.9% to 83.5% with overall mean scores, by definition, of 50%, while the classical method for analysis only produced the discrete scores 0–5. The item response models produced an adequate fit for the data as demonstrated by chi-square goodness of fit values/degrees of freedom of 0.86 and 0.64.

We conclude:

1. Quality of life assessments and diagnostic tests can be analyzed through item response modeling, and provide more sensitivity than do classical linear models.
2. Item response modeling can change largely qualitative data into fairly accurate quantitative data, and can, even with limited sets of items, produce fairly accurate frequency distribution patterns of quality of life, severity of disease, and other latent traits.

References

Anonymous (1991) Egret manual. Statistics and Epidemiology Research Computing. University of Seattle, Seattle
Baker FB, Kim SH (2004) Item response theory: parameter estimation techniques. Marcel Dekker, New York

Cleophas TJ, Zwinderman AH, Cleophas TF, Cleophas EP (2009a) Lack of sensitivity of quality of life (QOL) assessments. In: Statistics applied to clinical trials, 4th edn. Springer, Dordrecht, pp 323–329

Cleophas TJ, Zwinderman AH, Cleophas TF, Cleophas EP (2009b) Method 1: the chi-square goodness of fit test. In: Statistics applied to clinical trials, 4th edn. Springer, Dordrecht, pp 356–357

Cleophas TJ, Zwinderman AH, Cleophas TF, Cleophas EP (2009c) Method 2: the Kolmogorov-Smirnov goodness of fit test. In: Statistics applied to clinical trials, 4th edn. Springer, Dordrecht, pp 357–359

Conquest Generalized Item Response Modeling Software. www.rasch.org/rmt/rmt133o.htm. Accessed 15 Dec 2011

Cook KF, Teal CR, Bjorner JB, Celia D et al (2007) Item response theory health data analysis project: an overview and summary. Qual Life Res 16(s1):121–132

De Boeck P, Wilson M (2004) Explanatory item response models. A generalized linear and non-linear approach. Springer, New York

Douglas JA (1999) Item response models for longitudinal quality of life data in clinical trials. Stat Med 18:2917–2931

Fischer GH (1974) Einfuhrung in die Theorie psychologischer Tests. Huber, Bern

Full Lifecycle Unified Modeling Language Modeling Software. www.sparxsystems.eu/?gclid. Accessed 15 Dec 2011

Glas CA, Ellis J (1993) Rasch Scaling Program (RSP) I.E.C. University of Groningen, Groningen

Item Response Modeling with BILOG-MG and MULTILOG for Windows. www.eric.ed.gov/ERICWebPortal/custom/portlets/recorDetails/detailminii.jsp. Accessed 15 Dec 2011

Kessler RC, Mrocek DK (1995) Measuring the effects of medical interventions. Med Care 33:109–119

Rasch G (1980) Probabilistic models from intelligence and attainment tests, expanded edn. The University of Chicago Press, Chicago

Reeve BB, Hays RD, Chang CH, Perfetto E (2007) Applying item response theory to health outcomes. Qual Life Res 16(s1):1–3

Teresi JA, Fleishman JA (2007) Differential item functioning and health. Qual Life Res 16(s1):33–42

Uebersax J (2006) Free Software LTA (latent trait analysis) -2 (with binary items). www.john-uebersax.com/stat/Ital.htm. Accessed 15 Dec 2011

Uttaro T, Lehman A (1999) Graded response modeling of the quality of life interview. Program Plan 22:41–52

Van der Linden WJ, Veldkamp BP (2004) Constraining item exposure in computer adaptive testing with shadow tests. J Educ Behav Stat 29:273–291

Verhelst ND (1993) One parameter Logistic Model (OPLM). CITO, Arnhem

Zwinderman AH (1991) A generalized Rasch model with manifest predictors. Psychometrika 33:AS 109–AS 119

Zwinderman AH, Niemeijer MG, Kleinjans HA, Cleophas TJ (1998) Application of item response modeling for quality of life assessment. In: Kuhlmann J, Mrozikiewicz A (eds) Clinical Pharmacology, vol 16. What should a clinical pharmacologist know to start a clinical trial (phase I and II). Zuckschwerd Verlag, Munich, pp 48–55

Chapter 40
Statistical Analysis of Genetic Data

1 Introduction

In 1860, the benchmark experiments of the monk Gregor Mendel led him to propose the existence of genes. The results of Mendel's pea data were astoundingly close to those predicted by his theory. When we recently looked into Mendel's pea data and performed a chi-square test, we had to conclude the chi-square value was too small not to reject the null-hypothesis. This would mean that Mendel's reported data were so close to what he expected that we could only conclude that he had somewhat fudged the data (Table 40.1).

Though Mendel may have somewhat fudged some of his data, he started a novel science that now 140 years later is the largest growing field in biomedicine. This novel science, although in its first steps, already has a major impact on the life of all of us. For example, obtaining enough drugs, like insulin and many others, to treat illnesses worldwide was a problem that has been solved by recombinant DNA technology which enabled through genetic engineering of bacteria or yeasts the large scale production of various pharmaceutical compounds. The science of genes, often called genomics, is vast, and this chapter only briefly mentions a few statistical techniques developed for processing data of genetic research. We will start with the explanation of a few terms typically used in genomics.

T.J. Cleophas and A.H. Zwinderman, *Statistics Applied to Clinical Studies*, DOI 10.1007/978-94-007-2863-9_40, © Springer Science+Business Media B.V. 2012

Table 40.1 Chi-square-distribution not only has a right but also a left tail

Phenotype	A	a
B	AB 27	aB 271
b	Ab 9	ab 93

We reject the null-hypothesis of no difference with 1 degree of freedom if chi-square is larger than 3.84 or smaller than 0.004. In Mendel's data frequently very small chi-squares can be observed, as e.g., in the above example where it is as small as 0.0039. This means that the chi-square is too small not to reject the null-hypothesis. The results are closer to what can be expected than compatible with the assumption of a normal distribution. The obvious explanation is that Mendel somewhat mispresented his data

2   Some Terminology

Bayes' Theorem (Table 40.2)	Posterior odds = likelihood ratio × prior odds This approach is required for making predictions from genetic data. Although the general concept of including prior evidence in the statistical analysis of clinical trial data is appealing, this concept should not be applied in usual null-hypothesis testing, because we would have to violate the main assumption of null-hypothesis testing that H_0 and H_1 have the same frequency distribution.
Posterior odds (Table 40.2)	Prior odds adjusted for likelihood ratio.
Prior odds (Table 40.2)	Prior probability of being a carrier/prior probability of being no carrier.
Likelihood ratio (Table 40.2)	Probability for carriers of having healthy offspring/probability for non-carrier of having healthy offspring.
Genetic linkage	When two genes or DNA sequences are located near each other on the same chromosome, they are linked. When they are not close, crossing over occurs frequently. However, when they are close they tend to be inherited together. Genetic linkage is useful in genetic diagnosis and mapping because once you know that the disease gene is linked to a particular DNA sequence that is close, the latter can be used as a marker to identify the disease gene indirectly. Bayes' Theorem can be used to combine experimental data with prior linkage probabilities as established.
Autosomal	Not x- or y-chromosome linked.
Heterosomal	X- or y-chromosome linked.
Dominant gene	Gene that is expressed in the phenotype.
Recessive gene	Gene that is expressed in the phenotype only if it is present in two complementary chromosomes.
Haplotype	Group of genetic markers linked together on a single chromosome, such as a group of DNA-sequences.

(continued)

(continued)

Haploid genome	Chromosomes of haploid cell (23 chromosomes, 50,000–100,000 genes).
Diploid cell	Cell with 46 chromosomes.
Chromosome	2,000–5,000 genes.
Chromosomal microband	50–100 genes.
Gene	$1.5–2,000\cdot10^3$ base-pairs.
Genomic medicine	Use of genotypic analysis to enhance quality of care.
Complex disease traits	Multifactorial diseases where multiple genes and non-genetic factors interact.
Allele	Gene derived from one parent.
Homozygous	Having identical alleles.
Heterozygous	Having different alleles.
DNA- cloning	Isolation of DNA fragments and their insertion into the nucleic acid from another biologic vector for manipulation.
DNA probe	Cloned DNA fragment used for diagnostic or therapeutic purpose.
Hybridization of single stranded DNA	Double-stranded DNA is dissociated into single -stranded, which can then be used to detect complementary strands.
Blotting procedures	Southern, Northern, Immuno-, Western blotting are all procedures to hybridize target DNA in solution to known DNA-sequences fixed on a membrane support.
Polymerase chain reaction	Oligonucleotide of known nucleic acid sequence is incubated with the target DNA and then amplified with DNA polymerase.
DNA chips	Arrays of oligonucleotides on miniature supports developed for the analysis of unknown DNA sequences, taking advantage of the complementary nature of nucleic acid interaction.
Mutations	Changes in DNA either heritable or obtained.
Introns	Non-coding regions of the gene.
Exons	Coding regions of the gene.
Single gene disorders	One gene plays a predominant role in determining disease.
Genotype	Chemical structure of a gene.
Phenotype	Clinical characteristics of a gene.
Gene expression	Regulation of gene function is mediated at a transcriptional level through helix-turn-helix proteins and at a posttranscriptional level through various hormones, autacoids and many more factors.

3   Genetics, Genomics, Proteonomics, Data Mining

In the past two or three decades the role of genetic determinants have increased enormously in biomedical research. Of several monogenetic diseases the genetic foundation has been clarified almost completely (e.g. Huntington's disease), and of others the contribution of many genetic markers has been proved: for instance the

Table 40.2 Bayes' Theorem, an important approach for the analysis of genetic data: example

Based on historical data the chance for girls in a particular family of being carrier for the hemophilia A gene is 50%. Those who are carrier will have a chance of ½×½=¼=25% that two sons are healthy. Those who are no carriers will have a 100% chance of two healthy sons. This would mean that a girl from this population who had two healthy sons is 500/125=4 times more likely to be no carrier than to be carrier. In terms of Bayes' Theorem:		
Posterior odds=prior odds×likelihood ratio.		
Prior probability of being carrier=50%		
Prior odds=50: 50=1.0		
Likelihood ratio=probability for carrier of having two healthy sons/probability for non-carrier of having two healthy sons=25%/100%=0.25 posterior odds=1.0 times 0.25=25% or 1 in 4:		
if you saw many girls from this family you would see one carrier for every four non-carriers.		
Mothers with two sons who are:	Carrier n=500	No carrier n=500
Two sons healthy	n=125	n=500
Two sons not healthy	n=375	n=0

brca 1 and 2 genes in breast cancer (Cornelisse et al. 1996), and the mismatch gene mutations in coloncarcinoma (Wijnen et al. 1998). Simultaneously, the human genome project has been the catalyst for the development of several high-throughput technologies that have made it possible to map and sequence complex genomes. These technologies are used, and will be used increasingly in clinical trials for many purposes but predominantly to identify genetic variants, and differentially expressed genes that are associated with better or worse clinical efficacy in clinical trials. In addition, the proteins associated with these genes are being investigated to disentangle their roles in the biochemical and physiological pathways of the disease and the treatment that is being studied. Together these technologies are called (high-throughput) genetics, genomics, and proteomics.

The technological advancements have made it possible to measure thousands of genes/proteins of a single patient simultaneously, and the possibility to evaluate the role of each gene/protein in differentiating between e.g. responders and non-responders to therapy. This has increased the statistical problem of multiple testing hugely, but also has stimulated research into statistical methods to deal with it. In addition methods have been developed to consider the role of clusters of genes. In this chapter we will describe a number of these new techniques for the analysis of high throughput genetic data, and for the analysis of gene-expression data. We restrict the discussion to data that are typically sampled in clinical trials including unrelated individuals only. Familial data are extremely important to investigate genetic associations: their clustered structure requires dedicated statistical techniques but these fall outside the scope of this chapter.

4   Genomics

In the mid-1970s, molecular biologists developed molecular cloning and DNA sequencing. Automated DNA sequencing and the invention of the polymerase chain reaction (PCR) made it possible to sequence the entire human genome. This has

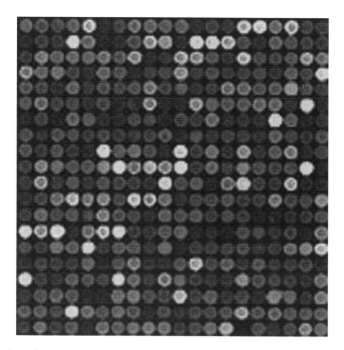

Fig. 40.1 Example of microarray of different expression of about 500 genes in tumour tissue of a single patient

lead to the development of microarrays, sometimes known as DNA-chip technology. Microarrays are ordered sets of DNA molecules of known sequence. Usually rectangular, they can consist of a few hundred to thousands of sets. Each individual feature goes on the array at a precisely defined location on the substrate, and thereafter, labeled cDNA from a test and a reference RNA sample are pooled and co-hybridized. Labeling can be done in several ways, but is usually done with different fluorescently labeled nucleotides (usually Cy5-dCTP for reference, and Cy3-dCTP for test RNA). After stimulation, the expression of these genes can be measured. This involves quantifying the test and reference signals of each fluorophore for each element on the array, traditionally by confocal laser scanning. The ratio of the test and reference signals is commonly used to indicate whether genes have differential expression. Many resources are available on the web concerning the production of microarrays, and about designing microarray experiments (e.g.: 123genomics. homestead.com). A useful textbook is that of Jordan (2001).

An example of a microarray is given in Fig. 40.1. This concerns the differential expression of about 500 genes in tumour tissue of a single patient with gastric tumour.

Each spot in this chip represents a different gene, and the ratio of the two fluorescent dyes indicates whether the genes are over-expressed (dark) or under-expressed (pale) in the tumor tissue with respect to normal tissue. The transformation of the image into gene expression numbers is not trivial: the spots have to be identified on

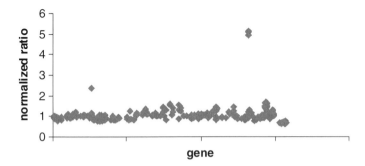

Fig. 40.2 Normalized ratios of the array from Fig. 40.1

the chip, their boundaries defined, the fluorescence intensity measured, and compared to the background intensity. Usually this 'image processing' is done automatically by the image analysis software, but sometimes laborious manual adjustments are necessary. One of the most popular systems for image analysis is ScanAlyze (http://rana.stanford.edu/software).

After the image analysis, differential expression is measured by a so-called normalized ratio of the two fluorescence signals, normalized to several experimental factors. The normalized ratios of the array in Fig. 40.1 are given in Fig. 40.2. On the x-axis are given the 500 genes, and on the y-axis is given the normalized ratio of each gene.

It is obvious that most genes have a ratio around unity, but three or four genes are highly over-expressed with ratios above two. It is typically assumed that ratios larger than 1.5 or 2.0 are indicative of a significant change in gene expression. These estimates are very crude, however, because the reliability of ratios depends on the two absolute intensities. On statistical grounds, moreover, we would expect a number of genes to show differential expression purely by chance (Claverie 2001).

One way of circumventing the multiple testing problem here, is to use a mixture model (McLachlan 2001). Usually, it is assumed that the sample of ratios consists of subgroups of genes with normal, under-, and over-expression. In each subgroup, the ratios are mostly assumed to be normally distributed. When the sample is large enough, the percentage of normal, under-, and over-expressed genes, and associated mean ratios and standard deviations can be estimated from the data. This can be done with the logarithmically transformed ratios. The histogram of the log-transformed ratios in Fig. 40.2 is given in Fig. 40.3, together with the three estimated normal distributions. In this model the probability of each gene of being over- of under-expressed can be calculated using Bayes' theorem.

Although under-expressed genes could not be identified in this case, over-expressed genes were clearly seen, represented by the second mode to the right. Actually it was estimated that 14% of the genes showed over-expression, corresponding with ratios larger than 1.3.

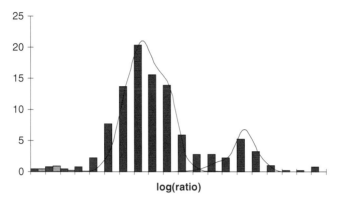

Fig. 40.3 The histogram of the log-transformed ratios from Fig. 40.2, calculated according to Bayes' Theorem

Above is illustrated how to look at the data of a single microarray. For the analysis of a set of microarrays several different approaches are used. Two distinctions can be used: supervised or unsupervised data analysis, and hypotheses-driven or data-mining. For supervised data analysis additional data must be available to which the expression data can be related. In clinical trials a major question is often how responders and non-responders can be distinguished. Relating such response data to expression data can be done using well known techniques such as discriminant-analysis, or logistic regression. Since there may be hundreds or thousands of expression variables, one must be careful in applying these techniques, and cross-validation is often extremely useful (Alizadeh et al. 2000). Unsupervised data analysis is usually done by cluster analysis or principal component analysis to find groups of co-regulated genes or related samples. These techniques are often applied without specific prior knowledge on which genes are involved in which case the analysis is a kind of data-mining. An example of a hypothesis driven analysis is to pick a potential interesting gene, and then find a group of similar or anti-correlated expression profiles.

Cluster-analysis is the most popular method currently used as the first step in gene expression analysis. Several variants have been developed: hierarchical (Eisen et al. 1998), and k-means (Tavazoie et al. 1999) clustering, self-organizing maps (Tamayo et al. 1999), and gene-shaving (Tibshirani et al. 1999), and there are many more. All aim at finding groups of genes with similar properties. These techniques can be viewed as a dimensionality reduction technique, since the many thousands of genes are reduced to a few groups of similarly behaving genes. Again many tools are available on the web, and a useful site to start searching is: www.microarray.org. We used Michael Eisen's package (Eisen et al. 1998) to cluster the expression data of 18 patients with gastric cancer. The typical output of a hierarchical clustering analysis is given in Fig. 40.4. This is a dendogram illustrating the similarities

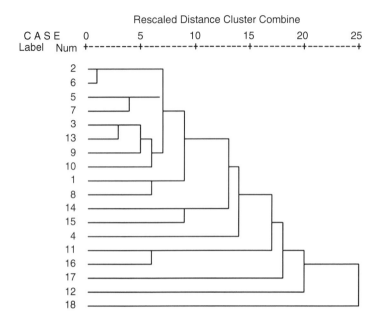

Fig. 40.4 The typical hierarchical clustering analysis of the expression data of 18 patients with gastric cancer

between patients, a similar graph can be obtained illustrating similarities between genes. In the present case one might conclude that patients 2, 6, 5, 7, 3, 13, 9, 10, 1 and 8 form a cluster, and patients 14, 15, 4, 11, 16, 17, 12, and 18 another cluster. But identifying more clusters may be meaningful too.

In a K-means cluster analysis the number of clusters must be specified a priori. When we specify two clusters, the same solution is found as above.

The above results illustrate that many subjective decisions need to be made in a cluster analysis, and such analysis cannot be regarded as hypothesis-driven; the primary output of a cluster analysis are new hypotheses concerning differential expressions.

5   Conclusions

Although high throughput methods are still relatively expensive, and are not used routinely in clinical trials, these methods undoubtedly will be used more often in the future. Their promise of identifying subgroups of patients with varying drug response is of major importance and is a major topic of pharmaco-genomics. In addition, differential expression profiles, and proteomics are of major importance of identifying new pathways for targeting new drugs. More sophisticated statistical methods are required, and will be developed.

References

Alizadeh AA et al (2000) Distinct types of diffuse large B-cell lymphoma identified by gene expression profiling. Nature 403:503–511

Claverie JM (2001) Computational methods for the identification of differential and coordinated gene expression. Hum Mol Genet 8(10):1821–1832

Cornelisse CJ, Cornelis RS, Devilee P (1996) Genes responsible for familial breast cancer. Pathol Res Pract 192(7):684–693

Eisen M et al (1998) Cluster analysis and display of genome-wide expression patterns. Proc Natl Acad Sci USA 95:14863–14867

Jordan B (ed) (2001) DNA microarrays: gene expression applications. Springer, Berlin

McLachlan G (2001) Mixture.model clustering of microarray expression data. Australian Biometrics and New Zealand Statistical Association Joint Conference. Christchurch, New Zealand

Tamayo P et al (1999) Interpreting patterns of gene-expression with self-organizing maps. Proc Natl Acad Sci USA 96:2907–2912

Tavazoie S et al (1999) Systematic determination of genetic network architecture. Nat Genet 22:281–285

Tibshirani R et al (1999) Clustering methods for the analysis of DNA microarray data. Technical report. Stanford University, Dept of Statistics, Stanford

Wijnen JT, Vasen HF, Khan PM, Zwinderman AH, van der Klift H, Mulder A, Tops C, Moller P, Fodde R (1998) Clinical findings with implications for genetic testing in families with clustering of colorectal cancer. N Engl J Med 339(8):511–518

Chapter 41
Relationship Among Statistical Distributions

1 Introduction

Samples of clinical data are frequently assessed through three variables:

The mean result of the data.
The spread or variability of the data.
The sample size.

Generally, we are primarily interested in the first variable, but mean or proportion does not tell the whole story, and the spread of the data may be more relevant. For example, when studying how two drugs reach various organs, the mean level may be the same for both, but one drug may be more variable than the other. In some cases, too little and, in other cases, dangerously high levels get through. The Chi-square-distribution, unlike the normal distribution, is used for the assessment of such variabilities. Clinical scientists although they are generally familiar with the concept of null-hypothesis testing of normally distributed data, have difficulties to understand the null-hypothesis testing of Chi-square-distributed data, and do not know how closely Chi-square is related to the normal-distribution or the T-distribution. The Chi-square-distribution has a relatively young history. It has been invented by K. Pearson (1900) 100 years ago, 300 years after the invention of the normal-distribution (A. de Moivre 1667–1754). The Chi-square-distribution and its extensions have become the basis of modern statistics and have provided statisticians with a relatively simple device to analyze complex data, including multiple groups and multivariable variables analyses. The present chapter was written for clinical investigators/scientists in order to better understand the relation between normal and chi-square distribution, and how they are being applied for the purpose of null-hypothesis testing.

2   Variances

Repeated observations exhibit a central tendency, the mean, but, in addition, exhibit spread or dispersion, the tendency to depart from central tendency. If measurement of central tendency is thought of as good bets, then measures of spread represent the poorness of central tendency otherwise called deviation or error. The larger such deviations are, the more do cases differ from each other and the more spread does the distribution show. What we need is an index to reflect this spread or variability. First of all, why not simply take the average of the deviations (d-values) about the mean as measure of variability:

$$\Sigma\left(d\,/\,n\right) \text{ where n = sample size.}$$

This, however, will not work, because when we add up negative and positive departures from the mean, our overall variance will equal zero. A device to get around this difficulty is to take the square of each deviation:

$$\Sigma\left(d^2\,/\,n\right) \text{ is defined the variance of n observations.}$$

Σ (d/n), although it can not be used as index to reflex variability, can be readily used to define the mean of a sample of repeated observations, if the size of observations is taken as distance from zero rather than mean. Suddenly, means and variances look a lot the same, and it is no surprise that statistical curves and tables used to assess either of them are closely related. A Chi-square-distribution is nothing else than the distribution of square values of a normal-distribution. Null-hypothesis-testing-of-variances is much similar to null-hypothesis-testing-of-means. With the latter we reject the null-hypothesis of no effect if our mean is more than 1.96 SEMs (standard errors of the mean) distant from zero. With the latter we reject the null-hypothesis of no effect if our standardized variance is more than 1.96^2 SEMs^2 distant from zero. Because variances are squared and, thus, non-negative values, the Chi-square approach can be extended to test hypotheses about many samples. When variances or add-up variances of many samples are larger than allowed for by the Chi-square-distribution-graphs, we reject the probability that our results are from normal distributions, and conclude that our results are significantly different from zero. The Chi-square test is not only adequate to test multiple samples simultaneously, but is also the basis of analysis of variance (ANOVA).

3   The Normal Distribution

The normal distribution curve can be drawn from the formula below.

$$f(x) = \frac{1}{\sqrt{2\pi s^2}}\, e^{-(x-m)^2/2s^2}$$

where s = standard deviation and m = mean value.

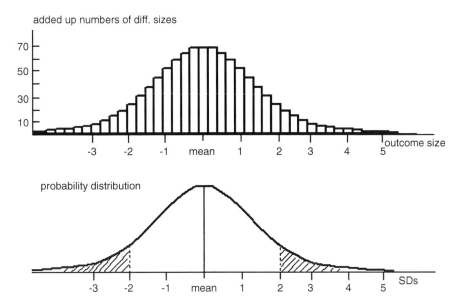

Fig. 41.1 *Upper graph* shows histogram: on the x-axis we have the individual data and on the y-axis we have "how often" (the mean value is observed most frequently, while the bars on both side of the mean gradually grew shorter). *Lower graph* shows normal distribution: the bars on the y-axis have been replaced with a continuous line, it is now impossible to read from the graph how many patients had a particular outcome. Instead, we infer that the total area under the curve (*AUC*) represents 100% of our data, AUC left from the mean represents 50%, left from −1 SD (standard deviation) approximately 15% of the data, and left from −2 SDs approximately 2.5% of the data. This curve although suitable for describing a sample of repeated observations, is not yet adequate for testing statistical hypotheses

Repeated observations in nature do not precisely follow this single mathematical formula, and may even follow largely different patterns. The formula is just an approximation. And so, it is remarkable that the approach works in practice, although the p-values obtained from it are sometimes given inappropriate emphasis. We should not forget that a p-value of <0.001 does not mean that we have proven something for the entire population, but rather that we have proven something on the understanding that our data follow a normal distribution and that our data are representative for the entire population. Frequently, the results as provided by clinical trials are much better than those observed in general practice, because the population follows a different frequency distribution or because the enrollees in a trial are selected groups not representative for the entire population. We wish that more often these possibilities would be accounted by the advocates of evidence-based medicine. If we are willing to accept the above limitations, the normal distribution can be used to try and make predictions, with the understanding that statistical testing cannot give certainties, only chances. How was the normal distribution invented? At first, investigators described their data in the form of histograms (Fig. 41.1 upper graph: on the x-axis the individual data and on the y-axis how often).

Fig. 41.2 Narrow and wide
normal curve: the wide one
summarizes the data of our
trial, the narrow one
summarizes the means of
many trials similar to our trial

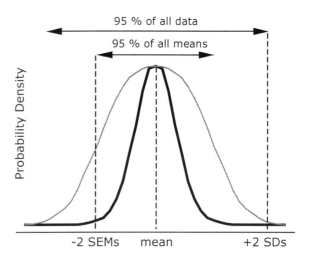

Often, the mean value is observed most frequently, while the bars on both side of
the mean gradually grow shorter. From this histogram to a normal distribution curve
is a short step (Fig. 41.1 lower graph). The bars on the y-axis have been replaced by
a continuous line. It is now impossible to read from the graph how many patients
had a particular outcome. Instead, relevant inferences can be made: the total area
under the curve (AUC) presents 100% of our data, AUC left from the mean presents
50%, left from −1 SD (standard deviation) approximately 15% of the data, and left
from −2 SDs approximately 2.5% of the data. This curve although suitable for
describing a sample of repeated observations, is not yet adequate for testing statistical hypotheses. For that purpose, a narrow normal curve is required (Fig. 41.2).

The narrow and wide curve from Fig. 41.2 are both based on the same data, but have
different meaning. The wide (with SDs on the x-axis) one summarizes the data of our
trial, the narrow one (with SEMs (standard errors of the mean) on the x-axis) summarizes the means of many trials similar to ours. This may be difficult to understand, but
our sample is representative, and it is easy to conceive that the distributions of means
of many similar samples from the same population will be narrower and have fewer
outliers than the distribution of the actual data. This concept is relevant, because we
want to use it for making predictions from our data to the entire population.

We should add here that there is only a small difference between the normal and
the t-distribution. The latter is a bit wider with small numbers. The chi-square distribution makes no difference between normally and t-like distributed data.

4   Null-Hypothesis Testing with the Normal or t-Distribution

What does "null-hypothesis" mean: we hypothesize that if the result of our trial is
not different from zero, we have a negative trial. What does the null-hypothesis look
like in graph? Figure 41.3 shows H_1, the graph based on the data of our trial with
SEMs on the x-axis (z-axis), and H_0, the same graph with a mean of 0.

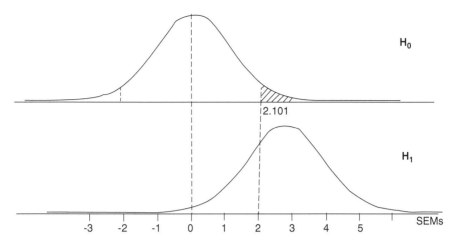

Fig. 41.3 H_1 is the graph based on the data of our trial with SEMs on the x-axis (z-axis), and H_0 is the same graph with mean 0 (mean $\pm$ SEM $= 0 \pm 1$)

Now we make a giant leap from our data to the entire population, and we can do so, because we assume, that our data are representative for the entire population. H_1 is also the summary of the means of many trials similar to our trial. If we repeated the trial, differences would be small and the summary would look alike. H_0 is also the summary of the means of many trials similar to our trial, but with an overall effect of 0. Our mean is not 0, but 2.9. Still it could be an outlier of may studies with an overall effect of 0. So, think from now on of H_0 as distribution of the means of many trials with overall effect 0. If hypothesis 0 is true, then the mean of our study is part of H_0. We can not prove this, but we can calculate the chance/probability of this possibility. A mean result of 2.9 is far distant from 0. Suppose it belongs to H_0. Only 5% of the H_0-trials are more than 2.1 SEMs distant from 0, because the AUC of $H_0 = 5\%$. Thus, the chance that it belongs to H_0 is less than 5%. We reject the null-hypothesis of no effect concluding that there is less than 5% chance to find this result. In usual terms, we reject the null-hypothesis of no effect at $p < 0.05$ or $< 5\%$.

5 Relationship Between the Normal Distribution and Chi-Square Distribution, Null-Hypothesis Testing with Chi-Square Distribution

The upper graph of Fig. 41.4 shows a normal distribution, on the x-axis individual data expressed as distances from the mean, and on the y-axis "how often" the individual data are being observed. The lower graph of Fig. 41.4 shows what happens of the x-values of this normal distribution is squared. We get no negative x-values

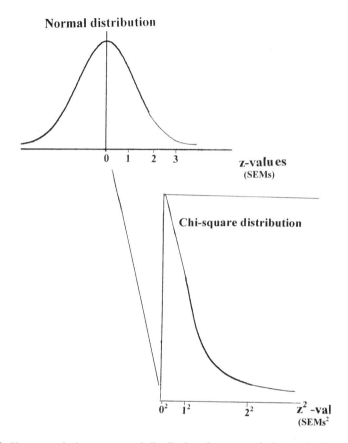

Fig. 41.4 *Upper graph* shows a normal distribution. *Lower graph* shows what happens if the x-values of this normal-like-curve are squared. The normal-curve changes into a Chi-square-curve

anymore, and the x-values 0 and 1 give rise to y-values twice the size, while the new curve is skewed to the right: the new curve is what we call a chi-square curve. The upper curve is used to test the null-hypothesis that the mean result of our trial is significantly different from zero, the lower one to test that our variance is significantly different from zero.

Figure 41.5 shows how things work in practice. The upper graph gives on the x-axis the possible mean result or our trial expressed in units of SEMs, otherwise called z-value, or, with t-test, t-value. On the y-axis we "how often this result will be obtained". If our mean result is more than approximately 2 SEMs (or with normal distribution precisely 1.96 SEMs) distant from zero, this will happen in 5% of the cases, because the AUC right from 1.96 SEMs is 5%. If more than 2.58 distant from zero, this will happen in 1% of the cases. With a result that far from

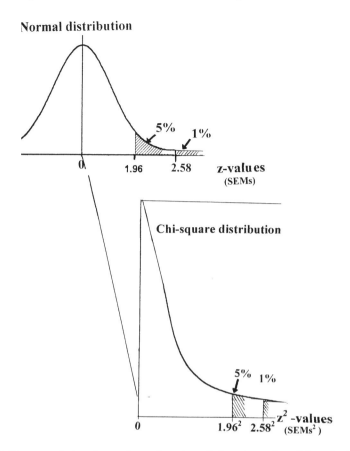

Fig. 41.5 *Upper graph* gives the x-values, otherwise called z-values, of a null-hypothesis of a real normal-distribution. *Lower graph* shows what happens when z-values are squared. The z-distribution turns into a non-negative Chi-square-distribution. *Upper graph*: with z >1.96 the *right-end* AUC <5%; *lower graph*: with $z^2 > (1.96)^2$ the *right-end* AUC <5%

zero we reject the null-hypothesis that our result is not different from 0, and conclude that, obviously, our data are significantly different from 0, at p <5% or 1% (<0.05 or <0.01).

Figure 41.5 lower graph gives a draft of the possible variances of our trial. On the x-axis we have the variance of our trial expressed in units $(SEMs)^2$, otherwise called z^2-values. On the y-axis we have again "how often this variance will be obtained". For example, if our variance is more than 1.96^2 $SEMs^2$ distant from zero, this will happen in less than 5% of the cases. This is so, because the AUC right from $z^2 = 1.96^2$ is 5% of the total AUC of 100%. If our variance is more than $z^2 = 2.58^2$ distant from zero, this chance is 1%. We reject the null-hypothesis that our variance is not significantly different from 0 and we do so at a probability of 1% (p<0.01).

6   Examples of Data Where Variance Is More Important Than Mean

The effects on circadian glucose levels of slow-release-insulin and acute-release-insulin are different. The mean glucose-level is the same for both treatment formulas, but the latter formula produces more low and high glucose levels. Spread or variance of the data is a more important determinant of treatment effect than is the mean glucose value.

A pill producing device is approved only if it will produce pills with a SD not larger than e.g. 6 mg. Rather than mean the variance of a test-sample is required to test the device.

People on selective serotonin reuptake inhibitors (SSRIs) may not only show a lower average of performance, but also a higher variability in performance relative to their counterparts. Variance, in addition to average of performance is required to allow for predictions on performances.

The variability in stay-days in hospital is more relevant than the mean stay-days, because greater variability is accompanied with a more demanding type of care.

Why should we statistically test such questions anyway? Or why not simply calculate the mean result and standard deviation of a sample of data, and, then, check if the SD is within a predefined area. We, subsequently, accept this as sufficient probability to make further predictions about future observations. However, by doing so we will never know the size of this probability. A statistical test rejects the null-hypothesis of no difference from 0 at a 5% or lower level of probability, and this procedure is widely valued as a powerful aid to erroneous conclusions. A more extensive overview of current routine methods to assess variability of data samples is given in Chap. 26.

7   Chi-Square Can Be Used for Multiple Samples of Data

7.1   Contingency Tables

The simplest extension of the chi-square test is the analysis of a two-by-two contingency table. With contingency tables we want to test whether two groups of binary data (yes/no data) are significantly different from one another. We have 4 cells ((1) group-1 yes, (2) group-1 no, (3) group-2 yes, (4) group-2 no). The null-hypothesis is tested by adding up:

$$\text{chi - square} = \frac{(O-E)^2_{cell\,1}}{E_{cell\,1}} + \frac{(O-E)^2_{cell\,2}}{E_{cell\,2}} + \frac{(O-E)^2_{cell\,3}}{E_{cell\,3}} + \frac{(O-E)^2_{cell\,4}}{E_{cell\,4}}$$

where O means observed numbers, and E means expected numbers per cell if no difference between the two groups is true (the null-hypothesis). The E-value in the denominator standardizes the test-statistic.

7.2 Pooling Relative Risks or Odds Ratios in a Meta-analysis of Multiple Trials

In meta-analyses the results of the individual trials are pooled in order to provide a more powerful assessment. Chi-square-statistic is adequate for testing a pooled result. The natural logarithms are used to approximate normality.

$$\text{Chi - square} = \frac{\left(\dfrac{\ln RR_1}{s_1^2} + \dfrac{\ln RR_2}{s_2^2} + \dfrac{\ln RR_3}{s_3^2} \cdots \right)^2}{\dfrac{1}{s_1^2} + \dfrac{1}{s_2^2} + \dfrac{1}{s_3^2} + \cdots}$$

where RR means relative risk and s means SD of this relative risk per sample. The $1/s^2$-term in the denominator takes care that a weighted average is calculated.

7.3 Analysis of Variance (ANOVA)

Unlike the normal-test or the t-test, the Chi-square-test can be extended to testing more than one sample of data simultaneously. Variances are non-negative values, and they can simply be added up. This is, actually, the way variance is defined, the add-up sum of squared distances from the mean. Any subsequent sample of data, if from a normal distribution or t-distribution can be simply added up to the first sample and the add-up sum can be analyzed simultaneously. And, so, with little more effort than demonstrated for 1 sample of data, multiple samples can be added to the model in order to test the null-hypothesis of no difference from zero. This is possible both for samples of continuous data and proportional data, including percentages, proportions, odds ratios, risk ratios etc. The only difference is the breadth of the chi-square curve: it gets wider and wider the more samples or the more proportions we add (Fig. 41.6).

A further extension of the use of the Chi-square-statistic is ANOVA. ANOVA makes use of the division-sum of two Chi-square-distributions. This division-sum, indeed, looks much like a usual Chi-square-distribution, as shown for example in Fig. 41.7.

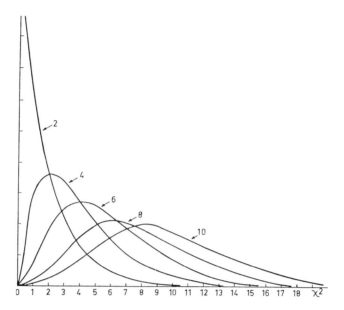

Fig. 41.6 The general form of the Chi-square distributions for larger samples of data

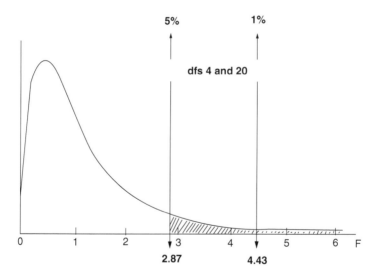

Fig. 41.7 Example of an F-distribution making use of the division-sum of two Chi-square-distributions with 4 and 20 degrees of freedom (dfs)

For example, ANOVA with k groups works as follows:

Total variation

| |

Between-group-variation   within-group-variation

Variations are expressed as sums of squares (SS) and can be added up to obtain the total variation.

We assess whether between-group-variation is large compared to within-group-variation.

Group	n patients	mean	sd
1	–	–	–
2	–	–	–
3	–	–	–
...			
k			

Grand mean $= (\text{mean } 1 + 2 + 3 + .. k)/ k$

$SS_{\text{between groups}} = n_1 (\text{mean}_1 - \text{grand mean})^2 + n_2 (\text{mean}_2 - \text{grand mean})^2 + ...$

$SS_{\text{within groups}} = (n_1 - 1)(sd_1^2) + (n_2 - 1)(sd_2^2) + ...$

$$F = \text{test - statistic} = \frac{SS_{\text{between groups}} / dfs^*}{SS_{\text{within groups}} / dfs}$$

*dfs means degrees of freedom (for SS between groups $dfs = k - 1$, for SS within groups $dfs = n_1 + n_2 + n_3 + ..n_k - k$).

The F-table gives p-value.

8   Discussion

The current chapter is not a cook-book-like instruction for the use of various statistical methods. It only briefly examines the connection between the Chi-square-distribution and other important statistical distributions. They form the basis of all statistical inferences, which are given so much emphasis in today's clinical medicine. The Chi-square-distribution is directly derived from the normal-distribution. The F-distribution is directly derived from the Chi-square distribution. Over and over again, these distributions have shown their utility in the solution of problems in statistical inference. However, none of these distributions is empirical in the sense that someone has taken a large number of samples and found that the sample values actually follow the same mathematical function. Of course, nature does not follow a single mathematical function. The function is an approximation, but it performs well and has proven to be helpful in making clinical predictions. The distribution is also based on assumptions, and, like other theory-based assessments, deals with "if-then" statements. That is why the assumptions about representative samples and normal-distribution in our sample are so important. If we apply the theory of statistics for making inferences from samples, we cannot expect this theory to provide us with adequate answers unless conditions specified in the theory hold true.

Apart from the general requirement of random sampling of independent observations, the most usual assumption made is that the population-distribution is normal. The Chi-square, the t -, and the F -distributions all rest upon this assumption. The normal-distribution can be considered the "parent" distribution to the others. Similarly, there are close connections between the F-distribution and both the normal- and the Chi-square-distributions. Basically, the F-statistic is the ratio of two independent Chi-square-statistics, each of which characterized by its own degrees of freedom. Since a Chi-square-statistic is defined in terms of a normal-distribution, the F-distribution also rests upon the same assumptions, albeit of two (or more than two) normal-distributions. The Chi-square-distribution focused on in this paper is, thus, just another approach of the bell-shape-like normal distribution and is also the basic element of the F-distribution. Having some idea of the interrelations of these distributions will be of help in understanding how the Chi-square is used to test a hypothesis-of-variance, and how the F-distribution is used to test a hypothesis-about-several-variances.

We conclude that the Chi-square-distribution and its extensions have become the basis of modern statistics and have provided clinical scientists with a relatively simple device to analyze complex data, including multiple groups/multiple variances. The present chapter was written for clinical investigators/scientists in order to better understand benefits and limitations of Chi-square-statistic and its many extensions for the analysis of experimental clinical data.

9   Conclusions

Statistical analyses of clinical data are increasingly complex. They often involve multiple groups and measures. Such data can not be assessed simply by differences between means but rather by comparing variances. The objective of this chapter was to focus on the Chi-square (χ^2)-test as a method to assess variances and test differences between variances. To give examples of clinical data where the emphasis is on variance. To assess interrelation between Chi-square and other statistical methods like normal-test (Z-test), T-test and Analysis-Of-Variance (ANOVA).

A Chi-square-distribution is nothing else than the distribution of square values of a normal-distribution. Null-hypothesis-testing-of-variances is much similar to null-hypothesis-testing-of-means. With the latter we reject the null-hypothesis of no effect if our mean is more than 1.96 SEMs (standard errors of the mean) distant from zero. With the latter we reject the null-hypothesis of no effect if our standardized variance is more than 1.96^2 SEMs^2 distant from zero. Because variances are squared and, thus, non-negative values, the Chi-square approach can be extended to test hypotheses about many samples. When variances or add-up variances of many samples are larger than allowed for by the Chi-square-distribution-graphs, we reject the probability that our results are from normal distributions, and conclude that our results are significantly different from zero. The Chi-square test is not only adequate to test multiple samples simultaneously, but is also the basis of ANOVA.

We conclude that the Chi-square-distribution focused on in this chapter is just another approach of the bell-shape-like normal-distribution and is also the basic element of the F-distribution as used in ANOVA. Having some idea about interrelations between these distributions will be of help in understanding benefits and limitations of Chi-square-statistic and its many extensions for the analysis of experimental clinical data.

Reference

Pearson K (1900) On a criterion that a given system of deviations from the probable in the case of a correlated system of variables is such that it cannot be reasonably supposed to have arisen from random sampling. Philos Mag 50:339–357

Chapter 42
Testing Clinical Trials for Randomness

1 Introduction

As it comes to well-balanced random sampling of representative experimental data, nature will be helpful to provide researchers with results that comply with the random property. It means that such data closely follow statistical frequency distributions. We continually make use of these statistical frequency distributions for analyzing the data and making predictions from them. However, we, virtually, never assess how close to the expected frequency distributions the data actually are. Unrandomness of the data may be one of the reasons for the lack of homogeneity in current research, and may jeopardize the scientific validity of research data (Cleophas 2004a, b; Cleophas and Cleophas 2001). Statistical tests used for the analysis of clinical trials assume that the observations represent a sample drawn at random from a target population. It means that any member of the population is as likely to be selected for the sampled group as the other. An objective procedure is required to achieve randomization. When other criteria are used to permit investigators to influence the selection of subjects, one can no longer conclude that the observed effects are due to the treatment rather than biases introduced by the process of selection. Also, when the randomization assumption is not satisfied, the logic underlying the distributions of the test statistics used to estimate that the observed effects are due to chance rather than treatment effect fails, and the resulting p-values are meaningless. Important causes for unrandomness in clinical trials include extreme exclusion criteria (Furberg 2002) and inappropriate data cleaning (Cleophas 2004a).

In the present chapter we review some methods to assess clinical data for their compliance with the random property.

2   Individual Data Available

If the individual data from a clinical trial are available, there are two methods to
assess the data for their compliance with the random property, the chi-square goodness of fit and the Kolmogorov-Smirnov goodness of fit tests. Both tests are based
on the assumption that differences between observed and expected experimental
data follow normal distributions. The two tests raise similar results. If both of them
are positive, the presence of unrandomness in the data can be assumed with confidence, and efficacy analysis of the data will be a problem. The tests can be used with
any kind of random data like continuous data, proportions or frequencies. In this
section two examples of continuous data will be given, in the next section an example
of frequencies will be given. Also, we briefly address randomness of survival data,
which are increasingly used as primary endpoint variable, e.g., of the 2003 volume
362 of the Lancet in 48% of the randomized trials published.

2.1   Method 1: The Chi-Square Goodness of Fit Test

In random populations body-weights follow a normal distribution. Is this also true
for the body-weights of a group of patients treated with a weight reducing compound? The example is modified from Levin and Rubin with permission from the
editor (Levin and Rubin 1998).

Individual weight (kg)

85	57	60	81	89	63	52	65	77	64
89	86	90	60	57	61	95	78	66	92
50	56	95	60	82	55	61	81	61	53
63	75	50	98	63	77	50	62	79	69
76	66	97	67	54	93	70	80	67	73

The area under the curve (AUC) of a normal distribution curve is divided into
five equiprobable intervals of 20% each, we expect approximately 10 patients per
interval. From the data a mean and standard deviation (sd) of 71 and 15 kg are calculated. Figure 42.1 shows that the standardized cut-off results (z-values) for the
five intervals are −0.84, −0.25, 0.25 and 0.84. The real cut-off results are calculated
according to

$$z = \text{standardized result} = \frac{\text{unstandardized result} - \text{mean result}}{\text{sd}}$$

and are given below (pts = patients).

Fig. 42.1 The standardized cut-off results (z-values) for the five intervals with an AUC of 20% are −0.84, −0.25, 0.25, and 0.84 (*AUC* area under the curve)

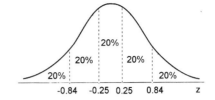

Intervals (kgs)	−∞	58.40	67.25	74.25	83.60	∞
As they are equiprobable, we expect per interval:		10 pts	10 pts	10 pts	10 pts	10 pts
We do, however, observe the following numbers:		10 pts	16 pts	3 pts	10 pts	11 pts

The chi-square value is calculated according to

$$\sum \frac{\left(\text{observed number} - \text{expected number}\right)^2}{\text{expected number}} = 8.6$$

This chi-square value means that for the given degrees of freedom of $5 - 1 = 4$ (there are five different intervals) the null-hypothesis of no-difference-between-observed-and-expected can not be rejected. However, our p-value is <0.10, and, so, there is a trend of a difference. The data may not be entirely normal, as expected. This may be due to lack of randomness.

2.2 Method 2: The Kolmogorov-Smirnov Goodness of Fit Test

In random populations plasma cholesterol levels follow a normal distribution. Is this also true for the plasma cholesterol levels of the underneath patients treated with a cholesterol reducing compound? This example is also modified from Levin and Rubin with permission from the editor (Levin and Rubin 1998).

Cholesterol (mmol/l)	<4.01	4.01–5.87	5.87–7.73	7.73–9.59	>9.59
Numbers of pts	13	158	437	122	20

The cut-off results for the five intervals must be standardized to find the expected normal distribution for these data according to

$$z = \text{standardized cut-off result} = \frac{\text{unstandardized result} - \text{mean result}}{\text{sd}}.$$

Fig. 42.2 The standardized
cut-off results (z-values) for
the five intervals are
calculated to be −2.25,
−0.75, 0.75, and 2.25.
Corresponding AUCs are
given in the graph (*AUC* area
under the curve)

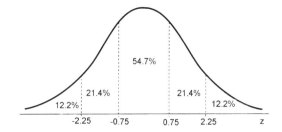

With a calculated mean (sd) of 6.80 (1.24) we find −2.25, −0.75, 0.75 and 2.25. Figure 42.2 gives the distribution graph plus AUCs. With 750 cholesterol-values in total the expected frequencies of cholesterol-values in the subsequent intervals are

$$12.2 \times 750 = 9.2$$
$$21.4 \times 750 = 160.8$$
$$54.7 \times 750 = 410.1$$
$$21.4 \times 750 = 160.8$$
$$12.2 \times 750 = 9.2$$

The observed and expected frequencies are, then, listed cumulatively (cumul = cumulative):

Frequency observed	Cumul	Relative (cumul/750)	Expected	Cumul	Relative (cumul/750)	Cumul observed-expected
13	13	0.0173	9.1	9.1	0.0122	0.0051
158	171	0.2280	160.9	170.0	0.2266	0.0014
437	608	0.8107	410.1	580.1	0.7734	0.0373
122	730	0.9733	160.8	740.9	0.9878	0.0145
20	750	1.000	9.1	750	1.000	0.0000

According to the Kolmogorov-Smirnov table (Table 42.1) the largest cumulative difference between observed and expected should be smaller than $1.36 / \sqrt{n} = 1.36 / \sqrt{750} = 0.0497$, while we find 0.0373. This means that these data are well normally distributed. We should add that a positive Kolmogorov-Smirnov test not only indicates that normal testing is not warranted, but also that rank testing (see also Chap. 23 and the next chapter) is not to be recommended, as Kolmogorow-Smirnov tests are based on a normal distribution of the data after cumulative ranking of the data.

2.3 Randomness of Survival Data

Cox regression is routinely used for the analysis of survival data. It assumes that randomly sampled human beings survive according to an exponential pattern. The presence of an exponential pattern can be confirmed by logarithmic transformation.

Table 42.1 Critical values of the Kolmogorov-Smirnov goodness of fit test

Sample size (n)	Level of statistical significance for maximum difference between cumulative observed and expected frequency				
n	0.20	0.15	0.10	0.05	0.01
1	0.900	0.925	0.950	0.975	0.995
2	0.684	0.726	0.776	0.842	0.929
3	0.565	0.597	0.642	0.708	0.828
4	0.494	0.525	0.564	0.624	0.733
5	0.446	0.474	0.510	0.565	0.669
6	0.410	0.436	0.470	0.521	0.618
7	0.381	0.405	0.438	0.486	0.577
8	0.358	0.381	0.411	0.457	0.543
9	0.339	0.360	0.388	0.432	0.514
10	0.322	0.342	0.368	0.410	0.490
11	0.307	0.326	0.352	0.391	0.468
12	0.295	0.313	0.338	0.375	0.450
13	0.284	0.302	0.325	0.361	0.463
14	0.274	0.292	0.314	0.349	0.418
15	0.266	0.283	0.304	0.338	0.404
16	0.258	0.274	0.295	0.328	0.392
17	0.250	0.266	0.286	0.318	0.381
18	0.244	0.259	0.278	0.309	0.371
19	0.237	0.252	0.272	0.301	0.363
20	0.231	0.246	0.264	0.294	0.356
25	0.21	0.22	0.24	0.27	0.32
30	0.19	0.20	0.22	0.24	0.29
35	0.18	0.19	0.21	0.23	0.27
Over 35	$\frac{1.07}{\sqrt{n}}$	$\frac{1.14}{\sqrt{n}}$	$\frac{1.22}{\sqrt{n}}$	$\frac{1.36}{\sqrt{n}}$	$\frac{1.63}{\sqrt{n}}$

If the transformed data are significantly different from a line, the exponential relationship can be rejected. Figure 42.3 shows the survivals of 240 patients with small cell carcinomas, and Fig. 42.4 shows the natural logarithms of these survivals. From Fig. 42.4 it can be observed that logarithmic transformation of the numbers of patients alive readily produces a close to linear pattern. A Pearson's correlation coefficient of these data at $p < 0.0001$ confirms that these data are closer to a line than could happen by chance. We can conclude that these survival data are compatible with a sample drawn at random.

3 Individual Data Not Available

3.1 Studies with Single Endpoints

If the actual data from the research are not available like in most clinical reports, it is harder to assess randomness of the data. However, it is not impossible to do so. Some criteria for assessing main endpoint results of published studies for such

Fig. 42.3 Survivals of 240 random patients with small cell carcinomas

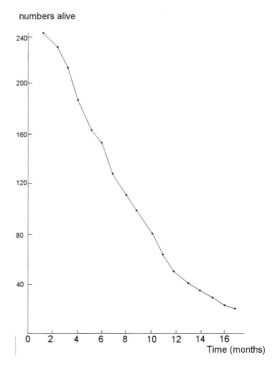

Fig. 42.4 The logarithmic transformation of the numbers of patients from Fig. 42.3 produces a close to linear pattern

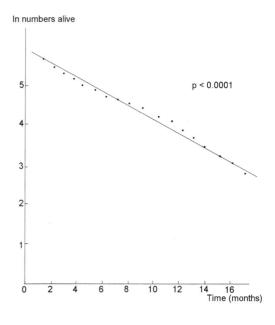

purpose have been recently proposed by us (Cleophas 2004a, b), and have already been addressed in Chap. 10.

1. An observed p-value of <0.0001 in a clinical trial.
   In statistics, a generally accepted concept is "the smaller the p-value, the better reliable the results". This is not entirely true with current randomized controlled trials. First, randomized controlled trials are designed to test small differences. A randomized controlled trial with major differences between old and new treatment is unethical because half of the patients have been given an inferior treatment. Second, they are designed to confirm prior evidence. For that purpose, their sample size is carefully calculated. Not only too small, but also too large a sample size is considered unethical and unscientific, because negative studies have to be repeated and a potentially inferior treatment should not be given to too many patients. Often in a study the statistical power is set at 80%. An expected power of 80% means a <10% chance of a p-value <0.0001 with normally distributed data (Hung et al. 1997) and a <5% chance of a p-value <0.0001 with t-distributed data and samples sizes under 50, (as often observed in, e.g., oncology trials).
2. An observed p-value of >95% in a clinical trial.
   P-values are generally used as a cut-off levels to indicate the chance of a difference from H_0 (the null-hypothesis-of-no-effect) in our data. The larger the p-value the smaller the chance of a difference from H_0. A p-value of 1.00 means 0% chance of a difference, while a p-value of 0.95 means a chance of a difference close to 0%. A p-value of >0.95 literally means that we have >95% chance of finding a result less close to H_0, which means a chance of <(1–0.95), i.e., <0.05 of finding a result this close or closer. Using the traditional 5% decision level, this would mean, that we have a strong argument that such data are closer to H_0 than compatible with random sampling.
3. An observed standard deviation (sd) <50% the sd expected from prior population data. From population data we can be pretty sure about sds to be expected. For example, the sds of blood pressures are close to 10% of their means, meaning that for a mean systolic blood pressures of 150 mmHg the expected sd is close to 15 mmHg, for a mean diastolic blood pressure of 100 mmHg the expected sd is close to 10 mmHg. If such sds can be assumed to follow a normal distribution, we will have <5% chance of finding sds <7.5 and <5 mmHg respectively.
4. An observed standard deviation (sd) >150% the sd expected from prior population data. With sds close to 10% of their means, we, likewise, will have <5% chance of finding sds >150% the size of the sds expected from population data.

3.2 Studies with Multiple Endpoints

A simple method to check the accuracy of multiple endpoints is to examine the distribution of the final digits of the results, using the chi-square goodness of fit test. In a clinical trial of cholesterol lowering treatment the results were presented mainly

Table 42.2 Multiple risk ratios as reported in a "statin" paper

Final digit or RR	Observed frequency	Expected frequency	$\sum \dfrac{(\text{observed} - \text{expected})^2}{\text{expected}}$
0	24	9.6	21.6
1	39	9.6	90.0
2	3	9.6	4.5
3	0	9.6	9.6
4	0	9.6	9.6
5	0	9.6	9.6
6	0	9.6	9.6
7	1	9.6	7.7
8	2	9.6	6.0
9	27	9.6	31.5
Total	96	96.0	199.7

in the form of relative risks (RR=risk of mortality during treatment/risk of mortality during control). In total 96 RRs were presented with many of them showing a 9 or 1 as final digit. For example, RRs of 0.99, 0.89, 1.01, and 1.11 etc were often reported. The accuracy of the multiple endpoints is checked according to Table 42.2.

If there were no tendencies to record only whole RRs, we would expect equal numbers of 0s, 1s, 2s,....9s for the final digit, that is 9.6 of each. The agreement between the observed and expected digits is, then, tested according to

$$\text{Chi - square} = \sum \frac{(\text{observed} - \text{expected})^2}{\text{expected}} = 199.7 \text{ for } 10 - 1 \text{ degrees of freedom}$$

(there are 10 different frequencies). For the given degrees of freedom a chi-square value >27.88 means that the null-hypothesis of no-difference-between-observed-and-expected can rejected at a p-value <0.001. The distribution of the final digits of the RRs in this study does not follow a random pattern. The presence of unrandomness in these results can be assumed with confidence, and jeopardizes the validity of this study.

4 Discussion

This chapter gives some simple statistical methods to assess trial data for their compliance with the random property. We should add that distribution-free statistical tests that are less dependent on random distributions, are available, but, in practice, they are used far less frequently than normal tests. Also, with slight departures from the normal distribution, normal tests are used even so. The same applies to the analysis of unrandomized studies: for their statistical analysis the same statistical tests are applied as those applied for randomized studies, although this, at the same time, is one of the main limitations of this kind of research. The issue of the current chapter is not the statistical analysis of unrandom data but rather the detection of it.

Regarding the studies with multiple endpoints, the problem is often a dependency of the endpoints in which case the presented method for the assessment of unrandomness is not adequate. For example endpoints like deaths, metastases, local relapses, etc in an oncology trial cannot be considered entirely independent. However, if the initial digits of the results are equally distributed, like, e.g., RRs 1.1/2.1/3.1/4.1/5.1, then little dependency is to be expected, and the presented method can be properly performed.

Important causes for unrandomness in clinical trials include extreme exclusion criteria (Furberg 2002) and inappropriate data cleaning (Cleophas 2004a). The first cause can be illustrated by the study of Kaariainen et al (1991) comparing the effect of strict and loose inclusion criteria on treatment results in 397 patients hospitalized for gastric ulcers. While under the loose inclusion criteria virtually none of patients had to be excluded, 71% of them had to be excluded under the strict inclusion criteria. Major complications of treatment occurred in 71 out of the 397 patients with the loose , in only two out of 115 patients with the strict inclusion criteria. These two major complications can hardly be considered representative results from a sample drawn at random from the target population. The second cause can be illustrated by Mendel's pea data. In 1860 Gregor Mendel performed randomized trials "avant la lettre" by using a selective samples of peas with different phenotypes. When we recently looked into Mendel's pea data, and performed a chi-square test, we had to conclude that the chi-square value was too small not to reject the null hypothesis (P > 0.99) (Cleophas and Cleophas 2001). This means that Mendel's reported data were so close to what he expected that we could only conclude that he somewhat misrepresented the data.

The current chapter is an effort to provide the scientific community with some simple methods to assess randomness of experimental data. These methods are routinely used in accountancy statistics for assessing the possibility of financial fraud, but they cannot be found in most textbooks of medical statistics.

Evidence-based medicine is under pressure due to the conflicting results of recent trials producing different answers to similar questions (Julius 2003; Cleophas and Cleophas 2003). Many causes are mentioned. As long as the possibility of unrandom data has not been addressed, this very possibility cannot be excluded as potential cause for the obvious lack of homogeneity in current research.

5 Conclusions

Well-balanced randomly sampled representative experimental data comply with the random property meaning that they follow statistical frequency distributions. We continually make use of these frequency distributions to analyze the data, but virtually never assess how close to the expected frequency distributions the data actually are. Unrandom data may be one of the reasons for the lack of homogeneity in the results from current research. The objective of this chapter was to propose some methods for routinely assessing clinical data for their compliance with the random property.

If the individual data from the trial are available, the chi-square goodness of fit and the Kolmogorov-Smirnov (KS) goodness of fit tests can be applied (both tests yield similar results and can be applied with any kind of data including continuous data, proportions, or frequencies), for survival data logarithmic transformation can be applied. It is wise to first perform a chi-square goodness of fit test. If positive, normal tests for data analysis will not be adequate. A subsequent KS test may be negative, and if so, rank testing will be no problem. If the individual data from the trial are not available, the following criteria may be used: observed p-values between 0.0001 and 0.95, observed standard deviations (sds) between 50% and 150% of the sd expected from population data. With multiple endpoints, the distribution of the final digits of the results may be examined using a chi-square goodness of fit test. In the current chapter some simple statistical tests and criteria are given to assess randomized clinical trials for their compliance with the random property.

References

Cleophas TJ (2004a) Research data closer to expectation than compatible with random sampling. Stat Med 23:1015–1017

Cleophas TJ (2004b) Clinical trials and p-values, beware of the extremes. Clin Chem Lab Med 42:300–304

Cleophas TJ, Cleophas GM (2001) Sponsored research and continuing medical education. J Am Med Assoc 286:302–304

Cleophas GM, Cleophas TJ (2003) Clinical trials in jeopardy. Int J Clin Pharmacol Ther 41:51–56

Furberg C (2002) To whom do the research findings apply? Heart 87:570–574

Hung HM, O'Neill RT, Bauer P, Köhne K (1997) The behavior of the p-value when the alternative hypothesis is true. Biometrics 53:11–22

Julius S (2003) The ALLHAT study: if you believe in evidence-based medicine, stick to it. J Hypertens 21:453–454

Kaaraininen I, Sipponen P, Siurala M (1991) What fraction of hospital ulcer patients is eligible for prospective drug trials? Scand J Gastroenterol 26:73–76

Levin RI, Rubin DS (1998) Statistics for management, 7th edn. Prentice-Hall International, Englewood Cliffs

Chapter 43
Clinical Trials Do Not Use Random Samples Anymore

1 Introduction

Current clinical trials do not use random samples anymore. Instead, they use convenience samples from selected hospitals, including only patients with strict characteristics, like cut-off laboratory values. This practice, although it improves the precision of the treatment comparison, raises the risk of non-normal data. This is a problem since the assumption of normality underlies many statistical tests. If this assumption is not satisfied, the logic underlying the distributions of the test statistics used to estimate whether the observed effects are due to chance rather than treatment effect, fails, and, consequently, the resulting p-values are meaningless. Evidence-based medicine is under pressure due to the heterogeneity of current trials (Cleophas 2004; Furberg 2002; Kaaraininen et al. 1991; Cleophas and Cleophas 2003). The possibility of non-normal data cannot be excluded as a contributing cause for this. The current chapter reviews and describes for a non-mathematical readership methods to assess data for compliance with normality, and summarizes solutions for the analysis of non-normal data.

2 Non-normal Sampling Distributions, Giving Rise to Non-normal Data

Figure 43.1 gives an example of sampling distributions of patients with heterozygous hypercholesterolemia. If all of the patients who genetically qualify are included, we will obtain an entirely normal frequency distribution of the individual LDL-cholesterol values. If, however, only patients with an LDL-cholesterol ≤5.7 or >3.4 mmol/l or between 3.4 and 5.7 mmol/l are included (Anonymous 2011), we will obtain non-normal distributions as shown in the Fig. 43.1. Figure 43.2 gives an example of patients with constitutional constipation before and after treatment with a laxative (Cleophas et al. 2006). Only patients with <3 stools per week were

T.J. Cleophas and A.H. Zwinderman, *Statistics Applied to Clinical Studies*,
DOI 10.1007/978-94-007-2863-9_43, © Springer Science+Business Media B.V. 2012

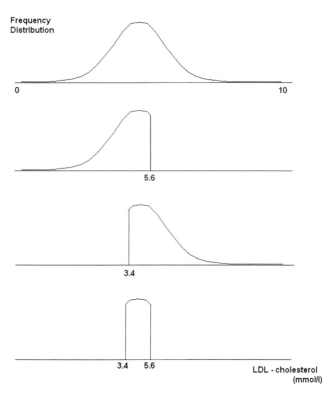

Fig. 43.1 Sampling distributions of patients with heterozygous hypercholesterolemia with on the x-axis individual results and on the y=axis "how often": (**1**) all of the patients that genetically qualify are included; (**2**) patients with an LDL-cholesterol ≤5.6 included; (**3**) patients with LDL-cholesterol >3.4 mmol/l included; (**4**) only patients with LDL-cholesterol between 3.4 and 5.6 mmol/l included

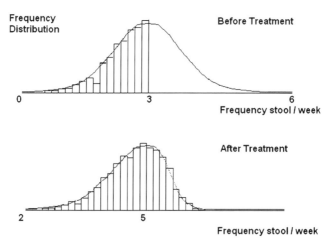

Fig. 43.2 Frequency distributions of patients with constitutional constipation before and after treatment with a laxative. Only patients with <3 stools per week were included

included. The Fig. 43.2 shows how a skewed sampling distribution may give rise to a non-normal trial result. This, obviously, happens not only to control groups and comparisons versus baseline, but also to active treatment groups, probably, due to the positive correlation between repeated observations in one subject.

3 Testing the Assumption of Normality

In trials with a single endpoint the chi-square goodness of fit test as discussed in Chap. 42 can be applied. In case of multiple endpoints a simple method to check the normality of multiple endpoints is to examine the distribution of the final digits of the results, also using the chi-square goodness of fit test. The example was modified from Kirkwood and Stern with permission from the editor (2003). In a clinical trial of cholesterol lowering treatment the results were presented mainly in the form of relative risks (RR = risk of mortality during treatment/risk of mortality during control). In total 96 RRs were presented with many of them showing a 9 or 1 as final digit. For example, RRs of 0.99, 0.89, 1.01, and 1.11 etc. were often reported.

The accuracy of multiple endpoints is checked as follows:

Final digit of RR	Observed frequency	Expected frequency	$\sum \dfrac{(\text{observed} - \text{expected})^2}{\text{expected}}$
0	24	9.6	21.6
1	39	9.6	90.0
2	3	9.6	4.5
3	0	9.6	9.6
4	0	9.6	9.6
5	0	9.6	9.6
6	0	9.6	9.6
7	1	9.6	7.7
8	2	9.6	6.0
9	27	9.6	31.5
Total	96	96.0	199.7

If there were no tendencies to record only whole RRs, we would expect equal numbers of 0s, 1s, 2s,...9s for the final digit, that is 9.6 of each. The agreement between the observed and expected digits is, then, tested according to

$$\text{chi - square} = \sum \frac{(\text{observed} - \text{expected})^2}{\text{expected}} = 199.7 \quad \text{for } 10 - 1 \text{ degrees of freedom}$$

(there are 10 different frequencies). For the given degrees of freedom a chi-square value >27.88 means that the null-hypothesis of no-difference-between-observed-and-expected can rejected at a p-value < 0.001. The distribution of the final digits of the RRs in this study does not follow a normal pattern. The presence of unrandomness in these results can be assumed, and jeopardizes the validity of this study.

4   What to Do in case of Non-normality

If the data are not normally distributed, they may be given ranknumbers and these ranknumbers often tend to look like normal distributions. For their analysis rank-sum tests have been developed, including the Mann-Whitney's and the Wilcoxon's tests. In order to assess whether the data are suitable for rank-testing a special goodness of fit test is available, the Kolmogorov-Smirnov test, as discussed in Chap. 42.

Also confidence intervals based on percentiles can be used if rank-testing is not warranted. Confidence intervals can be derived from the data without prior assumption about the type of distribution. The simplest way to do so is to take the range within which 95% of all possible outcomes lie. Medians rather than means should be used for calculation, because these data are skewed. The underneath method is correct for finding the 95% confidence interval of a difference between medians.

Group 1	Group 2
3.99	3.18
3.79	2.84
3.60	2.90
3.73	3.27
3.21	3.85
3.60	3.52
4.08	3.23
3.61	2.76
3.81	3.60
Median	
3.73	3.23
Difference in medians	
0.50	

All possible differences between the two groups ($9 \times 9 = 81$) lie between -0.64 and 1.24. After exclusion of 2.5% of the lowest and 2.5% of the highest differences, we will obtain a range containing 95% of the differences. This 95% confidence interval is between -0.25 and 1.15. This interval includes the value 0, which means that the difference between the two groups is not significantly different from 0 ($p > 0.05$).

A largely similar but more sophisticated method to obtain confidence intervals from your data is the bootstrap method (Levin and Rubin 1998; Carpenter and Bithell 2000). Bootstrapping, otherwise called jack-knifing, is a data based simulation process for statistical inference. The basic idea is sampling with replacement in order to produce random samples from the original data. The procedure is illustrated underneath for two bootstrap samples. In the first bootstrap sample observation 1 was picked up twice, while observations 2 and 4 were not picked. We repeat this procedure a large number of times, and record the difference in medians of each bootstrap sample. To derive confidence intervals, at least $n_{group\ 1} \times n_{group\ 2} = 9 \times 9 = 81$ bootstraps are required. To calculate the confidence intervals the percentile method like described above can be used. In this example a 95% confidence interval between -0.12 and 1.09 was obtained, again not significantly different from 0.

Original data			Bootstrap 1			Bootstrap 2		
Group 1		Group 2	Group 1		Group 2	Group 1		Group 2
1.	3.99	10. 3.18	1.	3.99	10. 3.18	1.	3.99	10. 3.18
2.	3.79	11. 2.84	1.	3.99	10. 3.18	2.	3.79	11. 2.84
3.	3.60	12. 2.90	3.	3.60	12. 2.90	2.	3.79	12. 2.90
4.	3.73	13. 3.27	5.	3.21	14. 3.85	2.	3.79	12. 2.90
5.	3.21	14. 3.85	6.	3.60	15. 3.52	4.	3.73	14. 3.85
6.	3.60	15. 3.52	8.	3.61	15. 3.52	5.	3.21	15. 3.52
7.	4.08	16. 3.23	8.	3.61	15. 3.52	7.	4.08	16. 3.23
8.	3.61	17. 2.76	9.	3.81	16. 3.23	7.	4.08	18. 3.60
9.	3.81	18. 3.60	9.	3.81	17. 2.76	8.	3.61	18. 3.60
Median group 1 = 3.73			Median group 1 = 3.61			Median group 1 = 3.79		
Median group 2 = 3.23			Median group 2 = 3.23			Median group 2 = 3.23		
Difference medians = 0.50			Difference medians = 0.38			Difference medians = 0.55		

5 Discussion

Current clinical trials do not, usually, use random samples, but rather convenience samples from selected hospitals, including only patients with strict characteristics, like cut-off laboratory values. This practice raises the risk of non-normal data. The assumption of normality underlies many statistical tests, including, among other tests, normal-, t-, chi-square-tests, analysis of variance, and regression analyses. With slight departures from the normal distribution, these tests can be used even so. They should not be used, however, if the chi-square goodness of fit is significant. Rank-testing is, then, an adequate alternative. But, sometimes, distributions do not allow for this approach either. This can be checked by the Kolmogorov-Smirnov test. If the latter test is also positive, rank-testing is not warranted, and confidence intervals can be derived from the data without prior assumption about the type of frequency distribution. This can be done by calculating the range within which 95% of all possible outcomes. We should add that medians, instead of means, are recommended for calculation, because the data are skewed. Another popular method for this purpose is bootstrapping, which resamples at random from the study's own data. The basic idea is simple: if we take repeated samples from the data themselves, we will mimick the way the data were sampled from the population in the way it should, namely at random. Although the theoretical properties of bootstrapping have not been well-understood, practical performance of this resampling method has been demonstrated in a number of simulation studies (Efron and Tibshirani 1993).

The current paper is just an introduction, and many aspects are not covered. SPSS (2011) uses, instead of the chi-square goodness of fit test, the Shapiro-Wilk (Royston 1993) test, which is mathematically more complicated, but performs otherwise largely similarly. We should add that, in clinical research, some data are, traditionally, non-normal, but have been recognized to follow a normal distribution after transformation. This is true for risk ratios, odds ratios, and hazard ratios that are analyzed after logarithmic transformations by simple normality tests. The final results can, then, be retrieved by taking the antilog term of the obtained result.

Well-balanced randomly sampled representative experimental data often comply with the so-called random property meaning that they follow normal or close to normal frequency distributions. We continually make use of these frequency distributions to analyze the data, but virtually never assess how close to the expected frequency distributions the data actually are. Unrandom data due to convenience sampling and extreme inclusion criteria may be one of the reasons for the lack of homogeneity in current research. We strongly believe that normality statistics, although the mainstay of statistical analysis for centuries, will rapidly be replaced with non-normal testing as the awareness of non-normal sampling distributions grows. Moreover, confidence intervals from data without prior assessment of frequency distributions are, currently, more easy to obtain than in the past, because computers can produce hundreds of random numbers from any set of experimental data within seconds. For example, with the function RANDBETWEEN, after giving the data ranknumbers, the EXCEL program (EXCEL 2011) can produce many random samples from any given population as well as their characteristics like medians, ranges, percentiles. We hope that this paper will strengthen the awareness of non-normal sampling distributions, and affect the design and analysis of future clinical trials.

6   Conclusions

Current clinical trials do not use random samples, but, instead, convenience samples. This raises the risk of non-normal data. This chapter reviews and describes for a non-mathematical readership common methods for testing the normal property, as well as methods for analyzing the data in case of non-normality.

With slight departures from the normal distribution, normality tests can be used even so. They include, among other tests, the normal-, t-, chi-square-tests, analysis of variance, and regression analyses. They should not be used, if the chi-square goodness of fit is significant. Rank-testing is, then, an alternative, but, sometimes, distributions do not allow for this approach either. This can be checked by the Kolmogorov-Smirnov test. If the latter test is also positive, rank-testing is not warranted, and confidence intervals can be derived from the data without prior assumption about the type of frequency distribution. This can be done by calculating the range within which 95% of all possible outcomes lie. Another popular method for this purpose is bootstrapping, which resamples at random from the study's own data.

This chapter reviews methods to assess data for compliance with normality, and summarizes solutions for the analysis of non-normal data. We, strongly, believe that normality statistics, although the mainstay of statistical analysis for centuries, will rapidly be replaced with non-normal testing as the awareness of non-normal sampling distributions grows, and hope that the chapter will strengthen this awareness, and affect the design and analysis of future clinical trials.

References

Anonymous KOWA Study Protocol. Pharmanet, Pharm@net. Accessed 15 Dec 2011

Carpenter J, Bithell J (2000) Bootstrap confidence intervals: when, which, what? A practical guide. Stat Med 19:1141–1164

Cleophas TJ (2004) Research data closer to expectation than compatible with random sampling. Stat Med 23:1015–1017

Cleophas GM, Cleophas TJ (2003) Clinical trials in jeopardy. Int J Clin Pharmacol Ther 41:51–56

Cleophas TJ, Zwinderman AH, Cleophas TF (2006) Example of crossover trial comparing efficacy of a new laxative versus bisacodyl. In: Statistics applied to clinical trials, 3rd edn. Springer, New York, pp 126–129

Efron B, Tibshirani RJ (1993) An introduction to the bootstrap. Chapman & Hall, New York

Excel Microsoft Office Online: EXCEL Home Page. Accessed 15 Dec 2011

Furberg C (2002) To whom do the research findings apply? Heart 87:570–574

Kaaraininen I, Sipponen P, Siurala M (1991) What fraction of hospital ulcer patients is eligible for prospective drug trials? Scand J Gastroenterol 26:73–76

Kirkwood BR, Sterne JA (2003) Medical statistics, 2nd edn. Blackwell Science, Oxford

Levin RI, Rubin DS (1998) Statistics for management, 7th edn. Prentice -Hall International, Englewood Cliffs

Royston P (1993) A toolkit for testing for non-normality in complete and censored samples. Statistician 42:37–43

SPSS Statistical Software. www.SPSS.com. Accessed 15 Dec 2011

Chapter 44
Clinical Data Where Variability Is More Important Than Averages

1 Introduction

In clinical studies, efficacies of new treatments are usually assessed by comparing averages of new treatment results versus control or placebo. However, averages do not tell the whole story, and the spread of the data may be more relevant. For example, when we assess how a drug reaches various organs, variability of drug concentrations is important, as in some cases too little and in other cases dangerously high levels get through. Also, for the assessment of the pharmacological response to a drug, variabilities may be important. For example, the effects on circadian glucose levels in patients with diabetes mellitus of a slow-release-insulin and acute-release-insulin formula are different. The latter formula is likely to produce more low and high glucose levels than the former formula. Spread or variability of the data is a determinant of diabetic control, and predictor of hypoglycaemic/hyperglycemic events. As an example, in a parallel-group study of $n = 200$ the former and latter formulas produced mean glucoses of 7.9 and 7.1 mmol/l, while standard deviations were 4.2 and 8.4 mmol/l respectively. This suggests that, although the slow-release formula did not produce a better mean glucose level, it did produce a smaller spread in the data. How do we test these kinds of data. Clinical investigators, although they are generally familiar with testing differences between averages, have difficulties testing differences between variabilities. The current chapter gives examples of situations where variability is more relevant than averages. It also gives simple statistical methods for testing such data. Statistical tests comparing mean values instead of variabilities are relatively simple and are one method everyone seems to learn. It is a service to the readership of this book to put more emphasis on variability.

2   Examples

2.1   Testing Drugs with Small Therapeutic Indices

Aminoglycosides like gentamicin and tobramicin are highly efficaceous against gram-negative bacilli, even pseudomonas. However, their therapeutic indices are small, and, particularly, irreversible nephrotoxicity requires careful monitoring of high plasma levels, while low levels lack therapeutic efficacy (Chambers and Sande 1996). For efficacy/safety assessments of such compounds, in addition to monitoring too high and too low averages, monitoring variability of plasma levels is relevant.

2.2   Testing Variability in Drug Response

In patients with hypertension the effects on circadian blood pressure levels of blood pressure lowering agents from different classes are different. For example, unlike beta-blockers, calcium channel blockers and angiotensin converting enzyme inhibitors amplified amplitudes of circadian blood pressure rhythms (Cleophas et al. 1998). Spread or variability of the data is a determinant of hypertensive control, and predictor of cardiovascular risks (Neutel and Smith 1997). Particularly, for the assessment of ambulatory blood pressure measurements variability in the data is important.

2.3   Assessing Pill Diameters or Pill Weights

A pill producing device is approved only if it will produce pill diameters with a standard deviation (SD) not larger than, e.g., 7 mm. Rather than the average diameter, the variability of the diameters is required for testing the appropriateness of this device.

2.4   Comparing Different Patient Groups for Variability in Patient Characteristics

Anxious people may not only show a lower average of performance, but also a higher variability in performance relative to their non-anxious counterparts. Variability assessment is required to allow for predictions on performances.

2.5 Assessing the Variability in Duration of Clinical Treatments

For hospital managers the variability in stay-days in hospital is more relevant than the mean stay-days, because greater variability is accompanied with a more demanding type of care.

2.6 Finding the Best Method for Patient Assessments

A clinician needs to know whether variability in rectal temperature is larger than variability in oral temperature in order to choose the method with the smaller variability.

Various fields of research, particularly in clinical pharmacology, make use of test procedures that, implicitly, address the variability in the data. For example, bioavailability studies consider variability through individual and population bioequivalence instead of just averages (Hauck and Anderson 1984; Tothfalusi and Endrenyl 2001). For the assessment of diagnostic estimators, repeatability tests and receiver operating (ROC) curves are applied (Almirall et al. 2004). Mann–Whitney tests for repeated measures consider whether treatment A is better than B (Petrie and Sabin 2000). However, none of such studies are especially designed to test variability. The current chapter reviews statistical methods especially designed for such purpose.

3 An Index for Variability in the Data

Repeated observations exhibit a central tendency, the mean, but, in addition, exhibit spread or dispersion, the tendency to depart from the mean. If measurement of central tendency is thought of as good bets, then measures of spread represent the poorness of central tendency, otherwise called deviation or error. The larger such deviations are, the more do cases differ from each other and the more spread does the distribution show. For the assessment of spread in the data we need an index to reflect variability. First of all, why not simply express variability as the departures of the individual data from the mean value. This, however, will not work, because the data will produce both negative and positive departures from the mean, and the overall variability will approach zero. A device to get around this difficulty is to take the add-up sum of the squares of deviations from the mean, and divide by $n-1$ (n = sample size):

$$\frac{\left(\text{datum } 1 - \text{mean}\right)^2 + \left(\text{datum } 2 - \text{mean}\right)^2 + \left(\text{datum } 3 - \text{mean}\right)^2 + \ldots}{n-1}$$

This formula presents the variance of n observations, and is widely used for the assessment of variability in a sample of data. The use of "n − 1" instead of "n" for denominator is related to the so-called degrees of freedom. Variances can be applied to assess data like those given in the above examples. The following tests are adequate for such purpose: the chi-square test for a single sample, the F-test for two samples, and the Bartlett's or Levene's tests for three or more samples. Additional methods for analyzing variability include (1) comparisons of confidence intervals, and (2) testing confidence intervals against prior defined intervals of therapeutic tolerance or equivalence. We should add that the variance is only one way to measure variability. Median absolute deviation (MAD) is another method not uncommonly used for pharmaceutical applications. It is found by taking the absolute difference of each datum from the sample median, and, then, taking the median of the total number of values. MADs will not be further discussed in this chapter.

4   How to Analyze Variability, One Sample

4.1 χ^2 Test

For testing whether the standard deviation (or variance) of a sample is significantly different from the standard deviation (or variance) to be expected the chi-square test is adequate. The chi-square test is closely related to the normal test or the t-test. The main difference is the use of squared values in the former. The underneath formula is used to calculate the chi-square value

$$\chi^2 = \frac{(n-1) \cdot s^2}{\sigma^2}$$

for n − 1 degrees of freedom
(n = sample size, s = standard deviation, s^2 = variance sample, σ = expected standard deviation, σ^2 = expected variance).

For example, in an ongoing quality control produced tablets are monitored for consistency in size. Samples of 50 tablets are only approved if the sample size standard deviation value is less than 0.7 mm. A 50 tablet sample has a standard deviation of 0.9 mm.

$$\chi^2 = (50-1)0.9^2 / 0.7^2 = 81$$

The chi-square table shows that, for 50 − 1 = 49 degrees of freedom, we find a p-value < 0.01 (one-sided test). This sample's standard deviation is significantly larger than that required. This means that this sample cannot be approved.

4.2   Confidence Interval

Instead of, or in addition to, the above chi-square test a confidence interval can be calculated. It can be more relevant than, simply, the above test, and it is considered good statistical practice to provide a confidence interval to accompany any estimates. The underneath formulas are used for calculation.

$$s\sqrt{\frac{(n-1)}{b}} \text{ and } s\sqrt{\frac{(n-1)}{a}}$$

n = sample size, s = standard deviation
b = cut-off value of left tail of χ^2 – distribution for given α and degrees of freedom
a = cut-off value of right tail of χ^2 – distribution for given α and given degrees of freedom
α = type I error

We use the above example, with a requested standard deviation (s) of 7 mm and observed s of 9 mm, to calculate 90% confidence interval (α = 10%). As the sample size = n = 50, the degrees of freedom is n − 1 = 49. The cut-off values, b and a, can be found in the left and right tail χ^2 tables, respectively available in Chap. 12, Table 12.2, and the Appendix, and the literature (Cleophas 2005).

$$s\sqrt{\frac{(n-1)}{b}} = 9 \times \sqrt{\frac{49}{37.69}} = 9 \times 1.14 \text{ mm} = 10.26$$

$$s\sqrt{\frac{(n-1)}{a}} = 9 \times \sqrt{\frac{49}{63.17}} = 9 \times 0.88 \text{ mm} = 7.92$$

The 90% confidence interval is, thus, between 7.9 and 10.3 mm, and it does not cross the required standard deviation of 7 mm. The device is not approved.

4.3   Equivalence Test

A limitation of the above methods is that a statistical difference is assumed based on normal standard deviations. To clinical pharmacologists a more appealing approach might be an equivalence test which uses prior defined boundaries of equivalence, and, subsequently, tests whether the 90 or 95% confidence intervals of a sample are within these boundaries. If entirely within, we accept equivalence, if partly within we are unsure, if entirely without, we conclude lack of equivalence. Furthermore, what is nice about equivalence intervals, is, that both mean and variability information are incorporated. Basic references are the guidelines given by Schuirmann and

Hahn (Schuirmann 1987; Hahn and Meeker 1991). As an example, the boundaries for demonstrating equivalence of the diameters of a pill could be set between 9.0 and 11.0 mm. A pill producing device produces a sample with a mean diameter of 9.8 mm and 90% confidence intervals of ± 0.7 mm. This would mean that the confidence intervals are between 9.1 and 10.5 mm, and that they are, thus, entirely within the set boundary of equivalence. We can state that we are 90% confident that at least 90% of the values lie between 9.1 and 10.5 mm (type I error 10%). According to this analysis, the pill producing device can be approved.

5   How to Analyze Variability, Two Samples

5.1   F Test

F tests can be applied to test if variability of two samples is significantly different. The division sum of the samples' variances (larger variance/smaller variance) is used for the analysis. For example, two formulas of gentamicin produce the following standard deviations of plasma concentrations:

	Patients (n)	Standard deviation (s) (μg/l)
Formula-A	10	3.0
Formula-B	15	2.0

$$F = s_{Formula-A}^{2} / s_{Formula-B}^{2} = 3.0^2 / 2.0^2 = 9 / 4 = 2.25$$

with degrees of freedom (dfs) for formula-A $10 - 1 = 9$ and for formula-B $15 - 1 = 14$.

The F-table shows that an F-value of at least 3.01 is required not to reject the null-hypothesis. Our F-value is 2.25 and, so, the p-value is >0.05. No significant difference between the two formulas can be demonstrated. This F-test is available in Excel. Approximate F-values can also be found in the F-table, Appendix.

5.2   Confidence Interval

Also for two samples the calculation of confidence intervals is possible. It will help to assess to what extent the two formulations actually have similar variances or whether the confidence interval is wide and, thus, the relationship of the two variances is really not known. The formulas for calculation are given.

$$(1 / \text{cut-off F-value}) \times \text{calculated F-value} \quad \text{and}$$

$$(\text{cut-off F-value}) \times \text{calculated F-value}$$

Cut-off F-value = F-value of F-table for given α and degrees of freedom
α = type I error

We calculate the 90% confidence interval from the above two sample example.

$$\left(1 / \text{cut-off F-value}\right) \times \text{calculated F-value} = 1 / 3.01 \times 2.25 = 0.75 \quad \text{and}$$

$$\left(\text{cut-off F-value}\right) \times \text{calculated F-value} = 3.01 \times 2.25 = 6.75$$

The 90% confidence interval for this ratio of variances is between 0.75 and 6.75. This interval crosses the cut-off F-value of 3.01. So, the result is not significantly different from 3.01. We conclude that no significant difference between the two formulations is demonstrated.

5.3   Equivalence Test

An equivalence test of two variances works largely similar to that of a single variance. We need to define a prior boundary of equivalence, and then, test whether our confidence interval is entirely within. A problem with ratios of variances is that they often have very large confidence intervals. Ratios of variances are, therefore, not very sensitive to test equivalence. Instead, we can define a prior overall boundary of equivalence and, then, test whether either of the two variances is within. For example, in the above two variances example the boundary of equivalence of plasma concentration of gentamicin for 90% confidence intervals had been set between 3.0 and 7.0 µg/l. The mean plasma concentrations were 4.0 for formula-A and 4.5 µg/l for formula-B.

Patients (n)	Standard deviation (s) (µg/l)	Mean (µg/l)	Standard error	90% confidence interval
Formula-A 10	3.0	4.0	0.9	2.5–5.5
Formula-B 15	2.0	4.5	0.6	3.5–5.5

As the 90% confidence interval for formula-A is not entirely within the set boundary, the criterion of equivalence is not entirely met. Based on this analysis, equivalence of the two formulas cannot be confirmed.

6   How to Analyze Variability, Three or More Samples

6.1   Bartlett's Test

Bartlett's test can be applied for comparing variances of three samples

$$\chi^2 = (n_1 + n_2 + n_3 - 3)\ln s^2 - \left[(n_1 - 1)\ln s_1^2 + (n_2 - 1)\ln s_2^2 + (n_3 - 1)\ln s_3^2\right]$$

where n_1 = size sample 1
s_1^2 = variance sample 1

$$s^2 = \text{pooled variance} = \frac{(n_1 - 1)s_1^2 + (n_2 - 1)s_2^2 + (n_3 - 1)s_3^2}{n_1 + n_2 + n_3 - 3} =$$

ln = natural logarithm

As an example, blood glucose variabilities are assessed in a parallel-group study of three insulin treatment regimens. For that purpose three different groups of patients are treated with different insulin regimens. Variabilities of blood glucose levels are estimated by group-variances:

	Group size (n)	Variance [(mmol/l)^2]
Group 1	100	8.0
Group 2	100	14.0
Group 3	100	18.0

$$\text{Pooled variance} = \frac{99 \times 8.0 + 99 \times 14.0 + 99 \times 18.0}{297} = 13.333$$

$$\chi^2 = 297 \times \ln 13.333 - 99 \times \ln 8.0 - 99 \times \ln 14.0 - 99 \times \ln 18.0$$
$$= 297 \times 2.58776 - 99 \times 2.079 - 99 \times 2.639 - 99 \times 2.890$$
$$= 768.58 - 753.19 = 15.37$$

We have three separate groups, and, so, $3-1=2$ degrees of freedom. The chi-square table shows that a significant difference between the three variances is demonstrated at $p < 0.001$. If the three groups are representative comparable samples, we may conclude that these three insulin regimens do not produce the same spread of glucose levels. In this study of parallel groups, variability in the data is assessed by comparison of between-subject variability. Other studies assess variability in the data by repeated measures within one subject.

6.2   Levene's Test

An alternative to the Bartlett's test is the Levene's test. The Levene's test is less sensitive than the Bartlett's test to departures from normality. If there is a strong evidence that the data do in fact come from a normal, or nearly normal, distribution, then Bartlett's test has a better performance. Both tests can be used for comparison of more than two variances. However, we should add that assessing significance of differences between more than two variances is, generally, not so relevant in clinical comparisons. In practice, clinical investigators are mostly interested in differences between two samples/groups rather than multiple samples/groups.

7 Discussion

For all tests discussed above we need to emphasize that the data come from a normal distribution. The tests can be quite misleading if applied to non-normal data. It would be good practice to look at the distribution of the data first, for example by drawing histograms or box plots, and to transform if needed. Also, non-parametric tests are available for the analysis of variances of non-normal data, for example the Kendall's test for the variance of ranks (Kendall and Stuart 1963; Siegel 1956; Tukey 1977).

In the current paper eight statistical methods are described for comparing variances of studies where the emphasis is on variability in the data. Clinical examples are given. The assessment of variability is, particularly, important in studies of medicines with a small therapeutic index. Table 44.1 gives an overview of such medicines, commonly used in practice. Their therapeutic ranges have been defined, and it is a prerequisite of many of them that peak and trough concentrations are carefully monitored in order to reduce toxicities and improve therapeutic efficacies. The development of such therapeutic ranges can benefit from variance-testing. For other medicines therapeutic indices may not be small, while plasma concentrations are not readily available. Instead of dose-concentration relationships, dose–response relationships are, then, studied in order to determine the best therapeutic regimens. This approach uses dose–response curves, and is based on the assumption that the mean response of many tests can be used for making predictions for the entire population. However, dose–response relationships may differ between individuals, and may depend on determinants like body mass, kidney function, underlying diseases, and other factors hard to control. Moreover, for the treatment of diseases like diabetes mellitus, hypercholesterolemia, hypertension etc., we are often more interested in the range of responses than we are in the mean response. Also for the study of such data variance-testing would, therefore, be in place.

Samples of observations are unpaired, if every patient is tested once, or paired, if every patient is tested repeatedly. In the case of repeated testing special statistical procedures have to be performed to adjust for correlations between paired observations. This is, particularly, required when analyzing averages, but less so when analyzing variances. Correlation levels little influence the comparison of variances, and, so, similar tests for the comparison of variances can be adequately used both for paired and for unpaired variances.

Table 44.1 Drugs with small therapeutic indices

1. Antibacterial agents	Gentamicin, vancomicin, tobramicin
2. Drugs for seizure disorders	Carbamazepine, phenytoine, phenobarbital, valproate
3. Cardiovascular and pulmonary drugs	Digoxin, theophylline, caffeine
4. Antidepressant drugs	Amitryptiline, nortriptyline, imipramine, clomipramine, maprotiline
5. Neuroleptic drugs	Clozapine

In conclusion, in clinical studies variability of the data may be a determinant more important than just averages. The current chapter provides eight straightforward methods to assess normally distributed data for variances, that can be readily used. The chi-square test for one sample and the F-test for two samples are available in Excel. The Bartlett's and Levene's test can be used for multiple variances, and are not in Excel, but can be found in statistical software programs. For the readers' convenience a reference is given (Anonymous 2011). Also, references are given for methods to analyze variances from non-normal data (Kendall and Stuart 1963; Siegel 1956; Tukey 1977).

8   Conclusions

Clinical investigators, although they are generally familiar with testing differences between averages, have difficulty testing differences between variabilities. The objective of this chapter was to give examples of situations where variability is more relevant than averages. Also to give simple methods for testing such data.

Examples include: (1) testing drugs with small therapeutic indices, (2) testing variability in drug response, (3) assessing pill diameters or pill weights, (4) comparing patient groups for variability in patient characteristics, (5) assessing the variability in duration of clinical treatments, (6) finding the best method for patient assessments. Various fields of research, particularly in clinical pharmacology, make use of test procedures that, implicitly, address the variability in the data. Tests especially designed for testing variabilities in the data include chi-square tests for one sample, F-tests for two samples, and Bartlett's or Levene's tests for three or more samples. Additional methods include (1) comparisons of confidence intervals, and (2) testing confidence intervals against prior defined intervals of therapeutic tolerance or equivalence. Many of these tests are available in Excel, and other statistical software programs, one of which is given.

We conclude that for the analysis of clinical data the variability of the data is often more important than the averages. Eight simple methods for assessment are described. It is a service to the readership of this book to put more emphasis on variability.

References

Almirall J, Bolibar I, Toran P et al (2004) Contribution of C-reactive protein to the diagnosis and assessment of severity of community-acquired pneumonia. Chest 125:1335–1342

Anonymoxus. http://www.itl.nist.gov/div898/handbook/eda/section3/eda35a.htm. Accessed 15 Dec 2011

Chambers HF, Sande MA (1996) Antimicrobial agents: the aminoglycosides. In: Goodman and Gillman's pharmacological basis of therapeutics, 9th edn. McGraw Hill, New York

Cleophas TJ (2005) Statistical tables to test data closer to expectation than compatible with random sampling. Clin Res Reg Affairs 22:83–92

Cleophas TJ, Van der Meulen J, Zwinderman AH (1998) Nighttime hypotension in hypertensive patients prevented by beta-blockers but not by angiotensin converting enzyme inhibitors or calcium channel blockers. Eur J Intern Med 9:251–257

Hahn GJ, Meeker WQ (1991) Statistical intervals: a guide for practitioners. Wiley, New York

Hauck WW, Anderson S (1984) A new statistical procedure for testing equivalence in two-group comparative bioavailability trials. J Pharmacokinet Biopharm 12:83–91

Kendall MG, Stuart A (1963) Rank correlation methods, 3rd edn. Griffin, London

Neutel JM, Smith DH (1997) The circadian pattern of blood pressure: cardiovascular risk and therapeutic opportunities. Curr Opin Nephrol Hypertens 6:250–256

Petrie A, Sabin C (2000) Medical statistics at a glance. Blackwell Science Ltd, London

Schuirmann DJ (1987) A comparison of the two one-sided test procedures and the proper approach for assessing the equivalence of average bioavailability. J Pharmacokinet Biopharm 15:657–680

Siegel S (1956) Non-parametric methods for behavioural sciences. McGraw Hill, New York

Tothfalusi L, Endrenyl L (2001) Evaluation of some properties of individual bioequivalence from replicate-design studies. Int J Clin Pharmacol Ther 39:162–166

Tukey JW (1977) Exploratory data analysis. Addison-Wesley, Reading

Chapter 45
Testing Reproducibility

1 Introduction

Poor reproducibility of diagnostic criteria is seldom acknowledged as a cause for low precision in clinical research. Also very few clinical reports communicate the levels of reproducibility of the diagnostic criteria they use. For example, of 11–13 original research papers published per issue in the ten last 2004 issues of the journal Circulation, none did, and of 5–6 original research papers published per issue in the ten last 2004 issues of the Journal of the American Association only 1 out of 12 did. These papers involved quality of life assessments, which are, notoriously, poorly reproducible. Instead, many reports used the averages of multiple measurements in order to improve the precision of the instruments used without further comment on reproducibility. For example, means of three blood pressure measurements, means of three cardiac cycles, average results of morphometric cell studies from two examiners, means of five random fields for cytogenetic studies were reported. Poor reproducibility of diagnostic criteria is, obviously, a recognized but rarely tested problem in clinical research. Evidence-based medicine is under pressure due to the poor reproducibility of clinical trials (Julius 2003; Cleophas and Cleophas 2003). As long as the possibility of poorly reproducible diagnostic criteria has not been systematically addressed, this very possibility cannot be excluded as a contributing cause for this. The current chapter reviews simple methods for routine assessment of reproducibility of diagnostic criteria/tests. These tests can answer questions like (1) do two techniques used to measure a particular variable, in otherwise identical circumstances, produce the same results, (2) does a single observer obtain the same results when he/she takes repeated measurements in identical circumstances, (3) do two observers using the same method of measurement obtain the same result.

T.J. Cleophas and A.H. Zwinderman, *Statistics Applied to Clinical Studies*,
DOI 10.1007/978-94-007-2863-9_45, © Springer Science+Business Media B.V. 2012

2   Testing Reproducibility of Quantitative Data (Continuous Data)

2.1   Method 1, Duplicate Standard Deviations (Duplicate SDs)

Reproducibility of quantitative data can be assessed by duplicate standard deviations. They make use of the differences between two paired observations. For example, ten patients are tested twice for their cholesterol-levels (mmol/l), (Fig. 45.1).

Patient	Test-1	Test-2	Difference (d)	d^2
1	5.4	5.5	−0.1	0.01
2	5.5	5.4	0.1	0.01
3	4.6	4.3	0.3	0.09
4	5.3	5.3	0.0	0.0
5	4.4	4.5	−0.1	0.01
6	5.5	5.4	0.1	0.01
7	6.6	6.4	0.2	0.02
8	5.4	5.6	−0.2	0.04
9	4.7	4.3	0.4	0.16
10	7.3	5.7	1.6	2.56
Mean	5.47	5.24	0.23	0.291
sd	0.892	0.677		

$$\text{Duplicate standard deviation} = \sqrt{\frac{1}{2}\sum\frac{d^2}{n}} = \sqrt{\frac{1}{2}\times 0.291} = 0.3814 \text{mmol/l}$$

d = differences between first and second measurements
n = sample size

$$\text{Relative duplicate standard deviation} = \frac{\text{duplicate standard deviation}}{\text{overall mean of data}}$$
$$= 0.3814 / \left[(5.47+5.24)/2\right]$$
$$= 0.0726 = 7.3\%$$

2.2   Method 2, Repeatability Coefficients

Repeatability coefficients equally make use of the differences between two paired observations.

The repeatability coefficient = 2 standard deviations (sds) of paired differences

$$= 2\sqrt{\sum\frac{\left(d-\bar{d}\right)^2}{n-1}} = 1.03$$

Fig. 45.1 Ten patients are
tested twice for their plasma
cholesterol levels

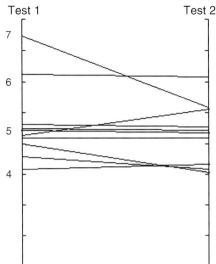

Plasma cholesterol (mmol/l)

d = differences between first and second measurements
d̄ = mean difference between first and second measurements
n = sample size

The advantage of the repeatability coefficient is that 95% limits of agreement can
be calculated from it. These are between d̄ ±2 sds = 0.23 ± 1.03 = between −0.80
and 1.26. Under the assumption of a normal distribution we can expect 95% of the
data to lie between these limits (Fig. 45.2).

2.3   Method 3, Intraclass Correlation Coefficients (ICCS)

Conceptually more complex is the calculation of intraclass correlation coefficients
(ICCs) for assessment of between-test agreement. It assesses reproducibility
between repeated measures within one subject by comparing the variability between
the repeated measures with the total variability in the data (Shrout and Fleiss 1979).
The formula is given by:

$$\text{Intraclass correlation coefficient (ICC)} = \frac{sd^2 \text{ between subjects}}{sd^2 \text{ between subjects} + sd^2 \text{ within subjects}}$$

The ICC ranges from 0 to 1, and it reflects the strength of association between
the first and second test. If it equals zero, no reproducibility can be expected. If 1,
then reproducibility is 100%. The ICC is otherwise called *proportion of variance* or
correlation ratio. If you are using SPSS (2011) to analyze the data, there is an easy

Fig. 45.2 Differences between first and second test for plasma cholesterol in the ten patients from Fig. 45.1. Nine of these ten patients have their differences within the 95% limits of agreement (*two horizontal lines*)

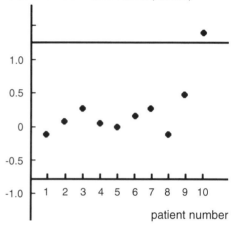

way to calculate the coefficient, which, additionally, provides you with a confidence interval and a p-value. A significant p-value is to be interpreted in terms of a proportion of total variance responsible for between-measurement variation significantly greater than 0. First command: Analyze/Scale/Reliability analysis. The dialog box allows you to include the two variables (results test-1 and results test-2). Next click the statistics box, and select the intraclass correlation coefficient, Model: one-way random, continue. The results for the above example are listed underneath:

Intraclass correlation coefficient = 0.7687
95% confidence intervals between 0.3386 and 0.9361
p-value 0.002
proportion of total variance responsible for between test variability = 77%.

ICCs can also be used for more than two repeated measures.

3   Testing Reproducibility of Qualitative Data (Proportions and Scores)

3.1   Cohen's Kappas

We use the example used by the Colorado Education Geography Center (Anonymous 2011). Suppose two observers assess the same patients for congenital heart disease, using Perloff's classification A–E (1991), and we wish to evaluate the extent to which they agree.

		Observer 1					
		A	B	C	D	E	Total
Observer 2	A	2	0	2	0	0	4
	B	0	1	0	0	0	1
	C	1	0	1	0	0	2
	D	0	0	0	2	1	3
	E	0	0	0	0	6	6
	Total	3	1	3	2	7	16 (N)

We present the results in a two-way contingency table of frequencies. The frequencies with which the observers agree are shown along the diagonal of the table (fat print). Note that all observations would be in the diagonal if they were perfectly matched. Then calculate the q-values, where q = the number of cases expected in the diagonal cells by chance.

$$q = n_{row} \times n_{column}/N$$
$$A = 4 \times 3/16 = 0.75$$
$$B = 1 \times 1/16 = 0.0625$$
$$C = 2 \times 3/16 = 0.375$$
$$D = 3 \times 2/16 = 0.375$$
$$E = 6 \times 7/16 = 2.625$$
$$q\ total = 4.1875 = 4.2$$

Then calculate kappa:

$$kappa = (d - q)/(N - q)$$
$$d = 12\ (the\ diagonal\ total\ of\ cells = 2 + 1 + 1 + 2 + 6 = 12)$$
$$N = total\ of\ columns\ or\ rows\ which\ should\ be\ equal$$
$$kappa = (12 - 4.2)/(16 - 4.2) = 0.66.$$

The closer the kappa is to 1.0, the better the agreement between the observers:

Poor if $k < 0.20$
Fair $0.21 < k < .040$
Moderate $0.41 < k < 0.60$
Substantial $0.61 < k < 0.80$
Good $k > 0.80$.

4   Incorrect Methods to Assess Reproducibility

4.1   Testing the Significance of Difference Between Two or More Sets of Repeated Measures

Instead of the repeatability coefficients or duplicate standard deviations, sometimes the significance of differences between two means or two proportions is used as method to assess reproducibility. For that purpose paired t-tests or

McNemar's tests are used. For more than two sets of repeated measures tests like the repeated-measures-analysis-of-variance or Friedman's tests are adequate. As an example, the significance of difference between the above two columns of cholesterol values are calculated as follows (sd = standard deviation, se = standard error):

$$\text{mean difference} \pm \text{sd} = 0.23 \pm 0.5165$$
$$\text{mean difference} \pm \text{se} = 0.23 \pm 0.1633$$
$$\text{t-value} = 0.23/0.1633 = 1.41$$
$$\text{according to the t-table } p > 0.05$$

This means that no significant difference between the first and second set of measurements is observed. This can not be taken equal to evidence of reproducibility. With small samples no evidence of a significant difference does not necessarily imply the presence of reproducibility. Yet, a test to preclude a significant difference is relevant within the context of reproducibility statistics, because it establishes the presence of a systematic difference. We are dealing with a biased assessment if we want to test the null-hypothesis of reproducibility.

4.2   Calculating the Level of Correlation Between Two Sets of Repeated Measures

If you plot the results from the first occasion against those from the second occasion, and calculate a Pearson's regression coefficient, a high level of correlation does not necessarily indicate a great reproducibility. For testing reproducibility we are not really interested in whether the points lie on a straight line. Rather we want to know whether they conform to the 45° line, which is the line of equality. This will not be established if we test the null-hypothesis that the correlation is zero.

5   Additional Real Data Examples

5.1   Reproducibility of Ambulatory Blood Pressure Measurements (ABPM)

Ambulatory blood pressure measurements (ABPM) are, notoriously, poorly reproducible. Polynomial curves of ABPM data may be better reproducible than the actual data. Figure 45.3 gives an example of data (Cleophas et al. 2001). Mean systolic ABPM blood pressures of ten untreated patients with mild hypertension ands their sds were recorded twice 1 week in-between. Figs 45.2 and 45.3 give 7th order polynomes of these data. Table 45.1 shows the results of the reproducibility assessment. Both duplicate sds and ICCs were used. Duplicate sds of means versus zero and versus grand mean were 15.9 and 7.2 mmHg, while of polynomes they were

Fig. 45.3 Mean values of ambulatory blood pressure data of ten untreated patients with mild hypertension and their sds, recorded twice, 1 week in-between

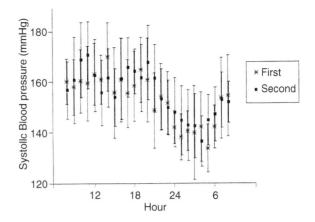

Table 45.1 Twenty four hour ambulatory blood pressure measurements in a group of ten patients with untreated mild hypertension tested twice: reproducibility of means of population

	Mean values variations vs zero	Mean values variations vs grand mean	Polynomes
Means (mmHg) (test 1/test 2)	153.1/155.4	153.1/155.4	–
Standard deviation (sd) (mmHg) (test 1/test 2)	21.9/21.1	15.7/13.8	–
95% CIs[a] (mmHg) (test 1/test 2)	139.4–166.8/ 142.2–168.6	143.3–163.9/ 146.8–164.0	–
Differences between means (sd) (mmHg)	−2.4 (22.4)	−2.3 (10.5)	–
P values differences between results tests 1 and 2	0.61	0.51	0.44
Duplicate sds (mmHg)	15.9	7.2	1.86
Relative Duplicate sds[b] (%)	66	31	7
Intra-class correlations (ICCs)	0.46	0.75	0.986
95% CIs	0.35–0.55	0.26–0.93	0.972–0.999
Proportion total variance responsible for between-patient variance (%)	46	75	99
95% CIs (%)	35–55	26–93	97–100

[a]*CIs* confidence intervals
[b]Calculated as 100% × [Duplicate sd/(overall mean − 130 mmHg)]

only 1.86 mmHg (differences in Duplicate sds significant at a P < 0.001 level). ICCs of means versus zero and versus grand mean were 0.46 and 0.75, while of polynomes they were 0.986 (differences in levels of correlation significant at a P < 0.001). Obviously, polynomes of ABPM data of means of populations produce significantly better reproducibility than do the actual data (Figs. 45.4 and 45.5).

Fig. 45.4 Polynome of corresponding ambulatory blood pressure recording (*first one*) from Fig. 45.3, reflecting a clear circadian rhythm of systolic blood pressures

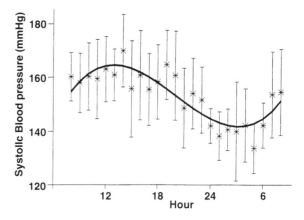

Fig. 45.5 Polynome of corresponding ambulatory blood pressure recording (*second one*) from Fig. 45.3, again reflecting a clear circadian rhythm of systolic blood pressures

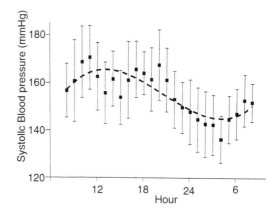

5.2 Two Different Techniques to Measure the Presence of Hypertension

Two different techniques are used in one group of patients to measure the presence of hypertension, namely (1) ambulatory blood pressure equipments and (2) self-assessed sphygmomanometers. Circumstances are, otherwise, identical.

		Ambulatory equipment		
		Yes	No	
Sphygmomanometer	Yes	184 (a)	54 (b)	218 (a+b)
	No	14 (c)	63 (d)	77 (c+d)
		198 (a+c)	117 (b+d)	315 (a+b+c+d)

We calculate kappa according to:

$$\text{expected value for cell (a)} = \frac{184+14}{315} \times 218 = 137$$

$$\text{expected value for cell (d)} = \frac{54+63}{315} \times 218 = 81$$

$$\text{kappa} = \frac{\dfrac{(218+77)}{315} - \dfrac{(137+81)}{315}}{1 - \dfrac{137+81}{315}} = 0.795$$

This would mean that we have a substantial level of agreement between the two techniques. However, McNemar's test shows a significant difference at $p<0.01$ between the two techniques indicating that a systematic difference exists, and that the reproducibility assessment is thus biased. The circumstances are not entirely identical.

6 Discussion

Any research profits from a reproducible challenge test to enhance sensitivity of the trial, and from a good interobserver agreement. The current paper gives some relatively simple methods for assessment. Reproducibility assessments are rarely communicated in research papers and this may contribute to the low reproducibility of clinical trials. We expected that reproducibility testing would, at least, be a standard procedure in clinical chemistry studies where a close to 100% reproducibility is generally required. However, even in a journal like the Journal of the International Federation of Clinical Chemistry and Laboratory Medicine out of 17 original papers communicating novel chemistry methods none communicated reproducibility assessments except for one study (Imbert-Bismut et al. 2004). Ironically, this very study reported two incorrect methods for that purpose, namely the assessment of significant differences between repeated measures, and the calculation of Pearson's correlation levels.

A more general explanation for the underreporting of reproducibility assessments in research communications is that the scientific community although devoted to the study of disease management, is little motivated to devote its energies to assessing the reproducibility of the diagnostic procedures required for the very study of disease management. Clinical investigators favor the latter to the former. Also the former gives no clear-cut career path, while the latter more often does so. And there are the injections from the pharmaceutical industry. To counterbalance this is a challenge for governments and university staffs.

We should add that textbooks of medical statistics rarely cover the subject of reproducibility testing: in only one of the 23 currently best sold textbooks for medical statistics the subject is briefly addressed (Petrie and Sabin 2000).

We conclude that poor reproducibility of diagnostic criteria/tests is, obviously, a well- recognized but rarely tested problem in clinical research. The current review of simple tests for reproducibility may be of some help to investigators.

7   Conclusions

Virtually no clinical papers communicate the levels of reproducibility of the diagnostic criteria/tests they use. Poor reproducibility cannot be excluded as a contributing cause for the poor reproducibility of clinical trials. The objective of this chapter was to review simple methods for reproducibility assessment of diagnostic criteria/tests.

Reproducibility of quantitative data can be estimated by (1) duplicate standard deviations, (2) repeatability coefficients, (3) intraclass correlation coefficients. For qualitative data Cohen's kappas are adequate. Incorrect methods include the test for a significant difference between repeated measures, and the calculation of levels of correlation between repeated measures.

Four adequate and two incorrect methods for reproducibility assessment of diagnostic criteria/tests are reviewed. These tests can also be used for more complex data like polynomial models of ambulatory blood pressure measurements. They may be of some help to investigators.

References

Anonymous Calculating Cohen's kappas. http://www.colorado.edu/geography/gcraft/notes/manerror/html/kappa.html. Accessed 15 Dec 2011

Cleophas GM, Cleophas TJ (2003) Clinical trials in jeopardy. Int J Clin Pharmacol Ther 41:51–6

Cleophas AF, Zwinderman AH, Cleophas TJ (2001) Reproducibility of polynomes of ambulatory blood pressure measurements. Perfusion 13:328–35

Imbert-Bismut F, Messous D, Thibaut V, Myers RB, Piton A, Thabut D, Devers L, Hainque B, Mecardier A, Poynard T (2004) Intra-laboratory analytical variability of biochemical markers of fibrosis and activity and reference ranges in healthy blood donors. Clin Chem Lab Med 42:323–33

Julius S (2003) The ALLHAT study: if you believe in evidence-based medicine. Stick to it. J Hypertens 21:453–4

Perloff JK (1991) The clinical recognition of congenital heart disease. Saunders, Philadelphia

Petrie A, Sabin C (2000) Assessing agreement. In: Medical statistics at a glance. Blackwell Science, London, p 93

Shrout PE, Fleiss JL (1979) Intraclass correlations: uses in assessing rater reliability. Psychol Bull 2:420–8

SPSS Statistical Software, Chicago, IL, www.SPSS.com. Accessed 15 Dec 2011

Chapter 46
Validating Qualitative Diagnostic Tests

1 Introduction

Clinical trials of disease management require accurate tests for making a diagnosis/patient follow-up. Whatever test, screening, laboratory or physical, investigators involved need to know how good it is. The goodness of a diagnostic test is a complex question that is usually estimated according to three criteria: (1) its reproducibility, (2) precision, and (3) validity. Reproducibility is synonymous to reliability, and is, generally, assessed by the size of differences between duplicate measures. Precision of a test is synonymous to the spread in the test results, and can be estimated, e.g., by standard deviations/standard errors. Validity is synonymous to accuracy, and can be defined as a test's ability to show which individuals have the disease in question and which do not. Unlike the first two criteria, the third is hard to quantify, first, because it is generally assessed by two estimators rather than one, namely sensitivity and specificity defined as the chance of a true positive and true negative test respectively. A second problem is, that these two estimators are severely dependent on one another. If one is high, the other is, as a rule, low, vice versa. Due to this mechanism it is difficult to find the most accurate diagnostic test for a given disease. In this chapter we review the current dual approach to accuracy and propose that it be replaced with a new method, called the overall accuracy level. The main advantage of this new method is that it tells you exactly how much information is given by the test under assessment. It, thus, enables you to determine the most accurate qualitative tests for making a diagnosis, and can also be used to determine the most accurate threshold for positive qualitative tests with results on a continuous scale.

T.J. Cleophas and A.H. Zwinderman, *Statistics Applied to Clinical Studies*,
DOI 10.1007/978-94-007-2863-9_46, © Springer Science+Business Media B.V. 2012

2   Overall Accuracy of a Qualitative Diagnostic Test

A test that provides a definitive diagnosis, otherwise called a gold standard test, is 100% accurate. But this test may be too expensive, impractical or simply impossible. Instead, inexpensive but less accurate screening tests, depending on the presence of a marker, are used. Prior to implementation, such tests must be assessed for level of accuracy against the gold standard test. Generally, such tests produce a yes/no result, and are, therefore, called qualitative tests, e.g., the presence of a positive blood culture test, a positive antinuclear antibody test, a positive leuco-esterase urine test, and many more. In order to assess accuracy of such tests, the overall accuracy level can be calculated from a representative sample of patients in whom the gold-standard result is known (Table 46.1).

The magnitude of the overall accuracy level in the example from Table 46.1 is 83.9%, which is between that of the sensitivity and specificity, 85.7% and 80%, but closer to the former than the latter. This is due to the larger number of patients with the disease than those without the disease. Obviously, the overall accuracy level, unlike sensitivity and specificity, adjusts for differences in numbers of patients with and without the disease as generally observed in a representative sample of patients. The overall accuracy level can be interpreted as the amount of information given by the test relative to the gold standard test: if the gold standard test provides 100% of information, the test will provide 83.9% of that information. An overall accuracy of 50% or less indicates that the information is not different from the information provided by mere guessing. Flipping a coin would do the job just as well as does this test. An example of a new test without information is given in Table 46.2. This new test has a specificity of only 20%, but a sensitivity of 60%, and so the investigators may conclude that it is appropriate to approve this new test, because it provides a

Table 46.1 Calculation of sensitivity, specificity, and overall accuracy level of qualitative test from a sample of patients

	Disease	Yes (n)	No (n)
Positive test	Yes (n)	180 a	20 b
Positive test	No (n)	30 c	80 d

n = number of patients
a = number of true positive patients
b = number of false positive patients
c = number of false negative patients
d = number of true negative patients

Sensitivity of the above test $= a/(a+c) = 180/210 = 85.7\%$

Specificity of the above test $= d/(b+d) = 80/100 = 80\%$

Overall accuracy level $= (a+d)/(a+b+c+d) = 260/310 = 83.9\%$

Table 46.2 Qualitative test providing no more information than mere guessing or tossing a coin

	Disease	Yes (n)	No (n)
Positive test	Yes	60 a	50 b
Positive test	No	40 c	10 d

n = number of patients

a = number of true positive patients

b = number of false positive patients

c = number of false negative patients

d = number of true negative patients

Sensitivity of the above test = $a / (a + c) = 60\%$

Specificity of the above test = $d / (b + d) = 20\%$

Overall accuracy level = $(a + d) / (a + b + c + d) = 70 / 160 = 43.8\%$

correct diagnosis in 60% of the patients who have the disease. However, given the overall accuracy of only 43.8% this diagnostic test does not provide more information than mere guessing or tossing a coin, and should not be approved.

3 Perfect and Imperfect Qualitative Diagnostic Tests

Qualitative diagnostic tests may produce results on a continuous scale, and the results of such tests can be displayed by two Gaussian curves (under the assumption that the data follow normal distributions), rather than simply by a two by two table. Figure 46.1 is an example of a perfect fit diagnostic test. The two curves show the frequency distribution with on the x-axis the individual patient results and on the y-axis "how often". The total areas under the curve of the two curves represent all of the patients, left graph those without the disease, and right graph those with the disease. The curves do not overlap. The test seems to be a perfect predictor for presence or absence of disease.

In Fig. 46.2 the situation is less than perfect, the two curves overlap, and, it is not obvious from the graphs where to draw the line between a positive and negative result. The decision made is shown as the vertical line. False positives/negatives are shown in the shaded areas under the curves. The above two examples are simplified, because they assume that in a random sample the total numbers of true positives and true negatives are equal in size, and have the same spread. In practice the numbers of patients with and without disease in a random sample have different sizes and spread, and this should be recognized in the distribution curves, complicating the assessment a little bit (Fig. 46.3).

The left and right graph are calculated from the mean erythrocyte sedimentation rate value and standard deviation of a random sample of patients with and without pneumonia. The areas under the curve represent 100% of either of the two groups. In order to assess accuracy of erythrocyte sedimentation rate as qualitative diagnostic test for pneumonia it is convenient to define a test positive if less than 2.5% of the true negative patients are negative in the test. Using this 2.5% as a threshold, the

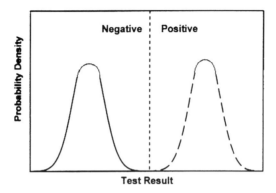

Fig. 46.1 Example of a perfect fit qualitative diagnostic test. The *two curves* show the frequency distributions with on the x-axis the individual patient results, and on the y-axis "how often". The patients with and without the disease do not overlap

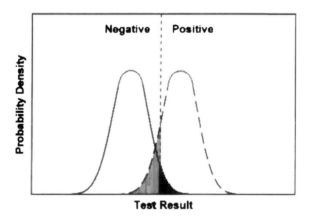

Fig. 46.2 Example of a less than perfect fit qualitative diagnostic test. The *two curves* show the frequency distributions with on the x-axis the individual patient results, and on the y-axis "how often". The patients with and without the disease overlap

results from Fig. 46.3 can now also be displayed in the form of a two by two table (Table 46.3). Sensitivity, specificity, and overall accuracy are calculated (Table 46.3).

4 Determining the Most Accurate Threshold for Positive Qualitative Tests

We would like to have a sensitivity and specificity close to 1 (100%), and thus an overall accuracy equally close to 1 (100%). However, in practice most diagnostic tests are far from perfect, and produce false positive and false negative results.

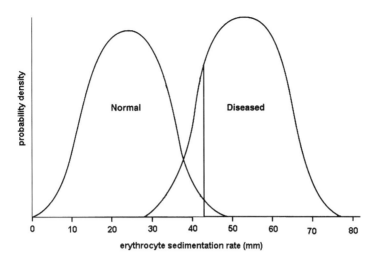

Fig. 46.3 Example of frequency distributions of erythrocyte sedimentation rate values in 200 patients with and 300 patients without pneumonia. On the x-axis are the individual erythrocyte sedimentation rate values of the normals and the diseased patients, and the areas under the curve represent 100% of either of the two groups. It is not obvious from the graphs where to draw the line between a positive and negative test: the decision made is shown by the *vertical line*

Table 46.3 Sensitivity, specificity, and overall accuracy level of qualitative test using the 2.5% threshold for true negative patients (Fig. 46.3)

	Disease	Yes ($n_1 = 300$)	No ($n_2 = 200$)
Positive test	Yes (%)	74% a	2.5% b
Positive test	No (%)	26% c	97.5% d

n = number of patients
a = number of true positive patients
b = number of false positive patients
c = number of false negative patients
d = number of true negative patients
Sensitivity of the above test = $a / (a + c) = 74\%$
Specificity of the above test = $d / (b + d) = 97.5\%$.
Overall accuracy level = $74 \left[n_1 / (n_1 + n_2) \right] + 97.5 \left[n_2 / (n_1 + n_2) \right] = 83.4\%$.

We can increase sensitivity by moving the vertical decision line between a positive and negative test (Fig. 46.3) to the left, and we can increase specificity by moving it in the opposite direction. Moving the above threshold further to the right would be appropriate, e.g., for an incurable deadly disease. You want to avoid false positives (cell b), meaning telling a healthy person he/she will die soon, while false negatives (cell c) aren't so bad since you can't treat the disease anyway. If, instead the test would serve for a disease fatal if untreated but completely treatable, it should provide

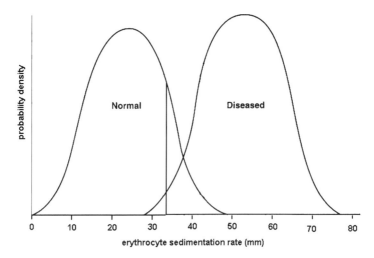

Fig. 46.4 Example of the frequency distributions of erythrocyte sedimentation rate values in 200 patients with and 300 patients without pneumonia. On the x-axis are the individual erythrocyte sedimentation rate values of the normals and the diseased patients, and the areas under the curve represent 100% of either of the two groups. It is not obvious from the graphs where to draw the line between a positive and negative test: the decision made is shown as the *vertical line*

a sensitivity better than 74%, even at the expense of a lower specificity. False-negative would be awful, as it means missing a case of a treatable fatal disease. For that purpose the threshold of such a test is set far more to the left (Fig. 46.4).

Sensitivity, specificity, and overall accuracy level can now be calculated (Table 46.4).

Sensitivity of the above test $= a / (a + c) = 97.5\%$

Specificity of the above test $= d / (b + d) = 77\%$

Overall accuracy level $= 97.5 \left(n_1 / (n_1 + n_2) \right) + 77 \left(n_2 / (n_1 + n_2) \right) = 89.3\%$

There are, of course, many diseases that do not belong to one of the two extremes described above. Also, there may be additional arguments for choosing a particular threshold. E.g., in non-mortality trials false negative tests, generally, carry the risk of enhanced morbidity, such as vision loss due to persistent glaucoma, hearing loss due to recurrent otitis etc. However, such risks may be small if repeat tests are performed in time. Also, false positive tests create here patient anxiety and costs. In situations like this, false positive tests are considered as important as false negative. Therefore, we might as well search for the threshold providing the best overall accuracy from our test. This is usually done by considering several cut-off points that give a unique pair of values for sensitivity and specificity, thus comparing the probabilities of a positive test in those with and those without the disease. A curve with "1-specificity" (= proportion of false positive tests) on the x-axis and sensitivity

Table 46.4 Calculation of sensitivity, specificity, and overall accuracy level of a qualitative test where the threshold is set according to Fig. 46.4

	Disease	Yes ($n_1 = 300$)	No ($n_2 = 200$)
Positive test	Yes (%)	97.5% a	23% b
Positive test	No (%)	2.5% c	77% d

n_x = number of patients
a = % true positive patients
b = % false positive patients
c = % false negative patients
d = % true negative patients

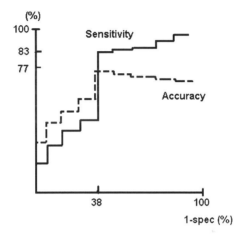

Fig. 46.5 The ROC (receiver operating characteristic) curve (*continuous curve*) of erythrocyte sedimentation rate values of patients with pneumonia plots the sensitivity values (true positives) against the "1-specificity" values (false positives). The accuracy "ROC" curve (*interrupted curve*) plots the overall accuracy values against the "1-specificity" values (false positives)

(= proportion of true positive tests) on the y-axis facilitates to choose cut-off levels with relatively high sensitivity/specificity. The continuous curve of Fig. 46.5, otherwise called a ROC (receiver operating characteristic) curve, is an example.

It shows the relationship between sensitivities and specificities of the erythrocyte sedimentation rate as a diagnostic test for the presence of pneumonia. The curve suggests that a relatively high sensitivity/specificity is obtained for the 83% sensitivity/38% "1-specificity". However, in many ROC curves more than a single cut-off value with relatively high sensitivity/specificity are observed, and it may, therefore, be difficult to choose the most accurate cut-off level from such curves. Also, ROC curves use sensitivity and specificity only, which means that they do not account for differences between the numbers of patients with and without the disease. These problems can be prevented by plotting, instead of the sensitivity, the overall accuracy level against "1-specificity". This is shown by the interrupted curve

Table 46.5 The calculation of positive and negative predictive values, and of likelihood ratios

	Disease	Yes (n)	No (n)
Positive test	Yes	a	b
Positive test	No	c	d

n = number of patients

Positive predictive value = a/(a + b)

Negative predictive value = d/(c + d)

Likelihood ratio for positive result = a/(a + c)/d/(b + d)

of Fig. 46.5. This accuracy "ROC" curve will unequivocally identify the cut-off threshold with the single best overall accuracy level.

ROC curves are only briefly addressed in this text. Details are beyond the scope of this chapter, but some advantages of accuracy "ROC" curves compared to the classic ROC curves are mentioned. In addition to ROC curves, accuracy is sometimes assessed by measure of concordance, the optimism corrected c-statistic of Young (Anonymous 2011). It is identical to the AUC (area under the curve) of the ROC curve, and varies between 0.5 and 1.0. The larger the AUC, the better the accuracy.

5   Discussion

Another approach to accuracy of diagnostic tests are the positive and negative predictive values and likelihood ratios, the calculation of which is shown in Table 46.5.

Just like the overall accuracy level, these estimators adjust for numbers of differences in patients with and without the disease, but they do not answer what proportion of patients has a correct test.

Riegelman (2005), recently, proposed another method for assessing accuracy of a qualitative diagnostic test, which he called the discriminant ability, defined as

$$\left(\text{sensitivity} + \text{specificity}\right) / 2.$$

Although this method avoids the dual approach to accuracy, it wrongly assumes equal importance and equal prevalence of sensitivity and specificity, and does neither answer what proportion of the patients has a correct test.

We should add that sensitivity, specificity and overall accuracy level are usually expressed as percentages. As with all estimates in clinical trials, we should calculate confidence intervals of these estimates in order to quantify the level of uncertainty involved in our results (see Chap. 47).

The advantage of the overall accuracy approach described in this chapter compared to the dual sensitivity/specificity approach is that it enables to determine not only the most accurate qualitative tests for making given diagnoses, but also the most accurate thresholds for positive qualitative tests with results on a continuous scale. The method is less adequate for the assessment of diagnostic tests for extreme disease like incurable deadly diseases and treatable but untreated deadly diseases for which diagnostic tests with either optimal sensitivity or optimal specificity are required.

For determining the most accurate threshold for a qualitative test we recommend to replace a ROC curve with an accuracy "ROC" curve, because the latter unlike the former accounts for possible differences in a random sample between the numbers of patients with and without the disease.

The overall accuracy level has four advantages compared to the sensitivity/specificity levels. It (1) adjusts for differences between numbers of patients with and without the disease, (2) is able to readily identify tests that give no information at all, (3) provides the amount of information given by the test relative to the gold standard test, (4) enables to draw ROC curves adjusted for the differences between numbers of patients with and without the disease.

6   Conclusions

Clinical trials of disease management require accurate tests for making a diagnosis/patient follow-up. Currently, accuracy of qualitative diagnostic tests is hard to quantify, because it is generally assessed by two estimators, sensitivity and specificity, that are severely dependent on one another. If one estimator is high, the other is, as a rule, low.

The objective of this chapter was to review the current dual approach to accuracy, and to propose that it be replaced with a new method, called the overall accuracy level.

The overall accuracy level is defined as the proportion of test results that are correct. Usage of this level, unlike sensitivity and specificity levels, enables (1) to adjust for differences between numbers of patients with and without the disease, (2) to readily identify tests that give no information at all, (3) to provide the entire amount of information given by the test relative to the gold standard test, (4) to draw receiver operating characteristic (ROC) curves adjusted for the differences between numbers of patients with and without the disease. The method is less adequate for the assessment of qualitative diagnostic tests for extreme diseases like incurable deadly diseases and treatable but untreated deadly diseases for which diagnostic tests with either optimal sensitivity or optimal specificity are required.

Due to the dual sensitivity/specificity approach to accuracy of qualitative diagnostic tests it is, currently, difficult to find the most accurate diagnostic test for a given disease. The overall accuracy level is more appropriate to that aim.

References

Anonymous. Chapter 8: statistical models for prognostication. In: Interactive textbook. http://symptomresearch.nih.gov.chapter_8. Accessed 15 Dec 2011

Riegelman RK (2005) Studying a study and testing a test. Lippincott Williams & Wilkins, Philadelphia

Chapter 47
Uncertainty of Qualitative Diagnostic Tests

1 Introduction

In clinical research gold standard tests for making a diagnosis are often laborious and sometimes impossible. Instead, simple and non-invasive tests are often used. A problem is that these tests have limited sensitivities and specificities. Levels around 50% means that no more information is given than flipping a coin. Levels substantially higher than 50% are commonly accepted as documented proof, that the diagnostic test is valid. However, sensitivity/specificity are estimates from experimental samples, and scientific rigor recommends that with experimental sampling amounts of uncertainty be included. Although the STARD (Standards for Reporting Diagnostic Accuracy) working party recently advised "to include in the estimates of diagnostic accuracy adequate measures of uncertainty, e.g., 95%-confidence intervals" (Bossuyt et al. 2003) , so far uncertainty is virtually never assessed in sensitivity/specificity evaluations of clinical diagnostic tests. This is a pity, because calculated levels of uncertainty can be used for statistically testing whether the sensitivity/specificity is significantly larger than 50%. The present chapter uses examples to describe (1) simple methods for calculating standard errors and 95% confidence intervals, and (2) how they can be employed for statistical testing whether the new test is valid. We do hope that this chapter will stimulate clinical investigators to more often assess the uncertainty of the diagnostic tests they apply.

2 Example 1

Two hundred patients are evaluated to determine the sensitivity/specificity of B-type Natriuretic Peptide (BNP) for making a diagnosis of heart failure.

		Heart failure (n)	
		Yes	No
Result diagnostic test	Positive	70 (a)	35 (b)
	Negative	30 (c)	65 (d)

The sensitivity (a/(a+c)) and specificity (d/(b+d)) are calculated to be 0.70 and 0.65 respectively (70% and 65%). In order for these estimates to be significantly larger than 50% their 95% confidence interval should not cross the 50% boundary.

The standard errors are calculated according to the equations given in Appendix 1. For sensitivity the standard error is 0.0458, for specificity 0.0477. Under the assumption of Gaussian curve distributions in the data the 95% confidence intervals of the sensitivity and specificity can be calculated using the equations

$$95\% \text{confidence interval of the sensitivity} = 0.70 \pm 1.96 \times 0.0458$$
$$\text{``} \qquad \text{``} \qquad \text{``} \qquad \text{specificity} = 0.65 \pm 1.96 \times 0.0477.$$

This means that the 95% confidence interval of the sensitivity is between 61% and 79%, for specificity it is between 56% and 74%. These results do not cross the 50% boundary and fall, thus, entirely within the boundary of validity. The diagnostic test can be accepted as being valid.

3   Example 2

Dimer tests have been widely used as screening tests for lung embolias.

		Lung embolia (n)	
		Yes	No
Dimer test	Positive	2 (a)	18 (b)
	Negative	1 (c)	182 (d)

The sensitivity (a/(a+c)) and specificity (d/(b+d)) are calculated to be 0.666 and 0.911 respectively (67% and 91%). In order for these estimates to be significantly larger than 50% the 95% confidence interval of them should again not cross the 50% boundary.

The standard errors as calculated according to the equations given in Appendix 1, are for sensitivity 3.672, for specificity 0.286. Under the assumption of Gaussian curve distributions the 95% confidence intervals of the sensitivity and specificity are calculated using the equations

$$95\% \text{ confidence interval of the sensitivity} = 0.67 \pm 1.96 \times 3.672$$
$$\text{``} \qquad \text{``} \qquad \text{``} \qquad \text{specificity} = 0.91 \pm 1.96 \times 0.286.$$

The 95% confidence interval of the sensitivity is between −5.4 and +7.8. The 95% confidence interval of the specificity can be similarly calculated, and is between 0.35 and 1.47. These intervals are very wide and do not at all fall within the boundaries of 0.5–1.0 (50–100%). Validity of this test is, therefore, not really demonstrated. The appropriate conclusion of this evaluation should be: based on this evaluation the diagnostic cannot be accepted as being valid in spite of a sensitivity and specificity of respectively 67% and 91%.

4   Example 3

A disadvantage of the sensitivity/specificity approach to validation is that it is dual and that the two estimates are severely dependent on one another. Instead, overall-validity is sometimes used. It is defined as the diagnostic test's ability to show which individuals have a true test either positive or negative $((a+d)/(a+b+c+d)$ where the letters indicate the numbers of patients in the four cells as demonstrated above).

As an example, for approval of C-reactive protein as a marker for a cardiovascular event a boundary of overall-validity is specified in the study protocol as being at least 85%. The 95% confidence interval of the overall validity level can be calculated from the data. If the confidence interval falls entirely within the specified boundary, overall validity is demonstrated.

The results are given underneath:

sensitivity = 80% with a standard error = 2%,
specificity = 90% with a standard error = 1%,
prevalence = 10% with a standard error = 3%.

With this information we can calculate the overall-validity using the method described in Appendix 2. The overall-validity equals 0.89 (89%), while its squared standard error, otherwise called variance, equals 0.000337.

The standard error of the overall-validity is, thus, the square root of its variance, and equals 0.01836 (1.836%). An overall-validity of 89% with a standard error of 1.836% means that the 95% confidence interval is between $0.89 - (1.96 \times 0.01836)$ and $0.89 + (1.96 \times 0.01836)$, and is thus between 85.4% and 92.6%. This interval falls entirely between the specified interval of validity of at least 85%. The overall-validity of this diagnostic test has been demonstrated.

5   Example 4

A methionine loading test is applied to assess cystathione-beta-synthase deficiency, an inborn error of metabolism causing homocystinuria. The gold standard test is the measurement of the intracellular lacking enzyme, a laborious method.

		Cystathione synthase deficiency (n)	
		Yes	No
Methionine loading test	Yes	18 (a)	17 (b)
	No	2 (c)	31 (d)

In this evaluation the sensitivity and specificity were adequate (0.90 and 0.65 respectively). However, in the protocol the investigators pre-specified their boundary of overall-validity between 0.5 and 1.0 (50% and 100%). For assessment of uncertainty and statistical testing the method of Appendix 2 was applied. Overall-validity equalled 0.7205, its standard error 0.1355. The 95% confidence intervals of the overall-validity were calculated to be between $0.7205 \pm (1.96 \times 0.1355)$ and is, thus, between 0.45 and 0.99. This confidence interval is wide, and does not entirely fall within the pre-specified boundaries. According to the presented assessment the validity of this test could not be confirmed. With larger samples this validation-procedure might have been more successful.

6 Discussion

The accuracy of cardiovascular diagnostic tests is often assessed by sensitivity, specificity, and sometimes by overall-validity, but the precision of these point estimates is rarely taken into account. Low precision means that the 95% confidence interval of them is wide, and, thus, that the diagnostic tests can not be reliably used for making predictions. In this paper it is shown that, by calculating the standard error of the diagnostic test, its precision can be assessed. From the standard errors 95% confidence can be calculated. If the 95% confidence intervals of the standard error fall entirely within pre-defined boundaries, the diagnostic test can be accepted as being valid. If not, the test should be rejected.

We should add that the sample size is, of course, a major determinant of the confidence intervals. For example, according to the above methods the 95% confidence intervals of the proportion of true positives (sensitivity) with:

$n = 10$ is between 0.410 and 0.990
$n = 100$ is between 0.610 and 0.790
$n = 1,000$ is between 0.671 and 0.729.

The validation samples should, therefore, largely match the sample sizes of the future clinical trials using the diagnostic test under study. If the size of your validation sample $n = 100$, then this diagnostic test is probably not adequately sensitive/specific for a clinical trial including a sample size of $n = 10$. In contrast, if clinical trials include many more patients than included in the validity assessment of their diagnostic tests, then the confidence intervals are underestimated, and the diagnostic test will perform even better than predicted by the calculated confidence intervals.

We conclude that adequate diagnostic tests are vital for the multitude of cardiovascular intervention studies of new therapies. For validation of diagnostic tests sensitivity/specificity/overall-validity are calculated. This practice is incomplete, because the number of true positives and true negatives in your assessment are estimates from experimental samples, and scientific rigor requires that with any estimate in clinical research standard errors/confidence intervals have to be included in order to quantify the level of uncertainty in your data. We provide simple methods for such purpose, and do hope that they be implied in future validation studies of cardiovascular diagnostic tests.

7 Conclusion

In clinical research simple and non-invasive tests are often used instead of the gold standard tests for making diagnoses. Because the sensitivity/specificity of the simple tests are limited, their magnitude is routinely accounted in validation procedures. These measures of validity are estimates from experimental samples, and their precision, otherwise called certainty, is rarely assessed. This chapter gives simple methods for establishing their uncertainty.

As with other estimates in clinical research the standard errors of the sensitivity and specificity can be calculated in order to quantify their uncertainty. From these standard errors confidence intervals can be calculated. In the study protocol validation boundaries of the confidence intervals should be pre-specified. Only, if the confidence intervals fall entirely within these validation boundaries, validity is demonstrated. We recommend that the lower level of the validation boundaries should never be set below 50%, because a sensitivity and specificity close to 50% gives no more information than tossing a coin.

An effort should be made to assess uncertainty of the sensitivity and specificity of diagnostic tests before accepting them for general use. Simple methods for that purpose are given.

Appendix 1

For the calculation of the standard errors (SEs) of sensitivity, specificity and overall-validity we make use of the Gaussian curve assumption in the data.

		Definitive diagnosis (n)	
		Yes	No
Result diagnostic test	Yes	a	b
	No	c	d

Sensitivity $= a/(a+c) =$ proportion true positives
Specificity $= d/(b+d) =$ proportion true negatives
1-specificity $= b/(b+d)$
Proportion of patients with a definitive diagnosis $= (a+c)/(a+b+c+d)$
Overall validity $= (a+d)/(a+b+c+d)$

In order to make predictions from these estimates of validity their standard deviations/errors are required. The standard deviation/error (SD/SE) of a proportion can be calculated.

$$SD = \sqrt{p(1-p)} \text{ where } p = \text{proportion.}$$

$$SE = \sqrt{\left[p(1-p)/n\right]} \text{ where } n = \text{sample size}$$

where p equals $a/(a+c)$ for the sensitivity. Using the above equations the standard errors can be readily obtained.

$$SE_{sensitivity} = \sqrt{ac/(a+c)^3}$$

$$SE_{specificity} = \sqrt{db/(d+b)^3}$$

$$SE_{1-specificity} = \sqrt{db/(d+b)^3}$$

$$SE_{proportion of patients with a definitive diagnosis} = \sqrt{(a+b)(c+d)/(a+b+c+d)^3}$$

Appendix 2

The equation of the SE of the overall-validity is less straightforward, but can be obtained using the Bayes' rule (Berger and Bernerdo 1989) and the delta method (Anonymous 2011). The calculations are given for the purpose of completeness (Var = variance = square root of the standard error; prevalence = proportion of patients with a definitive diagnosis).

$$\text{Overall - validity} = \text{sensitivity} \times \text{prevalence} + \text{specificity} \times (1 - \text{prevalence})$$

In order to calculate the standard error (SE), we make use of the equation (Var = variance, Cov = covariance)

$$Var(X+Y) = Var(X) + Var(Y) + 2\,Cov(X,Y)$$

If $X =$ sensitivity $\times$ prevalence, and $Y =$ specificity $\times (1 - \text{prevalence})$, then the equations can be combined to obtain an equation for the variance of the overall-validity (sens = sensitivity, spec = specificity, prev = prevalence)

$$Var_{overall - validity} = Var_{sens \times prev} + Var_{spec \times (1-prev)} + 2\,Cov_{sens \times prev,\ spec \times (1-prev)}$$

The variance of $X + Y$ may according to the delta-method (Anonymous 2011) be approached from:

$$\mathrm{Var}(X + Y) = Y^2 \mathrm{Var}(X) + X^2 \mathrm{Var}(Y)$$

By combining the equations we will end up finding:

$$\mathrm{Var}_{\text{overall - validity}} = \mathrm{prev}^2 \times \mathrm{Var}_{\text{sens}} + (1 - \mathrm{prev})^2 \times \mathrm{Var}_{1-\text{spec}} + (\mathrm{sens} - \mathrm{spec})^2 \times \mathrm{Var}_{\text{prev}}$$

The delta-method describes the variance of natural logarithm (ln) (X) as $\mathrm{Var}(\ln(x)) = \mathrm{Var}(x)/x^2$. The approach is sufficiently accurate if the standard errors of prevalence, sensitivity and specificity are small, which is true if samples are not too small. We should add that the delta method is very helpful for the statistical assessment of complex functions like those of standard errors. Second derivatives of parabolas with values similar to those of the complex functions are used to find the best fit parabolas (second order polynomes). Parabolas are easy, and produce a good fit of such complex functions. This methodology has developed tremendously, and terms commonly used for it are the quadratic approximation, eigenvectors, and the delta-method.

References

Anonymous Delta-method. http://en.wikidepia.org/wiki/Delta_method. Accessed 15 Dec 2011
Berger JO, Bernerdo J (1989) Estimating a product of normal means: Bayesian analysis with some priors. J Am Stat Assoc 84:200–207
Bossuyt PM, Reitsma JB, Bruns DE, Gatsonis CA, Glasziou PP, Irwig JG, Moher D, Rennie D, De Vet HC, for the STARD steering group (2003) Education and debate. Towards complete and accurate reporting of studies of diagnostic accuracy: the STARD initiative. BMJ 326:41–44

Chapter 48
Meta-Analysis of Qualitative Diagnostic Tests

1 Introduction

In the past few years many novel diagnostic methods have been developed, including multi-slice computer tomography, magnetic resonance, positive emission tomography and many more methods. Studies evaluating their respective sensitivities and specificities have been published, and meta-analyses of these studies can now be performed in order to establish whether the findings are consistent and can be generalized across populations and morbidity/treatment variations. Sensitivity and specificity are estimators of accuracy of diagnostic methods as explained in the underneath diagram.

	Gold standard test	Positive	Negative
Diagnostic test	Positive	TP	FP
	Negative	FN	TN

TP = number of true positive, FP of false positive, FN of false negative, and TN of true negative patients in a study.

$$\text{Sensitivity} = \text{true positive rate} \, (\text{TPR}) = \text{TP} / (\text{TP} + \text{FN})$$
$$\text{Specificity} = \text{true negative rate} \, (\text{TNR}) = \text{TN} / (\text{TN} + \text{FP}).$$

$$1 - \text{Specificity} = (\text{TN} + \text{FP}) / (\text{TN} + \text{FP}) - \text{TN} / (\text{TN} + \text{FP})$$
$$= \text{FP} / (\text{TN} + \text{FP}) = \text{FPR}$$

An intuitive approach to meta-analysis of diagnostic studies is to pool the odds of sensitivity (= TPR/(1 − TPR) and that of specificity (= TNR/(1 − TNR) of the separate studies. Sensitivities and specificities are, however, dependent on one another, and, in addition, in a non-linear manner as shown in the summary receiver operated characteristic (ROC) curve from Fig. 48.1. In order to account for these problems Moses and Wittemberg proposed diagnostic odds ratios of the sensitivities

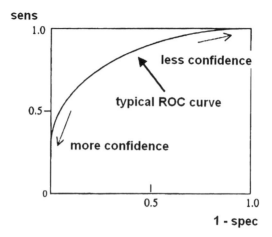

Fig. 48.1 Example of a summary receiver-operated-characteristic (ROC) curve, the proportion of true positive patients (= sensitivity) is drawn against the proportion of false positive patients (= 1 – specificity) using the results of multiple studies. *Sens* sensitivity, *1 – spec* 1 – specificity. With many diagnostic tests, tests results do not necessarily fall into one of two categories, but rather into categories with more or less confidence in the presence of a disease

versus the specificities (DORs) (Moses et al. 1993). In recent years this approach has been increasingly pursued (Hasselblad and Hedges 1995; Irwig et al. 1995; Walter 2002; Glas et al. 2003; Bipat et al. 2003). The current chapter using the results of a previously published review of diagnostic studies (Scheidler et al. 1997) as an example, reviews advantages and disadvantages of this novel method and discusses alternative possibilities.

2   Diagnostic Odds Ratios (DORS)

The accuracy of a diagnostic test is usually summarized by two statistics: the true-positive-rate (TPR) or sensitivity, and the true-negative-rate (TNR) or specificity. They are often used to draw ROC curves (Fig. 48.1). Instead of the dual approach of sensitivity and specificity, accuracy can also be summarized by the diagnostic odds ratio (DOR):

$$DOR = \frac{sensitivity \, / \, (1 - sensitivity)}{(1 - specificity) \, / \, specificity}$$

The DOR is an interesting term, since it compares the odds of true positive patients with that of false positives, and, thus, summarizes the overall accuracy of a diagnostic test.

Table 48.1 Example of meta-analysis of 17 diagnostic studies of lymphangiography for assessment of lymph node metastases

Study No.	tp	fp	fn	tn
1.	0	1	6	17
2.	12	3	3	7
3.	4	1	2	13
4.	10	4	3	25
5.	3	1	4	12
6.	9	3	3	29
7.	20	4	8	31
8.	17	5	7	21
9.	2	0	9	32
10.	3	1	9	38
11.	1	1	2	18
12.	5	2	2	61
13.	21	8	40	184
14.	4	3	9	42
15.	0	0	5	15
16.	7	11	22	158
17.	3	3	2	29

tp true positive, *fp* false positive, *fn* false negative, *tn* true negative

A problem is, that, like any odds ratio, it does not follow a Gaussian distribution, and a logarithmic transformation is required. For analysis a linear regression of the ln (DOR) on the statistic S is often applied.

$$\ln(DOR) = \ln\left(\frac{TPR}{1-TPR}\right) - \ln\left(\frac{FPR}{1-FPR}\right) \quad \text{and}$$

$$S - \ln\left(\frac{TPR}{1-TPR}\right) + \ln\left(\frac{FPR}{1-FPR}\right)$$

where TPR and FPR are the true and false positive rates and ln means the natural logarithm. The linear regression analysis is simply fitting a straigt line: ln (DOR)=a+b.S. Ln (DOR) is the dependent and S the independent variable. Although this is not obvious from the model as given, this method is often successful in producing a rather close linear fit for the data. The a-value is the intercept and the b-value the regression coefficient. If sensitivity equals specificity, then TPR=TNR=1−FPR and S reduces to 0. And so, the magnitude of the ln (DOR) at that point equals the a-value. The DOR can be calculated by back-log-transforming the calculated intercept.

As an example, the results of a previously published review of 44 diagnostic studies (Scheidler et al. 1997) of imaging techniques for lymph node metastases are used (Tables 48.1, 48.2, 48.3). For example, the ln(DOR) and S-values as calculated from the lymphangiography-studies are entered into the SPSS software program.

Table 48.2 Example of
meta-analysis of 17
diagnostic studies of
computerized tomography
(*CT*) imaging of lymph nodes
metastases

Study No.	tp	fp	fn	tn
1.	19	1	10	81
2.	8	9	2	13
3.	41	1	12	49
4.	5	1	2	18
5.	45	58	32	165
6.	8	6	2	32
7.	5	8	1	7
8.	15	17	11	52
9.	16	11	8	24
10.	4	8	2	25
11.	4	12	10	70
12.	10	4	4	55
13.	2	5	6	23
14.	7	10	7	30
15.	4	50	12	135
16.	8	3	1	37
17	4	3	0	14

tp true positive, *fp* false positive, *fn*
false negative, *tn* true negative

Table 48.3 Example of
meta-analysis of ten
diagnostic studies of
magnetic resonance imaging
(*MRI*) of lymph node
metastases

Study no.	tp	fp	fn	tn
1.	9	2	2	41
2.	3	6	5	32
3.	3	2	1	16
4.	3	1	12	44
5.	0	0	5	15
6.	7	2	22	167
7.	12	4	4	29
8.	23	5	14	230
9.	8	5	5	53
10.	16	2	2	22

tp true positive, *fp* false positive, *fn*
false negative, *tn* true negative

We command statistics; regression; linear. The program produces an a-value of 2.09
(standard error (SE)=0.35). The diagnostic odds ratio at the point S=0 is then found
by taking invert natural logarithm of 2.09=8.08 (SE=1.35). A summary of the
results of the regression analyses are in Table 48.4. The magnitude of DORs at S=0
can be used to estimate the level of overall accuracy of the diagnostic method.
Table 48.4 shows that MRI imaging is significantly more accurate than the other
two methods of cardiac imaging at p<0.001.

Table 48.4 Intercepts (a-values) and slopes (b-values) of the linear regression lines of the DORs of the three diagnostic modalities from Tables 48.1, 48.2 and 48.3

Diagnostic modality	Intercept (SE) (a-value)	Regression (SE) coefficient (b-value)	DOR at S=0 (SE) (p-values)
Lymphangiography	2.09 (0.30)	−0.35 (0.20)	8.08 (1.35) (<0.001 vs CT and MRI)
CT	2.84 (0.44)	0.23 (0.14)	17.16 (1.55) (<0.001 vs MRI and lymphangiography)
MRI	3.51 (0.56)	0.25 (0.17)	33.45 (1.75) (<0.001 vs CT and Lymphangiography)

3   Constructing Summary ROC Curves

The results of the separate studies are, thus, used to calculate the best fit a and b for the data. Subsequently, the underneath equation is adequate to construct the best fit summary ROC curve from the a- and b-values:

$$ \text{TPR} = \left[1 + e^{-a(1-b)} \left(\frac{1 - \text{FPR}}{\text{FPR}} \right)^{(1+b)(1-b)} \right]^{-1} $$

We enter the equation into Maple 9.5 software program for making graphs and fill out the a- and b-values. Then the software program produces the best fit ROC curves for the three diagnostic methods (Fig. 48.2). The curve closest to the top of the y-axis provides the best overall accuracy. A diagonal line from the top of the y-axis to the right end of the x-axis would contain all points on the summary ROC curves where sensitivity equals specificity, and thus S=0. Along this diagonal line the distance from the MRI curve would be shorter than that of the other curves, indicating a better accuracy of this diagnostic method. This is supported by a significantly larger DOR at p<0.001 as shown in Table 48.4 and discussed in the above section. The distances from the top of the y-axis to the MR/CT/lymphangiography summary ROC curves can be calculated using Pythagoras' equation for rectangular triangles,

$\sqrt{[(1 - \text{sensitivity})^2 + (1 - \text{specificity})^2]}$, and equals:
for the MR curv $(0.18^2 + 0.18_2) = 0.25$,
for the CT curv $\sqrt{(0.22^2 + 0.22^2)} = 0.31$,
for the lymphangiography curv $\sqrt{(0.26^2 + 0.26^2)} = 0.37$.

4   Discussion

The paper shows that diagnostic odds ratios (DORs) can be readily implemented in the meta-analyses of diagnostic research. An advantage of the DOR approach is that it accounts the special correlation between sensitivities and specificities of studies included. Another advantage is that it takes account of the heterogeneity between

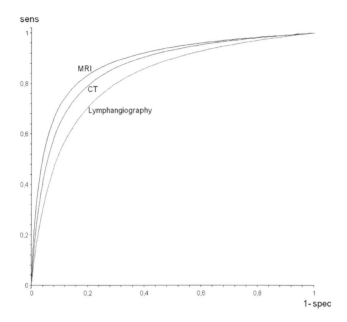

Fig. 48.2 The summary ROC curves for the three diagnostic modalities. A diagonal line drawn from the *top* of the y-axis to the *right* end of the x-axis contains the points of summary ROC curves where sensitivity equals specificity, and thus S = 0. Along this diagonal line the distance of the MRI curve to the *top* of the y-axis is shorter than that of the other curves, indicating a better accuracy of this diagnostic method. This is supported by a significantly larger DOR at p < 0.001 (Table 48.4). *Sens* sensitivity, *1 – spec* 1 – specificity

studies with respect to the different thresholds chosen by the investigators in the original studies: for particular reasons some investigators prefer large sensitivity and accept low specificity, while others prefer the reverse. These differences produce heterogeneity in DOR between studies, but that is taken into consideration by regression of ln(DOR) on S. A subsequent advantage is that it is easy to extend the model with covariates representing between-study differences in design. But this advantage is limited because in the summary ROC model these covariates are supposed to affect sensitivity and specificity in a similar manner, which need not be the case.

Some limitations have to be mentioned. First, as the outcome parameter is a summary estimate of both sensitivity and specificity, no summary estimates of sensitivity or specificity are available. Second, the magnitude of the studies included in the meta-analyses is not taken into account in the summary ROC method: it is impossible to weigh the true positives and false positives of the studies separately (Reitsma et al. 2005). However, it is common to report sensitivity and specificity from diagnostic studies without accounting the size of the sample from which they were calculated (Levin et al. 2008).

Other commonly used test indicators for diagnostic tests include positive predictive values, likelihood ratios, Youden's indexes. They are, in theory, useful for diagnostic meta-analyses, particularly from a bayesian perspective. However, they are rarely used, because they are not practical from a statistical viewpoint due to numerical and ceiling problems (Cleophas et al. 2007).

As an alternative, multivariate methods for pooling the meta-data accounting sensitivities and specificities, can be used. For example, multivariate methods like multivariate analysis of variance (MANOVA) with sensitivity and specificity as outcome variables and different diagnostic modalities as predictor variable can produce results similar to those of the DOR method, and, in addition, produce sensitivities and specificities separately and, at the same time, adjusted for their interaction (Reitsma et al. 2005). A limitation with this approach is that, again, the magnitude of the separate studies is not accounted, and that the numbers of studies included in the meta-analyses is often too small for reliable testing. A rule of thumb is that at least 10 studies per variable are required for multivariate analyses.

We should add, that, like with therapeutic meta-analyses, it is appropriate to account scientific rules including in any meta-analysis of diagnostic studies a thorough search of the literature, strict inclusion criteria and an assessment of the usual pitfalls of meta-analyses including publication bias, clinical heterogeneity, and lack of robustness (Cleophas and Zwinderman 2007).

5 Conclusions

Diagnostic reviews often include the sensitivity/specificity results of individual studies. A problem occurs when these data are pooled, because the correlation between sensitivity and specificity is generally strong negative, causing overestimation of the pooled results. The diagnostic odds ratio, defined as the odds of true positives versus that of false positives, may avoid this problem. This chapter reviews advantages and limitations of the diagnostic odds ratios (DORs).

A systematic review of 44 previously published diagnostic studies is used as an example.

DORs can be readily implemented in diagnostic research. Advantages include (1) that they adjust for the negative and curvilinear correlations between sensitivities and specificities, (2) that they take account of the heterogeneity between studies with respect to the different thresholds chosen by the investigators in the original studies, and (3) it is easy to extend the model with covariates representing between-study differences in design.

Limitations include (1) that the outcome parameter is a summary estimate of both sensitivity and specificity, and (2), that the magnitude of the studies included is not taken into account.

We conclude that reported sensitivities and specificities of different studies assessing similar diagnostic tests are not only negatively correlated, but also in a curvilinear manner. It is appropriate to take this negative curvilinear correlation into account in the data pooling of such meta-analyses. Diagnostic odds ratios can be applied for that purpose.

References

Bipat S, Glas AS, Van der Velden J, Zwinderman AH, Bossuyt PM, Stoker J (2003) Computed tomography and magnetic resonance imaging in staging of uterine cervical carcinoma: systematic review. Gynecol Oncol 91:59–66

Cleophas TJ, Zwinderman AH (2007) Primer in statistics: meta-analysis. Circulation 115:2870–2875

Cleophas TJ, Zwinderman AH, Van Ouwerkerk BM (2007) Log likelihood ratio tests for the assessment of cardiovascular events. Perfusion 20:79–82

Glas AS, Lijmer JG, Prins MH, Bonsel GJ, Bossuyt PM (2003) The diagnostic odds ratio: a single indicator of test performance. J Clin Epidemiol 56:1129–1135

Hasselblad V, Hedges LV (1995) Meta-analysis of screening and diagnostic tests. Psychol Bull 117:167–178

Irwig L, Macaskill P, Glasziou P, Fahey M (1995) Meta-analytic methods for diagnostic test accuracy. J Clin Epidemiol 48:119–130

Levin MD, Van de Bos E, Van Ouwerkerk BM, Cleophas TJ (2008) Uncertainty of diagnostic tests. Perfusion 21:42–48

Moses LE, Shapiro D, Littenberg B (1993) Combining independent studies of a diagnostic test into a summary ROC curve: data-analytic approaches and some additional considerations. Stat Med 12:1293–1316

Reitsma JB, Glas AS, Rutjes AW, Scholten RJ, Bossuyt PM, Zwinderman AH (2005) Bivariate analysis of sensitivity and specificity produces informative summary measures in diagnostic reviews. J Clin Epidemiol 58:982–990

Scheidler J, Hricak H, Yu KK, Subak L, Segal MR (1997) Radiological evaluation of lymph node metastases in patients with cervical cancer. A meta-analysis. JAMA 278:1096–1101

Walter SD (2002) Properties of the summary receiver operating characteristic (SROC) curve for diagnostic test data. Stat Med 21:1237–1256

Chapter 49
c-Statistic Versus Logistic Regression for Assessing the Performance of Qualitative Diagnostic Accuracy

1 Introduction

Clinical trials require adequate tests for making a diagnosis, and patient follow up. Whatever test, investigators need to know how good the test is. The performance of quantitative diagnostic tests, can be estimated from linear regression with the diagnostic result as predictor (independent) variable and the severities of disease as outcome (dependent) variable: the closer the outcome is to the best fit regression line the better the test is with a perfect test if R-square (the squared regression coefficient) equals 1. However, unfortunately, in clinical research many diagnostic tests have *qualitative* rather than quantitative outcome variables, e.g., a clinical event/ disease or not, and linear regression is not applicable for judging the goodness of such tests. Instead, sensitivity (chance of a true positive test) and specificity (chance of a true negative test) are usually calculated, but the problem is that these two estimators are inversely correlated, and that multiple thresholds for the definition of a positive test can be given. Figure 49.1 shows the frequency distributions of patients without (left half) and with the disease (right half) with on the x-axis the individual patient results and on the y-axis "how often observed".

With the threshold given by the vertical dotted line, we have here a perfect test, because the patients with and without disease do not overlap. However, this situation virtually never occurs in practice, and, generally, we will witness the situation of Fig. 49.2: the patients with and without the disease overlap, producing partly false positive and false negative results. The black and grey areas under the curve show the proportions of false positive and false negative patients.

$$\text{Sensitivity} = \left[\text{true positives} / \left(\text{false positive plus true positives}\right)\right]$$
$$\text{Specificity} = \left[\text{true negatives} / \left(\text{false negatives plus true negatives}\right)\right].$$

If you move the threshold indicated by the vertical dotted line in Fig. 49.2, you can observe, that, if one is high, the other, as a rule, is low, vice versa. A nice method for determining the relationship between different sensitivities and specificities is

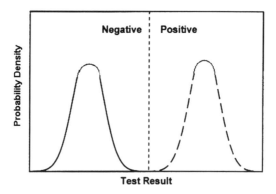

Fig. 49.1 Example of a perfect qualitative diagnostic test. The two frequency distributions of the patients without (*left half*) and with the disease (*right half*) have on the x-axis the individual patient results, and on the y-axis "how often observed". The curves do not overlap

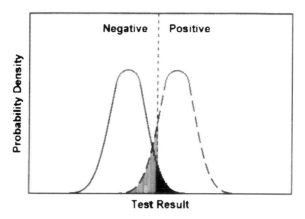

Fig. 49.2 Example of a less than perfect qualitative diagnostic test. The two curves show the frequency distributions of the patients without (*left curve*) and with disease (*right curve*). On the x-axis are the individual patient results, and on the y-axis "how often observed". The patient with and without the disease overlap. The vertical dotted line is the threshold chosen to distinguish between a negative and positive test

the ROC (receiver operated characteristic) curve with sensitivity on the y-axis and 1-specificity on the x-axis (Green and Swets 1966). A relatively new method is the smooth ROC-curve in which tests are no longer supposed to fall into one of two categories but, rather, into multiple categories with more or less confidence (Fig. 49.3) (Zou et al. 1997). The closer this smooth ROC curve approaches the top of the y-axis, the better the diagnostic test will be with an optimal area under curve of 1.0. In contrast, if the area under the curve is close to the 45 degree diagonal line, the area under the curve is close to 0.5, and the test is very poor. The area under curve of the smooth ROC curve is currently applied as an estimate of the goodness of a qualitative diagnostic test in a way similar to the R-square value for the quantitative

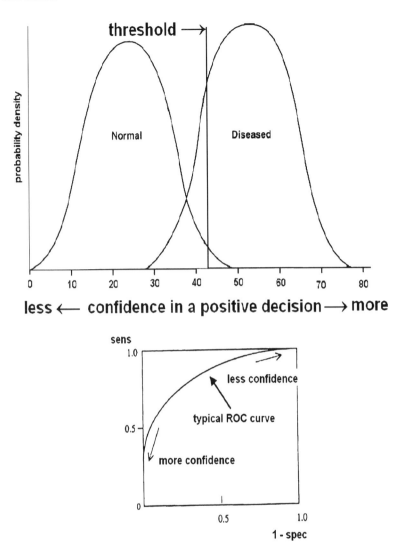

Fig. 49.3 A relatively new method is the smooth ROC-curve in which tests are no longer supposed to fall into one of two categories but, rather, into multiple categories with more or less confidence. The closer this smooth ROC curve approaches the top of the y-axis, the better precision the diagnostic test will provide with an optimal area under curve of 1.0 (*sens* sensitivity, *spec* specificity)

diagnostic tests. However, the area under curve method, nowadays commonly called the c-statistic (concordance-statistic), has limitations as summarized by Cook (2007): (1) the increase of area under the curve to judge a new (and better) diagnostic test is very small if the standard test already produced a large area under the curve, as commonly observed, and (2) the c-statistic assesses relative risk levels instead of absolute ones, while, in practice, the absolute risk levels are often more important.

Logistic regression with the odds of disease as outcome (dependent) variable and the test-scores as covariate (independent variable) could be used as an alternative method to model data files. The following reasoning can be used here. If we move the threshold for a positive test (Fig. 49.2) to the right, then the proportion of false positives will decrease. The steeper the logistic regression line, the faster this will happen. In contrast, if we move the threshold to the left, then the proportion of false negatives will decrease. The steeper the logistic regression line, the faster also this will happen. This would mean the steeper the logistic regression line, the fewer false positives and false negatives, and thus the better the diagnostic test. A pleasant aspect of this approach is that absolute instead of relative risks are measured. The current chapter uses as examples vascular lab scores to investigate the performance of logistic regression as compared to the current c-statistic.

2   The Performance of c-Statistics

Figure 49.4 shows the histograms of vascular lab scores in patients with peripheral vascular disease and healthy controls. The figure shows that the test is not perfect at all with considerable overlap between the patients with and without vascular

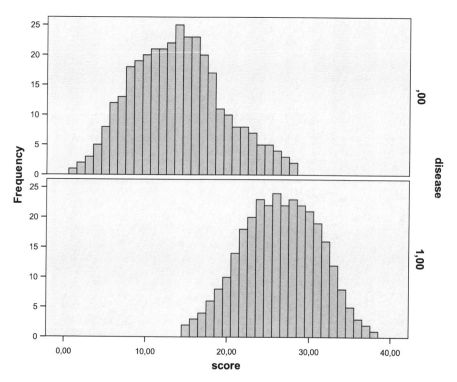

Fig. 49.4 Frequency distributions of a non-invasive test for the diagnosis of peripheral vascular disease (.00=no disease; 1.00=disease)

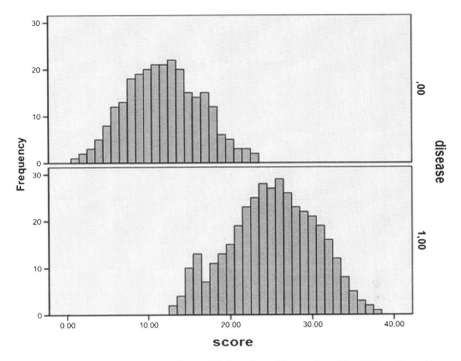

Fig. 49.5 Frequency distributions of a modified version of the test from Fig. 49.4 performed in a age-, sex-, and risk-factor-matched group (.00=no disease; 1.00=disease)

disease. Figure 49.5 shows the result of a modified and, possibly, improved test performed in patient group with similar characteristics. Again the test is not perfect, but the patterns of the curves have slightly changed. We can not observe from the figures which of the two tests is the best one. In order to find out c-statistic is performed.

SPSS 17.0 is used to calculate the c-statistic (SPSS 2011).
We command: Analyze....ROC curve....Test variable score....State variable disease.....value of state variable 1....ROC curve....standard error....OK.

The Figs. 49.6 and 49.7 give the ROC curves of the data from the Figs. 49.4 and 49.5 respectively. The software program produces area under the ROC curve values of respectively

0.954 and 0.969
with standard errors of 0.007 and 0.005.
The pooled standard error equal $\sqrt{(0.007^2+0.004^2)}=0.0086$.
The mean difference of the AUCs$=0.969-0.954=0.015$.

The t-test produces a t-value of
$0.015/0.0086=1.74$.
This corresponds with a p-value of 0.08,
which is larger than 0.05.

Fig. 49.6 The space of the
area under the curve,
otherwise called ROC space,
of the data from Fig. 49.4 is
calculated by the software to
be 0.954 (= 95.4%)

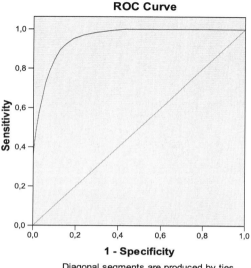

Fig. 49.7 The space of the
area under the curve of the
data from Fig. 49.5 is
calculated by the software to
be 0.969 (= 96.9%)

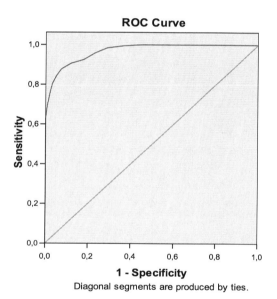

This means that no significant difference between the two tests is demonstrated.
C-statistic may underestimate the true difference between two smooth ROC curves
due to the phenomenon of overfitting. For adjustment bootstrap sampling was used
and this reduced the standard error to 0.0081. The adjusted t-value of 1.85 still did
not produce a significant difference between the two tests with a p-value of 0.065.

3   The Performance of Logistic Regression

Instead of the c-statistic logistic regression can be used to assess the performance of the new test compared to the standard test. For that purpose we use a model similar to the linear regression model used for assessing the goodness of quantitative diagnostic tests. However, because the outcome (dependent) variable is a binary rather than continuous variable, logistic regression instead of linear regression has to be applied.

Again SPSS 17.0 is used (SPSS 2011).

We command: regression...binary logistic.... Dependent variable disease...covariate score...ok.

The best fit regression equation for test 1 is given underneath:
log odds of having the disease$=-9.20+0.45$ times the score

The best fit regression equation for test 2 is below:
log odds of having the disease$=-9.31+0.58$ times the score.

Both regression equations produce highly significant regression coefficients with standard errors of respectively 0.04 and 0.05 and p-values of <0.0001. The two regression coefficients is tested for significance of difference using the z – test:

$$z=(0.58-0.45)/\sqrt{(0.04^2+0.05^2)}=0.13/0.064=2.03,$$
which corresponds with a p-value of 0.04.

Obviously, test 2 produces a significantly steeper regression model, which means that it is a better predictor of the risk of disease than test 1. We can, additionally, calculate the odds ratios of test 2 versus test 1. The odds of disease with test 1 equals $e^{0.45}=1.57$, and with test 2 it equals $e^{0.58}=1.79$. The odds ratio$=1.79/1.57=1.14$, meaning that the second test produces about a 1.14 times better chance of rightly predicting the disease than test 1 does.

4   Discussion

Comparing logistic regression coefficients between samples is not straightforward and is currently the subject of much discussion in the statistical literature as summarized in the recent article of Karlson et al. (2011). With quantitative diagnostic tests each individual score is associated with a single most probable severity of a disease. With qualitative diagnostic tests, however, each individual score is associated with four different possible outcomes: a false positive or negative outcome, a true positive or negative outcome. The meaning of the b-values of logistic equations is entirely different from those of linear equations. With the linear regression equation $y=bx$ the b-value estimates the ratio y/x. With logistic regression things are much more complex: it estimates log odds ratio of having a disease versus having no disease. This complex relationship is the main reason, that, so far, logistic regression has not been applied for assessing the performance of qualitative diagnostic tests, and that methods like c-statistic have been developed. The current paper shows that after redefinition of the term performance in terms of "odds ratio of having disease versus having no disease" logistic regression can adequately be used for performance assessments.

The current paper not only is the first one to show that logistic regression can be conveniently applied for assessing the performance of qualitative diagnostic tests, but also suggests that the method is better than c-statistic for that purpose.

Also longitudinal diagnostic tests can be assessed in this way. However, instead of logistic models Cox proportional hazard models are required. Log hazard instead of log odds and the corresponding regression coefficients, the b-values, will have to be used.

Recently, Pencina et al. (2008) proposed the method of reclassification as another alternative to c-statistic. This method uses logistic models like the ones described in this paper to find cut-off test-scores for predicting classes with different risk risks of disease. Hosmer-Lemeshow tests are used for comparing partitioned areas under the curves of different data samples. The problem with this method is that, unlike the method reviewed in this paper, it must be applied with paired data samples, which may be hard to obtain with large datasets required for meaningful assessment of small differences between two largely similar diagnostic tests.

Additional advantages of the logistic model compared to c-statistic have to be mentioned:

1. Absolute rather than relative risks of disease are assessed. The c-statistic uses sensitivities and specificities which are relative risks of being truly positive and truly negative, while logistic regression uses the absolute scores ad predictor of disease.
2. A limitation of c-statistic is the following. The increase of area under the curve, to judge a new (and better) diagnostic test is very small if the standard test already produced a large area under the curve, as commonly observed.

For performance assessment of quantitative diagnostic tests linear regression is adequate. The current paper shows that for performance assessment of qualitative diagnostic tests logistic regression is adequate, and seems to provide a better result than does the current c-statistics.

4.1   Conclusions

Logistic regression with presence of disease as outcome and scores as predictor variable is better than c-statistic for the purpose of comparing the performance of qualitative diagnostic tests. This finding may be relevant to future diagnostic research.

5 Conclusions

Qualitative diagnostic tests commonly produce false positive and false negative results. Smooth ROC (receiver operated characteristic) curves are used for assessing the performance of a new against a standard test. This method, called c-statistic (concordance statistic) has limitations. This chapter was written to assess whether logistic regression with the odds of disease as outcome and the test scores as covariate can be used as an alternative approach. Also, to compare the goodness of either of the two methods.

Using as examples vascular lab scores we assessed the performance of logistic regression as compared to c-statistic.

The c-statistic produced AUCs (areas under the curve) of respectively 0.954 and 0.969 (standard errors 0.007 and 0.005), means difference 0.015 with a pooled standard error of 0.0086. This meant that the new test was not significantly different from the standard test at $p = 0.08$. Logistic regression of these data with presence of disease as dependent and vascular lab scores as independent variable produced regression coefficients of 0.45 and 0.58 with standard errors of respectively 0.04 and 0.05. This meant that the new test was a significantly better predictor of disease than the standard test at $p = 0.04$.

We conclude that logistic regression with presence of disease as dependent and test scores as independent variable was better than c-statistic for assessing qualitative diagnostic tests. This may be relevant to future diagnostic research.

References

Cook NR (2007) Use and misuse of the receiver operating characteristic curve in risk prediction. Circulation 115:928–935

Green DM, Swets JM (1966) Signal detection theory and psychophysics. Wiley, New York

Karlson KB, Holm A, Breen R (2011) Comparing regression coefficients between models using logit and probit: a new method. Soc Methodol 42:1–43

Pencina MJ, D'Agostino RB, Vasan RS (2008) Evaluating the added predictive ability of a new marker: from area under the ROC curve to reclassification and beyond. Stat Med 27:157–172

SPSS Statistical Software, www.SPSS.com. Accessed 15 Dec 2011

Zou KH, Hall WJ, Shapiro DE (1997) Smooth receiver operated characteristic curves. Stat Med 116:2143–2156

Chapter 50
Validating Quantitative Diagnostic Tests

1 Introduction

Clinical research is impossible without valid diagnostic tests. The methods for validating *qualitative* diagnostic tests include sensitivity/specificity assessments and ROC (receiver operated characteristic) curves, and are generally accepted (Reid et al. 1995; Anonymous, 2011; Bossuyt et al. 2003; Delong and Delong 1988). In contrast, the methods for validating *quantitative* diagnostic tests have not been agreed upon by the scientific community (Delong and Delong 1988). This chapter, using real data examples, reviews the advantages and disadvantages of various methods that could be used for that purpose.

2 Linear Regression Testing a Significant Correlation Between the New Test and the Control Test

Regression methods are often used for that purpose, particularly, linear regression using a significant correlation as criterion for validation. In Fig. 50.1 an example is given. A positive correlation seems to exist between the new-test- and control-test-data given by the x-axis-data and the y-axis-data. We can draw a best fit regression line according to the equation

$$y = a + bx$$

For every x-axis-datum this line provides the best predictable y-axis-datum. The b-value is the regression coefficient (= direction coefficient), "a" the intercept, which is the place where the line crosses the y-axis. The values "a" and "b" from the equation $y = a + bx$ can be calculated:

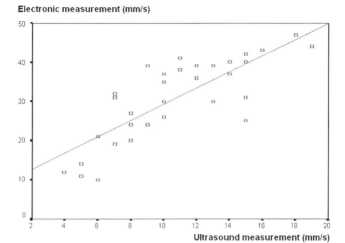

Fig. 50.1 Validity assessment with a linear regression model. The regression equation is given by $y = a + bx = 8.647 + 2.065x$ (a=intercept, b=regression coefficient, $p < 0.0001$). The x-axis-data, ultrasound estimates, are a very significant predictor of the y-axis-data, the electromagnetic measurements. However, the prediction, despite the high level of statistical significance, is very imprecise. For example, if $x = 6$, then y may be 10 or 21, if $x = 7$, y may be 19, 31 or 32

$$b = \text{regression coefficient} = \frac{\sum (x - \bar{x})(y - \bar{y})}{\sum (x - \bar{x})^2}$$

This equation is often described in a condensed way as
$b = \text{SP } xy/\text{SS } x$ (SP xy = sum of products of x- and y-data, SS x = sum of squared x-data)
$a = \text{intercept} = \bar{y} - b\bar{x}$.
Another important term for regression analyses is the r-value, the correlation coefficient,

$$r = \text{correlation coefficient} = \frac{\sum (x - \bar{x})(y - \bar{y})}{\sqrt{\sum (x - \bar{x})^2 \sum (y - \bar{y})^2}}$$

The term r gives the measure for strength of association between the x-data and the y-data. The stronger the association, the better the x-data predict the y-data. It varies from -1 to $+1$, $r = 0$ means no association at all, $r = -1$ or $= +1$ means 100% association (we can predict the y-values from the given x-values with 100% certainty).

The term r^2 is often more convenient, because it varies from 0 to $+1$. The r^2-value is used as a measure of the percentage certainty that has been obtained by the linear regression model. For example, an r^2-value of 0.36 means that we can predict the y-data with 36% certainty, if we know the corresponding x-data.

For statistical testing of linear regression lines we test with the Student's t-test whether the b-value is significantly larger than zero or with analysis of variance whether the r^2-value is significantly larger than zero. These tests are laborious, and, therefore, currently routinely performed by statistical software. For example, SPSS statistical software requires after entering the data the commands: statistics; regression; linear. In the given example (Fig. 50.1) the b-value is calculated to be 2.065 with a standard error of 0.276 and a t-value of 7.491, meaning that it is , indeed, significantly larger than zero at $p < 0.0001$, and that there is, thus, a strong significant association between the new-test-data and the control-test-data. Also the r^2-value of 0.63 as calculated is significantly larger than 0 at $p < 0.0001$. Both results, thus, indicate that a significant association exists between the x-data and the corresponding y-data. This means that the data are significantly closer to the regression line than could happen by chance. However, it does not mean that they are all situated exactly on the regression line. As can be observed in the Fig. 50.1, if, for example, x = 6 then y may be 10 or 21, if x = 7 then y may be 19, 31 or 32. Actually, given the r^2-value of 0.63, we may conclude that any particular x-datum can predict the corresponding y-datum only by 63%, while 37% remains uncertain. This percentage of uncertainty is rather large for accurate diagnostic tests. We have to conclude that the usual method for testing the strength of association between the x-data and y-data in a linear regression model, although widely applied for validating quantitative diagnostic tests, seems to be inaccurate. Obviously, stricter criteria have to be applied for validation.

3   Linear Regression Testing the Hypotheses That the a-Value = 0.000 and the b-Value = 1.000

A stricter method to test the association between the new-test-data (the x-data) and the control-test-data (y-values) was given by Barnett (1969). First, from the above equation y = a + bx it is tested whether the b-value is significantly different from zero like described above. Then, the hypothesis is tested that the a-value = 0.000 and the b-value = 1.000. As an example the graph from Fig. 50.1 is used once more. We need the b-value (or a-value) ± 1.96 times its standard error to calculate the 95% confidence intervals of b and a.

If the 95% confidence interval of the b-value (2.065 ± 1.96 × 0.276) contains 1.000,

and the a-value (8.647 ± 1.96 × 3.132) contains 0.000,

=> then validity can be accepted.

Here: the 95% confidence interval of the b-value is between 1.513 and 2.617,

and of the a-value is between 2.383 and 14.911,

=> the test can not be validated.

In the example of Fig. 50.2 the data are close to the "b = 1.000 and a = 0.000 line", otherwise called the identity line.

Fig. 50.2 Angiographic
cardiac volumes (liters) used
to predict cast cardiac
volumes (liters)

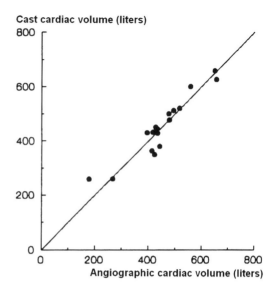

The 95% confidence interval of the b-value is between $0.917 \pm 1.96 \times 0.083$,
                                                    is between 0.751 and 1.083,
and it, thus, contains the number 1.000.
The 95% confidence interval of the a-value is between $39.340 \pm 1.96 \times 38.704$,
                                                    is between −38.068 and 116.748,
and it, thus, contains the number 0.000.

The diagnostic test of Fig. 50.2 is validated. If the hypothesis that $a = 0.000$ and
$b = 1.000$ can not be confirmed, and the b-value is significantly larger than 0, then
the underneath method can be applied for validation. A b-value significantly smaller
than 1.000 is an indicator for a diagnostic test that systematically overestimates the
gold standard test, and significantly larger than 1.000 it is so for a diagnostic test
that systematically underestimates the gold standard test.

4   Linear Regression Using a Squared Correlation Coefficient (r^2-Value) of >0.95

The previous method assumes that the best fit linear regression equation for the
diagnostic test is $y = x$. A diagnostic test with the best fit equation $y = a + bx$, rather
than $y = x$ like in the example from Fig. 50.1 is not necessarily useless, and could be
approved as a valid test if it is precise, that means if the x-data precisely predict the
$(y - a)/b$- data rather than the y-data. If we apply such a test, the result of the x-data
will, of course, have to be transformed into $a + bx$ to find the y-data. Validation is
accomplished by determining whether the regression line precisely predicts the

Fig. 50.3 The relative residual variance is calculated from the add-up sum of the least squared distances from the points to the regression line

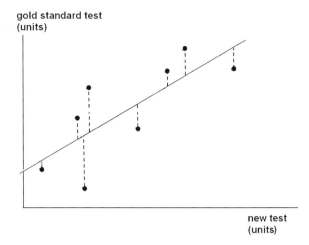

control test from the new test, and we recommend to use for that purpose as criterion a squared correlation-coefficient $r^2 > 95\%$. This can be calculated from

$$r^2 = SP^2xy / (SSx \cdot SSy).$$

In the example from Fig. 50.1 $r^2 = 63\%$, much smaller than 95%, and, so, the results can not be validated. In the literature often the term *intraclass correlation* is applied instead of the r^2-value, but its meaning is the same.

$$\text{Intraclass correlation} = \frac{\text{SS regression}}{\text{SS regression} + \text{SS residual}} = \frac{SP^2xy / SSx}{SSy}.$$

A largely similar approach is given by the calculation of the *relative residual variance* of the linear regression. The relative residual variance is calculated from the add-up sum of the least squared distances from the regression line (Fig. 50.3) and is equal to $(1 - r^2)$. The larger it is, the poorer the validity of the test. A residual variance smaller than 5% is adequate for validation.

$$\text{Relative residual variance} = \frac{\text{SS residual}}{\text{SS regression} + \text{SS residual}}$$

$$SS\ residual = SSy - \left(SP^2xy / SSx \right)$$

$$\text{Relative residual variance} = \frac{SSy - \left(SP^2xy / SSx \right)}{SSy} = \frac{SSy}{SSy} - \frac{\left(SP^2xy / SSx \right)}{SSy} = \left(1 - r^2 \right)$$

$$= 37\% \text{ in the example from Fig.1.}$$

The levels 95% and 5% are, of course, arbitrarily chosen. However, they are consistent with the cut-off for type I errors as commonly chosen in clinical research.

When using the linear model for testing validity, it is recommended to test the linear hypothesis, i.e. to test that the relationship between the new-test-data and control-test-data are, indeed, linear, rather than curvilinear. This can be done by testing the hypothesis that a second order correlation exists between the x- and y-data. For that purpose the equation $y = a + bx^2$ is used. If the data are modeled according to this equation and the b-value is significantly larger than the b-value of the linear model $y = a + bx$, then the linear model has to be rejected, and the data should be modelled according to a second order relationship between the new-test-values (x-values) and the control-test-values (y-values). If a log linear relationship between the diagnostic test and the gold standard test better fits the data than a linear relationship, then a so-called pseudo-R2 or R2-like measure instead of r^2 value can be calculated (Hoetker 2007).

5   Alternative Methods

All of the methods discussed so far assume uncertainty in the new test, but not in the control test. Two assessments, that assume uncertainty of both the new-test- and the control-test-data, are the paired Student's t-test and the Altman-Bland plot or method. The first uses the average difference between the new-test-values and the old-test-values as estimate of bias, and the standard error of the mean difference as estimate of precision (McGee et al. 2007). The second (Bland and Altman 1986) uses the spread of the subtraction sums of the new-test- and old-test-data and their standard deviation. If 95% of the subtraction sums fall within the limits of agreements, as calculated by the mean differences ±1.96 times its standard deviation, then the test is validated. It may, generally, be perfectly all right to assume no uncertainty in the control test, particularly, if it is the gold standard test, for which there is no better alternative. The gold standard test, then, simply produces the truth. In this situation the additional amount of uncertainty assumed in the control test causes loss of sensitivity of testing. Even if the control test is not 100% accurate, we are, generally, merely interested in the validation against the control test, no matter its accuracy. A second problem with the above two methods is that, unlike linear regression, they assume Gaussian-like sampling distributions of the subsequent x- and y-values. This assumption is not always appropriate, since the data are, generally, not randomly sampled, but obtained from selected groups.

If we want to account the uncertainty of a control test, which is not a gold standard test, then a better approach will be to test both the new and the control test against the gold standard test. This will unmask which of the two tests performs better. In the situation where there is no certain gold standard test and where it is decided to account uncertainty of the control test to be used, Deming (Linnet 1998) and Passing-Bablok (Passing and Bablok 1983) regression are sometimes used instead. They are methods based on linear regression and mathematically more complex than simple linear regression. Deming regression, just like the paired t-test and the Altman-Bland plot, assumes normal distributions of the subsequent x- and y-data. In contrast, Passing-Bablok regression does not. It is a non-parametric method using the Kendall's rank-correlation test to assess the above-described hypotheses that b = 1.000, and a = 0.000. First, one should produce a ranked sequence of all possible slope-values between two x and two y-values (Sij values). We, then, compare the Sij values >1 with those <1, and test whether there is a significant difference using Kendall's standard error equation, SE (standard error) = $\sqrt{ }$ n(n − 1) (2n + 5) /18 with n = number of paired values. If, after continuity correction (add −1 to the difference as calculated), the SE is smaller than half the size of the calculated difference, then the b-value is not significantly different from 1.000. The a-value is calculated from the medians of x and y using the calculated b, its SE from the upper and lower limit of the confidence intervals of the b-value. The method is laborious, particularly, with large samples, but available through S-plus, Analyse-it, EP Evaluator, and MedCalc and other software programs.

6 Discussion

Simple linear regression testing the presence of a significant correlation between the new-test-data (x-axis-data) and the control-test-data (y-axis-data) is not accurate for testing the validity of a novel quantitative diagnostic test. Accurate methods using linear regression include the following.

1. From y = a + bx, test the hypothesis that b is statistically significantly larger than zero, than test the hypothesis that b = 1.000 and a = 0.000.
2. If "the b = 1.000 and a = 0.000 hypothesis" cannot be confirmed, then use as criterion for validation a squared correlation-coefficient r^2 or intraclass correlation of >95%, or a relative residual variance of <5%. If the new test is validated this way, then the predicted control-test-values are calculated from the equation y = a + bx.

Altman-Bland plots, paired t-tests, Deming regression and Passing-Bablok regression assume uncertainty of both the new test and the control test. This is rarely a condition for validation, and carries the risk of unneeded loss of sensitivity of testing. However, if there is no gold standard test and it is decided to account the uncertainty of the control test, then Passing-Bablok regression is the only method adequate for non-normal data as often present in practice.

When using a data plot with one test on the x- and one on the y-axis, sometimes non-linear or curvilinear or exponential patterns can occur. The diagnostic test may, then, be useful even so. But, we will first have to find the best fit equation for the data, which is generally the equation producing the largest regression coefficient, and may, for example, look like y = log x, y = a + bx^2 and many more forms. Such a test can be approved as valid, if it is a precise predictor of the control test, even if the x-data do not predict y, but rather something like antilog y or $\sqrt{ }$ [(y − a)/b]. In practice, however, linear relationships are the most common pattern observed with quantitative diagnostic tests.

7   Conclusions

Clinical research is impossible without valid diagnostic tests. The methods for validating *quantitative* diagnostic tests have not been agreed upon by the scientific community. This chapter reviews the advantages and disadvantages of methods that could be used for that purpose. Using real data examples we review seven possible methods.

Simple linear regression testing the presence of a significant correlation between the new-test-data (x-axis-data) and the control-test-data (y-axis-data) is not accurate for testing the validity of a novel quantitative diagnostic test. Accurate methods using linear regression include the following. First, from $y = a + bx$, test the hypothesis that b is statistically significantly larger than zero, than test the hypothesis that $b = 1.000$ and $a = 0.000$. Second, if "the $b = 1.000$ and $a = 0.000$ hypothesis" cannot be confirmed, then use as criterion for validation a squared correlation-coefficient r^2 or intraclass correlation of >95%, or a relative residual variance of <5%. If the new test is validated this way, then the predicted control-test-values are calculated from the equation $y = a + bx$.

The above three methods assume uncertainty of the new-test-data, but not of the control-test-data. Deming regression, Passing-Bablok regression, paired Student's t-tests, and Altman-Bland plots assume uncertainty of both the new test and the control test. This is rarely a condition for validation, and carries the risk of unneeded loss of sensitivity of testing. However, if the control test is not the gold standard test and it is decided to account the uncertainty of the control test, then Passing-Bablok regression is the only method that adjusts for non-normal data as frequently observed in practice.

More information on accuracy assessments of quantitative diagnostic tests is given by the CLSI protocols published by the Clinical and Laboratory Standards Institute, particularly the protocols EP9 and EP14 (Guidelines for global application developed by the Clinical and Laboratory Standards Institute 2011).

References

Anonymous The quality of diagnostic tests statement, the CONSORT statement. www.consort-statement.org. Accessed 15 Dec 2011

Barnett DV (1969) Simultaneous pairwise linear structural relationships. Biometrics 28:129–142

Bland JM, Altman DG (1986) Statistical methods for assessing agreement between two methods of clinical measurement. Lancet i:307–310

Bossuyt PM, Reitsma JB, Bruns DE, Gatsonis CA, Glasziou PP, Irwig JG, Moher D, Rennie D, De Vet HC, for the STARD steering group (2003) Education and debate. Towards complete and accurate reporting of studies of diagnostic accuracy: the STARD initiative. BMJ 326:41–44

Delong ER, Delong DM (1988) Comparing the areas under two or more correlated receiver operated characteristic curves; a nonparametric approach. Biometrics 44:837–845

Guidelines for global application developed by the Clinical and Laboratory Standards Institute. www.techstreet.com. Accessed 15 Dec 2011

Hoetker G (2007) The use of logit and probit models in strategic management research. Strat Manage J 28:331–343

Linnet K (1998) Performance of Deming regression analysis in case of miss-specified analytical error in method comparison studies. Clin Chem 44:1024–1031

McGee WT, Horswell JL, Calderon J, Janvier G, Van Severen T, Van den Berghe G, Kozikowski L (2007) Validation of a continuous arterial pressure-based cardiac output measurement: a multicenter, prospective trial. Crit Care 11:R105, 1–7

Passing H, Bablok W (1983) A new biometrical procedure for testing the equality of measurements from two different analytical methods. J Clin Chem Clin Biochem 21:709–720

Reid MC, Lachs MS, Feinstein AR (1995) Use of methodological standards in diagnostic test research. Getting better but still not good. JAMA 274:645–650

Chapter 51
Summary of Validation Procedures for Diagnostic Tests

1 Introduction

Clinical studies are impossible without adequate diagnostic tests, and diagnostic tests can, therefore, be considered the real basis of evidence-based medicine. In 1995 Reid et al. (1995) stated after a search of 1,302 diagnostic studies that most diagnostic tests are inadequately appraised. Efforts to improve the quality of diagnostic tests are given by initiatives like those of the CONSORT (Consolidated Standard Randomized Trials) (Anonymous, 2011) movement and the STARD (Standards for Reporting Diagnostic Accuracy) (Bossuyt et al. 2003) group launching quality criteria statements for diagnostic tests in 2002 and 2003. In spite of such initiatives the evaluation of diagnostic tests prior to implementation in research programs, continues to be lacking (Morgan et al. 2007). A diagnostic test can be either qualitative, e.g., the presence of an elevated erythrocyte sedimentation rate to demonstrate pneumonia, or quantitative, e.g., the ultrasound flow velocity to estimate the invasive electromagnetic flow velocity. For both qualitative and quantitative diagnostic tests three determinants of validity have been recommended by working parties:

Assess accuracy: the test shows who has the disease and how severe it is.
Assess reproducibility: when a subject is tested twice, the second test produces the same result as the first test.
Assess precision: there is a small spread in a random sample of test results.

The methods of assessment have, however, not been defined so far. The current chapter reviews correct and incorrect methods and new developments.

2   Qualitative Diagnostic Tests

2.1   Accuracy

Assessing accuracy is probably most important. Accuracy is synonymous to valid-ity, and can here be defined as a test's ability to show which individuals have the disease and which do not. It is, generally, assessed by sensitivity and specificity, defined as the chance of a true positive and true negative test respectively.

How do we calculate accuracy

Disease	Yes (n)	No (n)
Positive test	a	b
Negative test	c	d

n = number of patient
a = number of true positive patients
b = false positive patients
c = false negative patients
d = true negative patients

Sensitivity of the above test = a/(a + c)

Specificity = d/(b + d)

In addition to sensitivity and specificity sometimes overall accuracy is given

Overall accuracy = (a + d)/(a + b + c + d)

It is important to realize that a sensitivity/specificity close to 50% gives no more information than does flipping a coin, and that such a result is not a basis for valida-tion. Often qualitative diagnostic tests have multiple sensitivities/specificities dependent on normal values used. In the example of the Figs. 46.3 and 46.4 in Chap. 46 the erythrocyte sedimentation rate (ESR) is used as an estimator of pneumonia with chest x-ray as gold standard test. The sample population consists of two Gaussian distributions of patients, one with and the other without pneumonia.

Figure 46.1 in Chap. 46 shows that, if a normal value of the ESR is defined as < 43 mm, many healthy subjects are rightly diagnosed. However, many diseased are missed. The test, thus, produces a high specificity, but low sensitivity: we have many false negatives. If, in contrast, an ESR of >32 mm is used as level between health and disease (Fig. 46.2, Chap. 46), then we do not miss many diseased, but we will misdiagnose many healthy subjects. Our test will have a low specificity: we will have many false positives. The question is what normal ESR value is best in order to miss as few diagnoses as possible, and obtain both a high sensitivity and high specificity. ROC (receiver operating) curves are helpful for finding both (Fig. 51.1). First, we calculate for several tentative normal values sensitivity/specificity. Then, we draw a curve with sensitivities on the y-axis and specificities or 1-specificities (producing a somewhat prettier curve) on the x-axis. A perfect test reaches the top of the y-axis where both sensitivity and 1-specificity are 100%. The given example does not produce a perfect test, but we can readily observe from the graph that an

Fig. 51.1 The ROC (receiver operating characteristic) curve of the erythrocyte sedimentation rate (*ESR*) values of the patients with pneumonia from the Figs. 51.1 and 51.2 plot the sensitivity values against the "1-specificity"values (*sens* sensitivity, *spec* specificity)

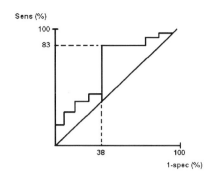

ESR of 38 mm produces the shortest distance to the top of the y-axis. If you want proof, you may wish to measure the distance between the top of the y-axis and the curve or calculate it using rectangular triangles and Pythagoras' equation.

ROC curves are very popular, but have some limitations. First, sometimes more than 1 shortest distance to the top of the y-axis is observed. Second, ROC curves close to the diagonal provide no more information than tossing a coin (overall accuracy is only 50%). Third, often two different diagnostic tests are compared for identifying the better of the two using areas under the curve of the ROC curves. A problem is, that such ROC curves often cross, which means, that a diagnostic test may perform better in one interval, worse in another.

2.2 Reproducibility

Cohen's kappas are used for assessing reproducibility of qualitative diagnostic tests. As an example 30 patients are assessed twice for a positive test for brain natriuretic peptide for a diagnosis of heart failure.

		1st time positive test		
		Yes	No	
2nd time positive test	Yes	10	5	15
	No	4	11	15
		14	16	30

It can be demonstrated that, if the test were not reproducible at all,

$$\text{you would find}\,(14 \times 15 / 30 =)\,7 \times \text{twice yes}$$
$$\text{and}\,(16 \times 15 / 30 =)\,\underline{8 \times \text{twice no} +}$$
$$15 \times \text{twice the same.}$$
In fact, we do find $21 \times$ twice the same.

The kappa estimator is calculated according to:

$$\text{Kappa} = \frac{\text{observed} - \text{minimal}}{\text{maximal} - \text{minimal}} = \frac{21 - 15}{30 - 15} = 0.4$$

The result is interpreted as follows: a kappa value of 0 means a very poor reproducibility, a value of 1 an excellent reproducibility. In our example the reproducibility is moderate.

2.3 Precision

The STARD (standards for reporting diagnostic accuracy) working party (Barnett 1969) has proposed to include a "measure of uncertainty" in any validation procedure. Standard deviations/errors (SDs/SEs) can be used for that purpose.

Disease	Yes (n)	No (n)
Positive test	a	b
Negative test	c	d

$$SE_{sensitivity} = \sqrt{ac / (a+c)^3}$$

$$SE_{specificity} = \sqrt{db / (d+b)^3}$$

$$SE_{overall\ accuracy} = \sqrt{prev^2 \times var_{sensitivity} + (1 - prev)^2 \times var_{1-specificity} + (sens - spec)^2}$$
$$\times var_{prev}$$

where prev = prevalence = $(a+d)/(a+b+c+d)$ and var = variance = SD^2.

A small sensitivity with a relatively wide spread, for example, a sensitivity of 55% with a $SE_{sensitivity}$ larger than 2.5% means that the sensitivity is not significantly different from 50%, a result that does not give more information than tossing a coin. This diagnostic test is not adequately precise for validation. Many diagnostic tests have been erroneously validated in the past based on sensitivities/specificities higher than 50%, without assessment for uncertainty (see Chap. 47).

3 Quantitative Diagnostic Tests

3.1 Accuracy

Linear regression with the gold standard test as dependent and the new diagnostic test as independent variable (respectively y- and x-variable) is very popular for assessing accuracy of quantitative diagnostic tests. If a statistically significant

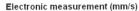

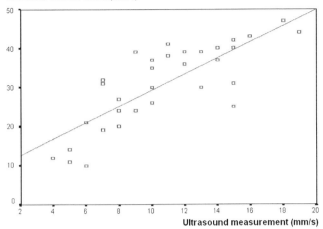

Fig. 51.2 Accuracy assessment with a linear regression model. The regression equation is given by $y = a + bx = 8.647 + 2.065$ x (a = intercept, b = regression coefficient, $p < 0.0001$). The x-variable, ultrasound estimate, is a very significant predictor of the y-variable, the electromagnetic measurement. However, the prediction, despite the high level of statistical significance, is very imprecise. For example, if $x = 6$, then y may be 10 or 21, if $x = 7$, y may be 19, 31 or 32

association between y and x is established, this is generally considered sufficient evidence for validation. This approach is incorrect. For example, in Fig. 51.2 an example is given where flow velocity (mm/s) as estimated by ultrasound is used to predict the standard electromagnetic measurements (mm/s). The regression equation calculated from the SPSS Statistical Software program is given by $y = a + bx = 8.647 + 2.065$ x (a = intercept, b = regression coefficient). The standard error of the regression coefficient $b = Se_b = 0.276$. This means that the t-value = 2.065/0.276, equaling 7.491, and the p-value is thus <0.0001. The x-variable, ultrasound estimate, is a very significant predictor of the y-variable, the electromagnetic measurement. However, the graph shows that the prediction despite the high level of statistical significance, is very imprecise. For example, if $x = 6$, then y may be 10 or 21, if $x = 7$, y may be 19, 31 or 32. A significant correlation is, thus, not good enough to validate a quantitative diagnostic test. A more adequate method for validation was given by Barnett (1969). Test the hypotheses $a = 0.000$, and $b = 1.000$. If the 95% confidence intervals of the calculated a and b include the numbers 0.000 and 1.000 respectively, then the test can be accepted as validated. Confidence intervals can be calculated several ways, but here we use the Gaussian approach:

95% confidence interval of $a = a \pm 2\ Se_a\ (8.647 \pm 2 \times 3.132)$
95% confidence interval of $b = b \pm 2\ Se_b\ (2.065 \pm 2 \times 0.276)$
$a \pm 2\ Se_a$ = between 2.383 and 14.911.
$b \pm 2\ Se_b$ = between 1.513 and 2.617

The numbers 0.000 and 1.000 are not included in the 95% confidence intervals. No validity has been established.

Fig. 51.3 Angiographic
cardiac volumes (liters) used
to predict cast cardiac
volumes (liters)

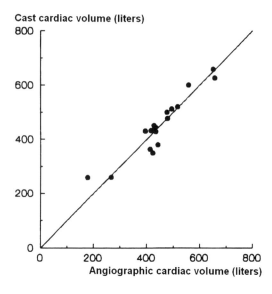

Another example is given in Fig. 51.3. Angiographic cardiac volumes (liters) are
used to predict cast cardiac volumes (liters). When testing the hypotheses $a=0.000$
and $b=1.000$, SPSS will produce the following results.
95% confidence intervals of $a = a \pm 2\ Se_a = 39.340 \pm 2 \times 38.704$
95% confidence intervals of $b = b \pm 2\ Se_b = 0.917 \pm 2 \times 0.083$

$a \pm 2\ Se_a$ = between -38.068 and 116.748
$b \pm 2\ Se_b$ = between 0.751 and 1.083

The 95% confidence intervals include 0.000 and 1.000 respectively. The diagnostic can be accepted as validated.

3.2   Reproducibility

Reproducibility is often calculated incorrectly. The first commonly used incorrect
method is given in the example underneath. The individual differences between test
1 and 2 per patient are calculated. If the mean difference is small, it is concluded
that the test is well reproducible.

Patient no	Test 1	Test 2	Difference
1	1	11	−10
2	10	0	10
3	2	11	−9
4	12	2	10
5	11	1	10
6	1	12	−11
	Mean difference		0

As can be observed from the above example of flow velocities (mm/s), the mean difference between test 1 and test 2 is zero. Yet, the tests are very poorly reproducible, because the range of differences is no less than 21 (differences vary from −11 to +10) mm/s.

The second commonly used incorrect method is the following. A regression line is drawn with test 1 data on x-axis and test data on y-axis. If the data are close to the line, it is concluded that reproducibility is good. There are two problems with this approach. First, testing twice introduces a regression to the mean phenomenon: patients scoring low the first time, have a better chance of scoring higher next time vice versa. A second problem is that only good reproducibility is an adequate conclusion if the direction coefficient of the regression line has a direction of 45°.

The correct methods for assessing reproducibility with quantitative diagnostic tests are summarized.

1. Duplicate standard deviation
2. Repeatability coefficient
3. Intraclass correlation

1. *Duplicate standard deviation (SD)*
The duplicate standard deviation is used in the underneath example.

Patient no	Test 1	Test 2	Difference (d)	(difference)^2
1	1	11	−10	100
2	10	0	10	100
3	2	11	−9	81
4	12	2	10	100
5	11	1	10	100
6	1	12	−11	121
Average	6.17	6.17	0	100.3

$$\text{Duplicate SD} = \sqrt{\ \tfrac{1}{2}\Sigma d^2\ /\ n} = \sqrt{(1/2 \times 100.3)} = 7.08$$

$$\text{Duplicate SD \%} = \frac{\text{duplicate SD}}{\text{overall mean}} \times 100\% = \frac{7.08}{6.17} \times 100\% = 115\%$$

An adequate reproducibility corresponds to a duplicate SD of 10–20%.

2. *Repeatability coefficient*
The repeatability coefficient is applied in the underneath example.

Patient no	Test 1	Test 2	Difference
1	1	11	−10
2	10	0	10
3	2	11	−9
4	12	2	10
5	11	1	10
6	1	12	−11
Mean	6.17	6.17	0
Standard deviation (SD)			10.97

The repeatability coefficient = mean difference ± 2 SD $_{\text{difference}}$ = 0 ± 21.95
The interpretation is as follows. A repeatability coefficient must be < than the largest measured difference between test 1 and test 2.

3. *Intraclass correlation*

The intraclass correlation is applied in this example (SD = standard deviation, SS = sum of squares).

Patient	Test 1	Test 2	Average	SD^2
1	1	11	6	50
2	10	0	5	50
3	2	11	6.5	40.5
4	12	2	7	32
5	11	1	6	50
6	1	12	6.5	60.5
Mean	6.17	6.17		
Overall mean	6.17			

$$SS_{\text{between subjects}} = (\text{mean subject 1} - \text{grand mean})^2 + (\text{mean subject 2} - \text{grand mean})^2$$
$$+ \ldots\ldots = 3.0134$$
$$SS_{\text{within subjects}} = SD_1^2 + SD_2^2 + SD_3^2 + SD_4^2 + \ldots = 283$$

The intraclass correlation (ICC) is given be the equation =

$$\frac{SS_{\text{between subjects}}}{SS_{\text{between subjects}} + SS_{\text{within subjects}}} = 0 - 1$$

If $SS_{\text{between}} = 0$, then the test will be poorly reproducible; if $SS_{\text{within}} = 0$, then the test will be excellently reproducible. Here the intraclass correlation = 0.01051, and, so, the test is very poorly reproducible.

3.3   Precision

A good precision can be interpreted as a small spread in the data, for example, estimated by a small SD or SE (standard error). If the spread in a data sample is wide, some legitimate statistical methods are available to reduce the size of the SDs/SEs, such as data modeling (massage) using multiple regression or logarithmic transformation, exponential modeling, polynomial modeling or other methods. Figure 51.4 gives an example of data modeled using a multiple linear regression model. On the x-axis the baseline Ldl-cholesterol levels of the patients in a cholesterol-study are given, on the y-axis the decreases of Ldl-cholesterol after treatment is given. The upper graph gives the results without, the lower with modeling. It can be

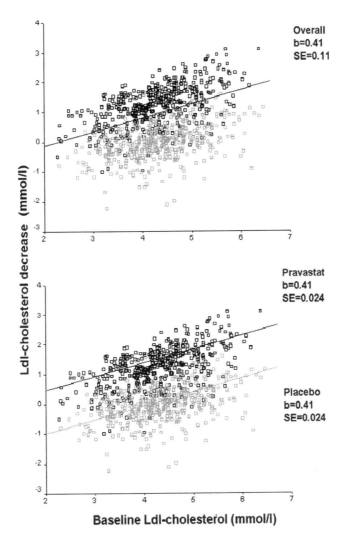

Fig. 51.4 Example of data modeling for increasing precision using a multiple linear regression model. On the x-axis the baseline Ldl-cholesterol level of the patients in a cholesterol-study are given, on the y-axis the decrease of Ldl-cholesterol after treatment is given. The *upper graph* gives the results without, the lower with modeling. It can be observed in the figure that the treatment efficacy given by the b-values are similar but that the SEs are smaller in the *modeled graph*, and so this modeling produced a better precision

observed in the figure that the treatment efficacy given by the b-values is unchanged, but that the spread in the data given by the SEs is smaller with the multiple linear regression models.

Another example is in Fig. 51.5 showing the ambulatory blood pressure measurements (ABPMs) of ten subjects; both means and SDs and 7th order polynomial

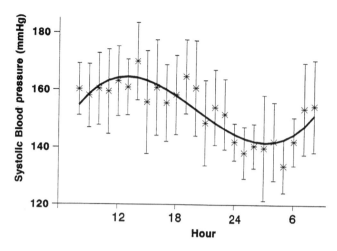

Fig. 51.5 Ambulatory blood pressure measurements (ABPMs) of ten subjects; both means and SDs and 7th order polynomial regression models of the data are drawn. The SPSS program calculates the spread in the data using either of the two methods. The pooled SD of the ABPM values using the means equals 17 mmHg (pooled departure from all means). The SD of the polynomial model is much smaller and equals 7 mmHg (pooled departure from the polynomial curve). Obviously, this curvilinear regression model provides a much better precision, and is, therefore, a more precise model for analyzing the differences between the ABPM recordings of different blood pressure reducing therapies than simply the use of averages and their SDs

regression models of the data are drawn. The SPSS program calculates the spread in the data using either of the two methods. The Pooled SD of the means equals 17 mmHg. The SD of the polynomial model is much smaller and equals 7 mmHg. Obviously, this curvilinear regression model provides a better precision, and is, therefore, a more precise model for analyzing the effects on the ABPM recordings of different blood pressure reducing therapies than simply using the averages and their SDs.

4   Additional Methods

Three relatively new methods for the accuracy assessment of diagnostic tests are available.

1. *Continuous receiver operated characteristic (ROC) curves* (Delong and Delong 1988; Hanley and McNeil 1982)

   In the use of many diagnostic tests, test results do not necessarily fall into one of two categories, but rather into categories with more or less confidence in the presence of disease (Fig. 51.6). While using multiple thresholds for making a diagnosis, a continuous ROC curve can be obtained (Fig. 51.7). The closer this

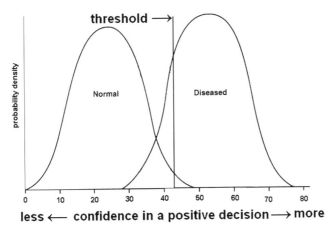

Fig. 51.6 Diagnostic test where results do not fall into one of two categories but rather into categories with more or less confidence

Fig. 51.7 Continuous receiver operated characteristic (*ROC*) curve

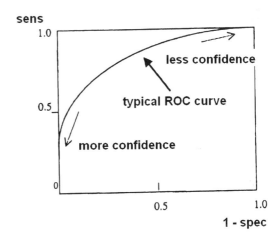

ROC curve approaches the top of the y-axis, the better accuracy the diagnostic test will provide with an optimal AUC of 1.0. In contrast, if the ROC curve is close to the 45° diagonal line, the AUC is close to 0.5, and the test is very inaccurate. The simplest method for calculating the AUC is summing the areas of the trapezoids formed by the curve and the x-axis. Various statistical software programs including SPSS can be used to calculate the area under the curve of continuous ROC curves, otherwise called c-statistics (concordance statistics) (Chap. 49). It is used to estimate the performance of qualitative diagnostic tests. However, as demonstrated in Chap. 49 simply binary logistic regression with the odds of disease as outcome and the test score as independent variable can be equally well used for the purpose.

2. *Intraclass correlation (ICC) for agreement with the gold standard test* (Lee et al. 1989)

The Intraclass correlation has recently been used not only for assessing reproducibility of diagnostic tests, but also as an alternative method for accuracy assessments. It is given by the equation (SS = sum of squares)

$$ICC = \frac{SS_{\text{between techniques}}}{SS_{\text{between techniques}} + SS_{\text{within techniques}}}.$$

The interpretation is similar to that of the intraclass correlation method for reproducibility assessment as explained above. It can be demonstrated that this method is less sensitive in demonstrating disagreement between the diagnostic test and the gold standard test than the previously mentioned methods. Also the Bland-Altman method, which will be discussed next, performs better.

3. *Bland-Altman method* (Bland & Altman 1995)

Bland and Altman recommended the following approach. Calculate the individual differences between the diagnostic test results and the gold standard test results and, subsequently, the standard deviation of these differences. If this standard deviation is less than or equal to the standard deviation of the both the diagnostic test results and the gold standard test results, then the two difference tests are exchangeable and, therefore, equivalent. The diagnostic test is, then, accurate.

5 Discussion

The current chapter gives some relatively simple methods for assessment. Validity assessments of diagnostic tests are rarely communicated in research papers and this may contribute to the low reproducibility of clinical trials. We expected that validation would, at least, be a standard procedure in clinical chemistry studies where a close to 100% accuracy/reproducibility is not unusual. However, even in a journal like the Journal of the International Federation of Clinical Chemistry and Laboratory Medicine out of 17 original papers publishing novel chemistry methods in 2006 none of the papers communicated validity assessments except for one study (Imburt-Bismut et al. 2004). Ironically, this very study reported two incorrect methods for assessing reproducibility, namely the assessment of significant differences between repeated measures, and the calculation of Pearson's correlation levels.

A more general explanation for the underreporting of validation procedures for diagnostic tests in research communications is that the scientific community although devoted to the study of disease management, is little motivated to devote its energies to assessing the validity of the diagnostic procedures required for the very study of disease management. Clinical investigators favor the latter to the former. Also the former gives no clear-cut career path, while the latter more often does so. And there is the injections from the pharmaceutical industry. To counterbalance this

Table 51.1 Summary of correct methods for validation of both quantitative and qualitative diagnostic tests

Accuracy	Reproducibility	Precision
Qualitative diagnostic test		
Sensitivity	Kappas	Confidence intervals
Specificity		
Overall accuracy		
ROC curves		
Logistic regression		
Quantitative diagnostic test		
Barnett's test	Duplicate standard deviation	Confidence intervals
Intraclass correlation vs gold test	Repeatability coefficient	
Bland-Altman test	Intraclass correlation vs duplicate test	

is a challenge for governments and university staffs. Correct methods for validation of both quantitative and qualitative diagnostic methods are summarized in Table 51.1.

6   Conclusions

Clinical developments of new treatments are impossible without adequate diagnostic tests. Several working parties including the Consolidated Standard Randomized Trials (CONSORT) movement and the Standard for Reporting Diagnostic Accuracy (STARD) group have launched quality criteria for diagnostic tests. Particularly, accuracy-, reproducibility- and precision-assessments have been recommended, but methods of assessment have not been defined so far.

This chapter summarizes correct and incorrect methods and new developments for that purpose.

A diagnostic test can be either qualitative like the presence of an elevated erythrocyte sedimentation rate to demonstrate pneumonia, or quantitative like ultrasound flow velocity to estimate invasive electromagnetic flow velocity.

Qualitative diagnostic tests can be assessed for:

- *accuracy* using sensitivity/specificity/overall accuracy, and receiver operated (ROC) curves,
- *reproducibility* using Cohen's kappas,
- *precision* using confidence intervals of sensitivity/specificity/overall accuracy.

Quantitative diagnostics tests can be assessed for

- *accuracy* using a linear regression line $(y = a + bx)$ and testing $a = 0.00/b = 1.00$,

– *reproducibility* using duplicate standard errors, repeatability coefficients or intraclass correlations,
– *precision* by calculating confidence intervals. Improved confidence intervals can be obtained by data modeling.

A significant linear correlation between the diagnostic test and the gold standard test does not correctly indicate adequate accuracy. A small mean difference between repeated measures or a significant linear relationship between repeated measures does not indicate adequate reproducibility.

New developments include continuous ROC curves, intraclass correlations, and Bland-Altman agreement tests for the accuracy assessments of quantitative diagnostic tests.

References

Anonymous The quality of diagnostic tests statement, the CONSORT statement. www.consort-statement.org. Accessed 15 Dec 2011

Barnett DV (1969) Simultaneous pairwise linear structural relationships. Biometrics 28:129–142

Bland JM, Altman DG (1995) Comparing two methods of clinical measurement: a personal history. Int J Epidemiol 24:s7–s14

Bossuyt PM, Reitsma JB, Bruns DE, Gatsonis CA, Glasziou PP, Irwig JG, Moher D, Rennie D, De Vet HC, for the STARD steering group (2003) Education and debate. Towards complete and accurate reporting of studies of diagnostic accuracy: the STARD initiative. BMJ 326:41–44

Delong ER, Delong DM (1988) Comparing the areas under two or more correlated receiver operated characteristic curves; a nonparametric approach. Biometrics 44:837–845

Hanley JA, McNeil BJ (1982) The meaning and use of the area under curve under a receiver operating characteristic (ROC) curve. Diagn Radiol 143:29–36

Imburt-Bismut F, Messous D, Thibaut V, Myers RB, Piton A, Thabut D, Devers L, Hainque B, Mecardier A, Poynard T (2004) Intra-laboratory analytical variability of biochemical markers of fibrosis and activity and reference ranges in healthy blood donors. Clin Chem Lab Med 42:323–333

Lee J, Koh D, Ong CN (1989) Statistical evaluation of agreement between two methods for measuring a quantitative variable. Comput Biol Med 19:61–70

Morgan TM, Krumholz HM, Lifton RP, Spertus JA (2007) Nonvalidation of reported genetic risk factors for acute coronary syndrome in a large scale replication study. JAMA 297:1551–1561

Reid MC, Lachs MS, Feinstein AR (1995) Use of methodological standards in diagnostic test research. Getting better but still not good. JAMA 274:645–650

Chapter 52
Validating Surrogate Endpoints
of Clinical Trials

1 Introduction

Clinical trials are often constructed with surrogate endpoints for practical or cost considerations, for example, lipid levels as a surrogate for arteriosclerosis, arrhythmias for coronary artery disease, and cervical smears for tubal infections (Pratt and Moye 1995; Canner et al. 1986; Riggs et al. 1990; Fleming and DeMets 1996; Boissel and Hc 1992). Such trials make inferences from surrogate observations about the effect of treatments on the supposed true endpoints without accounting the strength of association between the surrogate and true endpoints. The main problem with this practice is that the surrogate endpoint may lack sufficient validity to predict the true endpoint, giving rise to misleading trial results. The International Conference of Harmonisation (ICH) Guideline E9 Statistics Principles for Clinical Trials (Philips and Haudiquet 2003) recommends that, for the approval of a surrogate marker, (1) a statistical relationship with the true endpoint in observational studies be demonstrated, (2) evidence be given from clinical trials that treatment effects on the surrogate correspond to those on the true clinical endpoint, and (3) the surrogate marker like a diagnostic test be tested for sensitivity and specificity to predict the true endpoint. There is, thus, considerable consensus to routinely assess the accuracy of surrogate markers, but not specifically how to do so. Problems with the current sensitivity-specificity approach to validity is, that it is dual and that an overall level of validity is, therefore, hard to give (Cleophas 2005). Also, it can be used for binary (yes/no) endpoints only. As an alternative, regression-models have been proposed (Philips and Haudiquet 2003; Chen et al. 2003). However, a correlation of borderline statistical significance between the surrogate and the true endpoint is not enough to indicate that the surrogate is an accurate predictor. The current chapter underscores the need for accuracy assessment of surrogate endpoints by comparing the required sample sizes of trials with and without surrogate endpoints, and describes two novel procedures for assessment. The first makes use of an overall level of accuracy with confidence intervals and a prespecified boundary of accuracy. The second uses a regression model that accounts both the association between the

T.J. Cleophas and A.H. Zwinderman, *Statistics Applied to Clinical Studies*,
DOI 10.1007/978-94-007-2863-9_52, © Springer Science+Business Media B.V. 2012

surrogate and the true endpoint, and the association between either of these variables and the treatments to be tested.

2   Some Terminology

Surrogate marker/ endpoint/test	Laboratory measurement or physical sign used as a substitute for a clinically meaningful endpoint that measure directly how a patient feels, functions, or survives, otherwise called the true endpoint.
Validity of a surrogate test	The surrogate test's ability to show which individuals have a true test either positive or negative. We sometimes use the term overall validity to emphasize that the approach is different from assessing sensitivity and specificity separately.
Sensitivity	Chance of a true positive surrogate test.
Specificity	Chance of a true negative surrogate test.
Odds ratio (OR)	Odds of the clinically meaningful endpoint in the treatment group/ odds of it in the control group.
Alpha (α)	Type I error, chance of finding a difference where there is none.
Beta (β)	Type II error, chance of finding no difference where there is one.
Null-hypothesis	The study is negative, the treatment does not work. The null-hypothesis of no treatment effect is rejected when the difference from a zero effect is significant.
Variance	Estimate of spread or precision in the data. Variance of proportion $p = p\,(1-p)$
Standard error (SE)	$\sqrt{(\text{variance}/n)}$, where n = sample size.
Confidence interval (CI)	It covers a percentage of the results that can be expected if the study would be repeated many times. For example, 95% CI between an OR of 1.10 and 1.86 means that 95% of many similar studies would produce an OR between 1.10 and 1.86. 95%CI of a proportion be calculated according to: proportion $\pm 1.96 * \text{SE}_{\text{proportion}}$, where * is the sign of multiplication.
Prespecified boundary of validity	It is often chosen on clinical grounds, and covers the range of results that are accepted by the investigators as sufficiently valid to use the surrogate test for its purpose. Currently, it is considered good statistical practice to define a prespecified boundary of your expected validity, and, then, test whether the confidence interval of your calculated level of validity falls entirely within the prespecified boundary. If so, you accept, if not you reject the presence of validity.
Dependent variable	y-variable in a regression analysis.
Independent variable	x-variable in a regression analysis.
Correlation coefficient squared (r^2)	Estimate of strength of association between paired observations. If $r^2 = 0$, there is no association, if $r^2 = 1$, there is 100% association. If $r^2 = 0.5$, there is 50% association. One variable determines the other by 50%, and there is 50% uncertainty. The r^2 value expresses the proportion of variability in the y-variable determined by the variability in the x-variable.
Regression coefficient (b)	Estimate of strength of association between paired observations particularly used in the case of multiple regression.

3   Surrogate Endpoints and the Calculation of the Required Sample Size in a Trial

The validity or accuracy of a surrogate marker can be expressed in terms of sensitivity and specificity to predict the true endpoint, e.g. healings.

	Healings	Non-healings
New treatment (group1)	170 (E)	140 (F)
Control treatment (group 2)	190 (G)	230 (H)

odds of healing E/F and G/H,

$$\text{odds ratio}\,(\text{OR}) = E\,/\,F\,/\,G\,/\,H$$
$$= (170\,/\,140)\,/\,(190\,/\,230) = 1.47.$$

Figure 52.1 shows that a true endpoint test for the assessment of the above data has a 95% confidence interval between 1.09 and 1.99, and that it can reject the null-hypothesis of no difference between the two treatments at $P < 0.02$. If a surrogate test for the assessment of the same data has a sensitivity of 80% and specificity of 100%, the OR will diminish, because the observed numbers of healings will fall by 20%, and those of the non-healings will rise correspondingly (OR = 1.38; 95% confidence interval 1.10–1.86, P = 0.05). If it has a sensitivity of 80% and specificity of only 90%, the OR can be calculated to further fall to 1.31 (95% confidence interval −0.029–1.77, p = 0.10), and a significance of difference between the two treatments can no longer be demonstrated (Fig. 52.1). Obviously, with surrogate markers rapidly less certainty is provided to estimate the chance of healing or no-healing. In order to maintain a close to true endpoint level of certainty the sample size will have to be increased.

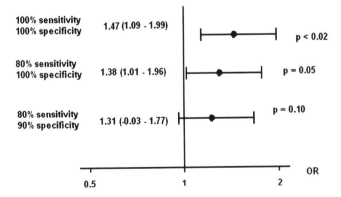

Fig. 52.1 Effect of sensitivity and specificity levels on odds ratios and their 95% confidence intervals (odds ratio = odds of healing of the new treatment/odds of healing of the control treatment)

The effect on sample size requirement of a reduced sensitivity or specificity is illustrated in the underneath hypothesized example.

In a parallel study 10% healings are expected in group 1, and 20% healings in group 2.

The required sample size can be calculated according to:

$$\text{required sample size} = \text{power index}^* \frac{p_1\left(1-p_1\right)+p_2\left(1-p_2\right)}{\left(p_1-p_2\right)^2}\text{subjects per group}$$

$$= 195 \text{ subjects per group}$$

p_1 = expected proportion of healings in group 1, p_2 = expected proportion of healings in group 2, power index for $\alpha=0.05$ and $\beta=0.20$ equals 7.8, $*$ = the sign of multiplication.

If the surrogate test provides 80% sensitivity, then in group 1 not 10% but $80\% \times 10\% = 8\%$ healings will be observed, in group 2 not 20% but $80\% \times 20\% = 16\%$. The required sample size will rise to:

$$= 254 \text{ subjects per group.}$$

If sensitivity = 80% and specificity = 90%, it can be similarly calculated that the required sample size will further rise to no less than:

$$= 515 \text{ subjects per group.}$$

In trials using surrogate endpoints the sample size has to be based not only on the expected treatment efficacy but also on the validity of the surrogate marker used. We will now describe two procedures that can be readily applied for validating the surrogate marker. The first is adequate for binary variables, the second both for continuous and binary variables. The first can also be chosen after the assignment of continuous data to binary ones.

4   Validating Surrogate Markers Using 95% Confidence Intervals

The validity of a surrogate marker can, like a diagnostic test, be assessed by sensitivity and specificity to predict the true endpoint. In addition to this dual approach to accuracy, an overall validity can be calculated as illustrated below.

		Observed surrogate endpoint (n)	
		Yes	No
Observed true endpoint	Yes	a	b
	No	c	d

Sensitivity = a/(a+c)
Specificity = d/(b+d)
1-specificity = b/(b+d)
Prevalence of true endpoint = (a+b)/(a+b+c+d)

The variance of sensitivity is given by $ac/(a+c)^3$.
For the specificity the variance $= db/(d+b)^3$.
Also for 1-specificity the variance $= db/(d+b)^3$
For the prevalence of the true endpoint the variance $= (a+b)(c+d)/(a+b+c+d)^3$
Overall validity = sensitivity * prevalence + specificity * (1-prevalence).
* = the sign of multiplication.

For approval of a surrogate marker a boundary of validity is prespecified in the study protocol, e.g., 85% < validity < 100%, and a confidence interval of the overall validity level is calculated. If the confidence interval falls entirely between the pre-specified boundary, validity is demonstrated. For example, the true endpoint is a cardiovascular event, the surrogate endpoint is an elevated C-reactive protein level, currently a widely used marker for cardiovascular disease.

For the calculation of the confidence intervals standard errors (SEs) are required. In order to calculate the standard error (SE) ($= \sqrt{\text{(variance)}}$) of the overall validity, we make use of the formula:

$$Var(X+Y) = Var(X) + Var(Y) + 2\,Cov(X,Y).$$

$$Var(\text{overall validity}) = Var(\text{sens} * \text{prev}) + Var(\text{spec}) * (1-\text{prev})$$
$$+ 2Cov(\text{sens} * \text{prev}, \text{spec} * (1-\text{prev})).$$

Var = variance; sens = sensitivity; spec = specificity; prev = prevalence; cov = covariance. The variance of X*Y may be approached from

$$Var(X*Y) = Y^2 Var(X) + X^2 Var(Y).$$

Using this formula we will end up finding:

$$Var(\text{overall validity}) = \text{prev}^2 * Var(\text{sens}) + (1-\text{prev})^2 * Var(1-\text{spec})$$
$$+ (\text{sens} - \text{spec})^2 * Var(\text{prev}).$$

If, e.g.,

sensitivity = 80% with SE = 2%,
specificity = 90% with SE = 1%,
prevalence = 10% with SE = 3%,

then we can calculate:

$$\text{overall validity} = 0.8 * 0.1 + (0.9) * (1-0.1) = 0.89$$

and

$$Var(\text{overall validity}) = 0.1^2 * 0.02^2 + (1-0.1)^2 * 0.02^2 + (0.8-0.9)^2 * 0.03^2$$
$$= 0.000337.$$

The SE of the overall validity is the square root of the variance, and equals $0.018356 = 1.8356\%$.

This approach makes use of the so-called delta-method which describes the variance of natural logarithm (ln) (X) as $Var(\ln(x)) = Var(x)/x^2$. The approach is sufficiently accurate if the standard errors of prev, sens and spec are small which is true if samples are large.

An overall validity of 89% with SE 1.8356% means that the 95% confidence interval is between

$$0.89 - 1.96 * 0.018356 \text{ and}$$
$$0.89 + 1.96 * 0.018356,$$

and is thus between 85.4 and 92.6%. This interval falls entirely between the pre-specified interval of validity of $85\% < \text{validity} < 100\%$. This surrogate endpoint is, thus, validated.

5 Validating Surrogate Endpoints Using Regression Modeling

Table 52.1 shows the total and LDL cholesterol levels being used as tentative surrogate endpoints for coronary artery diameter. For the validation of the two surrogate endpoints the following linear model is used:

$$y = a + b_1 x_1 + b_2 x_2$$

y = true endpoint,
x_1 = treatment modality (0 = placebo, active treatment = 1)
x_2 = surrogate endpoint

$$y = a + b_1 x_1$$

r^2 of this equation = proportion variability in y explained by x_1

$$y = a + b_1 x_1 + b_2 x_2$$

r^2 of this equation = proportion variability in y explained by x_1 and x_2.

The subtraction sum of the two r^2-values = proportion variability y explained by the surrogate endpoint x_2; the larger the subtraction sum the better the surrogate endpoint. Table 52.2 gives a summary of the calculations. Both LDL-cholesterol and total cholesterol levels are significant predictors of the true endpoint in the multiple regression model with respectively $b = 0.891$, $se = 0.003$, $p = <0.0001$ and $b = 0.685$, $se = 0.018$, $p < 0.0001$. However, the subtraction sum of the r^2-values is $0.75 - 0.25 = 0.50$ for total cholesterol and $0.98 - 0.25 = 0.73$ for LDL-cholesterol. If the surrogate endpoint is made the dependent variable instead of the true endpoint,

Table 52.1 Total cholesterol and LDL-cholesterol levels are used as tentative surrogate endpoints for coronary artery diameter

Pt no.	Cor art (mm)	Treat	Tchol (mmol/l)	LDLchol (mmol/l)
1	24	0	4.0	2.4
2	30	0	6.5	3.2
3	25	0	7.5	2.4
4	35	1	5.0	3.6
5	39	1	4.5	3.8
6	30	0	5.0	3.0
7	27	0	4.0	2.6
8	14	0	2.5	1.6
9	39	1	6.5	4.0
10	42	1	7.5	4.2
11	41	1	5.5	4.0
12	38	1	5.5	3.8
13	39	1	6.0	3.6
14	37	1	5.0	3.4
15	47	1	9.0	4.8
16	30	0	6.5	2.8
17	36	1	6.0	3.8
18	12	0	2.0	1.0
19	26	0	5.0	2.8
20	20	1	4.0	2.0
21	43	0	8.0	4.4
22	31	0	7.5	3.0
23	40	1	7.0	3.8
24	31	0	3.5	3.2
25	36	1	6.0	3.4
26	21	0	3.0	2.0
27	44	0	9.5	4.6
28	11	1	2.5	1.0
29	27	0	4.0	2.6
30	24	0	4.5	2.6
31	40	1	7.5	3.8
32	32	1	3.5	3.4
33	10	0	3.0	0.8
34	37	1	7.0	3.2
35	19	0	3.5	2.0

Pt no. patient number, *Cor art* coronary artery diameter, *Treat* treatment modality (0=placebo. 1=active treatment), *Tchol* total cholesterol level, *LDLchol* LDL-cholesterol level

then LDL-cholesterol performs better than does total cholesterol. For LDL-cholesterol $r^2 = 0.20$, p-values <0.01, power approximately 80%; for total cholesterol $r^2 = 0.04$, $p = 0.226$.

We can conclude that in order to establish a powerful correlation between treatment modality and a surrogate endpoint ($p < 0.01$, power $> 80\%$), the proportion variability in y explained by the surrogate endpoint should be close to 70% or more for accurate predictions.

Table 52.2 Analysis of associations between true endpoint, treatment modality and surrogate endpoints from Fig. 52.1

		r²-value	F-value	p-value	
True vs treat		0.250	10.9	0.002	
LDL-chol vs treat		0.202	8.3	0.007	
Tchol vs treat		0.044	105	0.266	
True vs LDL-chol		0.970	1052.9	0.000	
True vs Tchol		0.630	56.1	0.000	
		b-value	standard error	p-value	r²
True vs treat and LDL-chol	treat	0.0135	0.006	0.032	0.98
	LDL-chol	0.891	0.003	0.000	
True vs treat and Tchol	treat	0.375	0.005	0.000	0.75
	Tchol	0.685	0.018	0.001	

True true endpoint, *treat* treatment modality (0 or 1 for placebo and active treatment), *LDL-chol* surrogate endpoint LDL-cholesterol level, *Tchol* surrogate endpoint total cholesterol level, *r²* Pearson's correlation coefficient squared, *b* regression coefficient

A wrong method is to accept as a valid result a surrogate endpoint that is a significant determinant of the true endpoint but not of the treatment modality.

We should add that different regression models are more convenient for different data like logistic regression models for odds ratios and Cox regression for survival data, but that the approach, otherwise, is similar.

6   Discussion

In trials using surrogate endpoints the sample sizes have to be based not only on the expected treatment efficacy but also on the validity of the surrogate marker used. A method for calculating adjusted samples sizes is given.

Binary surrogate endpoints can be validated by calculating sensitivity and specificity to predict the true endpoint. However, overall validity is hard to quantify using this dual approach. Instead, an overall validity can be expressed by the proportion of patients that have a true surrogate test, either positive or negative, which we called the overall validity level. Still other approaches to the validity of surrogate tests are the so-called positive and negative predictive values and likelihood ratios. Just like the overall validity level, these estimators adjust for numbers of differences in patients with and without the true endpoint, but unlike the overall validity level they do not answer what proportion of patients has a correct test. Riegelman (2005), recently, proposed as method for assessing validity of diagnostic tests the discriminant ability, defined as (sensitivity + specificity)/2. Although this method avoids the dual approach to validity, it wrongly assumes equal importance and equal prevalence of true positive and true negatives, and does neither answer what proportion of the patients has a correct test. We, therefore, decided to use an overall validity level, expressed as the percentage of patients with a true surrogate test, either positive or negative. We calculated confidence intervals of this estimate in order to quantify the level of uncertainty involved in the trial results. If the 95% confidence interval of the data is entirely within a previously set interval of validity, then the surrogate marker can be validated for use in subsequent trials.

In case of continuous surrogate tests regression models are adequate for testing validity. Not only the association between surrogate and true endpoint must be accounted, but also the associations between either of these variables and the treatment modality to be tested. Interaction assessments are not necessary, if there are no clinical arguments for the presence of interaction. A surrogate test can be validated only, if the proportion of variability in the surrogate endpoint explains the true endpoint by 70% or more, because the power of the surrogate endpoint to determine the treatment effect is then about 80%. A wrong conclusion would be to accept adequate validity if the surrogate test is an independent determinant of the true endpoint but not of the treatment modality.

Validating surrogate endpoints can only be done in a trial where a sufficient number of patients reaches both the surrogate and the true endpoint. With mortality or major cardiovascular events as true endpoint large randomized trials with long term follow-up are needed for that purpose. Chen et al. (2003) proposed as an alternative a semi-large study with a validation and non-validation set of patients, but this approach is not really different from two separate studies in a single framework. Another interesting alternative was recently proposed by Kassaï et al. They meta-analyzed multiple small studies, but their effort was limited by its post-hoc nature and the heterogeneity of the studies included (Kassaï et al. 2005).

If the required sample size or length of follow-up cannot be accomplished, then validity testing of surrogates for true endpoints will be impossible. We will have to look for alternative research methods like looking for intermediate endpoints such as morbidity instead of mortality. We should add that there are additional problems with a true endpoint like mortality: (1) for estimating the effects of preventive medicine that is begun when subjects are middle-aged this endpoint will be statistically weak, because at such ages the background noise of mortality due to other conditions associated with senescence is high, (2) to individual patients low morbidity and high quality of life, generally, means more than does a few additional years of survival. Fortunately, in other research the true endpoint is very well possible, and the surrogate endpoint is pursued because of practical and costs considerations. This applies, e.g., to the example described in the above section. This paper was, particularly, written for the latter purpose. It is to be hoped that the paper will affect the validity of future clinical trials constructed with surrogate endpoints.

7 Conclusions

The International Conference of Harmonisation (ICH) Guideline E9 Statistics Principles for Clinical Trials recommends that surrogate endpoints in clinical trials be validated using either (1) the sensitivity-specificity approach or (2) regression analysis. The problem with (1) is that an overall level of validity is hard to give, and with (2) that a significant correlation between the surrogate and true endpoint is not enough to indicate that the surrogate is a valid predictor. This chapter provides for a nonmathematical readership procedures that avoid the above two problems.

(1) Instead of the sensitivity-specificity approach we used an overall validity level, expressed as the percentage of patients with a true surrogate test, either positive or negative. We calculated confidence intervals of this estimate, and assessed whether they were entirely within the prespecified interval of validity. If so, the surrogate marker was validated for use in subsequent trials. (2) For validating continuous surrogate variables, regression analysis was used, accounting both the correlation between the surrogate and true endpoints, *and* the associations between these two variables and the treatment modalities to be tested. If the proportion of variability in the surrogate endpoint explained the true endpoint by 70% or more, the surrogate test was validated. A wrong conclusion would be here to accept validity if the surrogate endpoint was an independent determinant of the true endpoint, but not of the treatment modality. It is to be hoped that this chapter will affect the validity of future clinical trials constructed with surrogate endpoints.

References

Boissel JP, Hc C (1992) Surrogate endpoints: a basis for a rational approach. Eur J Clin Pharmacol 43:235–244

Canner PL, Berg KG, Wenger NK, Stamler J, Friedman L, Prineas RJ, Friedewald F (1986) Fifteen year mortality of the coronary drug project. J Am Coll Cardiol 8:1245–1255

Chen SX, Leung DH, Qin J (2003) Information recovery in a study with surrogate endpoints. J Am Stat Assoc 10:7–18

Cleophas TJ (2005) Clinical trials: a new method for assessing accuracy of diagnostic tests. Clin Res Regul Aff 22:93–101

Fleming TR, DeMets DL (1996) Surrogate end points in clinical trials: are we being misled? Ann Intern Med 125:605–613

Kassaï B, Shah NR, Leizorovicz A, Cucherat M, Gueyffier F, Boissel JP (2005) The true treatment benefit is unpredictable in clinical trials using surrogate outcome measures with diagnostic tests. J Clin Epidemiol 58:1042–1051

Philips A, Haudiquet V (2003) The international conference of harmonisation (ICH) guideline E9, statistics principles for clinical trials. Stat Med 22:1–11

Pratt Cm, Moye LA (1995) The cardiac arrhythmias suppression trial. Circulation 91:245–247

Riegelman RK (2005) Studying a study and testing a test. Lippincott Williams & Wilkins, Philadelphia

Riggs P et al (1990) Osteoporosis in postmenopausal women. N Engl J Med 32:802–809

Chapter 53
Binary Partitioning

1 Introduction

One of the most important and original applications of binary partitioning was to develop data-based decision cut-off levels that can assist physicians in diagnosing patients potentially suffering heart attacks (Wasson et al. 1985). Traditionally, the physicians made decisions based on their clinical experience. Also, laboratories developed diagnostic tests with normal values based on rather intuitive grounds. Classifications based on representative historical data has the advantage of added empirical information from large numbers of patients. This is, particularly, important if symptoms, signs and diagnostic procedures give rise to a substantial number of false positive and false negative results as often observed in clinical practice. The main purpose of the data-based methods is to reduce the latter number. The book by Breiman et al. (1984) on classification and regression trees is a milestone on binary partitioning and closely related cut-off decision trees, otherwise called CART (classification and regression) trees. The associated CART program has become a commercial software (www.salford-systems.com), but simple partitions and decision trees can also be performed on a pocket calculator. This chapter was written to familiarize the research community with this important methodology for improving the diagnostic accuracy of clinical decision trees.

2 Example

Several vascular labs have defined their estimators for peripheral vascular disease as shown underneath (Jaff and Dorros 1998).

T.J. Cleophas and A.H. Zwinderman, *Statistics Applied to Clinical Studies*,
DOI 10.1007/978-94-007-2863-9_53, © Springer Science+Business Media B.V. 2012

1. Ankle blood pressure	> brachial blood pressure
2. Ankle pressure after 5 min treadmill	>20% reduction from baseline
3. Proximal thigh pressure	>30 mmHg above brachial pressure
4. Segmental pressures (thigh, calf, ankle)	<20 mmHg difference between 2 levels
5. Toe pressure	<40% different from brachial pressure.

Considering the rounded pattern of the above "normal" values for predicting the presence of vascular disease, we may assume that the values as given are based on empiricism and agreement rather than calculated averages, but we can do better. Although the accumulated evidence of the assessment may give rise to a sensitivity close to 95% and a specificity close to 95%, both sensitivity and specificity may increase to 98 or 99% if we fine-tune the cut-off levels of the contributory estimators using representative historical data.

For that purpose a representative sample of patients has to be assessed against a golden standard, i.e., angiography in the given example. The entire sample can be split into patients with a higher and those with an equal or lower ankle blood pressure than their brachial blood pressure, because we know that this is a major symptom of vascular disease. The procedure of splitting is less straightforward, if the estimators are quantitative and multiple cut-off levels are possible like the above no. 2–5 estimators show.

3 ROC (Receiver Operating Characteristic) Method for Finding the Best Cut-Off Level

A hypothesized example of a cut-off level is given in Fig. 53.1. If a fall of ankle blood pressure after 5 min treadmill exercise of >26% is used as threshold for a positive test, then the number of patients with a true positive test are "a", true negative "b", false positive "c", and false negative "d". The ratio "a/(a+c)" is called the sensitivity of the test, the ratio "b/(d+b)" the specificity of the test.

Underneath, an overview is given of the calculated sensitivities and specificities if different cut-off levels are applied.

Cut-off level	Sensitivity	Specificity
22%	1.000	0.723
23%	0.997	0.701
24%	0.990	0.855
25%	0.980	0.908
26%	**0.960**	**0.950**
27%	0.940	0.972
28%	0.910	0.986
29%	0.860	0.993
30%	0.800	1.000

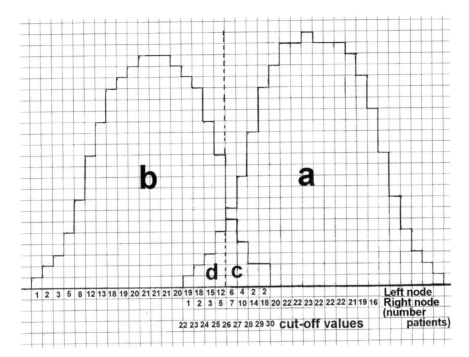

Fig. 53.1 Histogram of a patients' sample assessed for peripheral vascular disease; "a" summarizes the patients with a positive test and the presence of disease, "b" the patients with a negative test and the absence of disease, "c" and "d" are the false positive and false negative patients respectively, if 26 is used as a cut-off value between a positive and a negative test

We would like to have a sensitivity and specificity close to 100%. However, in practice most diagnostic tests are far from perfect and produce false positive and false negative effects. With qualitative tests there is little we can do. With quantitative tests we can increase the sensitivity by moving the vertical decision line between a positive and negative test to the left (Fig. 53.1), and we can increase specificity by moving it in the opposite direction. Figure 53.2 shows the relationship between sensitivities and specificities. The curve suggests a high sensitivity and at the same time high specificity, if 26% or 27% are used as cut-off levels for a positive test. The best cut-off level is obtained if the distance from the curve at that point to the top of the y-axis is closest. The 26% cut-off level can be calculated to provide the closest distance: Pythagoras's equation for right angular triangles shows a distance of $\sqrt{(3^2+5^2)}=\sqrt{41}$ which is closer than the shortest distance next to it $\sqrt{(6^2+3^2)}=\sqrt{45}$. This result is, thus, a better predictor for vascular disease than the value of 20% as previously agreed in the vascular laboratory on intuitive grounds (Jaff and Dorros 1998). In this manner the ROC method can be used for determining the best cut-off level to be included in a decision tree of diagnostic procedures like the above one.

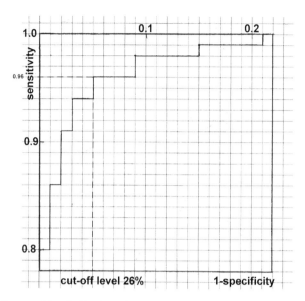

Fig. 53.2 ROC curve of threshold values of positive tests for vascular disease based on the% ankle blood pressure reduction after 5 min treadmill. The shortest distance to the top of the y-axis, and, thus, the best predictive test is obtained with 26% blood pressure reduction as cut-off value

The problem with ROC method is that the sample sizes of the positive and negative tests are not taken into account, reducing the power of this approach. This is, particularly, a problem if the numbers of positive and negative tests are largely different in size. The entropy method is helpful in this situation.

4   Entropy Method for Finding the Best Cut-Off Level

The entropy method has an interesting history. It received its name, because it makes use of an equation that was formerly applied in science to estimate the amount of energy loss in thermodynamics, but, otherwise, has no connection with its application to science. A pleasant thing about this method is that, unlike the ROC method, the result can be easily adjusted for magnitude of the samples. This is also the reason that the result of the ROC method often slightly differs from that of the entropy method.

In entropy-method-terminology the entire sample of patients (Fig. 53.1) is called the parent node, which can, subsequently, be repeatedly split, partitioned if you will, into binary internal nodes. Mostly, internal nodes contain false positive or negative patients, and are, thus, somewhat impure. The magnitude of their impurity is assessed by the log likelihood method, previously explained (Cleophas et al. 2007). Impurity equals the maximum log likelihood of the y-axis-variable by assuming that the x-axis-variable follows a Gaussian (i.e. binomial) distribution and is expressed in units, sometimes called bits (a short-cut for "binary digits"). All this sounds rather complex, but it works smoothly.

The x – axis variable for the right node = x_r = a/(a + b),

The x – axis variable for the left node   = x_l = d/(d + c).

If the impurity equals 1.0 bits, then it is maximal, if it equals 0.0, then it is minimal.

Impurity node either right or left = $- x \ln x - (1 - x) \ln(1 - x)$,

where ln means natural logarithm.

The impurities of the right and left node are calculated separately. Then, a weighted overall impurity of each cut-off level situation is calculated according to (*= sign of multiplication):

Weighted impurity cut-off =

[(a + b)/(a + b + c + d)* impurity-right-node] +

[(d + c)/(a + b + c + d)* impurity-left-node].

Underneath, an overview is given of the calculated impurities at the different cut-off levels. The cut-off percentage of 27 gives the smallest weighted impurity, and is, thus, a better predictor for vascular disease than the value of 20% as previously agreed on intuitive grounds (Wasson et al. 1985).

Cut-off	Impurity right node	Impurity left node	Impurity weighted
22%	0.5137	0.0000	0.3180
23%	0.4392	0.0559	0.3063
24%	0.4053	0.0982	0.2766
25%	0.3468	0.1352	0.2711
26%	0.1988	0.1688	0.1897
27%	**0.1352**	**0.2268**	**0.1830**
28%	0.0559	0.3025	0.1850
29%	0.0559	0.3850	0.2375
30%	0.0000	0.4690	0.2748

Also, it should be a better predictor of vascular disease than the 26% value as established by the ROC method, because, unlike the ROC method, the entropy method takes into account and adjusts the differences in sample sizes of the nodes.

5   Discussion

The best cut-off level for making optimal predictions from diagnostic tests can be calculated from the ROC and entropy methods. The next step is, of course, to include multiple tests in order to further increase accuracy of making predictions.

Decision trees can help making rapid clinical decisions, and these decisions are more accurate if they are based on calculation instead of intuition. The cut-off levels used in the example of this paper could, after the decision tree procedure, look somewhat like the levels shown below with accompanying sensitivities/specificities of 99% instead of 95%.

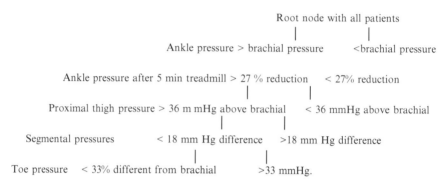

We should add that, in addition to mathematical arguments, there may be clinical arguments for setting the cut-off levels for sensitivity and specificity. For example, for incurable deadly diseases, you may want to avoid false positives, meaning telling a healthy person he/she will die soon, while false negatives are not so bad since you can not treat the condition anyway. If, instead, the test would serve as a first screening for a fatal condition if untreated but completely treatable, it should provide a better sensitivity even at the expense of a lower specificity.

We conclude that the binary partition and its closely related decision trees may become one of the standard analytic choices in clinical disease, but they likely complement rather than replace the classic statistical methods. For assessing the level of statistical significance of assumed differences and effects the classic statistical methods are more suitable.

6   Conclusions

Binary partitioning can assist physicians in diagnosing patients potentially suffering heart attacks and other clinical conditions. Traditionally, the physicians made decisions based on their clinical experience. Classifications based on representative historical data has the advantage of added empirical information from large numbers of patients. This chapter is to familiarize the research community with this important methodology for improving the diagnostic accuracy of prognostic cardiovascular decision analysis.

An example is used to explain The ROC (receiver operating characteristic) and entropy methods for simple partitions.

ROC curves are used for finding the best cut-off levels in a decision tree of diagnostic procedures. The problem with ROC curves is that the sample sizes of the positive and negative tests are not taken into account, reducing the power of this approach. This is, particularly, a problem if the numbers of positive and negative tests are largely different in size. The entropy method based on log likelihood statistics is helpful in this situation. The theory sounds rather complex, but the equations work smoothly, and can be performed even on a pocket calculator.

We conclude that binary partition and its closely related decision trees may become one of the standard analytic choices in clinical research, but they likely complement rather than replace the classic statistical methods. For assessing the level of statistical significance of assumed differences and effects the classic statistical methods are more suitable.

References

Breiman L, Friedman JH, Olshen RA, Stone CJ (1984) Classification and regression trees. Chapman @ Hall (Wadsworth Inc), New York

Cleophas TJ, Zwinderman AH, Van Ouwerkerk BM (2007) Log likelihood ratio tests for the assessment of cardiovascular events. Perfusion 20:79–82

Jaff MR, Dorros G (1998) The vascular laboratory: a critical component required for successful management of peripheral arterial occlusive disease. J Endovasc Surg 5:146–158

Wasson JH, Sox HC, Neff RK, Goldman L (1985) Clinical prediction rules: applications and methodologic standards. N Engl J Med 313:793–799

Chapter 54
Methods for Repeated Measures Analysis

1 Introduction

Repeated measures of the same kind, like, for example, blood pressures obtained from a single subject at subsequent times, are different from single measures of separate subjects, because repeated measures in a single subject are generally more similar to one another than those obtained from entirely different subjects, and statistical analyses have to take this difference into account. For that purpose there are paired and unpaired t-tests, repeated and non-repeated measures analysis of variance (ANOVA) (Chaps. 1 and 2), paired and unpaired tests for binary data (Chap. 3), and paired and unpaired non-parametric tests (Chap. 2). Paired data or repeated measures means that multiple observations are performed in a single subject with the advantage that less subjects are required for answering a scientific question. A special type of repeated measures are longitudinal data including times series and survival data. They have been discussed in the Chaps. 16 and 43.

The most important reason for writing this chapter is the fact that repeated measures are frequently analyzed inappropriately. A linear regression or unpaired t-test or non-repeated measures ANOVA using repeated values does not take into account the repeated nature of the data, and, is therefore, likely to overestimate the magnitude of differences in the data. For example, drug-elimination curves (Benet et al. 1997) and R2-like models (Hoetker 2007) for predicting probabilities of events are usually assessed with linear regression in spite of the repeated measures character of the data.

The current chapter reviews methods for repeated measures of continuous data. Particular attention will be given to (1) summary measures and (2) repeated measures ANOVA with and (3) without between-subjects covariates.

2   Summary Measures

It is appropriate when possible to use a summary estimate of repeated data. For example, the area under the curve of drug concentration-time curves is used in clinical pharmacology as an estimate of bioavailability of a drug. Also, maximal values, mean values, changes from baseline are applied. The disadvantage of these measures is, that they do not use the data fully, because they use summary measures instead, and, therefore, may lose precision, but, otherwise, they are unbiased, and can be used perfectly well.

3   Repeated Measures ANOVA Without Between-Subjects Covariates

Summary measures are impossible if we want to assess the differences between the separate measures.

The study in Table 54.1 shows that a repeated measure ANOVA can be performed in a sample size as small as four subjects. The study compares the effects of three different treatments to reduce vascular resistance and contains only 12 data. A condensed version of this example was already presented in Benet et al. (1997).

$$SS_{\text{within subj}} = 147.95 + 77.05 + \dots$$
$$SS_{\text{treatment}} = (17.58 - 11.63)^2 + (7.73 - 11.63)^2 + \dots$$
$$SS_{\text{residual}} = SS_{\text{within subject}} - SS_{\text{treatment}}$$

We use SPSS statistical software: command: analyze; general linear model; repeated measurements.

Mauchly's test of sphericity chi-square $= 2.07$, 2 dfs, $p = 0.355$. No inequality of variance is in the data.

	SS	dfs	Mean square	F	p-value
Within subject	127.2	1	127.2	$127.2/7.0 = 18.2$	0.024
Residual	20.964	3	7.0		

SS sum of squares, dfs degrees of freedom

Table 54.1 Repeated measures ANOVA, effects of three treatments on vascular resistance (blood pressure/cardiac output)

Subject	Treatment 1	Treatment 2	Treatment 3	SD^2
1	22.2	5.4	10.6	147.95
2	17.0	6.3	6.2	77.05
3	14.1	8.5	9.3	18.35
4	17.0	10.7	12.3	21.4
Treatment mean	17.58	7.73	9.60	
Grand mean $= 11.63$				

According to the data-analysis there is a significant difference between the three treatments with F = 18.2 and p = 0.024. In order to assess the appropriateness of the linear assumption of the model a quadratic relationship between indicator and outcome variables is assessed, but the F-value and, thus, the p-value was smaller (11.01 and p = 0.045), and, so the linear assumption seems to be appropriate. Between subjects differences are assumed not to influence the treatment-comparisons, and are, therefore, not taken into account in the data analysis.

4   Repeated Measures ANOVA with Between-Subjects Covariates

In the study of Table 54.2 an example is given of a study where both repeated and non-repeated factors are combined. Three treatment modalities for the treatment of exercise tachycardias are assessed in both male and female subjects of different age classes, 20–30, 30–40, and 40–60 years of age. The variable 1 gives the age class (respectively 1, 2, and 3). The variable 5 gives the genders (respectively 1 and 2).

SPSS statistical software (2000): command: analyze; general linear model; repeated measurements.

Mauchly's test of sphericity chi-square = 30.7, 2 dfs, p < 0.0001. Inequality of variance in the data cannot be excluded.

Therefore, the Greenhouse-Geisser adjustment is used.

	SS	dfs	Mean square	F	p-value
1. Within-subjects	281,916.3	1.35	208,537.9	2,814.9	0.000
2. VAR 1 (age class)	4,681.0	2	2,340.5	3.045	0.057
3. VAR 5 (gender)	26,373.0	1	26,373.0	34.3	0.000
4. VAR 1 × VAR 5	2,155.4	2	1,077.7	1.402	0.256
5. Within-subjects × VAR 1	241.7	2.70	89.4	1.206	0.313
6. Within-subjects × VAR 5	1,034.8	1.35	765.4	10.332	0.001
7 Within-subjects x VAR 1 × VAR 5	1,481.9	2.70	548.1	7.398	0.000

SS sum of squares, dfs degrees of freedom

The variables 2, 3, and 4 give the exercise heart rate during treatment with respectively high dose, low dose and very low dose beta-blocker in beats/min. The study tries to answer seven research questions:

1. Does treatment modality influence exercise heart rate?
2. Do subjects from different age classes have different heart rates?
3. Do males have different heart rates from females?
4. Does the pattern of differences between pulse rates for the age class groups change between the genders?
5. Does the pattern of differences between pulse rates for the age class groups change between the treatment modalities?
6. Does the pattern of differences between pulse rates for genders change between the treatment modalities?

Table 54.2 Repeated measures ANOVA with between-subjects covariates, data-file of 54 subjects, the variables are explained in the text

Subject	VAR 1	VAR 2	VAR 3	VAR 4	VAR 5
1.	1,00	112,00	166,00	215,00	1,00
2.	1,00	111,00	166,00	225,00	1,00
3.	1,00	89,00	132,00	189,00	1,00
4.	1,00	95,00	134,00	186,00	2,00
5.	1,00	66,00	109,00	150,00	2,00
6.	1,00	69,00	119,00	177,00	2,00
7.	2,00	125,00	177,00	241,00	1,00
8.	2,00	85,00	117,00	186,00	1,00
9.	2,00	97,00	137,00	185,00	1,00
10.	2,00	93,00	151,00	217,00	2,00
11.	2,00	77,00	122,00	178,00	2,00
12.	2,00	78,00	119,00	173,00	2,00
13.	3,00	81,00	134,00	205,00	1,00
14.	3,00	88,00	133,00	180,00	1,00
15.	3,00	88,00	157,00	224,00	1,00
16.	3,00	58,00	99,00	131,00	2,00
17.	3,00	85,00	132,00	186,00	2,00
18.	3,00	78,00	110,00	164,00	2,00
19.	1,00	112,00	166,00	215,00	1,00
20.	1,00	111,00	166,00	225,00	1,00
21.	1,00	89,00	132,00	189,00	1,00
22.	1,00	95,00	134,00	186,00	2,00
23.	1,00	66,00	109,00	150,00	2,00
24.	1,00	69,00	119,00	177,00	2,00
25.	2,00	125,00	177,00	241,00	1,00
26.	2,00	85,00	117,00	186,00	1,00
27.	2,00	97,00	137,00	185,00	1,00
28.	2,00	93,00	151,00	217,00	2,00
29.	2,00	77,00	122,00	178,00	2,00
30.	2,00	78,00	119,00	173,00	2,00
31.	3,00	81,00	134,00	205,00	1,00
32.	3,00	88,00	133,00	180,00	1,00
33.	3,00	88,00	157,00	224,00	1,00
34.	3,00	58,00	99,00	131,00	2,00
35.	3,00	85,00	132,00	186,00	2,00
36.	3,00	78,00	110,00	164,00	2,00
37.	1,00	112,00	166,00	215,00	1,00
38.	1,00	111,00	166,00	225,00	1,00
39.	1,00	89,00	132,00	189,00	1,00
40.	1,00	95,00	134,00	186,00	2,00
41.	1,00	66,00	109,00	150,00	2,00
42.	1,00	69,00	119,00	177,00	2,00
43.	2,00	125,00	177,00	241,00	1,00
44.	2,00	85,00	117,00	186,00	1,00
45.	2,00	97,00	137,00	185,00	1,00

(continued)

Table 54.2 (continued)

Subject	VAR 1	VAR 2	VAR 3	VAR 4	VAR 5
46.	2,00	93,00	151,00	217,00	2,00
47.	2,00	77,00	122,00	178,00	2,00
48.	2,00	78,00	119,00	173,00	2,00
49.	3,00	81,00	134,00	205,00	1,00
50.	3,00	88,00	133,00	180,00	1,00
51.	3,00	88,00	157,00	224,00	1,00
52.	3,00	58,00	99,00	131,00	2,00
53.	3,00	85,00	132,00	186,00	2,00
54.	3,00	78,00	110,00	164,00	2,00

The SPSS file uses commas instead of dots
VAR variable

7. Does the pattern of differences between pulse rates for treatment modalities change in a subgroup with a particular gender and age class?

The above research questions given in research terms are the following:

1. Is there a within-subjects main effect?
2. Is there a between-subjects main gender effect?
3. Is there a between-subjects main age class effect?
4. Is there a between-subjects interaction
5–7. Is there a within-subjects by between-subjects interaction effect?

Because the test for non-equality of the variances can not be rejected, the usual ANOVA-model is inappropriate. Either an adjusted ANOVA, e.g., Greenhouse-Geisser adjusted univariate repeated measures ANOVA, or Multivariate Analysis of Variance (MANOVA) has to be applied. MANOVA is, conceptually, different, because it assumes multiple outcome variables instead of a single-one-with-multiple-levels. SPSS produces an analysis of both approaches. In our example the results of the two were virtually the same. According to the data-analysis there was a significant difference between the three treatments with $F = 2814.9$ and $p = 0.000$. In order to assess the appropriateness of the linear assumption of the model a quadratic relationship between indicator and outcome variables, but the F-value and thus p-value were smaller, and, so the linear assumption seems appropriate.

It can be hard to interpret the results of interactions. For example, the above 7th question is confirmed: there is a significant interaction between treatment modality and gender and age class. Averages of the subgroups can be examined in order to understand what is going on (Fig. 54.1). The Fig. 54.1 shows that gender differences do not remain the same but seem to increase with subsequent treatment modalities. There is, obviously, interaction between treatment modality and gender. However, this is only true in the younger, but not in the older age classes.

Generally, a significant interaction is a disaster for a comparative study of different treatment modalities, because an overall comparison of the treatment modalities becomes meaningless. In the given example the magnitude of the interaction is limited, and an overall treatment differences can still be observed (Fig. 54.1). The overall result can be reported, at least, in a qualitative manner.

Fig. 54.1 Gender differences do not remain the same but seem to increase with subsequent treatment modalities. There is interaction between treatment modality and gender. However, this is only true in the younger, but not in the older age classes

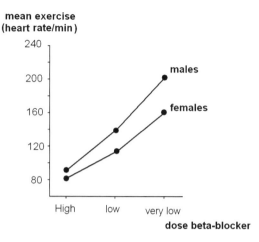

5 Conclusions

1. Repeated measures in a single subject are generally more similar to one another than data obtained from entirely different subjects, and statistical analyses have to take this into account.
2. It is appropriate when possible to use a summary estimate if the repeated data. For example, the area under the curve of drug time-concentration and time-effi-cacy curves, maximal values, mean values, change from baseline.
3. In parallel-group studies the level of statistical significance of between-subjects differences is usually assessed. In repeated measures within-subjects differences are usually assessed for that purpose. The general linear model available in SAS, SPSS and other statistical software programs provides repeated measures ANOVA appropriate for that purpose.
4. Repeated measures ANOVA can also adequately include subgroup factors like gender differences and age class differences into the analysis.
5. Like any type of ANOVA equality of variances and linearity in the data have to be checked. Most software programs routinely do so, and present alternative approaches in case these requirements can not be satisfied.

References

Benet LZ, Kroetz DL, Sheiner LB (1997) Pharmacokinetics. In: Goodman and Gilman's pharma-cologic basis therapeutics, 9th edn. McGraw-Hill, New York, pp 5–27
Hoetker G (2007) The use of logit and probit models in strategic management research: critical issues. Strateg Manage J 28:331–343
SPSS Statistical Software 13.0 (2000) Chicago, IL, USA

Chapter 55
Mixed Linear Models for Repeated Measures

1 Introduction

In current clinical research repeated measures in a single subject are common. The problem with repeated measures is that they are more close to one another than unrepeated measures. If this is not taken into account, then data analysis will lose power. The classical general linear analysis of variance (ANOVA) model for the analysis of such data has been recently supplemented by a novel method, mixed linear modeling. Mixed modeling was first described by Henderson et al. (1959) in the early 1960s as a linear model for making predictions from longitudinal observations in a single subject. It first became popular in the early 1990s by the work of Robinson (1991) and McLean et al. (1991) who improved the model by presenting consistent analysis procedures. In the past decade user-friendly statistical software programs like SAS (2011) and SPSS (2011) have enabled the application of mixed models even by clinical investigators with limited statistical background.

With mixed models repeated measures *within* subjects receive fewer degrees of freedom than they do with the classical general linear model, because they are nested in a separate layer or subspace. In this way better sensitivity is left in the model to demonstrate differences *between* subjects. Therefore, if the main aim of your research is to demonstrate differences *between* subjects, then the mixed model should be more sensitive. However, the two methods should be equivalent if the main aim of your research is to demonstrate differences between repeated measures, for example different treatment modalities in a single subject. A limitation of the mixed model is that it includes additional variances, and is, therefore, more complex. More complex statistical models are, ipso facto, more at risk of power loss, particularly, with small data.

The current chapter uses examples to demonstrate how the mixed model performs in practice. The examples show that the mixed model, unlike the general linear, produced a very significant effect in a parallel-group study with repeated measures, and that the two models were approximately equivalent for analyzing a crossover study with three treatment modalities. We hope this explanatory chapter will be helpful to researchers assessing repeated measures.

2   A Placebo-Controlled Parallel Group Study of Cholesterol Treatment

A placebo-controlled parallel group study cholesterol is used as first example. Each patient is measured for HDL-cholesterol level for 5 weeks once a week. Table 55.1 gives the data file. A significant difference between the two treatments is expected. The graph of the summaries of the data (Fig. 55.1) shows, indeed, that already after 2 weeks the treatment-1 group (active treatment group) starts to perform better than the treatment-0 group (placebo-group). Multiple unpaired t-tests of treatment-0 versus treatment-1 demonstrate significant differences with p-values as small as 0.08 at the weeks 3, 4 and 5 (analysis not shown). However, this analysis is not entirely appropriate, because it does not take the repeated nature of the data into account. A repeated measurements analysis of variance using the classical

Table 55.1 Two parallel groups of ten patients are assessed five times for their HDL-cholesterol

Patient no	Week 1	Week 2	Week 3	Week 4	Week 5	Treatment modality
1	1,66	1,62	1,57	1,52	1,50	0,00
2	1,69	1,71	1,60	1,55	1,56	0,00
3	1,92	1,94	1,83	1,78	1,79	0,00
4	1,95	1,97	1,86	1,81	1,82	0,00
5	1,98	2,00	1,89	1,84	1,85	0,00
6	2,01	2,03	1,92	1,87	1,88	0,00
7	2,04	2,06	1,95	1,90	1,91	0,00
8	2,07	2,09	1,98	1,93	1,94	0,00
9	2,30	2,32	2,21	2,16	2,17	0,00
10	2,36	2,35	2,26	2,23	2,20	0,00
11	1,57	1,82	1,83	1,83	1,82	1,00
12	1,60	1,85	1,89	1,89	1,85	1,00
13	1,83	2,08	2,12	2,12	2,08	1,00
14	1,86	2,11	2,16	2,15	2,11	1,00
15	2,80	2,14	2,19	2,18	2,14	1,00
16	1,92	2,17	2,22	2,21	2,17	1,00
17	1,95	2,20	2,25	2,24	2,20	1,00
18	1,98	2,23	2,28	2,27	2,24	1,00
19	2,21	2,46	2,57	2,51	2,48	1,00
20	2,34	2,51	2,55	2,55	2,52	1,00

SPSS uses commas instead of dots
Treatment modality 0 = placebo, 1 = active treatment

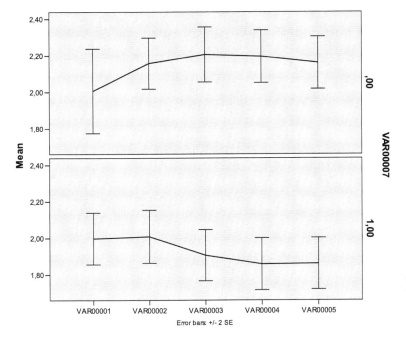

Fig. 55.1 Two parallel groups treated for hypercholesterolemia for 5 weeks (0,00 = placebo treatment; 1,00 = active treatment) (Treatment outcome (HDL-cholesterol level, mmol/l) Week of treatment (1–5))

general linear model is performed (full factorial design). SPSS statistical software is used (2011).

We command:

Analyze – General linear model – Repeated Measurements – Define factors – Within-subjects factor names: week – number levels: 5 – add – Define – enter week 1, 2, 3, 4, 5 in box: "Within-subjects Variables" – enter treatment in box between-subjects covariates – ok.

The above Table 55.2 gives the results. As the test for sphericity (equal standard errors) had to be rejected (not shown), sphericity could not be assumed, and the Huynh-Feldt test was the next best for demonstrating a difference between the repeated measures (Table 55.2: source week). With p = 0.115 no significant difference between the repeated measures could be demonstrated (upper part of Table 55.2). The subsequent between-subjects comparison of the two treatments showed a borderline effect with p-value of 0.048 (lower part of Table 55.2).

As an alternative a mixed linear model is applied using the same version of SPSS. For that purpose the data file has to be adapted. Every week must be given a separate row (Table 55.3).

Table 55.2 Repeated measures ANOVA using the classical general linear model for the analysis of the data from Table 55.1. As the test for sphericity was rejected (not shown), sphericity could not be assumed, and the Huynh-Feldt test was the next best for demonstrating a difference between the repeated measures (source: week). With p = 0.115 no significant difference between the repeated measures was demonstrated (*upper table*). The subsequent between-subjects comparison showed a borderline effect with p-value of 0.048 (*lower table*)

Tests of with-subjects effects

Measure: MEASURE_1

Source		Type III sum of squares	df	Mean square	F	Sig.
Week	Sphericity assumed	,089	4	,022	2,692	,038
	Greenhouse-Geisser	,089	1,022	,087	2,692	,117
	Huynh-Feldt	,089	1,086	,082	2,692	,115
	Lower-bound	,089	1,000	,089	2,692	,118
Week*treatment	Sphericity assumed	,380	4	,095	11,460	,000
	Greenhouse-Geisser	,380	1,022	,372	11,460	,003
	Huynh-Feldt	,380	1,086	,350	11,460	,003
	Lower-bound	,380	1,000	,380	11,460	,003
Error (week)	Sphericity assumed	,597	72	,008		
	Greenhouse-Geisser	,597	18,396	,032		
	Huynh-Feldt	,597	19,550	,031		
	Lower-bound	,597	18,000	,033		

Tests of between-subjects effects

Measure: MEASURE_1

Transformed variable: average

Source	Type III sum of squares	df	Mean square	F	Sig.
Intercept	414,530	1,1,18	414,530	1573,798	,000
Treatment	1,188		1,188	4,511	,048
Error	4,741		,263		

We command:

Analyze – mixed models – linear – specify subjects and repeated – variable 1 – continue – linear mixed model – dependent: variable 3 – factors: variable 2, variable 4 – fixed – build nested term – variable 4 – add – variable 2 – add – variable 2 build term by* variable 4 – variable 4 * variable 2 – add – continue – ok (*=sign of multiplication).

Table 55.4 gives the results. With the mixed model analysis the treatment modality has become a very significant predictor of treatment outcome with p < 0.0001. This result is in agreement with our prior expectation, and it is also more similar to the above unpaired t-tests than the general linear model is.

We can now conclude that, after adjustment for the repeated nature of the data, there is a very significant difference between the effect of the placebo and the active treatment on HDL cholesterol a p < 0.0001.

Table 55.3 The data from Table 55.1 adapted for mixed linear modeling, each patient is now included five times (five rows)

1	2	3	4
Patient	Week	Outcome	Treatment
1,00	1,00	1,66	,00
1,00	2,00	1,62	,00
1,00	3,00	1,57	,00
1,00	4,00	1,52	,00
1,00	5,00	1,50	,00
2,00	1,00	1,69	,00
2,00	2,00	1,71	,00
2,00	3,00	1,60	,00
2,00	4,00	1,55	,00
2,00	5,00	1,56	,00
3,00	1,00	1,92	,00
3,00	2,00	1,94	,00
3,00	3,00	1,83	,00
3,00	4,00	1,78	,00
3,00	5,00	1,79	,00
4,00	1,00	1,95	,00
4,00	2,00	1,97	,00
4,00	3,00	1,86	,00
4,00	4,00	1,81	,00
4,00	5,00	1,82	,00
5,00	1,00	1,98	,00
5,00	2,00	2,00	,00
5,00	3,00	1,89	,00
5,00	4,00	1,84	,00
5,00	5,00	1,85	,00
6,00	1,00	2,01	,00
6,00	2,00	2,03	,00
6,00	3,00	1,92	,00
6,00	4,00	1,87	,00
6,00	5,00	1,88	,00
7,00	1,00	2,04	,00
7,00	2,00	2,06	,00
7,00	3,00	1,95	,00
7,00	4,00	1,90	,00
7,00	5,00	1,91	,00
8,00	1,00	2,07	,00
8,00	2,00	2,09	,00
8,00	3,00	1,98	,00
8,00	4,00	1,93	,00
8,00	5,00	1,94	,00
9,00	1,00	2,30	,00
9,00	2,00	2,32	,00
9,00	3,00	2,21	,00
9,00	4,00	2,16	,00
9,00	5,00	2,17	,00

(continued)

Table 55.3 (continued)

1	2	3	4
Patient	Week	Outcome	Treatment
10,00	1,00	2,36	,00
10,00	2,00	2,35	,00
10,00	3,00	2,26	,00
10,00	4,00	2,23	,00
10,00	5,00	2,20	,00
11,00	1,00	1,57	1,00
11,00	2,00	1,82	1,00
11,00	3,00	1,83	1,00
11,00	4,00	1,83	1,00
11,00	5,00	1,82	1,00
12,00	1,00	1,60	1,00
12,00	2,00	1,85	1,00
12,00	3,00	1,89	1,00
12,00	4,00	1,89	1,00
12,00	5,00	1,85	1,00
13,00	1,00	1,83	1,00
13,00	2,00	2,08	1,00
13,00	3,00	2,12	1,00
13,00	4,00	2,12	1,00
13,00	5,00	2,08	1,00
14,00	1,00	1,86	1,00
14,00	2,00	2,11	1,00
14,00	3,00	2,16	1,00
14,00	4,00	2,15	1,00
14,00	5,00	2,11	1,00
15,00	1,00	2,80	1,00
15,00	2,00	2,14	1,00
15,00	3,00	2,19	1,00
15,00	4,00	2,18	1,00
15,00	5,00	2,14	1,00
16,00	1,00	1,92	1,00
16,00	2,00	2,17	1,00
16,00	3,00	2,22	1,00
16,00	4,00	2,21	1,00
16,00	5,00	2,17	1,00
17,00	1,00	1,95	1,00
17,00	2,00	2,20	1,00
17,00	3,00	2,25	1,00
17,00	4,00	2,24	1,00
17,00	5,00	2,20	1,00
18,00	1,00	1,98	1,00
18,00	2,00	2,23	1,00
18,00	3,00	2,28	1,00
18,00	4,00	2,27	1,00
18,00	5,00	2,24	1,00

(continued)

Table 55.3 (continued)

1	2	3	4
Patient	Week	Outcome	Treatment
19,00	1,00	2,21	1,00
19,00	2,00	2,46	1,00
19,00	3,00	2,57	1,00
19,00	4,00	2,51	1,00
19,00	5,00	2,48	1,00
20,00	1,00	2,34	1,00
20,00	2,00	2,51	1,00
20,00	3,00	2,55	1,00
20,00	4,00	2,55	1,00
20,00	5,00	2,52	1,00

SPSS uses commas instead of dots
1 = patient number, 2 = week of treatment (1–5), 3 = outcome (HDL cholesterol), 4 = treatment modality (0 or 1).

Table 55.4 Mixed model analysis of the data from Table 55.2 with treatment modality and week of treatment as predictors, and treatment outcome as dependent variable. The treatment modality is a very significant predictor of treatment outcome

Type III tests of fixed effects[a]

Source	Numerator df	Denominator df	F	Sig.
Intercept	1	76,570	6988,626	,000
Week	4	31,149	,384	,818
Treatment	1	76,570	20,030	,000
Week * treatment	4	31,149	1,337	,278

[a]Dependent variable: outcome

3   A Three Treatment Crossover Study of the Effect of Sleeping Pills on Hours of Sleep

A three treatment crossover study of the effect of sleeping pills on hours of sleep is used as a second example. Table 55.5 gives the data file. Ten patients are given three different sleeping pills in a randomized double-blind fashion. The hours of sleep after treatment are the outcome variable. A significant difference between the three treatment outcomes is expected. Figure 55.2 is a graph of the summaries of the treatment effects. The third treatment seems to perform significantly worse than the other two treatments as indicated by the error bars giving 95% confidence intervals of the means. However, this conclusion is not entirely appropriate, because it does not take the repeated nature of the data into account.
We command:

Analyze – General linear model – Repeated Measurements – Define factors – Within-subjects factor names: treatment – number levels: 3 – add – Define – enter

Table 55.5 A single group is assessed for three different treatments (hours of sleep) in a crossover fashion, age and gender are in the columns five and six

Patient no	Treatment 1	Treatment 2	Treatment 3	Age	Gender
1	6,10	6,80	5,20	55,00	0,00
2	7,00	7,00	7,90	65,00	0,00
3	8,20	9,00	3,90	74,00	0,00
4	7,60	7,80	4,70	56,00	1,00
5	6,50	6,60	5,30	44,00	1,00
6	8,40	8,00	5,40	49,00	1,00
7	6,90	7,30	4,20	53,00	0,00
8	6,70	7,00	6,10	76,00	0,00
9	7,40	7,50	3,80	67,00	1,00
10	5,80	5,80	6,30	66,00	1,00

SPSS uses commas instead of dots

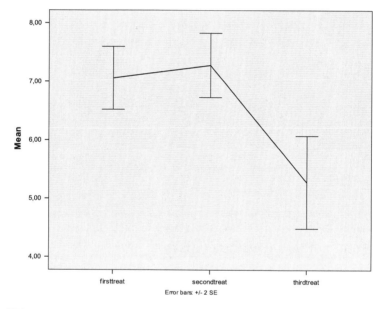

Fig. 55.2 Crossover study of the effect on hours of sleep of three sleeping pills in a single group of patients (Treatment outcome (hours of sleep/night) treatment modality (1–3))

treatment 1, 2, 3 in box: "Within-subjects Variables" – enter gender in box between-subjects covariates – ok.

Table 55.6 gives the results. As the test for sphericity (equal standard errors) had to be rejected again (not shown), sphericity could not be assumed, and the Huynh-Feldt test was the next best for demonstrating a difference between the repeated measures (Table 55.6: source treatment). With p=0.010 a very significant difference

Table 55.6 Repeated measures ANOVA using the classical general linear model for the analysis of the data from Table 55.5. As the test for sphericity was rejected (not shown), sphericity could not be assumed, and the Huynh-Feldt test was the next best for demonstrating a difference between the repeated measures (source: treat number). A significant difference between the repeated measures was demonstrated with p=0.010 (*upper table*). The subsequent between-subjects comparison did not show a significant effect of gender with p-value of 0.65 (*lower table*)

Tests of with-subjects effects

Measure: MEASURE_1

Source		Type III sum of squares	df	Mean square	F	Sig.
Treatment	Sphericity assumed	24,056	2	12,028	9,642	,002
	Greenhouse-Geisser	24,056	1,024	23,494	9,642	,014
	Huynh-Feldt	24,056	1,181	20,369	9,642	,010
	Lower-bound	24,056	1,000	24,056	9,642	,015
Treatment * gender	Sphericity assumed	,392	2	,196	,157	,856
	Greenhouse-Geisser	,392	1,024	,383	,157	,708
	Huynh-Feldt	,392	1,181	,332	,157	,742
	Lower-bound	,392	1,000	,392	,157	,702
Error (treatment)	Sphericity assumed	19,959	16	1,247		
	Greenhouse-Geisser	19,959	8,191	2,437		
	Huynh-Feldt	19,959	9,448	2,112		
	Lower-bound	19,959	8,000	2,495		

Tests of between-subjects effects

Measure: MEASURE_1

Transformed variable: average

Source	Type III sum of squares	df	Mean square	F	Sig.
Intercept	1283,148	1	1283,148	1472,063	,000
Gender	,192	1	,192	,220	,651
Error	6,973	8	,872		

between the repeated measures, the treatments, could be demonstrated (upper part of Table 55.2). The subsequent between-subjects comparison of the two genders did not produces a significantly different effect of the genders on the treatment outcome with a p-value of 0.65 (lower part of Table 55.6).

As an alternative a mixed linear model is applied using the same version of SPSS. For that purpose the data file has to be adapted. Each treatment (3) must be given a separate row. Table 55.7 gives the adapted data file made adequate for mixed linear modeling.

We command:

Analyze – mixed models – linear – specify subjects and repeated – variable 1 – continue – linear mixed model – dependent: variable 3 – factors: variable 2, variable 4 – fixed – build nested term – variable 4 – add – variable 2 – add – variable 2 build term by* variable 4 – variable 4 * variable 2 – add – continue – ok (*=sign of multiplication).

Table 55.7 The data from Table 55.5 adapted for mixed linear modeling, each patient is included three times (three rows)

Variable			
1	2	3	4
1,00	1,00	6,10	0,00
1,00	2,00	6,80	0,00
1,00	3,00	5,20	0,00
2,00	1,00	7,00	0,00
2,00	2,00	7,00	0,00
2,00	3,00	7,90	0,00
3,00	1,00	8,20	0,00
3,00	2,00	9,00	0,00
3,00	3,00	3,90	0,00
4,00	1,00	7,60	1,00
4,00	2,00	7,80	1,00
4,00	3,00	4,70	1,00
5,00	1,00	6,50	1,00
5,00	2,00	6,60	1,00
5,00	3,00	5,30	1,00
6,00	1,00	8,40	1,00
6,00	2,00	8,00	1,00
6,00	3,00	5,40	1,00
7,00	1,00	6,90	0,00
7,00	2,00	7,30	0,00
7,00	3,00	4,20	0,00
8,00	1,00	6,70	0,00
8,00	2,00	7,00	0,00
8,00	3,00	6,10	0,00
9,00	1,00	7,40	1,00
9,00	2,00	7,50	1,00
9,00	3,00	3,80	1,00
10,00	1,00	5,80	1,00
10,00	2,00	5,80	1,00
10,00	3,00	6,30	1,00

SPSS uses commas instead of dots
1 = patient number, 2 = treatment number, 3 = outcome, 4 = gender

Table 55.8 gives the results. With the mixed model analysis the treatment number is a very significant predictor of treatment outcome with p = 0.005. This result is in agreement with our prior expectation, and it is also rather similar to the above general linear model analysis (p = 0.010).

We can now conclude that after adjustment for the repeated nature of the data there is a significantly different effect of the three treatment modalities on the hours of sleep with a p-value of 0.005.

Table 55.8 Mixed model analysis of the data from Table 55.6 with treatment number as predictor, and treatment outcome as dependent variable. The treatment number is a very significant predictor of the treatment outcome

Type III tests of fixed effects[a]

Source	Numerator df	Denominator df	F	Sig.
Intercept	1	17,574	1143,456	,000
Gender	1	17,574	,171	,684
Treatment number	2	11,628	8,470	,005
Treatment number * gender	2	11,628	,202	,820

4 Discussion

The examples given in the current report confirm the primary hypothesis of this paper. In the first example the aim of the research was to demonstrate a difference between the two treatment modalities given to two parallel groups of patients, while the differences between the repeated measures in a single patient was less important. Indeed, the mixed model produced a much better result than did the general linear model with overall p-values of <0.0001 versus only 0.048 for treatment effect. In the second example the main aim was to demonstrate a significant difference between the repeated measures in a single patient. The general linear model produced a significant p-value at 0.010, compared to a much similar p-value of 0.005 in the mixed model. Mixed models do, indeed, seem to produce better sensitivity of testing, when there are small within-subject differences and large-between subject-differences.

As indicated in the introduction, a disadvantages of the novel model is, that it is more complex, and, therefore, may require a larger sample size than the general linear model. Yet, as demonstrated in the examples, it may perform well even with samples as small as 10–20, that is, if the model being used is not too complex.

Apart from the advantage that it can sometimes handle between-subject differences with more sensitivity, it may provide a number of additional advantages including:

1. the general linear model will drop cases with missing entirely, whereas the mixed model can include incomplete cases in the analysis;
2. the general linear model assumes that all subjects are measured at the same point of time, whereas the mixed model allows subjects to be measured at different points of time;
3. the general linear model requires subjects to have equal numbers of repeated measurements, whereas the mixed model allows unequal repetitions;
4. the presence of sphericity (equal standard errors) is not a requirement of the mixed models.

We conclude that the mixed model is a welcome supplement to the commonly-used general linear models for the overall analysis of studies with repeated measures. Unfortunately, although widely discussed in methodology papers (Milliken and Johnson 1992; West et al. 2007; Breslow and Clayton 1993; Engel and Keen 1994; Littell et al. 1996), the mixed model is little used by clinical researchers in practice so far. This may be due to its obvious complexity. Yet, the current paper shows that with modern user-friendly statistical software its use is straightforward, and its software commands are no more complex than they are with standard methods for data analysis. We do hope that this paper will encourage clinical researchers to more often make use of the benefits of the mixed model.

We have to add that current statistical terminology is somewhat chaotic. Alternative terms used to express mixed linear model methodologies include: hierarchical linear model, cluster analysis, multidimensional scaling, nearest neighbor search, structural data analysis, latent class analysis, data mining, data stream clustering, adjusted mutual information.

5 Conclusion

In current clinical research repeated measures in a single subject are common. The problem with repeated measures is, that they are more close to one another than unrepeated measures. If this is not taken into account, then data analysis will lose power. In the past decade user-friendly statistical software programs like SAS and SPSS have enabled the application of mixed models as an alternative to the classical general linear model for repeated measures with, sometimes, better sensitivity. This chapter assesses whether in studies with repeated measures, designed to test between-subject differences, the mixed model performs better than does the general linear model.

In a parallel group study of cholesterol reducing treatments with five evaluations per patient, the mixed model performed much better than did the general linear model with p-values of respectively 0.0001 and 0.048. In a crossover study of three treatments for sleeplessness the mixed model and general linear model produced similarly well with p-values of 0.005 and 0.010.

We conclude that mixed models do, indeed, seem to produce better sensitivity of testing, when there are small within-subject differences and large-between subject-differences, and when the main objective of your research is to demonstrate between- rather than within-subject differences.

The novel mixed model may be more complex. Yet, with modern user-friendly statistical software its use is straightforward, and its software-commands are no more complex than they are with standard methods. We hope that this chapter will encourage clinical researchers to more often make use of its benefits.

References

Breslow NE, Clayton DG (1993) Approximate inferences in generalized linear mixed models. J Am Stat Assoc 88:9–25

Engel B, Keen A (1994) A simple approach for the analysis of generalized linear mixed models. Statist Neerlandica 48:1–22

Henderson CR, Kempthorne O, Searle SR, Von Krosigk CM (1959) The estimation of environmental and genetic trends from records subject to culling. Biometrics 15:192–218

Littell RC, Milliken GA, Stroup WW, Wolfinger RD (1996) SAS system for mixed models. SAS Instit Inc, Cary

McLean RA, Sanders WL, Stoup WW (1991) A unified approach to mixed linear models. Am Stat 45:54–64

Milliken GA, Johnson DE (1992) Analysis of messy data. Designed experiments. Chapman and Hall, New York

Robinson GK (1991) That best linear unbiased predictions (BLUP) is a good thing. Stat Sci 6:15–32

SAS statistical software, www.sas.com. Accessed 15 Dec 2011

SPSS statistical software, www.spss.com. Accessed 15 Dec 2011

West BT, Welch KB, Galecki AT (2007) Linear mixed models: a practical guide to using statistical software. Chapman and Hall, New York

Chapter 56
Advanced Analysis of Variance, Random Effects and Mixed Effects Models

1 Introduction

In clinical trials it is common to assume a fixed effects research model. This means that the patients selected for a specific treatment are assumed to be homogeneous and have the same true quantitative effect and that the differences observed are residual, meaning that they are caused by inherent variability in biological processes, rather than some hidden subgroup property. If, however, we have reasons to believe that certain patients due to co-morbidity, co-medication, age or other factors will respond differently from others, then the spread in the data is caused not only by the residual effect but also by between patient differences due to some subgroup property. It may even be safe to routinely treat any patient effect as a random effect, unless there are good arguments no to do so. Random effects research models require a statistical approach different from that of fixed effects models (Anonymous 2006; Campbell 2006; Gao 2003).

With the fixed effects model the treatment differences are tested against the residual error, otherwise called the standard error. With the random effects models the treatment effects may be influenced not only by the residual effect but also by some unexpected, otherwise called random, factor, and so the treatment should no longer be tested against the residual effect. Because both residual and random effect constitute a much larger amount of uncertainty in the data, the treatment effect has to be tested against both of them (Anonymous 2011a; Anonymous 2011b).

Random effects models have been used in several studies recently published (Brier and Aronoff 1996; Dalla Costa et al. 1997; Mahmood 2003; Meibohm and Derendorf 1997; Lima et al. 2005; Lotsch et al. 2004; Mueck et al. 2007). They are a very interesting class of models, but even a partial understanding is fairly difficult to achieve. This chapter was written to explain random effects models in analysis of variance and to give examples of studies qualifying for them.

T.J. Cleophas and A.H. Zwinderman, *Statistics Applied to Clinical Studies*,
DOI 10.1007/978-94-007-2863-9_56, © Springer Science+Business Media B.V. 2012

2   Example 1, a Simple Example of a Random Effects Model

In a particular study the data may be different from one assessing doctor to the other due to differences in personality, education, or other doctor-factors. The example in

The computations are:

$$\text{SS total} = \sum (y - \bar{y})^2 = \sum y^2 - \frac{\left(\sum y\right)^2}{n} = 1,455.94 - \frac{(240.8)^2}{40} = 6.32$$

$$\text{SS between} = \frac{(44.0)^2 + ...(49.3)^2}{8} - \frac{(240.8)^2}{40} = 3.48$$

$$\text{SS within} = \text{SS total} - \text{SS between} = 6.32 - 3.48 = 2.84.$$

Notice that the SS within is calculated differently from the usual way (e.g., pages 26 and 32).

Source	SS	df	MS	F	p-value
Between assessors	3.48	5−1=4	0.87	0.87/0.08=10.72	<0.01
Within assessors	2.84	40−5=35	0.08		

SS sum of squares, *df* degree of freedom, *MS* mean square, *F* test statistic for F-test

Table 56.1 gives the data of the above study where a random sample of five doctors assess eight different patients each. The data consist of individual health scores per patient. This example was modified from an example used by Hays (1988).

The scientific question is: "are the differences between the doctors larger than could happen by chance". We have no prior theory that one or two particular assessing doctors will produce higher health scores than the rest, but rather expect that in the population of assessing doctors at large there may be heterogeneity for whatever reason. This means that a random effects model applies to this situation. We test whether between doctor variability compared to within doctor variability is large. On top of this page are the results of the analysis. For 4 and 35 degrees of freedom the F-test exceeds the F of 3.25, and the hypothesis of no difference between the doctors is rejected. Indeed, there is a significant difference between the doctors. More in general the conclusion of this result should be that we can expect differences within any random sample of assessing doctors.

The calculations for a fixed effects model analysis of these data would produce the same result. The inference from it would, however, be entirely different: we would conclude that while we do not know anything about the population of assessing doctors at large, we definitely found a significant difference within this particular set of assessing doctors. It should be emphasized that the calculations for a fixed

Table 56.1 Example 1, a simple example of a random effects model

Assessing doctor no	1	2	3	4	5	
Patient	5.8	6.0	6.3	6.4	5.7	
	5.1	6.1	5.5	6.4	5.9	
	5.7	6.6	5.7	6.5	6.5	
	5.9	6.5	6.0	6.1	6.3	
	5.6	5.9	6.1	6.6	6.2	
	5.4	5.9	6.2	5.9	6.4	
	5.3	6.4	5.8	6.7	6.0	
	5.2	6.3	5.6	6.0	6.3 +	
	44.0	49.7	47.2	50.6	49.3	Add-up sum = 240.8

effect and a random effect are similar, but the interpretation is different. The choice between the fixed and random effect model is dependent on the statistical question. Both situations may be encountered in real life.

3 Example 2, A Random Interaction Effect Between Study and Treatment Efficacy

In clinical trials the observed differences between treatment modalities are compared to the differences caused by residual effects otherwise called noise. In studies with unexpected subgroup effects, this method is not appropriate and the increased variability in the data due to the subgroup effect has to be accounted. Random effects models are adequate for that purpose. An example is given underneath.
The computations are:

$$\text{SS total} = 52^2 + 48^2 + \ldots 35^2 - \frac{(52 + 48 + + \ldots 35)^2}{40} = 1,750.4$$

$$\text{SS treat by study} = \frac{464^2 + \ldots 378^2}{10} - \frac{(52 + 48 + + \ldots 35)^2}{40} = 1,327.2$$

$$\text{SS residual} = \text{SS total} - \text{SS treat by study} = 423.2$$

$$\text{SS rows} = \frac{766^2 + 746^2}{20} - \frac{(52 + 48 + + \ldots 35)^2}{40} = 10.0 \, (= \text{SS gender})$$

$$\text{SS columns} = \frac{832^2 + 680^2}{20} - \frac{(52 + 48 + + \ldots 35)^2}{40} = 577.6 \, (= \text{SS treatment})$$

$$\text{SS interaction} = \text{SS treat by study} - \text{SS rows} - \text{SS columns}$$
$$= 1327.2 - 10.0 - 577.6 = 739.6$$

Source	SS	df	MS	F	p-value
Fixed effects analysis of variance					
Rows (study effect)	10.0	1			
Columns (treatment effect)	577.6	1	577.6	577.6/11.76=49.1	<0.0001
Interaction	739.6	1	739.6	739.6/11.76=62.9	<0.0001
Residual	423.2	36	11.76		
Total					
Random effects analysis of variance					
Rows (study effect)	10.0	1			
Columns (treatment effect)	577.6	1	577.6	577.6/739.6=0.781	ns
Interaction	739.6	1	739.6	739.6/11.76=62.9	<0.0001
Residual	423.2	36	11.76		
Total					

SS sum of squares, *df* degree of freedom, *MS* mean square, *F* test statistic for F-test, *ns* not significant

The effects of two compounds on the numbers of episodes of paroxysmal atrial fibrillation is assessed in two rather similar parallel-group trials of 20 patients each. For the purpose of power the two studies are analyzed simultaneously. The data are given in Table 56.2. Overall metoprolol scores better than verapamil, but this is only true for the patients in study-1. There seems to be interaction between the study number and the treatment efficacy. The data are entered in the SPSS Software program (2011) commanding: statistics, general linear model, univariate. Choose as dependent variable numbers of episodes of paroxysmal atrial fibrillation, and as independent variables (1) treatment modality and (2) study number. The software program enables to treat the independent variables either as fixed or random variable. On top of this page are the results of the two assessments. If study-number is treated as a fixed effects variable, both treatment effect and interaction effect are compared to the residual effect. With 1 and 36 degrees of freedom the F-tests exceed the F of 5.57. Both a significant treatment effect and interaction effect is in the data. If treatments have different efficacies across studies, then an overall effect is not relevant anymore since the treatment effects cannot be interpreted independently of the interaction effect. The treatment efficacy of the treatment modalities is determined not only by the treatment modality but also by the study number. The information given by the random effect model is more adequate. The interaction effect is compared to the residual effect. With 1 and 36 degrees of freedom the F-test exceeds the F of 5.57. Subsequently, the treatment effect is compared not to the residual effect but rather to the interaction effect. With 1 and 1 degrees of freedom an F-value of 648 is required. The hypothesis of no treatment effect cannot be rejected. Thus, a significant interaction exists and the overall treatment efficacy is not significant anymore. This result is

		Verapamil	Metoprolol	
Table 56.2 Example 2, a random interaction effect between the study number and treatment efficacy	Study 1	52	28	
		48	35	
		43	34	
		50	32	
		43	34	
		44	27	
		46	31	
		46	27	
		43	29	
		49	25	
		464	302	766
	Study 2	38	43	
		42	34	
		42	33	
		35	42	
		33	41	
		38	37	
		39	37	
		34	40	
		33	36	
		34	35	
		368	378	746
		832	680	

obtained because the difference in the data due to different treatments is not compared with the residual differences but rather with the differences due to the interaction (which in this model includes the residual differences).

4   Example 3, A Random Interaction Effect Between Health Center and Treatment Efficacy

The computations are:

$$SS \text{ total} = 4^2 + \ldots + 13^2 - \frac{(342)^2}{36} = 245$$

$$SS \text{ treatment by center} = \frac{10^2 + \ldots + 27^2}{2} - \frac{(342)^2}{36} = 224$$

$$SS \text{ error} = SS \text{ total} - SS \text{ ab}$$
$$= 245 - 224 = 21$$

$$\text{SS columns} = \frac{99^2 + 105^2 + 138^2}{12} - \frac{342^2}{36} = 73.5$$

$$\text{SS rows} = \frac{49 + \ldots + 65^2}{6} - \frac{342^2}{36} = 30.67$$

$$\text{SS interaction} = \text{SS treat by center} - \text{SS rows} - \text{SS columns}$$
$$= 224 - 30.67 - 73.5 = 119.8$$

Source	SS	df	MS	F	p-value
Fixed effects analysis of variance					
Rows (center effect)	30.67	6−1=5			
Columns (treatment effect)	73.5	3−2=1	36.75	36.75/1.17=31.49	<0.0001
Interaction (treatment×center)	119.8	2×5=10	11.98	11.98/1.17=10.24	<0.0001
Residual	21	18×(2−1)=18	1.17		
Total	245	35			
Random effects analysis of variance					
Rows (center effect)	30.67	6−1=5			
Columns (treatment effect)	73.5	3−2=1	36.75	36.75/11.98=3.07	ns
Interaction (treatment×center)	119.8	2×5=10	11.98	11.98/1.17=10.24	<0.0001
Residual	21	18×(2−1)=18	1.17		
Total	245	35			

SS sum of squares, *df* degrees of freedom, *MS* mean square, *F* test statistic for F-test, *ns* not significant

The effect of three compounds on the frequency of anginal attacks in patients with stable angina pectoris is assessed in a three group parallel-group study (Table 56.3). Current clinical trials of new treatments often include patients from multiple health centers, national or international. Differences between centers may affect local results. We might say these data are at risk of interaction between centers and treatment efficacy. Patients were randomly selected in six health centers, six patients per center, and every patient was given one treatment at random, and so in each center two patients were given one of the three treatments.

When looking into the data we observe something special and unexpected. Metoprolol performs well in groups 4–6, i.e., better than in groups 1–3, and better than verapamil. This is unexpected, and may be due to interaction between the efficacy of treatment and the presence of particular health centers. There may be something about the combination of a particular health center with a particular treatment that accounts for differences in the data. For the analysis, as given on top of this page, SPSS statistical software (2011) is used again using the commands: statistics, general linear model, univariate. The numbers of anginal attacks are the dependent variable, dependent variables are (1) treatment modalities and (2) health center. If health

Table 56.3 Example 3, a random interaction effect between the health center and treatment efficacy

Treatment	Verapamil	Metoprolol	Isosorbide mononitrate	Total number of attacks per patient
Health center				
1	4	10	10	
	6	9	10 +	
	10	19	20	49
2	5	9	11	
	7	11	10 +	
	12	20	21	53
3	4	11	10	
	7	12	13 +	
	11	23	23	57
4	9	6	11	
	10	8	11 +	
	19	14	22	55
5	12	7	12	
	12	7	13 +	
	24	14	25	63
6	11	7	14	
	12	8	13 +	
	23	15	27	65
Total	99	105	138	342

center is treated as a fixed effect variable, again both treatment effect and interaction effect are compared to the residual effect. With respectively 2 vs 18 and 10 vs 18 degrees of freedom the F values of 4.46 and 2.77 are exceeded. Both a significant treatment effect and interaction effect is in the data. In multiple health centers we may have multiple treatment effects. The random effects method is more appropriate. With health center as random independent variable the analysis shows that with 10 vs 18 degrees of freedom the F-value of 2.77 is exceeded. A significant interaction exists. Subsequently, the treatment effect is tested against the interaction effect. With 2 and 10 degrees of freedom an F of 5.46 is required for significance, so that the hypothesis of no treatment effect cannot be rejected. The overall treatment efficacy is not significant anymore. This result is, like in the above example, obtained, because the difference in the data due to different treatments is not compared with the residual differences but rather with the differences due to the interaction. The following inference is adequate. Within the health centers, treatment differences apparently exist. Perhaps the capacity of a treatment to produce a certain result in a given patient depends on his/her health center background. Explanations include environmental factors like social and ethnic factors, investigator factors.

5 Example 4, a Random Effects Model for Post-hoc Analysis of Negative Crossover Trials

Source	SS	df	MS	F	p-value
Fixed effects analysis of variance					
Between-patients	81.4	$12-1=11$			
Within-patients	226.6	$3 \times 12 = 36$	6.29		
Treatment	24.0	$4-1=3$	8	$8/6.14 = 1.30$	ns
Residual	202.6	$3 \times 11 = 33$	6.14		
Total	308.0	47			
Random effects analysis of variance					
Within-patients	226.6	$12-1=11$			
Treatment	24.0	$4-1=3$	8	$8/1.74 = 4.60$	<0.05
Subjects×treatments	57.5	$3 \times 11 = 33$	1.74		
Total	308.0	47			

SS sum of squares, *df* degrees of freedom, *MS* mean square, *F* test statistic for F-test, *sd* standard deviation, *ns* not significant

In a crossover study different treatments are assessed in one and the same subject. An example of four treatments is given in Table 56.4. This example was also modified from an example used by Hays (1988). A real difference between the treatments is expected and this is tested by comparing the observed differences between the treatment with the residual error, estimated from the subtraction of the sum of squares (SS) within-patients minus the SS treatment. Obviously, none of the treatments produced an effect significantly different from that of another treatment. If a difference is not established like in this example, this may be due to random subgroup effects. In some patients one or more treatments may outperform the others, while in other patients other treatments may do so.

Because the study result was, thus, negative, we perform a post-hoc random effects analysis, testing treatment effect against treatments x patients interaction (SPSS statistical software (2011); command: mixed model, linear). This assessment shows that the four treatments appear to be having different effects to different subsets. Some patients seem to respond better than the others to one or more treatments. This may due to personal factors like a genetic characteristic, a societal and/or developmental factor etc. Note that, although in the first analysis the SS within-patients has 36 degrees of freedom [number of patients × (number of treatment modalities − 1)], in the second analysis it only has 11 degrees of freedom (number of patients − 1). This is, because in the latter analysis the factors defining the treatment effects are considered to be fixed, while the subjects are viewed as randomly sampled.

Table 56.4 Example 4, a random effects model for crossover trials

Patient no.	Treatment 1	Treatment 2	Treatment 3	Treatment 4	sd²
1	49	48	49	45	
2	47	46	46	43	
3	46	47	47	44	
4	47	45	45	45	
5	48	49	49	48	
6	47	44	45	46	
7	41	44	41	40	
8	46	45	43	45	
9	43	41	44	40	
10	47	45	46	45	
11	46	45	45	42	
12	45	40	40	40	
	552	540	540	528	Add-up sum = 2,160

6 Discussion

In this chapter research models are discussed that account for variables with random rather than fixed effects. These models are often called type 2 models if they include random exposure variables and type 3 models if they include both fixed and random exposure variables. For example, the example 1 in this chapter gives a type 2 model while the last three examples are type 3 models, otherwise called mixed effects models. Another example of mixed effects models is the non-linear mixed effects (non-mem) modeling, increasingly for the development of pharmacokinetic parameters (Dalla Costa et al. 1997; Meibohm and Derendorf 1997; Lotsch et al. 2004; Mueck et al. 2007; Boeckman et al. 1992). It is a program for nonlinear regression modeling that makes use of analysis of variance methods similar to those described in this chapter.

The work-up of the advanced research models is sometimes largely the same as that of simple research models. But, inferences made are quite different. All inferences made under the simple model mostly concern means and differences between means. In contrast, the inferences made using advanced models deal with variances, and involve small differences between subsets of patients or between individual patients. This type of analysis of variance answers questions like: do differences between assessors, between classrooms, between institutions, or between subjects contribute to the overall variability in the data?

We should consider some limitations of the methods. If the experimenter chooses the wrong model, he/she may suffer from a loss of power. Also the standards of homogeneity/heterogeneity in the data must be taken seriously. The patients in the subsets should not be sort of alike, rather they should be exactly alike on the variable to be assessed. Often this assumption can not be adequately met, raising the risk of a biased interpretation of the data.

The random effects research models enable to assess the entire sample for the presence of possible differences between subgroups without need to, actually, split the data into subgroups. This very point is a major argument in their favor. Also they are, of course, more appropriate if variables can be assumed to be random rather than fixed. A potential disadvantage is that the sensitivity to detect a significant difference in the data is generally somewhat reduced as explained in this paper. However, the reduction of sensitivity should not be regarded as a disadvantage, but rather an advantage, since the chance to make a correct conclusion is increased. Data should be analyzed according to the correct procedure, not according to the procedure that gives the largest chance to demonstrate a significant difference.

Only the simplest examples have been given in the present paper. The Internet provides an overwhelming body of information on the advanced research models including the type 2 and 3 research models as discussed here. For example, the Google data system provides 495,000 references for explanatory texts on this subject. This illustrates the enormous attention currently given to these upcoming techniques. Yet in clinical research these models are little known. We hope that this chapter will stimulate clinical investigators to more often apply them.

7   Conclusions

In clinical trials a fixed effects research model assumes that the patients selected for a specific treatment have the same true quantitative effect and that the differences observed are residual error. If, however, we have reasons to believe that certain patients respond differently from others, then the spread in the data is caused not only by the residual error but also by between patient differences. The latter situation requires a random effects model. This chapter explains random effects models in analysis of variance and to give examples of studies qualifying for them.

1. If in a particular study the data are believed to be different from one assessing doctor to the other, and if we have no prior theory that one or two assessing doctors produced the highest scores, but rather expect there may be heterogeneity in the population of doctors at large, then a random effect model will be appropriate. For that purpose between doctor variability is compared to within doctor variability.
2. If the data of two separate studies of the same new treatment are analyzed simultaneously, it will be safe to consider an interaction effect between the study number and treatment efficacy. If the interaction is significant, a random effects model with the study number as random variable, will be adequate. For that purpose the treatment effect is tested against the interaction effect.
3. In a multi-center study the data are at risk of interaction between centers and treatment efficacy. If this interaction is significant, a random effects model with

the health center as random variable, will be adequate. The treatment effect is tested not against residual but against the interaction.

4. If in a crossover study a treatment difference is not observed, this may be due to random subgroup effects. A post-hoc random effects model, with patients effect as random variable, testing the treatment effect against treatments x patients interaction, will be appropriate.

Random effects research models enable the assessment of an entire sample of data for subgroup differences without need to split the data into subgroups. Clinical investigators are generally hardly aware of this possibility and, therefore, wrongly assess random effects as fixed effects leading to a biased interpretation of the data.

References

Anonymous (2006) Distinguishing between random and fixed variables, effects and coefficients. Newson, USP 656 Winter 2006, pp 1–3

Anonymous (2011a) Random effects models. Wikipedia, the free encyclopedia. en.wikipedia.org/wiki/random-effects_models.html. Accessed 15 Dec 2011

Anonymous (2011b) Variance components and mixed models. http://www.statsoft.com/textbook/stvarcom.html. Accessed 15 Dec 2011

Boeckman AJ, Sheiner LB, Beal SL (1992) NONMEM user's guide. NONMEM Project Group, University of California, San Francisco

Brier ME, Aronoff GR (1996) Application of artificial neural networks to clinical pharmacology. Int J Clin Pharmacol Ther 34:510–514

Campbell MJ (2006) Random effects models. In: Campbell MJ (ed) Statistics at square two, 2nd edn. Blackwell Publishing/BMJ Books, Oxford/Malden, pp 67–83

Dalla Costa T, Nolting A, Rand K, Derendorf H (1997) Pharmacokinetic-pharmacodynamic modelling of the in vitro antiinfective effect of piperacillin-tazobactam combinations. Int J Clin Pharmacol Ther 35:426–433

Gao S (2003) Special models for sampling survey. In: Lu Y, Fang J (eds) Advanced medical statistics, 1st edn. World Scientific, River Edge, pp 685–709

Hays WL (1988) Random effects and mixed models. In: Statistics, 4th edn. Holt, Rhinehart and Winnston Inc, Chicago, pp 479–543

Lima JJ, Beasley BN, Parker RB, Johnson JA (2005) A pharmacodynamic model of the effects of controlled-onset extended-release verapamil on 24-hour ambulatory blood pressure. Int J Clin Pharmacol Ther 43(4):187–194

Lotsch J, Kobal G, Geisslinger G (2004) Programming of a flexible computer simulation to visualize pharmacokinetic-pharmacodynamic models. Int J Clin Pharmacol Ther 42:15–22

Mahmood I (2003) Center specificity in the limited sampling model (LSM): can the LSM developed from healthy subjects be extended to disease states? Int J Clin Pharmacol Ther 41:517–523

Meibohm B, Derendorf H (1997) Basic concepts of pharmacokinetic/pharmacodynamic (PK/PD) modelling. Int J Clin Pharmacol Ther 35:401–413. Review

Mueck W, Becka M, Kubitza D, Voith B, Zuehlsdorf M (2007) Population model of the pharmacokinetics and pharmacodynamics of rivaroxaban–an oral, direct factor xa inhibitor–in healthy subjects. Int J Clin Pharmacol Ther 45:335–344

SPSS Statistical Software. http://www.spss.com. Accessed 15 Dec 2011

Chapter 57
Monte Carlo Methods for Data Analysis

1 Introduction

For more than a century statistical tests based on Gaussian curves have been applied in clinical research, like t-tests, chi-square tests, analysis of variance and most regression analyses methods. Current clinical trials often make use of convenience samples and small samples that do not follow Gaussian curves. This raises the risk of false negative results (Zwinderman et al. 2006). Alternatively, samples can be analyzed using the Monte Carlo method. Basically, the Monte Carlo method uses random numbers from your own study rather than assumed Gaussian curves to assess the data. It was invented by the physicist Stanislaw Ulam and Ulam (1949) in the post-world-war-II era, and was called by him after the city of the roulette, because roulette is a simple generator of random numbers. The Monte Carlo method is, actually, very general: all it requires is the use of random numbers. It allows you to examine complex issues more easily than advanced mathematical methods, including integrals and matrix algebra. It is currently found in everything from economics to regulating flow of traffic to quantum mechanics. In clinical research the Monte Carlo method has been recently applied, for example, for the analysis of brachytherapy data (Vieira et al. 2002), computer tomographic images (Haidekker 2005), pharmacological data (Upton and Ludbrook 2005), and observational data (Nijhuis et al. 2006). Overall, however, the Monte Carlo method is little used in clinical research. This is a pity given the great potential of this relatively new method. This chapter was written to elucidate its principle and gives some real data-examples for a non-mathematical readership. The body of ongoing clinical research is huge, and clinical investigators tend to perform basic statistics without the help from a statistician. This chapter was written for their benefit. It is to be hoped that the chapter will stimulate them to use the Monte Carlo method more often, particularly in case of convenience samples and small samples.

T.J. Cleophas and A.H. Zwinderman, *Statistics Applied to Clinical Studies*,
DOI 10.1007/978-94-007-2863-9_57, © Springer Science+Business Media B.V. 2012

2   Principles of the Monte Carlo Method Explained from a Dartboard to Assess the Size of Π

The basics of the Monte Carlo method was explained by Woller (1996) using a dartboard for the purpose of assessing the size of π. Figure 57.1 simply pictures one quadrant of a circle. We assume that a very poor dart player throwing darts at it produces the same result as that obtained by throwing darts randomly at the figure. In this case the number of darts in the circle quadrant is proportional to the area of that part of the Figure. This would mean:

number darts in circle quadrant/total number darts = area circle quadrant/total area of graph.

High school geometry told us (r = radius of circle):

$$\text{area circle quadrant / total area of graph} = \tfrac{1}{4}\pi r^2 / r^2 = \tfrac{1}{4}\pi.$$

If at random a dart lands somewhere inside the graph, the ratio of hits in the circle quadrant will be one-fourth the value of π. Throwing many darts can thus be used as a method to assess the size of π.

$$\pi = 4 \times (\text{area circle quadrant / total area of graph})$$

$$= 4 \times (\text{number darts in circle quadrant / total number darts})$$

However, if you actually use this type of experiment for the assessment of π, you will observe that it will take a large number of throws to obtain a reliable value of π... well over 1,000. Yet, it is a straightforward alternative to the advanced mathematical methods commonly used to solve the problem. In clinical data analysis the Monte Carlo method can serve a similar purpose.

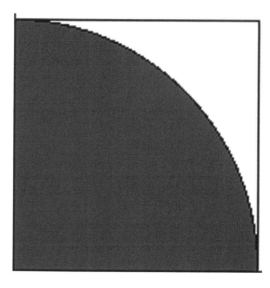

Fig. 57.1 A very poor dart player is assumed to have equal chances of throwing darts inside and outside the circle area, a situation which simulates throwing darts randomly (r radius of the dartboard) (StatsDirect 2011, with permission from the author)

3   The Monte Carlo Method for Analyzing Continuous Data

Table 57.1 gives an example of a parallel-group study assessing the effect of two cholesterol-reducing treatments on low density lipoprotein (LDL)-cholesterol. Small samples like those given here often do not follow a Gaussian curve. Non-parametric testing can restore a Gaussian curve. However, sometimes it is not good enough. SPSS Software (2011) is helpful. In the main box for two-samples-non-parametric testing the possibility of a test for the adequacy of non-parametric testing is given: the Kolmogorov-Smirnov (KS) test. If you click the KS test and then ok, a p-value of 0.037 is given, indicating that the KS test is positive and that non-parametric testing is, indeed, not good enough. If we, subsequently, click "exact" in the main dialog box, another dialog box will occur. It gives you the possibility to use either an exact test or the Monte Carlo method. Exact tests make use of rank numbers, i.e., all individual results are given a rank-number in ascending order, and these ranks are added up to determine the exact chance of finding an overall result in your data. The problem with rank testing is that it rapidly runs into numerical problems that even modern computers have difficulty to solve. SPSS statistical software is helpful regarding this problem. When clicking "exact" for the second time, the program will highlight the text "exact method will be used instead of Monte Carlo when computa-tional limits allow". You should set your computational time limits, e.g. 5 or 10 min, and the program will automatically use the Monte Carlo method if your requested time limits can not be met. In our particular example, the exact test required only 2 min and produced a p-value of 0.010 while the Monte Carlo method took less than a few seconds and produced a p-value of 0.011, virtually the same.

For the continuous data as given in this example a special type of Monte Carlo method is used, called the bootstrap method (Efron and Tibshirani 1993). The name bootstrap derives from the saying "pull yourself up by your boot-straps" meaning that you can continue what you are doing but in a much faster way. It works essentially as follows. A patient is randomly picked up from the given samples while replacing the picked-up patient so that the sample from which to choose remains unchanged. In mathematical terms this method of sam-pling is called "sampling with replacement". By doing so, we can produce ran-dom samples from the original data.

The procedure is illustrated in Table 57.1. In the first random sample observation-1 was picked up twice, while the observations no 2 and 4 were not. We repeat the procedure a large number of times, and record the difference between medians every time. To derive reliable confidence intervals, at least 1,000 repetitions are required. Medians rather than means are used, because with extreme high (or low) values the mean value is less representative of the data average than the median. The null hypothesis is, that no real difference exists between the data from group 1 and 2. This null hypothesis is rejected if the median of group 1 is larger than that of group 2 at least 95% of the times. All of the 1,000 differences between the medians as calculated from the bootstraps lay between −0.12 and 1.09, while 98.9% of the dif-ferences lay between 0.00 and 0.844. In this example the bootstrap medians from

Table 57.1 The bootstrap method is a data based simulation process for statistical inference. The basic idea is randomly picking up a patient from a given sample while replacing the picked-up patient so that the sample from which to choose remains unchanged

Original data

LDL-cholesterol (mmol/l)				Bootstrap 1				Bootstrap 2			
Group1		Group 2		Group1		Group 2		Group 1		Group 2	
1.	3.99	10.	3.18	1.	3.99	10.	3.18	1.	3.99	10.	3.18
2.	3.79	11.	2.84	1.	3.99	10.	3.18	2.	3.79	11.	2.84
3.	3.60	12.	2.90	3.	3.60	12.	2.90	2.	3.79	12.	2.90
4.	3.73	13.	3.27	5.	3.21	14.	3.85	2.	3.79	12.	2.90
5.	3.21	14.	3.85	6.	3.60	15.	3.52	4.	3.73	14.	3.85
6.	3.60	15.	3.52	8.	3.61	15.	3.52	5.	3.21	15.	3.52
7.	4.08	16.	3.23	8.	3.61	15.	3.52	7.	4.08	16.	3.23
8.	3.61	17.	2.76	9.	3.81	16.	3.23	7.	4.08	18.	3.60
9.	3.81	18.	3.60	9.	3.81	17.	2.76	8.	3.61	18.	3.60

Median group 1=3.73	Median group 1=3.61	Median group 1=3.79
Median group 2=3.23	Median group 2=3.23	Median group 2=3.23
Difference medians=0.50	Difference medians=0.38	Difference medians=0.55

group1 are indeed larger than those from group 2 over 95% of the times. We, therefore, reject the null hypothesis at $p < (1 - 0.95)$ or $p < 0.05$. There is a significant difference between the groups at $p < 0.05$ ($p = 0.011$ to be precise).

4   The Monte Carlo Method for Analyzing Proportional Data

Table 57.2 gives an example of a population-based cohort study assessing the effect of a prophylactic treatment on the number of cardiac events. For proportional data, including fractions and percentages, the chi-square test is a standard method of analysis. The data are usually displayed in 2×2 contingency tables (Table 57.2). However, the cells of a 2×2 contingency table must not be too small, 5–10 patients are required in each of its four cells. If smaller, the Fisher's exact test is an alternative, but with proportions from large groups computational problems will rapidly arise, because it uses faculties: "995 faculty" $= 995\ != 995 \times 994 \times 993 \times 992 \times 991$ …etc. These kinds of calculations are time-consuming even for modern computers. The SPSS program is helpful again. If you click "exact" in the main dialog box, then another dialog box will occur. You should set your computational time limits, e.g. 5 min, and the program will automatically use the Monte Carlo method if your requested time limits will exceed.

The Monte Carlo method to calculate is, then, less labour-intensive, and works essentially as follows. The question is answered: are the observed cells significantly different from the cells expected from the population data base. If the proportion of patients-with-event in the target population can be expected to be 10 out of 1,000, then the ratio 10:1,000 will be observed most frequently when randomly sampling from such a target population. How great is the chance of finding a ratio 5:1,000 if 10:1,000 is to be expected. This chance will be small. We can randomly

Table 57.2 2×2 contingency table of a population-based cohort study assessing the effect of a prophylactive treatment on the numbers of cardiac events

Proportion	Patients with an event		Patients without an event	
Observed 5/1,000	Cell 1	5	Cell 2	955
Expected from target population 10/1,000	Cell 3	10	Cell 4	990

pick up a patient 1,000 times from a sample of 1,000, 10 of which have the code "event", and 990 of which have the code "no-event", while replacing the picked-up patient, so that the sample from which to choose remains unchanged (sampling with replacement).

	Patients with an event
The first 1,000 patients chosen produced the following result	9
Second 1,000 patients	10
Third 1,000 patients	8
.....	4
....	...
.....	...
Thousandth 1,000 patients	12

The null hypothesis is, that the difference between observed and expected is due to chance rather than a statistically significant effect. This null hypothesis is rejected at p<0.05 if in 95% of the times the expected number of patients with an event is larger than the observed number 5. In this example all of the 1,000 pick-up procedures produced results between 4 and 16, while 95% of them were between 6 and 14, which is consistently larger than the observed number 5. We can, therefore, reject the null hypothesis at p<0.05.

5   Discussion

The Monte Carlo method is a scientifically safe alternative approach to data analysis. It, essentially, derives confidence intervals from the data without prior assessment of the type of frequency distribution. Other advantages of this method include:

- It does not require equal standard deviations of groups in paired or parallel-group treatment comparisons.
- It is often less time-consuming than exact methods.

Disadvantages include:

– Although less laborious than many standard methods, it is still rather laborious without a computer.
– Samples must not be very small. With a sample of say four, there are only 16 distinct re-samplings equally likely. The median of such a sample will take one of the four sample values. This is not a very strong basis for constructing a 95% confidence interval. The above examples show that rather small samples are generally no problem. The p-value produced by the Monte Carlo method in the first study comparing 9 versus 9 patients was only slightly larger than the p-value produced by the exact test, with p-values of 0.011 and 0.010 respectively.

Nowadays Monte Carlo methods can be carried out with computer programs for statistical analyses, like SPSS, S-plus, StatsDirect, StatXact, SAS etc. (SPSS 2011; S-plus 2011; StatsDirect 2011; StatXact 2011; True Epistat 2011; BUGS y WinBUGS 2011; R 2011; SAS 2011). The current paper gives only the simplest examples of the Monte Carlo method for the analysis of clinical data. Several books have been written providing more complex models (Gardner and Altman 2000; Shao and Tu 1995; Fishman 1996). However, all of the models are based on the same simple principle. We do hope that this paper will strengthen the awareness the great potential of the Monte Carlo method for the analysis of research data.

6   Conclusions

For more than a century statistical tests based on Gaussian curves have been applied in clinical research. Current clinical trials often make use of convenience samples and small samples that do not follow Gaussian curves. This raises the risk of false negative results. This chapter elucidates the Monte Carlo method as an alternative method for the assessment of such data.

The Monte Carlo method derives confidence intervals from the data without prior assumption about the presence of Gaussian curves in the data. For 2-parallel-groups studies with continuous data the basic idea is to produce multiple random samples from your own 2 parallel groups. If in at least 95% of these random samples the first group scores better than the second, then a statistically significant difference between the two groups will be accepted at $p < 0.05$.

Also for population-based cohort studies with proportional data multiple random samples can be produced from your own observed data. If in at least 95% of these random samples the expected proportion exceeds the observed proportion, then a statistically significant difference between the observed and expected data will be accepted at $p < 0.05$.

Advantages of the Monte Carlo method include:

– It does not depend upon Gaussian curves.
– It is less time-consuming than many standard methods.

A disadvantages is that, although less time-consuming than many standard methods, it is still rather laborious without a computer. We do hope that this chapter will strengthen the awareness of the Monte Carlo method as an often more reliable alternative for analysis of clinical research.

References

BUGS y WinBUGS. http://www.mrc-bsu.cam.ac.uk/bugs. Accessed 15 Dec 2011

Efron B, Tibshirani RJ (1993) An introduction to the bootstrap. Chapman & Hall, New York

Fishman GS (1996) Monte Carlo, concepts, algorithms and applications. Springer, New York

Gardner MJ, Altman DG (2000) Statistics with confidence. Book with diskette edited by BMJ, London, UK

Haidekker YG (2005) Trans-illumination optical tomography of tissue-engineered blood vessels: a Monte Carlo simulation. Appl Opt 44:4265–4271

Nijhuis RL, Stijnen T, Peeters A, Witteman JC, Hofman A, Hunink MG (2006) Apparent and internal validity of a Monte Carlo-Markow model for cardiovascular disease in a cohort follow-up study. Med Decis Making 26:134–144

R. http://cran.r-project.org. Accessed 15 Dec 2011

S-plus. http://www.mathsoft.com/splus. Accessed 15 Dec 2011

SAS. http://www.prw.le.ac.uk/epidemiol/personal/ajs22/meta/macros.sas. Accessed 15 Dec 2011

Shao J, Tu D (1995) The jackknife and bootstrap. Springer, New York

SPSS Statistical Software. http://www.spss.com. Accessed 15 Dec 2011

StatsDirect. http://www.camcode.com. Accessed 15 Dec 2011

StatXact. http://www.cytel.com/products/statxact/statact1.html. Accessed 15 Dec 2011

True Epistat. http://ic.net/~biomware/biohp2te.htm. Accessed 15 Dec 2011

Ulam N, Ulam S (1949) The Monte Carlo method. J Am Stat Assoc 44:335–341

Upton RN, Ludbrook GL (2005) Pharmacokinetic-pharmacodynamic modelling of the cardiovascular effects of drugs-method development and application in sheep. BMC Pharmacol 5:1471–1481

Vieira JW, Lima FR, Kramer R (2002) A Monte Carlo approach to calculate dose distribution around the lineal brachytherapy sources. Cell Mol Biol 48:445–450

Woller J (1996) The basics of Monte Carlo simulation. http://www.chem.unl.edu/zeng/joy/mclab/mcintro.html. Accessed 15 Dec 2011

Zwinderman AH, Cleophas TJ, Van Ouwerkerk B (2006) Clinical trials do not use random samples anymore. Clin Res Regul Aff 23:85–95

Chapter 58
Artificial Intelligence

1 Introduction

Artificial intelligence is an engineering method that simulates the structures and operating principles of the human brain. Much is unknown of how the brain trains itself to process information, but we do know that brain cells, called neurons, can be activated to send an electric signal through long thin stands called axons. At the end of the axon a structure called the synapse connects the axon with a connected neuron, and provides it with excitatory/inhibitory imput or when the signal is too weak no imput at all. Learning processes in the brain is thought to take place by repeated similar electric signals at similar places giving rise to similar outcomes observed by the brain. This principle can be modeled by artificial neural networks software using observed variables as artificial signals. Software is available in SPSS, MATLAB and so forth: in the current paper SPSS version 17.0, with neural network add-on has been applied (WWW.SPSS.COM). Artificial neural networks are different from traditional statistics that usually assumes Gaussian curve distributions for making predictions from the data. In practice the data, sometimes, do not follow Gaussian distributions, and, for that purpose, distribution-free methods, like non-parametric tests and Monte Carlo methods, have been developed. The artificial neural network is another distribution-free method based on layers of artificial neurons that transduce imputed information. It has been recognized to have a number of advantages including the possibility to process imperfect data, and complex non linear data (Stergiou and Siganos 2004). The current chapter reviews the principles, procedures, and limitations of BP artificial neural networks for a non-mathematical readership.

2 Historical Background

Artificial intelligence was first proposed by the group of neurophysiologist McCulloch in the 1950s (Andrew 2004). Initially, it was merely to explore and simulate informational processing of the human brain. In the 1960s Rosenblatt (1962)

T.J. Cleophas and A.H. Zwinderman, *Statistics Applied to Clinical Studies*, DOI 10.1007/978-94-007-2863-9_58, © Springer Science+Business Media B.V. 2012

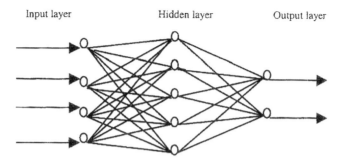

Fig. 58.1 A simple three-layer neural network: each layer of neurons after having received a signal beyond some threshold propagates it forward to the next layer

developed a three-layer perceptron model (Fig. 58.1), that, with the help of a traditional digital computer system, was capable to process experimental data samples. In the mid-1970s Minsky (1974) showed that models with more than three layers were generally required to perform with the precision of current multiple regression models. Particularly, perceptrons with learning samples, otherwise called back propagation (BP) models (Rumbelhart et al. 1986), have been successful in the past two decades, and have been applied for various purposes including sales forecasting, process control, and target marketing (Stergiou and Siganos 2004). Also in clinical research it has been increasingly applied. In oncology research it has been used for diagnostic purposes (Simpson et al. 1995; Naguib et al. 1996; Sherman et al. 1997; Mango and Valente 1998; Doornewaard et al. 1999; Prismatic Project Management Team 1999; Finne et al. 2000; Gamito et al. 2000) and survival analysis (Bugliosi et al. 1994; Kothari et al. 1996; Glas and Reddick 1998; Bryce et al. 1998), in critical care medicine for patient monitoring (Stock et al. 1994; Si et al. 1998; Zernikow et al. 1998; Zernikow et al. 1999; Eftekbar et al. 2005), and in cardiovascular medicine for making diagnoses, including the presence of myocardial infarction (Selker et al. 1995; Baxt and Skora 1996; Ellenius et al. 1997) and coronary artery disease (Goodenday et al. 1997; Polak et al. 1997; Lindahl et al. 2000), and cardiovascular risk predictions (Patil and Smith 2009).

3 The Back Propagation (BP) Neural Network: The Computer Teaches Itself to Make Predictions

The BP neural networks software include one imput layer, one or more hidden layers and one output layer. Each layer consists of various artificial neurons taking on two phases: activity or inactivity. Figure 58.1 gives a simple example with a single hidden layer. Each neuron in the imput layer after having received a signal

Table 58.1   Part of weights matrix of transferred signals to the first hidden layer

−0.040	0.370	0.117	0.066	−0.082	−0.227	0.36	−0.321
−0.288	0.070	0.178	−0.190	−0.275	0.283	−0.467	0.032
−0.128	−0.052	−0.305	−0.237	0.442	0.350	0.077	−0.378
−0.585	−0.247	0.271	−0.045	−0.213	0.272	0.403	0.383
0.248	−0.221	−0.149	0.152	−0.012	0.204	−0.233	−0.007
−0.108	−0.338	0.523	−0.046	−0.321	0.309	0.433	−0.068
0.068	0.142	−0.346	0.014	−0.154	−0.052	−0.048	0.160

Table 58.2   Part of weights matrix of transferred signals to the second hidden layer

−0.148	0.602	−0.571	−0.207	0.256	−0.495
0.098	0.684	−0.559	−0.731	1.364	0.097
0.336	−0.541	0.505	−0.241	0.632	−0.188
−0.287	−0.108	0.186	0.124	−0.458	−0.215
0.710	−0.002	−0.387	−0.301	0.735	−0.500

beyond some threshold propagates it forward to the next layer. This process will not stop until the signal reaches the output layer sending out the processed signal. The magnitude of the imput values and output values is determined by the structure and functioning of the network. The network is also provided with previously observed outcome data, the socalled learning sample. The computer will find, by modifying the weights for all signal-transfers, an outcome as close to the observed outcome as possible. In other words, the neural network tries to find the best-fit outcome for making predictions about the observed outcome data from the imputed data, in a way, similar to regression models. However, unlike regression models no Gaussian distribution models are required, but rather weighted signal-transfers from one layer to another. The Tables 58.1 and 58.2 give examples of weights matrices of imputed signals in the first and second hidden layer of a real data example which will be used in the next section. For finding the best-fit weights the computer uses a technique called iteration or bootstrapping, which means it makes maximally 2,000 guesses, depending on the setting when running the neural network, and then picks out the combination of guesses with the best-fit. The output activity is determined by all imput activities times their weights, and, subsequently, the various hidden layer activities times their weights. The BP principle is, that all imput produces error. Error is assessed, in the usual way, by taking the sums of squared difference from the means of the observed variables. The result with the smallest error is the one with the best-fit. At present, there is no matured theory on how to select the numbers of artificial neurons and hidden layers. The precision of the neural network is improved by feedback signaling (negative weights in the matrices).

4   A Real Data Example

Body surface area is a better indicator for metabolic body mass than body weight, because it is less affected by adipose mass. In laboratory medicine it is used for adjusting oxygen, CO_2 transport parameters, blood volumes, urine creatinine clearance, protein/creatinine ratios and other parameters. The predicting factors of body surface consist of gender, age, weight and height. The body surfaces of 90 persons (Table 58.3) were calculated using direct photometric measurements (Mitchell et al. 1971).

The Fig. 58.2 shows the nonlinear relationship between the weights, heights, and measured body surfaces. Using SPSS 17.0 with the neural network add-on module, we assess whether a neural network with two hidden layers would be able to adequately predict the measured body surfaces, and whether it would perform better than the Haycock equation (* = sign of multiplication) (Haycock et al. 1978) :

$$\text{body surface} = 0.024265 * \text{height}^{0.3964} * \text{weight}^{0.5378}.$$

The data file consists of a row for each person with different factors and one dependent variable, the measured body surface (Table 58.3). We command: neural networks; multilayer perceptron. Select the dependent variable, the measured body surface, factors, body height and weight, and covariates, age and gender, in the main dialog box. Here are also various dialog boxes that can be assessed from the main dialog box:

1. the dialog box partitioning: set the training sample (70), test sample (20)
2. the dialog box architecture: set the numbers of hidden layers (2)
3. the dialog box activation function: click hyperbolic tangens
4. the dialog box output: click diagrams, descriptions, synaptic weights
5. the dialog box training: maximal time for calculations 15 min, maximal numbers of iterations 2,000.

Then press ok, and synaptic weights and body surfaces predicted by the neural network are displayed as well as the smallest error. The results are in Table 58.3. Also, the values obtained from the Haycock equation are included in the table.

Both the predicted values from the neural network and from the Haycock equation are close to the measured values. When performing a linear regression with neural network as predictor, the r-square value was 0.983, while the Haycock produced an r-square value of 0.995.

In order to assess the robustness of the neural network result, smaller training samples, fewer iterations and a single hidden layer were assessed, but all of these changes produced smaller r-square values indicating less precision. Models with more than two hidden layers were not assessed, because the SPSS software add-on program does not allow for these models.

Considering the usual requirement for accurate diagnostic testing (Atiqi et al. 2009) of r-square values larger than 0.95, we have to conclude that both methods perform adequately, although the Haycock model was slightly better. The example still illustrates the potential of the neural network as an exact technique for predicting body surfaces.

Table 58.3 Ninety persons' physical measurements and body surfaces (one row is one person) predicted by mathematical equation and the best-fit result from a two hidden layer neural network. The best-fit result as presented had an error as small as 0.0035 obtained after maximally 2,000 iterations

Gender	Age	Weight	Height	Body surface measured	Predicted from equation	Predicted from neural network
Var 1	Var 2	Var 3	Var 4	Var 5		
1,00	13,00	30,50	138,50	10072,90	10770,00	10129,64
0,00	5,00	15,00	101,00	6189,00	6490,00	6307,14
0,00	0,00	2,50	51,50	1906,20	1890,00	2565,16
1,00	11,00	30,00	141,00	10290,60	10750,00	10598,32
1,00	15,00	40,50	154,00	13221,60	13080,00	13688,06
0,00	11,00	27,00	136,00	9654,50	10001,00	9682,47
0,00	5,00	15,00	106,00	6768,20	6610,00	6758,45
1,00	5,00	15,00	103,00	6194,10	6540,00	6533,28
1,00	3,00	13,50	96,00	5830,20	6010,00	6096,53
0,00	13,00	36,00	150,00	11759,00	12150,00	11788,01
0,00	3,00	12,00	92,00	5299,40	5540,00	5350,63
1,00	0,00	2,50	51,00	2094,50	1890,00	2342,85
0,00	7,00	19,00	121,00	7490,80	7910,00	7815,05
1,00	13,00	28,00	130,50	9521,70	10040,00	9505,63
1,00	0,00	3,00	54,00	2446,20	2130,00	2696,17
0,00	0,00	3,00	51,00	1632,50	2080,00	2345,39
0,00	7,00	21,00	123,00	7958,80	8400,00	7207,74
1,00	11,00	31,00	139,00	10580,80	10880,00	8705,10
1,00	7,00	24,50	122,50	8756,10	9120,00	7978.52
1,00	11,00	26,00	133,00	9573,00	9720,00	9641,04
0,00	9,00	24,50	130,00	9028,00	9330,00	9003,97
1,00	9,00	25,00	124,00	8854,50	9260,00	8804,45
1,00	0,00	2,25	50,50	1928,40	1780,00	2655,69
0,00	11,00	27,00	129,00	9203,10	9800,00	9982,77
0,00	0,00	2,25	53,00	2200,20	1810,00	2582,61
0,00	5,00	16,00	105,00	6785,10	6820,00	7017,29
0,00	9,00	30,00	133,00	10120,80	10500,00	9762,62
0,00	13,00	34,00	148,00	11397,30	11720,00	12063,78
1,00	3,00	16,00	99,00	6410,60	6660,00	6370,21
1,00	3,00	11,00	92,00	5283,30	5290,00	5372,90
0,00	9,00	23,00	126,00	8693,50	8910,00	8450,32
1,00	13,00	30,00	138,00	9626,10	10660,00	11196,58
1,00	9,00	29,00	138,00	10178,70	10460,00	10445,87
1,00	1,00	8,00	76,00	4134,50	4130,00	3952,50
0,00	15,00	42,00	165,00	13019,50	13710,00	13056,80
1,00	15,00	40,00	151,00	12297,10	12890,00	12094,26
1,00	1,00	9,00	80,00	4078,40	4490,00	4520,18
1,00	7,00	22,00	123,00	8651,10	8620,00	8423,78
0,00	1,00	9,50	77,00	4246,10	4560,00	3750,54

(continued)

Table 58.3 (continued)

Gender	Age	Weight	Height	Body surface measured	Predicted from equation	Predicted from neural network
Var 1	Var 2	Var 3	Var 4	Var 5		
1,00	7,00	25,00	125,00	8754,40	9290,00	8398,58
1,00	13,00	36,00	143,00	11282,40	11920,00	11104,75
1,00	3,00	15,00	94,00	6101,60	6300,00	6210,85
0,00	0,00	3,00	51,00	1850,30	2080,00	2345,39
0,00	1,00	9,00	74,00	3358,50	4360,00	3788,70
0,00	1,00	7,50	73,00	3809,70	3930,00	3800,02
0,00	15,00	43,00	152,00	12998,70	13440,00	13353,48
0,00	13,00	27,50	139,00	9569,10	10200,00	9395,76
0,00	3,00	12,00	91,00	5358,40	5520,00	6090,37
0,00	15,00	40,50	153,00	12627,40	13050,00	12622,94
1,00	5,00	15,00	100,00	6364,50	6460,00	6269,19
1,00	1,00	9,00	80,00	4380,80	4490,00	4520,18
1,00	5,00	16,50	112,00	7256,40	7110,00	7430,72
0,00	3,00	12,50	91,00	5291,50	5640,00	5487,65
1,00	0,00	3,50	56,50	2506,70	2360,00	3065,52
0,00	1,00	10,00	77,00	4180,40	4680,00	3914,55
1,00	9,00	25,00	126,00	8813,70	9320,00	8127,39
1,00	9,00	33,00	138,00	11055,40	11220,00	10561,80
1,00	5,00	16,00	108,00	6988,00	6900,00	6413,58
0,00	11,00	29,00	127,00	9969,80	10130,00	9471,79
0,00	7,00	20,00	114,00	7432,80	7940,00	7299,95
0,00	1,00	7,50	77,00	3934,00	4010,00	4042,95
1,00	11,00	29,50	134,50	9970,50	10450,00	10408,70
0,00	5,00	15,00	101,00	6225,70	6490,00	6307,14
0,00	3,00	13,00	91,00	5601,70	5760,00	5623,51
0,00	5,00	15,00	98,00	6163,70	6410,00	6296,79
1,00	15,00	45,00	157,00	13426,70	13950,00	13877,81
1,00	7,00	21,00	120,00	8249,20	8320,00	8445,74
0,00	9,00	23,00	127,00	8875,80	8940,00	9023,25
0,00	7,00	17,00	104,00	6873,50	7020,00	6935,27
1,00	15,00	43,50	150,00	13082,80	13450,00	13508,38
1,00	15,00	50,00	168,00	14832,00	15160,00	13541,31
0,00	7,00	18,00	114,00	7071,80	7510,00	7161,82
1,00	3,00	14,00	97,00	6013,60	6150,00	6200,79
1,00	7,00	20,00	119,00	7876,40	8080,00	7606,17
0,00	0,00	3,00	54,00	2117,30	2130,00	2559,28
1,00	1,00	9,50	74,00	4314,20	4490,00	4531,14
0,00	15,00	44,00	163,00	13480,90	13990,00	13612,74
0,00	11,00	32,00	140,00	10583,80	11100,00	10401,88
1,00	0,00	3,00	52,00	2121,00	2100,00	2337,69

(continued)

Table 58.3   (continued)

Gender	Age	Weight	Height	Body surface measured	Predicted from equation	Predicted from neural network
Var 1	Var 2	Var 3	Var 4	Var 5		
0,00	11,00	29,00	141,00	10135,30	10550,00	10291,93
0,00	3,00	15,00	94,00	6074,90	6300,00	6440,60
0,00	13,00	44,00	140,00	13020,30	13170,00	12521,73
1,00	5,00	15,50	105,00	6406,50	6700,00	6532,15
1,00	9,00	22,00	126,00	8267,00	8700,00	8056,85
0,00	15,00	40,00	159,50	12769,70	13170,00	12994,08
1,00	1,00	9,50	76,00	3845,90	4530,00	4240,36
0,00	13,00	32,00	144,00	10822,10	11220,00	10964,35
1,00	13,00	40,00	151,00	12519,90	12890,00	12045,33
0,00	9,00	22,00	124,00	8586,10	8650,00	8411,62
1,00	11,00	31,00	135,00	10120,60	10750,00	9934,60

Var means variable

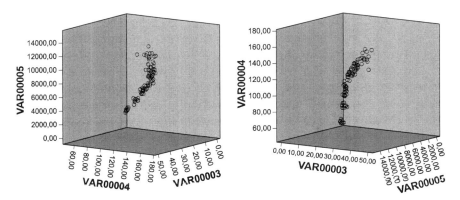

Fig. 58.2 *VAR00003* weight, *VAR00004* height, *VAR00005* measured body surface. The three dimensional scatter plot shows the nonlinear relationship between the variables

5   Discussion

In our example of 90 persons a four layer BP neural network accurately predicted body surface though not as exact as did the usual mathematical equation. Similar results were recently observed by Eftekbar et al. (2005): neural network predicted head trauma mortality accurately, but not as exact as logistic models. Neural networks were sometimes better than alternative procedures. For example, in 331 adults with chest pain for making a diagnosis of acute infarction than were the attending emergency room physicians (sensitivity and specificity 97% and 96% versus 78% and 85%) (Baxt and Skora 1996). Also, in 1,107 patients BP neural networks was more sensitive to detect anterior and inferior infarctions than conventional automated electrocardiogram interpretation (81% and 78% versus 68 and 66%) (Heden et al. 1994). Nowadays, intelligent computing techniques, mimicking the brain, receive a great deal of attention from the scientific world: e.g., the Google database system gives approximately 10 million hits for the search term "artificial intelligence". Yet, many questions are unanswered. For example, artificial intelligence does not possess human brain-characteristics like tolerance, robustness, and levels of consciousness. Also, methods that are more prone to generalization, such as the BP based neural network techniques and their computational systems are generally unable to provide a definite explication of the outcome, sometimes leading to incorrect conclusions, and, if used for the classifications of single cases, to questionable results.

We should add that data driven analyses are, generally, not a sound basis for scientific research, and a major source of misunderstandings due to results based on chance rather than true effects. Neural network by its very nature of black box modeling is at risk of being abused for that purpose. When applied for clinical research, particularly diagnostic research, it should be based on appropriate prior hypotheses and prior knowledge. Fortunately, this has been recognized and emphasized by several investigators (Redding et al. 1993; Sperduti and Starita 1993; Wnek and Michalski 1994; Lytton 2002).

Regarding the potential users of neural network methods, we believe that, despite the requirement of basic statistical knowledge, current user-friendly statistical software like the SPSS add-on module "Neural Network" (WWW.SPSS.COM) can be used by clinical and laboratory investigators without the help of a statistician. After all, those who invented artificial intelligence were neurologists and neurophysiologists, rather than statisticians (Stergiou and Siganos 2004).

Although artificial intelligence may *approximately* correspond to the intelligence of human beings, it is, probably, also largely different from the brain, and should, currently, be interpreted as just another non-Gaussian method for data assessment. Moreover, its mathematical basis is not fully recognized. Also, traditional statistical methods like regression methods have to be added for testing its accuracy against alternative methods. Nonetheless, it has great potential through its ability to learn by example instead of learning by theory, making it very flexible and powerful.

6   Conclusions

Back propagation (BP) artificial neural networks is a distribution-free method for data-analysis based on layers of artificial neurons that transduce imputed information. It has been recognized to have a number of advantages compared to traditional methods including the possibility to process imperfect data, and complex nonlinear data. This chapter reviews the principles, procedures, and limitations of BP artificial neural networks for a non-mathematical readership

A real data sample of 90 persons' weights, heights and measured body surfaces was used as an example. SPSS 17.0 with neural network add-on was used for the analysis. The predicted body surfaces from a two hidden layer BP neural network were compared to the body surfaces calculated by the Haycock equation. Both the predicted values from the neural network and from the Haycock equation were close to the measured values. A linear regression analysis with neural network as predictor produced an r-square value of 0.983, while the Haycock equation produced a value of 0.995 (r-square >0.95 is a criterion for accurate diagnostic-testing).

BP neural networks may, sometimes, predict clinical diagnoses with accuracies similar to those of other methods. However, traditional statistical procedures like regression analyses have to be added for testing their accuracies against alternative methods. Nonetheless, BP neural networks has great potential through its ability to learn by example instead of learning by theory.

References

Andrew AM (2004) Work of Warren McCulloch. Kybernetes 33:141–146

Atiqi R, Van Iersel C, Cleophas TJ (2009) Accuracy of quantitative diagnostic tests. Int J Clin Pharmacol Ther 47:153–159

Baxt WG, Skora J (1996) Prospective validation of artificial neural network trained to identify acute myocardial infarction. Lancet 347:12–15

Bryce TJ, Dewhirst MW, Floyd CE, Hars V, Brizel DM (1998) Artificial neural networks of survival in patients treated with irradiation with and without concurrent chemotherapy for advanced carcinoma of the head and neck. Int J Radiat Oncol Biol Phys 41:339–345

Bugliosi R, Tribalto M, Avvisati G, Boccardoro M, De Martinis C, Friera R, Mandelli F, Pileri A, Papa G (1994) Classificiation of patients affected by multiple myeloma using neural network software. Eur J Haematol 52:182–183

Doornewaard H, Van der Schouw YT, Van der Graaf Y, Bos AB, Habbema JD, Van den Tweel JG (1999) The diagnostic value of computer assisted primary smear screening: a longitudinal cohort study. Mod Pathol 12:995–1000

Eftekbar B, Mohammad K, Ardebilli HE, Ghodsi M, Ketabchi E (2005) Comparison of artificial neural network and regression models for prediction of mortality in head trauma based on clinical data. BMC Med Inform Decis Mak 5:3–9

Ellenius J, Groth T, Lindahl B (1997) Neural network of biochemical markers for early assessment of acute myocardial infarction. Stud Health Technol Inform 43:382–385

Finne P, Finne R, Auvinen A, Juusela H, Aro J, Maattanen L, Hakama M, Ranniko S, Tammela TL, Stenman U (2000) Predicting the outcome of prostate biopsy in screen positive men by a multilayer perceptron network. Urology 56:418–422

Gamito EJ, Stone NN, Batuello JT, Crawford ED (2000) Use of artificial neural networks in the clinical staging of prostate cancer. Tech Urol 6:60–63

Glas JO, Reddick WE (1998) Hybrid artificial neural netwwork segmentation and classification of dynamic contrast enhanced MR imaging of osteosarcoma. Magn Reson Imaging 16:1075–1083

Goodenday LS, Cios KJ, Shin L (1997) Identifying coronary stenosis using an image recognition neural network. IEEE Eng Med Bio Mag 16:139–144

Haycock GB, Schwarz GJ, Wisotsky DH (1978) Body surface area calculated from the height and weight. J Pediatr 93:62–66

Heden B, Edenbrandt L, Hasity WK, Pahlm O (1994) Artificial neural networks for electrocardiographic diagnosis of healed myocardial infarction. Am J Cardiol 74:5–8

Kothari R, Cualing H, Balachander T (1996) Neural network analysis of flow cytometry immunophenotype data. IEEE Biomed Eng 43:803–810

Lindahl D, Toft J, Hesse B, Palmer J, Ali S, Lundin A, Edenbrandt L (2000) Scandinavian test of artificial neural network for classification of myocardial perfusion images. Clin Physiol 20:253–261

Lytton WW (2002) From artificial neural network to realistic neural network. In: From computer to brain. Springer, New York, pp 259–268

Mango LJ, Valente PT (1998) Neural networks assisted analysis and microscopic rescreening in presumed negative cervical cytologic smears. Acta Cytol 42:227–232

Minsky M (1974) A framework for representing knowledge. Technical Report Massachusetts Institute of Technology, AIM-306, Cambridge MA, USA

Mitchell D, Strydom NB, Van Graan CH, Van der Walt H (1971) Human surface area: comparison of the du Bois formula with direct photometric measurement. Eur J Physiol 325:188–190

Naguib RN, Adams AE, Horne CH, Angus B, Sherbet GV, Lennard TW (1996) The detection of nodal metastasis in breast cancer using neural networks. Physiol Meas 17:297–303

Patil N, Smith TJ (2009) Neural network analysis speeds disease risk predictions, innovative clinical models transform cardiovascular assessment algorithms. Sci Comput; Rockaway NJ 07866. www.scientificcomputing.com. Accessed 15 Dec 2011

Polak MJ, Zhou SH, Rautaharju PM, Armstrong WW, Chaitman BR (1997) Using automated analysis of resting twelve lead ECG to identify patients at risk of developing transient myocardial ischaemia. Physiol Meas 18:317–325

Prismatic Project Management Team (1999) Assessment of automated primary screening on PAPNET of cervical smears in the PRISMATIC trial. Lancet 353:1381–1385

Redding NJ, Kowalczyk A, Downs T (1993) Constructive higher order network algorithms that is polynomial time. Neural Netw 6:997–1010

Rosenblatt F (1962) Principles of neurodynamics: perceptrons and the theory of brain mechanisms. Spartan, Washington, DC

Rumbelhart DE, Hinton GE, Williams RJ (1986) Learning representations by back-propagating errors. Nature 323:533–536

Selker HP, Griffith JL, Patil S, Long WJ, D'Agostino RB (1995) A comparison of performance of mathematical predictive methods for medical diagnosis: identifying acute cardiac ischemia among emergency department patients. J Investig Med 43:468–476

Sherman ME, Schiffman MH, Mango LJ, Kelly D, Acosta D, Cason Z, Elgert P, Zaleski S, Scot DR, Kurman R, Stoler M, Lorincz AT (1997) Evaluation of PAPNET testing as an ancillary tool to clarify the status of the atypical cervical smear. Mod Pathol 10:564–567

Si Y, Gotman J, Pasupathy A, Flanagan D, Rosenblatt B, Gottesman R (1998) An expert system for EEG monitoring in the pediatric intensive care. Electroencephalogr Clin Neurophysiol 106:488–500

Simpson JH, McArdle C, Pauson AW, Hume P, Turkes A, Griffiths K (1995) A non-invasive test for the pre-cancerous breast. Eur J Cancer 31A:1768–1772

Sperduti A, Starita A (1993) Speed up learning and network optimization with extended back propagation. Neural Netw 6:365–383

Stergiou C, Siganos D (2004) Neural networks. www.doc.ic.ac.uk. Accessed 15 Dec 2011

Stock A, Rogers MS, Li A, Chang AM (1994) Use of neural networks for hypothesis generation in fetal surveillance. Baillieres Clin Obstet Gynaecol 8:533–548

Wnek J, Michalski RS (1994) Hypothesis driven constructive induction in AQ17-HCI: a method and experiments. Mach Learn 14:139–168

Zernikow B, Holtmannspotter K, Michel E, Theilhaber M, Pielemeier W, Hennecke KH (1998) Artificial neural network for predicting intracranial haemorrhage in preterm neonates. Acta Paediatr 87:969–975

Zernikow B, Holtmannspotter K, Michel E, Hornschuh F, Groote K, Hennecke KH (1999) Predicting length of stay in preterm neonates. Eur J Pediatr 158:59–62

Chapter 59
Fuzzy Logic

1 Introduction

Lofti Zadeh, professor of science at Berkeley, published in 1964 the concept of fuzzy truths, as answers that may be "yes" at one time and "no" at the other, or that may be partially true and partially untrue (Zadeh 1965). He developed an analytical model based on this concept. When you think of real life, you can imagine many things that are not entirely certain, and it is remarkable, therefore, that it took over 20 years before this analytical model became successfully implemented in science (Zadeh 1965). Nowadays Tokyo subway traffic uses fuzzy logic running and braking systems, and Maserati sportscars have a fuzzy logic automatic transmission with one position for forward instead of the usual three or four, and with much better performance (Hirota 1993).

In the field of medicine fuzzy logic is little used in spite of the, typically, uncertain character of this branch of science. When searching for published papers we found a few papers on diagnostic imaging (Fournier et al. 2003) and clinical decision analysis (Catto et al. 2003; Bates and Young 2003; Caudrelier et al. 2004). In clinical pharmacology fuzzy logic has been applied for pharmacological treatment decision analyses (Naranjo et al. 1997; Helgason and Jobe 2005; Helgason 2004), and structure-activity modeling (Russo and Santagati 1998). However, we found no papers on fuzzy logic and pharmacodynamic modeling. Often the basic molecular mode of action of a drug is unknown, and pharmacodynamics is, then, used as a surrogate for studying the pharmacological response to a drug of the body. By its very nature pharmacodynamics can be argued to be particularly fuzzy. For example, the answer to the question "does a patient respond or not to a particular thiopental induction dose", or questions like "does propranolol cause the same effects at the same time in the same subject or not" are typically questions of a fuzzy nature, and might, thus, benefit from an analysis based on fuzzy logic.

In the present chapter we study whether fuzzy logic can improve the precision of predictive models for pharmacodynamic data, i.e., models that better fit the observed

T.J. Cleophas and A.H. Zwinderman, *Statistics Applied to Clinical Studies*,
DOI 10.1007/978-94-007-2863-9_59, © Springer Science+Business Media B.V. 2012

data, and, thus, better predict future data. We hope that the examples given will stimulate researchers analyzing pharmacodynamic data to more often apply fuzzy methodologies.

2 Some Fuzzy Terminology

Universal space.
Defined range of input values, defined range of output values.

Fuzzy memberships.
The universal spaces are divided into equally sized parts called membership functions

Linguistic membership names.
Each fuzzy membership is given a name, otherwise called linguistic term.

Triangular fuzzy sets.
A common way of drawing the membership function with on the x-axis the input values, on the y-axis the membership grade for each input value.

Fuzzy plots.
Graphs summarizing the fuzzy memberships of (for example) the input values (Fig. 59.2 upper graph).

Linguistic rules.
The relationships between the fuzzy memberships of the input data and those of the output data (the method of calculation is shown in the underneath examples).

3 First Example, Dose–Response Effects of Thiopental on Numbers of Responders

We will use as an example the quantal pharmacodynamic effects of different induction dosages of thiopental on numbers of responding subjects (Table 59.1, left two columns). It is usually not possible to know what type of statistical distribution the experiment is likely to follow, sometimes Gaussian, sometimes very skewed. A pleasant aspect of fuzzy modeling is that it can be applied with any type of statistical distribution and that it is particularly suitable for uncommon and unexpected non linear relationships. Quantal response data are often presented in the literature as S-shape dose-cumulative response curves with the dose plotted on a logarithmic scale, where the log transformation has an empirical basis. We will, therefore, use a logarithmic regression model. SPSS Statistical Software 17.0 (2011) is used for analysis.

Table 59.1 Quantal pharmacodynamic effects of different induction dosages of thiopental on numbers of responding subjects

Input values	Output values	Fuzzy-modeled output
Induction dosage of thiopental (mg/kg)	Numbers of responders (n)	Numbers of responders (n)
1	4	4
1.5	5	5
2	6	8
2.5	9	10
3	12	12
3.5	17	14
4	17	16
4.5	12	14
5	9	12

Command: Analyze…regression…curve estimation…dependent variable: data second column…independent variable: data first column…logarithmic…ok.

The analysis produces a moderate fit of the data (Fig. 59.1 upper curve) with an r-square value of 0.555 (F-value 8.74, p-value 0.024).

We, subsequently, fuzzy-model the input and output relationships (Fig. 59.2).
First of all, we create linguistic rules for the input and output data.
For that purpose we divide the universal space of the input variable into fuzzy memberships with linguistic membership names:

input-*zero, -small, -medium, -big, -superbig.*

Then we do the same for the output variable:

output-*zero, -small, -medium, -big.*

Subsequently, we create linguistic rules.
Figure 59.2 shows that input-*zero* consists of the values 1 and 1.5.

The value 1 (100% membership) has 4 as outcome value (100% membership of output-*zero*).
The value 1.5 (50% membership) has 5 as outcome value (75% membership of output-*zero*, 25% of output-*small*).

The input-*zero* produces $100\% \times 100\% + 50\% \times 75\% = 137.5\%$ membership to output-*zero*, and $50\% \times 25\% = 12.5\%$ membership to output-*small*, and so, output-*zero* is the most important output contributor here, and we forget about the small contribution of output-*small*.
Input-*small* is more complex, it consists of the values 1.5, and 2.0, and 2.5.

The value 1.5 (50% membership) has 5 as outcome value (75% membership of output-*zero*, 25% membership of output-*small*).
The value 2.0 (100% membership) has 6 as outcome value (50% membership of outcome-*zero*, and 50% membership of output-*small*).

Fig. 59.1 Pharmacodynamic relationship between induction dose of thiopental (x-axis, mg/kg) and number of responders (y-axis). The un-modeled curve (*upper curve*) fits the data less well than does the modeled (*lower curve*) with r-square values of 0.555 (F-value = 8.74), and 0.852 (F-value = 40.34) respectively

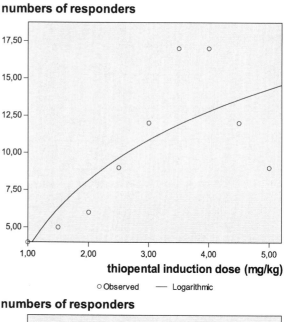

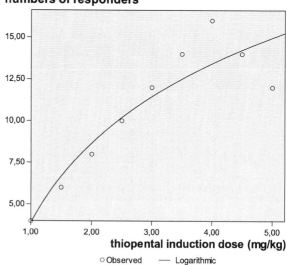

The value 2.5 (50% membership) has 9 as outcome value (75% membership of output-*small* and 25% of output-*medium*).

The input-*small* produces $50\% \times 75\% + 100\% \times 50\% = 87.5\%$ membership to output-*zero*, $50\% \times 25\% + 100\% \times 50\% + 50\% \times 75\% = 100\%$ membership to output-*small*,

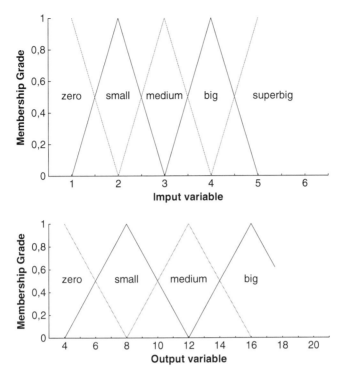

Fig. 59.2 Fuzzy plots summarizing the fuzzy memberships of the input values (*upper graph*) and output values (*lower graph*) from the thiopental data (Table 59.1 and Fig. 59.1)

and $50\% \times 25\% = 12.5\%$ membership to output-*medium*. And so, the output-*small* is the most important contributor here, and we forget about the other two.

For the other input memberships similar linguistic rules are determined:

Input-*medium* → output-*medium*
Input-*big* → output-*big*
Input-*superbig* → output-*medium*

We are, particularly interested in the modeling capacity of fuzzy logic in order to improve the precision of pharmacodynamic modeling.

The modeled output value of input value 1 is found as follows.

Value 1 is 100% member of input-*zero*, meaning that according to the above linguistic rules it is also associated with a 100% membership of output-*zero* corresponding with a value of 4.

Value 1.5 is 50% member of input-*zero* and 50% input-*small*. This means it is 50% associated with the output-*zero* and –*small* corresponding with values of $50\% \times (4 + 8) = 6$.

For all of the input values modeled output values can be found in this way. Table 59.1 right column shows the results. We perform a logarithmic regression on the fuzzy-modeled outcome data similar to that for the un-modeled output values. The fuzzy-modeled output data provided a much better fit than did the un-modeled output values (Fig. 59.2, lower curve) with an r-square value of 0.852 (F-value = 40.34) as compared to 0.555 (F-value 8.74) for the un-modeled output data.

4 Second Example, Time-Response Effect of Propranolol on Peripheral Arterial Flow

The pharmacodynamic effect of a single oral dose of 120 mg of propranolol on peripheral arterial is used as a second example (Table 59.2 left two columns). The magnitude of the pharmacodynamic response is estimated as absolute change of fore arm flow using a venous occlusion plethysmograph. Like with quantal dose response curves it is, usually, impossible to know what statistical distribution the curves are likely to follow. This is no problem for fuzzy modeling. But we use a quadratic regression model (second order model), because it is the simplest model after the linear model and fits many nonlinear data. SPSS Statistical Software 17.0 (2010) is used for analysis.

Command: Analyze...regression...curve estimation...dependent variable: data second column...independent variable: data first column...quadratic...ok.

The analysis produces a good fit of the data (Fig. 59.3 upper graph) with an r-square value as large as 0.977 with an F-value of 168.

Table 59.2 Time-response effect of single oral dose of 120 mg propranolol on peripheral arterial flow

Input values	Output values	Fuzzy-modeled output
Hours after oral administration of 120 mg propranolol	Peripheral arterial flow (ml/100 ml tissue/min)	Peripheral arterial flow (ml/100 ml tissue/min)
1	20	20
2	12	14
3	9	8
4	6	6
5	5	4
6	4	4
7	5	4
8	6	6
9	9	8
10	12	14
11	20	20

fore arm flow (ml/100ml tissue/min)

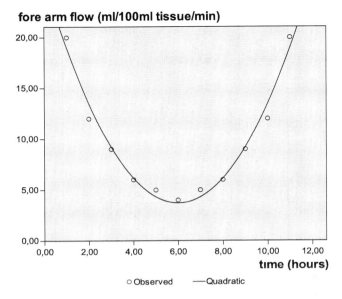

fore arm flow (ml/100ml tissue/min)

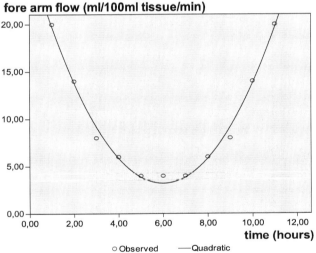

Fig. 59.3 Pharmacodynamic relationship between the time after oral administration of 120 mg of propranolol (x-axis, hours) and absolute change in fore arm flow (y-axis, ml/100 ml tissue/min). The un-modeled curve (upper curve) fits the data slightly less well than does the modeled (lower curve) with r-square values of 0.977 (F-value=168), and 0.990 (F-value=416) respectively

We, subsequently, fuzzy-model the input and output relationships.

First of all, we create linguistic rules for the input and output data.

For that purpose we divide the universal space of the input variable into fuzzy memberships with linguistic membership names:

input-*null, -zero, -small, -medium, -big, -superbig.*

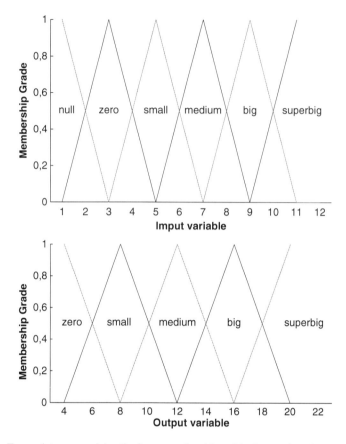

Fig. 59.4 Fuzzy plots summarizing the fuzzy memberships of the input values (*upper graph*) and output values (*lower graph*) from the propranolol data (Table 59.2 and Fig. 59.3)

Then we do the same for the output variable:

    output-*zero, -small, -medium, -big, -superbig.*

Subsequently, we will create linguistic rules.

Input-*null* consists of the values 1 and 2 (Fig. 59.4).

The value 1 (100% membership) has 20 as outcome value (100% membership of output-*superbig*)

The value 2 (50% membership) has 12 as outcome value (100% membership of output-*medium*).

    The input-*null* produces $100\% \times 100\% = 100\%$ membership to output-*superbig*, $50\% \times 100\% = 50\%$ membership to output-*medium*. And so, output-*superbig* is the most important contributor here, we forget about the other one.

Input-*zero* consists of the values 2,3,4.

The value 2 (50% membership) has 12 as outcome value (100% membership of output-*medium*).

The value 3 (100% membership) has 9 as outcome value (75% membership of outcome-*small*, and 25% membership of output-*medium*).

The value 4 (50% membership) has 6 as outcome value (50% membership of output-*small* and 50% of output-*zero*).

The input-*zero* produces $50\% \times 100\% + 100\% \times 25\% = 125\%$ membership to output-*medium*, $100\% \times 75\% + 50\% \times 50\% = 100\%$ membership to output-*small*, and $50\% \times 50\% = 25\%$ membership to output-*zero*. And so, output-*medium* is the most important contributor here, and we forget about the other two.

For the other input memberships similar linguistic rules are determined:

Input-*small* → output-*zero*
Input-*medium* → output-*zero*
Input-*big* → output-*small*
Input-*superbig* → output-*superbig*

We are, particularly, interested in the modeling capacity of fuzzy logic in order to improve the precision of pharmacodynamic modeling.

The modeled output value of input value 1 is found as follows.

Value 1 is 100% member of input-*null*, meaning that according to the above linguistic rules it is also associated with a 100% membership of output-*superbig* corresponding with a value of 20.

Value 2 is 50% member of input-*null* and 50% input-*zero*. This means it is 50% associated with the output-*superbig* and –*small* corresponding with values of $50\% \times (8+20) = 14$.

For all of the input values modeled output values can be found in this way. Table 59.2 right column shows the results. When performing a quadratic regression on the fuzzy-modeled outcome data similar to that shown above, the fuzzy-modeled output values provided a better fit than did the un-modeled output values (Fig. 59.3, upper and lower curves) with r-square values of 0.990 (F-value=416) and 0.977 (F-value=168).

5 Discussion

Biological processes are full of variations. Statistical analyses do not provide certainties, only chances, particularly, the chances that prior hypotheses are true or untrue. Fuzzy statistics is different from conventional statistical methods, because it does not asses the chance of entire truths, but, rather, the presence of partial truths. The advantage of fuzzy statistics compared to conventional statistics is that it can answer questions to which the answers are "yes" and "no" at different times, or partly "yes" and "no" at the same time. Additional advantages are that it can be used to match any set of in- and output data, including incomplete and imprecise data, and nonlinear functions of unknown complexity as sometimes observed with pharmacodynamic data. The current paper suggests, indeed, that fuzzy logic may better fit and, thus, better predict pharmacodynamic data than conventional methods.

We have only shown the simplest method of fuzzy modeling with a single input and a single output variable. Just like with multiple regression, multiple input variables are possible, and are capable of adequately modeling complex chemical and engineering processes (Ross 2004). To date, complex fuzzy models are rarely applied in medicine, but one recent clinical study successfully used 10 input variables including sex, age, smoking, and clinical grade, to predict tumor relapse time (Catto et al. 2003). The problem is that such calculations soon get very complex and can not be carried out on a pocket calculator like in our examples. Statistical software is required. Fuzzy logic is not yet widely available in statistical software programs, and it is not in SPSS (2011) or SAS (2011), but several user-friendly programs do exist (FuzzyLogic 2011; Fuzzy logic 2011; Defuzzification methods 2011).

We conclude.

1. Fuzzy logic is different from conventional statistical methods, because it does not asses the chance of entire truths but rather the presence of partial truths.
2. The advantage of fuzzy statistics compared to conventional statistics is that it can answer questions to which the answers are "yes" and "no" at different times, or partly "yes" and "no" at the same time.
3. Additional advantages are that it can be used to match any set of in- and output data, including incomplete and imprecise data, and nonlinear functions of unknown complexity as sometimes observed with pharmacodynamic data.
4. Fuzzy modeling may better than conventional statistical methods fit and predict quantal dose response and time response data.

We hope that the examples given will stimulate researchers analyzing pharmacodynamic data to more often apply fuzzy methodologies.

6 Conclusions

Fuzzy logic can handle questions to which the answers may be "yes" at one time and "no" at the other, or may be partially true and untrue. Pharmacodynamic data deal with questions like "does a patient respond to a particular drug dose or not", or "does a drug cause the same effects at the same time in the same subject or not". Such questions are typically of a fuzzy nature, and might, therefore, benefit from an analysis based on fuzzy logic. This chapter assesses whether fuzzy logic can improve the precision of predictive models for pharmacodynamic data.

1. The quantal pharmacodynamic effects of different induction dosages of thiopental on numbers of responding subjects was used as the first example. Regression analysis of the fuzzy-modeled outcome data on the input data provided a much

better fit than did the un-modeled output values with r-square values of 0.852 (F-value = 40.34) and 0.555 (F-value 8.74) respectively.

2. The time-response effect propranolol on peripheral arterial flow was used as a second example. Regression analysis of the fuzzy-modeled outcome data on the input data provided a better fit than did the un-modeled output values with r-square values of 0.990 (F-value = 416) and 0.977 (F-value = 168) respectively.

We conclude that fuzzy modeling may better than conventional statistical methods fit and predict pharmacodynamic data, like, for example, quantal dose response and time response data. This may be relevant to future pharmacodynamic research.

References

Bates JH, Young MP (2003) Applying fuzzy logic to medical decision making in the intensive care. Am J Respir Crit Care Med 167:948–952

Catto JW, Linckens DA, Abbod MF, Chen M, Burton JL, Feeley KM, Hamdy FC (2003) Artificial intelligence in predicting bladder cancer outcome: a comparison of fuzzy modelling and artificial intelligence. Clin Cancer Res 9:4172–4177

Caudrelier JM, Vial S, Gibon D, Kulik C, Swedko P, Boxwala A (2004) An authoring tool for fuzzy logic based decision support systems. Medinfo 9:1874–1879

Defuzzification methods. www.mathworks.com. Accessed 15 Dec 2011

Fournier C, Castelain B, Coche-Dequeant B, Rousseau J (2003) MRI definition of target volumes using logic method for three-dimensional conformal radiation therapy. Int J Radiat Oncol 55:225–233

Fuzzy logic: flexible environment for exploring fuzzy systems. www.wolfram.com. Accessed 15 Dec 2011

FuzzyLogic. fuzzylogic.sourceforge.net. Accessed 15 Dec 2011

Helgason CM (2004) The application of fuzzy logic to the prescription of antithrombotic agents in the elderly. Drugs Aging 21:731–736

Helgason CM, Jobe TH (2005) Fuzzy logic and continuous cellular automata in warfarin dosing of stroke patients. Curr Treat Options Cardiovasc Med 7:211–218

Hirota K (1993) Subway control. In: Hirota K (ed) Industrial applications of fuzzy technology. Springer, Tokyo, pp 263–269

Naranjo CA, Bremmer KE, Bazoon M, Turksen IB (1997) Using fuzzy logic to predict response to citalopram in alcohol dependence. Clin Pharmacol Ther 62:209–224

Ross J (2004) Fuzzy logic with engineering applications, 2nd edn. Wiley, Chichester

Russo M, Santagati NA (1998) Medicinal chemistry and fuzzy logic. Inform Sci 105:299–314

SAS Statistical Software. www.SAS.com. Accessed 15 Dec 2011

SPSS Statistical Software. www.SPSS.com. Accessed 15 Dec 2011

Zadeh LA (1965) Fuzzy sets. Inf Control 8:338–353

Chapter 60
Physicians' Daily Life and the Scientific Method

1 Introduction

Physicians' daily life largely consists of routine, with little need for discussion. However, there are questions physicians simply do not know the answer of. Some will look for the opinions of their colleagues or the experts in the field. Others will try and find a way out by guessing what might be the best solution. The benefit of the doubt doctrine (Ordronaux 1869) is often used as a justification for unproven treatment decisions, and, if things went wrong, another justification is the expression: clinical medicine is an error-ridden activity (Paget 1990). So far, few physicians have followed a different approach, the scientific method. The scientific method is, in a nutshell: reformulate your question into a hypothesis and try to test this hypothesis against control observations. In clinical settings this approach is not impossible, but rarely applied by physicians, despite their lengthy education in evidence based medicine, which is almost entirely based on the scientific method. This chapter was written to give simple examples of how the scientific method can be implied in a physician's daily life, and to explain its advantages and limitations. We do hope that this chapter will stimulate physicians to more often apply the scientific method for a better outline of their patients' best possible treatment options.

2 Example of Unanswered Questions of a Physician During a Single Busy Day

We assumed the numbers of unanswered questions in the physicians' daily life would be large. But just to get of impression, one of the authors of this paper (TC) recorded all of the unanswered answers he asked himself during a single busy day. Excluding the questions with uncertain but generally accepted answers, he included nine questions.

During the hospital rounds 8.00–12.00 h.

1. Do I continue, stop or change antibiotics with fever relapse after 7 days treatment?
2. Do I prescribe a secondary prevention of a venous thrombosis for 3, 6 months or permanently?
3. Should I stop anticoagulant treatment or continue with a hemorrhagic complication in a patient with an acute lung embolia?
4. Is the rise in falling out of bed lately real or due to chance?
5. Do I perform a liver biopsy or wait and see with liver function disturbance without obvious cause?

During the outpatient clinic 13.00–17.00 h.

6. Do I prescribe aspirin, hydroxy-carbamide or wait and see in a patient with a thrombocytosis of $800 \times 10^{12}/l$ over 6 months?
7. Are fundic gland polyps much more common in females than in males?

During the staff meeting 17.00–18.00 h

8. Is the large number of physicians with burn out due to chance or the result of a local problem?
9. Is the rise in patients' letters of complaints a chance effect or a real effect to worry about?

Many of the above questions did not qualify for a simple statistical assessment, but others did. The actual assessments, that were very clarifying for our purposes, are given underneath.

3 How the Scientific Method Can Be Implied in a Physician's Daily Life

3.1 Falling Out of Bed

Falling out of bed is the prime cause of injury in hospitalized patients, and the prevention of it is a high priority and criterion for quality care (Lambert 1992; Anonymous 2001). If more patients fall out of bed than expected, a hospital department will put much energy in finding the cause and providing better prevention. If, however, the scores tend to rise, another approach is to first assess whether or not the rise is due to chance, because daily life is full of variations. To do so the numbers of events observed is compared the numbers of event in a sister department. The pocket calculator method is a straightforward method for that purpose.

	Patients with fall out of bed	Patients without	
Department 1	16 (a)	26 (b)	42 (a+b)
Department 2	5 (c)	30 (d)	35 (c+d)
	21 (a+c)	56 (b+d)	77 (a+b+c+d)

Pocket calculator method:

$$\text{chi - square} = \frac{(ad-bc)^2\,(a+b+c+d)}{(a+b)(c+d)(b+d)(a+c)} = 5.456.$$

If the chi-square value is larger than 3.841, then a statistically significant difference between the two departments will be accepted at $p<0.05$. This would mean that in this example, indeed, the difference is larger than could be expected by chance and that a further examination of the measures to prevent fall out of bed is warranted.

3.2   Evaluation of Fundic Gland Polyps

A physician has the impression that fundic gland polyps, an otherwise rather benign condition, are more common in females than it is in males. Instead of reporting this subjective finding, he decides to follow the next 2 months every patient in his program.

	Patients with fundic gland polyps	Patients without	
Females	15 (a)	20 (b)	35 (a+b)
Males	15 (c)	5 (d)	20 (c+d)
	30 (a+c)	25 (b+d)	55 (a+b+c+d)

Pocket calculator method:

$$\text{chi - square} = \frac{(ad-bc)^2\,(a+b+c+d)}{(a+b)(c+d)(b+d)(a+c)} = 5.304$$

The calculated chi-square value is again larger than 3.841. The difference between males and females is significant at $p<0.05$. We can be for about 95% sure that the difference between the genders is real and not due to chance. The physician can report to his colleagues that the difference in genders is to be taken into account in future work-ups.

3.3   Physicians with a Burn-Out

Two partnerships of specialists have the intention to associate. However, during meetings, it was communicated that in one of the two partnerships there were three specialists with burn-out. The meeting decided not to consider this as chance finding, but requested a statistical analysis of this finding under the assumption that unknown factors in partnership 1 may place these specialists at an increased risk of obtaining a burn-out.

	Physicians with burn out	Without burn out	
Partnership 1	3 (a)	7 (b)	10 (a+b)
Partnership 2	0 (c)	10 (d)	10 (c+d)
	3 (a+c)	17 (b+d)	20 (a+b+c+d)

Pocket calculator method

$$\text{chi - square} = \frac{(ad - bc)^2 \ (a+b+c+d)}{(a+b)(c+d)(b+d)(a+c)} = \frac{(30-0)2(20)}{10 \times 10 \times 17 \times 3} = \frac{900 \times 20}{\cdots\cdots} = 3.6$$

The chi-square value was between 2.706 and 3.841. This means that no significant difference between the two partnerships exists, but there is a trend to a difference at $p < 0.10$. This was communicated back to the meeting and it was decided to disregard the trend. Ten years later no further case of burn-out had been observed.

3.4   Patients' Letters of Complaints

In a hospital the number of patients' letters of complaints was twice the number in the period before. The management was deeply worried and issued an in-depth analysis of possible causes. One junior manager recommended that prior to this laborious exercise it might be wise to first test whether the increase might be due to chance rather than a real effect.

	Patients with letter of complaints	Patients without	
Year 2006	10 (a)	1,000 (b)	1,010 (a+b)
Year 2005	5 (c)	1,000 (d)	1,005 (c+d)
	15 (a+c)	2,000 (b+d)	2,015 (a+b+c+d)

$$\text{chi - square} = \frac{(ad - bc)^2 \ (a+b+c+d)}{(a+b)(c+d)(b+d)(a+c)} = 1.64..$$

The chi-square was smaller than 2.706, and so the difference could not be ascribed to any effect to worry about but rather to chance. No further analysis of the differences between 2006 and 2005 were performed.

There are of course many questions in physicians' daily life that are less straightforward and cannot be readily answered with a pocket calculator. For example, the effects of subgroups and other covariates in a patient group will require t-tests, analyses of variance, likelihood ratio tests, and regression models. Fortunately, in the past 15 years user-friendly statistical software (SPSS 2011; S plus 2011; StatsDirect 2011; StatXact 2011; True Epistat 2011; BUGS y WinBUGS 2011; SAS 2011; Cleophas et al. 2002) and self-assessment programs (Cleophas et al. 2002) have been developed that can help answering complex questions. Nowadays, many clinical investigators already use them without the help of a statistician. However, we as authors of this paper are not aware of any physician who is not involved in a research program and still assesses his/her every-day questions in the way illustrated in the above examples.

4 Discussion

Since the era of Hippocrates, 500 years BC, physicians have had an ethical obligation not only to provide the best possible care for their patients but also to enhance health to the entire population. Statistical tests have been recognized to produce the best evidence you can get from your data, and physicians applying them thus serve their population in the best possible way. A second point is that most practicing physicians are not avid readers of clinical trials. The information of new treatments is, instead, often brought to them by the media, the pharmaceutical industry and even the patients. This is not necessarily a criticism of well-trained and hard-working doctors. The problem is that the language of the published reports is such that physicians are almost as lost as a layperson, particularly, when it comes to the core sections of the report, the statistical analysis and result sections. It follows that either the results are accepted with too little of scepticism or rejected with too much of it. Particularly, the former may take place if a pharmaceutical representative communicates overstated the benefits and understated the risks. Being actively involved in the scientific method is a strong antidote against these hazards. Also, physicians start better reading the published clinical research and understanding its strengths and limitations, and, most important, its implications to health.

Do we have guarantees that the result is true if statistically significant. No, but it is the best evidence from your data you can get. There is, of course, the chance of type I errors of finding an effect which is a non-effect. This chance is particularly large with multiple testing. Then there is the chance of a type II error of finding no effect where there is one. This chance is particularly large with small samples. Third, you may be mistaking because you can not predict with full confidence if your target population is older, younger, from a different gender, or from any other sampling distribution than that of your test sample. But there are more limitations with the application of the scientific method. Hard-working doctors tend to have a full agenda, and, usually, do not have the leisure to write a study protocol, and rewrite it several times as required by their institutions' ethic committees, and find it hard to complete an entire informed consent procedure. Instead, many study protocols, particularly, those of observational studies, do not necessarily require ethic approval and written informed consent. None of the examples given needed the latter. A subsequent limitation is the limited validity of the chi-square test with samples smaller than 5. A final limitation is the possible damage in the patient-doctor relationship sometimes attributed to scientific activities in a daily practice. Indeed, many patients may expect from their doctor a more personal relationship based on thrust and sympathy, and in addition the best possible treatment. Telling a patient of the risks of being in a placebo-control group and thus receiving nothing for his condition is not a typical basis for thrust. We should add that observational studies in this context are more patient-friendly than clinical trials. At least in observational studies patients are not recruited for a randomized treatment, but rather treated following their voluntary clinical visits.

5   Conclusions

So far, few physicians have followed the scientific method for answering practical questions they simply do not know the answer of. The scientific method is, in a nutshell: reformulate your question into a hypothesis and try to test this hypothesis against control observations. This chapter gives simple examples of how the scientific method can be implied in a physician's daily life.

Of nine unanswered daily questions, four qualified for simple statistical assessments, which were very clarifying for the physicians involved. Additional advantages of the scientific method include: (1) since the scientific method has been recognized to produce the best evidence you can get from your observations, physicians applying it serve their population in the best possible way; (2) being actively involved in the scientific method is a strong antidote against the hazards of accepting published studies from others with too little of scepticism or rejecting them with too much of it.

Limitations of the scientific method include: (1) type I and II errors; (2) misinterpretations due to different frequency distributions, (3) lack of leisure time on the part of the physicians to write a study protocol, (4) the risk of a damaged patient-doctor relationship.

References

Anonymous (2001) Beds in hospital, nursing homes and home health care. Drugs Health Prod (May issue):2–6
BUGS y WinBUGS. http://www.mrc-bsu.cam.ac.uk/bugs. Accessed 15 Dec 2011
Cleophas TJ, Zwinderman AH, Cleophas TF (2002) In: Cleophas TJ (ed) Statistics applied to clinical trials: self-assessment book. Kluwer, Boston
Lambert V (1992) Improving safety, reducing use. FDA Consum (October issue):1–5
Ordronaux J (1869) The jurisprudence of medicine in relation to the law of contracts, torts and evidence. The Lawbook Exchange, LTD, Clark, London, UK
Paget MA (1990) The unity of mistakes, a phenomenological interpretation of medical work. Contemp Sociol 19:118–119

R http://cran.r-project.org SAS. http://www.prw.le.ac.uk/epidemiol/personal/ajs22/meta/macros.sas. Accessed 15 Dec 2011

S-plus. http://www.mathsoft.com/splus. Accessed 15 Dec 2011

SPSS Statistical Software. http://www.spss.com. Accessed 15 Dec 2011

StatsDirect. http://www.camcode.com. Accessed 15 Dec 2011

StatXact. http://www.cytel.com/products/statxact/statact1.html. Accessed 15 Dec 2011

True Epistat. http://ic.net/~biomware/biohp2te.htm. Accessed 15 Dec 2011

Chapter 61
Incident Analysis and the Scientific Method

1   Introduction

In the past two decades incidents in clinical care are increasingly analyzed in a systematic manner in order to establish organisational, technical and human causal factors responsible. Initially experts tended to look for an event directly preceding the incident, and, subsequently, declared it as the most probable cause. Meanwhile, this method has been largely superseded, because experts often disagreed, and came to the insight that many incidents are caused by a cascade of events. For example, a fatal hemorrhage in hospital can, doubtlessly, be caused by an overdose of anticoagulant treatment, but in many situations more factors are possible, including a weakened patient's condition, an operational error, concomitant morbidities and medications, a wrong dosage time, a wrong laboratory test, a flawed treatment such as a delayed transfusion policy etc.

The PRISMA (Prevention and Recovery System for Monitoring and Analysis) (www.medsight.nl) -, CIA (Critical Incident Analysis) (www.healthsystem.virginia. edu/Internet/ciag/) -, CIT (Critical Incident Technique) (www.en.wikipedia.org/ wiki/Critical_Incident_Technique) -, TRIPOD (method based on the so-called tripod-theory that looks at underlying organisational factors) (www.tripodsolutions.net) – methods are modern approaches to incident – analysis, generally providing seven or more usable causes for explaining a single incident. Health facilities routinely use them in their struggle for improved health care quality, and are, in this way, able to adjust treatment protocols and treatment policies for the obtained results from such incident – analyses. This could mean in the given example: in future a lower dosage of anticoagulant treatment, only in patients without co – morbidities, no more operation of the same kind or, alternatively, an operation of a more safe type, another dosage time of medication, double-checks on laboratory errors, rewriting treatment protocols etc. It is clear that each one of these measures, however well-intentioned, can also lead to deleterious effects. For, lower dosages will lead to more morbidity, thromboses in the given example, other operations will lead to new complications, double checks will lead to overburdening and loss of sight on the

T.J. Cleophas and A.H. Zwinderman, *Statistics Applied to Clinical Studies*,
DOI 10.1007/978-94-007-2863-9_61, © Springer Science+Business Media B.V. 2012

part of the health professionals, and, subsequently, to new human errors etc. It is remarkable that the above – mentioned methods of incident – analysis ignore categorically the so-called scientific method, which, otherwise, is quite well used for health care questions for which there is no simple answer. The scientific method consists, in a nutshell, of reformulating your question into a hypothesis, and, subsequently, trying to test this hypothesis against control observations (Anonymous 2011). It is unclear to the writers of this chapter why the scientific method has been systematically ignored in incident – analysis. This was the most important reason for writing this chapter.

2   The Scientific Method in Incident-Analysis

As an example we will use the case of the fatal hemorrhage in a hospital during an observational period of 1 year. In case of a fatal hemorrhage the physician in charge of the analysis will first make an inventory of how many fatal hemorrhages of the same kind have occurred in the period of 1 year. The number seems to be ten.

The null – hypothesis is that 0 hemorrhages will occur per year, and the question is whether 10 is significantly more than 0. A one – sample – z – test is used for that purpose: $z = 10/\sqrt{10} = 3.16$. This z – value is larger than 3.080. It means that the p – value is <0.002, and that the number 10 is, thus, much larger than a number that could occur by accident. Here an avoidable error could very well be responsible. However, a null – hypothesis of 0 hemorrhages is probably not correct, because a year without fatal hemorrhages, actually, never happens, not even if health care quality was optimal. Therefore, we will compare the number of fatal hemorrhages in the given year with that of the year before. There were five fatal hemorrhages then. The z – test produces the following result: $z = (10-5)/\sqrt{(10+5)} = 1.29$ This result is not statistically significant, because z is <1.96.

We can, however, question whether both years are representative for a longer period of time. Epidemiological data have established that an incident-reduction of 70% is possible with optimal quality health care. We test whether 10 is significantly different from $(10 - (70\%) \times 10) = 3$. The z-test now shows that $z = (10-3)/\sqrt{(10+3)} = 1.94$, which is just below the value of 1.96. It means that here also no significant effect has been demonstrated.

A more sensitive mode of testing will be obtained, if we take into account the entire number of admissions per year. In the given hospital there were 10,000 admissions in either of the 2 years. A chi-square test can now be performed according to the 2×2 contingency table in Table 61.1. With one degree of freedom this value ought to have been at least 3.84 in order to demonstrate whether a significant difference is in the data. And, so, again there is no significant difference between the 2 years.

Finally, a log – likelihood – ratio – test is performed, a test which falls into the category of exact – tests, and is, therefore, still somewhat more sensitive. The result is in Table 61.2. It is close to 3.84, but still somewhat smaller. Also this test shows

Table 61.1 Rates of fatal hemorrhages in a hospital during 2 subsequent years of observation

	Year 1	Year 2
Number fatal hemorrhages	10	5
Number control patients	9,990	9,995

$$\text{Chi - square} = \frac{(10 \times 9995 + 5 \times 9990)^2 \, (20000)}{10 \times 9990 + 5 \times 9995} = 1.62$$

According to the chi-square statistic <3.84 the difference in rates is not significant

Table 61.2 Log – likelihood – ratio – test of the data from Table 61.1. Also this test is not significant with a chi-square value smaller than 3.84

$$\text{Log - likelihood - ratio} = 5 \log\left(\frac{10/9990}{5/9995}\right) + 9995 \log\left(\frac{1-10/9990}{1-5/9995}\right)$$

$$= 3.468200 - 5.008856 = -1.540656$$

$$\text{Chi - square} = -2 \log - \text{likelihood - ratio} = 3.0813$$

log natural logarithm

no significant difference between the frequencies of deadly fatal hemorrhages in the 2 years of observation. Based on the above analyses the conclusion is justified, that the hemorrhages are more due to random factors than avoidable ones. Biological processes are full of variations, and fatal events can occur sporadically without an avoidable or blameable causal factor. This would mean a great chance that a profound investigation of possibly responsible mechanisms will reveal nothing, and that changes in future treatment protocols and policies do not seem to be warranted.

The analyst in charge takes the decision to perform one last test, making use of epidemiological data that have shown that with optimal health care quality in a facility similar to ours we may accept with 95% confidence that the number of fatal hemorrhages will remain below 17 per 10,000 admissions. With 10 deadly bleedings the 95% confidence interval can be calculated to be 10 ± 6.20, and, thus, between 3.80 and 16.2. This result is just under 17. Also from this analysis it can be concluded that a profound research of the fatal hemorrhages is not warranted. The number of hemorrhages falls under the boundary of optimal quality care.

3 Discussion

It is not obvious to the writers of this chapter, why, so far, the scientific method has not been applied in incident – analysis of health care. Maybe that the very sophisticated PRISMA method originated from the petrochemical industry and propagated in health care circles, for example by former SHELL president Rein Willems was thought – provoking to the extent that health professionals started to think statistical analysis to be superfluous (Anonymous 2006). Of course, if you are working with extremely inflammable compounds, safety is a goal where priorities are evident, and an untested system of incident prevention can be justified. If the causal factors are obvious, then a statistical test is not required anymore. In health care terms, you do not have to statistically prove that penicillin can cure a pneumonia. Many health care effects in human beings are, however, small and multi – causal. Therefore, statistical testing is the method par excellence to demonstrate small effects and con-comitant effects. For the evaluation of therapeutic modalities this way of testing is currently considered an essential first step. We do not see why this evidence – based method can not be equally applied with incident – analysis in health care.

Moreover, there is a very dark side to the untested use of various recently devel-oped methods for incident-analysis. Mostly this incident – analysis will lead to more complex procedures at work with as many or even larger chances of incidents and lack of safety, the risk that people drop out, make new mistakes, procedures become more time – consuming and expensive.

We have to mention the limitations of the scientific method. A negative test may be due to a type II error as a consequence of lack of power. Also confounding and interaction may give rise to false positive and negative tests. Nonetheless, the scientific method, in spite of limitations of its own, can be helpful in giving a clue to which incidents are based on randomness and which ones are not.

The latter category, subsequently, deserves all attention, and a profound study and measures being taken for improvement. In this manner high quality health care can progress in a way largely parallel to the way that has been successfully applied in evidence – based medicine. In conclusion, we recommend that the scientific method be applied in incident – analysis.

4   Conclusions

Incidents in clinical care are analyzed in a systematic manner in order to establish organisational, technical and human causal factors responsible. The PRISMA (Prevention and Recovery System for Monitoring and Analysis) and other software programs are modern approaches, and produce seven or more usable causes for explaining single incidents. These methods ignore the so – called scientific method, which is well – used for other health care questions. This chapter reviews examples of how the scientific method can be implemented in incident – analysis.

Using the case of a fatal hemorrhage in hospital we demonstrate that the following tests can be used:

z – tests, chi - square tests, log likelihood ratio tests, and confidence intervals against established boundaries of high quality health care.

We conclude that there is a dark side to the untested use of current methods for incident – analysis. Mostly, it will lead to more complex procedures at work with at least similar chance of incidents, lack of safety, the risk of overburdening people causing new mistakes, procedures becoming more time – consuming and expensive. We recommend that the scientific method be applied in incident – analysis.

References

Anonymous. Scientific method. http://en.wikipedia.org/wiki/Scientific_method, Accessed 15 Dec 2011

Anonymous (2006) Safety expertise shell can make health care considerably safer. Incidents can drop by 75%. In: Getting better more rapidly. Bosboom, The Hague

Chapter 62
Clinical Trials: Superiority-Testing

1 Introduction

One of the flaws of modern statistics is that it can produce statistically significant results even if treatment effects are very small. For example, a sub-analysis of the SOLVD study (Yusuf et al. 1992) found symptoms of angina pectoris in 85.3% of the patients on enalapril and in 82.5% of the patients on placebo, difference statistically significant at $p < 0.01$. In a situation like this one has to question about the clinical relevance of the small difference. Another problem of clinical trials is that the statistics is increasingly complex, and that clinicians are at a loss to understand it. This is not, necessarily, a criticism of well-trained and hard-working doctors, but it does have a very dark side. Studies are, generally, accepted if the magic p-values are <0.05, and the disappointment about the small benefit to individual patients comes later. The problem is that a p-value of 0.05 means that the power of finding a true positive effect is only 50%, and, more important, the chance of not finding it is equally 50%. Such a result is hardly acceptable for reliable testing.

The objectives of the current chapter were (1) to give some examples of studies that have been published as unequivocally positive studies, although the treatment effects were substantially smaller than they were expected to be, (2) to introduce superiority-testing as a novel statistical approach avoiding the risk of statistically significant but clinically irrelevant results. Superiority-testing defines a priori in the protocol clinically relevant boundaries of superiority of the new treatment. If the 95% confidence interval of the study result is entirely within the boundary, then superiority is accepted, and we do not have to worry about the p-values anymore.

T.J. Cleophas and A.H. Zwinderman, *Statistics Applied to Clinical Studies*,
DOI 10.1007/978-94-007-2863-9_62, © Springer Science+Business Media B.V. 2012

2   Examples of Studies Not Meeting Their Expected Powers

The Lancet publishes benchmark research. We extracted from recent volumes of the Lancet six original articles of controlled clinical trials that were reported as being positive studies, although they did not meet their expected power. The studies produced only 53–83% of the statistical power expected, while the new treatments produced only 46–86% of the magnitude of response expected (Table 62.1). For example, in the PROSPER study (Shepherd et al. 2002) the new treatment only produced half the benefit that was expected (10% instead of 20% relative reduction in events). In the Andrews study (Andrews et al. 2004) the new treatment produced less than half the benefit expected (an average of 1.6 instead of 3.5 months of survival). These results, although statistically significant at the $p < 0.05$ level, may not unequivocally demonstrate clinical superiority, and may not be good enough for accepting the new treatment for general use.

Table 62.1 Discrepancies between expected and observed statistical powers and treatment efficacies of six controlled clinical trials recently published in the Lancet

Study observ	Sample size	Comparison	Expect/observ power (%)	Expect/observ effect size	Observ p-value
1. PPP study (Collaborative Group of Primary Prevention Project 2001)	4,495	Aspirin vs placebo	90/48	From 5.4% to 2.9%/absolute risk reduction from 2.8% to 2.0%	0.055[a]
2. Staedke et al. (2001)	400	Amiodiaquine vs sulfadioxine-pyrimethamine	80/66	15%/7% absolute reduction treatment failures	0.023[b]
3. PROSPER (Shepherd et al. 2002)	5,804	Statin vs placebo	92/73	20%/10% relative reduction events	0.015
4. ESTEEM (Wallenstein et al. 2003)	1,883	Ximelagatran vs warfarin	80/56	27%/22% relative reduction events	0.036
5. Jochan et al. (2004)	379	Adjuvant chemother vs no	90/63	2.10/1.58 hazard ratios	0.020
6. Andrews et al. (2004)	333	Stereotactic radiosurgery vs no	80/53	3.5/1.6 months of survival	0.040

vs versus, *expect* expected; *observ* observed, *chemother* chemotherapy

[a]composite endpoint, this study was yet reported as a positive study, because separate endpoints were significant at 0.035–0.049

[b]the largest difference of the three main endpoints, the other two were not significant

3 How to Assess Clinical Superiority

The PROSPER study (Shepherd et al. 2002) included 5,804 patients to test whether in elderly pravastatin performed better than placebo in preventing cardiovascular morbidity/mortality. The sample size in this study was based on an expected statistical power of 92% to observe a relative reduction of events of 20% (absolute reduction of 3.2%) with an absolute risk of events of 16% at baseline. Statistical power can be best described as the chance of finding a significant effect in your data, if there is a real effect. It means that the expected chance that any real effect in the data is not detected (the type II error) is only 8%. However, it turned out that the relative reduction in events was only 10% (absolute reduction 1.6%).

Figures 62.1, 62.2, and 62.3 give the relationships between statistical power, p-values, and t-values (two-sided t-tests with samples sizes >200). The curves are approximately similar to the curves for the z-test (the test for normal distributions). T-values can be best interpreted as standardized measures of treatment efficacy; t-values larger than approximately 2 SEMs (standard errors of the mean) indicate that there is a significant effect at $p < 0.05$ in the data. From the Figs. 62.1, 62.2, and 62.3 it can be extrapolated that the main endpoint result of the PROSPER study corresponded with a power of only 73%, instead of 92%, and, consequently, a type II error of 27% instead of the expected 8%. In spite of this disappointing result, the study reported that an unequivocal superiority of the new treatment had been demonstrated. However, the risk reduction observed was only half that expected, and the chance of a type II error of finding no difference next time, was 3.4 times that expected. This may not be good enough a result for implementing the new treatment, particularly not, if potential adverse effects of the new treatment are taken into account.

Traditionally, in clinical trials a significant efficacy of a new treatment is accepted if the null-hypothesis of no treatment effect is rejected at $p = 0.05$, corresponding with a type II error of no less than 50%. This would mean for the PROSPER study a relative risk reduction of only approximately 5% (absolute risk reduction of 0.7%), which is not what one would call an impressive result. Instead of a p-value of 0.05 as cut-off criterion for demonstrating superiority a stricter criterion seems to be welcome. For that purpose an approach similar to that of equivalence-testing and non-inferiority-testing may be applied (Fig. 62.4, upper two graphs). With equivalence/non-inferiority -testing we have prior arguments to assume little difference between the new treatment and control treatment, and we are more interested in similarity and non-inferiority of the new treatment versus control than in a statistically significant difference between the new treatment and control. A boundary of similarity or non-inferiority is a priori defined in the protocol. If the 95% confidence interval of the study turns out to be entirely within these boundaries, then similarity or non-inferiority is accepted.

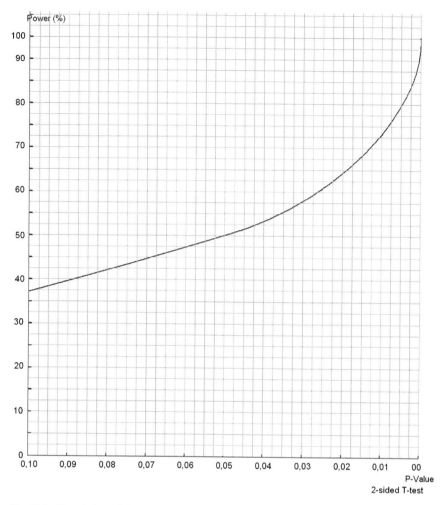

Fig. 62.1 The relationship between power and p-values (two sided *t*-test with samples sizes >200). The curve is approximately similar to the curve for the z-test (normal distribution)

Also for superiority-testing a prior boundary of superiority has to be defined in the study protocol. For example, a boundary producing 10% less the power of the study's expected power could be chosen. Figure 62.5 shows what will happen if this boundary is applied in the PROSPER study. The 95% confidence interval of the PROSPER study crosses this boundary and this means that the study is be unable to demonstrate superiority, and that the result is, therefore, negative.

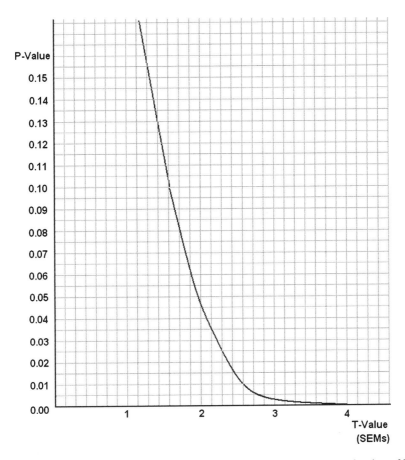

Fig. 62.2 The relationship between p-values and t-values (two sided *t*-test with samples sizes >200). The curve is approximately similar to the curve for the z-test (normal distribution)

4 Discussion

Routinely replacing the assessment of p-values with superiority testing in comparative trials will have some advantages:

1. Studies with large type II errors will no longer be interpreted as positive studies, because small and irrelevant treatment efficacies, producing large type II errors, will no longer meet the criterion of superiority.
2. The general incentive to produce as small a p-value as possible, even if the study effect is very small will be gone. Specific methods for producing small p-values have been developed. They include the use of very large samples and composite

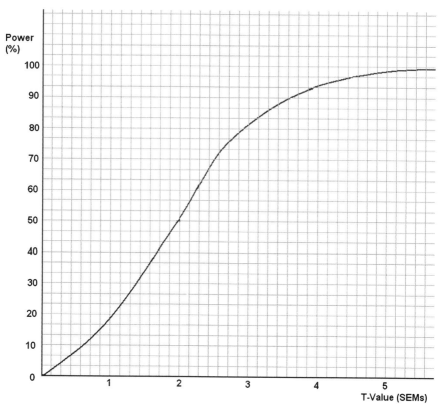

Fig. 62.3 The relationship between power and t-values (two sided *t*-test with samples sizes >200). The curve is approximately similar to the curve for the z-test (normal distribution)

endpoints. Very large samples will almost certainly show a statistically significant difference in the data, but this difference will be questionably clinically relevant. Composite endpoints produce small p-values, but are frequently complicated by large gradients in importance to patients result in misleading impressions of the impact of treatment (Ferreira-Gonzalea et al. 2007). With superiority-testing as introduced in this paper, the p-values are no longer the criterion for a positive study.

3. P-values are, traditionally, applied for testing the null-hypotheses of no effect in the data. However, in current clinical trials the issue is not *any* effect in the data, but rather a *clinically relevant* effect or not. This latter question can never be answered by null-hypothesis testing, and requires a different approach. For that purpose clinical relevance has to be quantitatively defined, e.g. in the form boundaries of superiority, as introduced in the present paper.

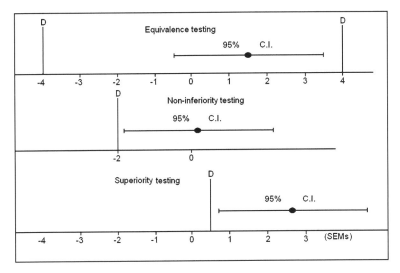

Fig. 62.4 Examples of equivalence, non-inferiority- and superiority studies: any 95% confidence interval (*C.I.*) that does not cross the pre-specified range of equivalence, inferiority, or superiority as indicated by the D boundaries presents the presence of equivalence, non-inferiority, or superiority respectively

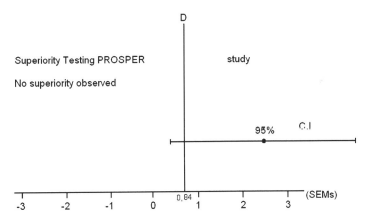

Fig. 62.5 The 95% confidence interval (*C.I.*) of the PROSPER study crosses the D boundary. With the given D boundary this study is unable to demonstrate superiority

We come to some important recommendations in this study. We recommend that investigators consider replacing testing null-hypotheses of comparative clinical trials with testing a priori defined boundaries of clinical superiority of new treatments. A similar approach is already common in equivalence-studies and non-inferiority-studies, but could very well be applied to the "normal" comparative studies usually performed for establishing the clinical superiority of one treatment over another. Nowadays, too many borderline significant studies are being reported as convincingly positive studies. This is a misleading practice as it produces overestimated expectations from new treatments (Horng and Grudy 2003; Fetting et al. 1990; Anonymous 1995). Superiority-testing, as introduced in this paper, is a simple method to avoid this problem.

5   Conclusions

One of the flaws of modern statistics is that it can produce statistically significant results even if treatment effects are very small. The objective of the current chapter was (1) To give some examples of studies that have been published as unequivocally positive studies, although the treatment effects were substantially smaller than they were expected to be. (2) To introduce superiority-testing as a novel statistical approach avoiding the risk of statistically significant but clinically irrelevant results.

We extracted from recent volumes of the Lancet six original articles of controlled clinical trials that were reported as being positive studies, although they did not meet their expected power. The studies produced only 53–83% of the statistical power expected, while the new treatments produced only 46–86% of the magnitude of response expected. Instead of a p-value of 0.05 as cut-off criterion for demonstrating superiority a stricter criterion seems to be welcome. For that purpose, similar to equivalence-testing and non-inferiority-testing, prior boundaries of superiority have to be defined in the protocol. If the 95% interval of the study turns out to be entirely within these boundaries, then superiority is accepted.

Nowadays, too many borderline significant studies are being reported as convincingly positive studies. This is a misleading practice, as it produces overestimated expectations from new treatments. Superiority-testing, as introduced in this paper, is a simple method to avoid this problem.

References

Andrews DW, Scott CB, Speranto PW et al (2004) Whole brain irradiation therapy with or without stereotactic radiosurgery boost for patients with 1–3 brain metastases. Lancet 363:1665–1672
Anonymous (1995) Patients' demands for prescriptions in primary care. Br Med J 310:1084–1085
Collaborative Group of Primary Prevention Project (2001) Low dose aspirin and vitamin E in people at cardiovascular risk: a randomised trial in general practice. Lancet 357:89–95
Ferreira-Gonzalea I, Busse JW, Heels-Ansdell D et al (2007) Problems with use of composite end points in cardiovascular trials: systematic review of randomised controlled trials. BMJ 334:786–788
Fetting JH, Siminoff CA, Piantadosi S et al (1990) Effects of patients' expectations of benefit with standard breast cancer adjuvant therapy on participants in clinical trials. J Oncol 8:1476–1482
Horng S, Grudy C (2003) Misunderstanding of clinical research. Ethics Hum Res 25:11–16

Jochan D, Richter A, Hofmann L et al (2004) Adjuvant autologous renal tumour cell vaccine and risk of tumor progression in patients with renal cell carcinoma. Lancet 362:594–599

Shepherd J, Blauw GJ, Murphy MB, et al, on behalf of the PROSPER study group (2002) Pravastatin in elderly individuals at risk of vascular disease: a randomised trial. Lancet 360:1623–1630

Staedke SG, Kanga MR, Dorsey G et al (2001) Amiodaquine, sulfadioxone/pyrimethamine and combination therapy for treatment of falciparum malaria in Kampala, Uganda: a randomised trial. Lancet 358:368–374

Wallenstein L, Wilcox RG, Weaver WD, et al, for the ESTEEM investigators (2003) Oral ximela-gatran for secondary prophylaxis after myocardial infarction. Lancet 362:789–797

Yusuf S, Pepine CJ, Garces C et al (1992) Effect of enalapril on myocardial infarction and angina pectoris in patients with low ejection fraction. Lancet 340:1173–1178

Chapter 63
Noninferiority Testing

1 Introduction

Traditionally, noninferiority studies have been designed to demonstrate that the efficacy of a new compound is not inferior to a standard compound documentedly efficacious. A major argument for performing noninferiority studies is, that a direct comparison versus placebo of the new compound is less ethical with an efficacious standard treatment already available, because half of the patients in such a trial is given an inferior treatment. The solution is given by a direct comparison of the new versus standard treatment. However, the comparison versus standard is at risk of establishing little difference, and, thus, a negative result. Non-inferiority studies are based on arbitrary margins of noninferiority. Generally, there are three possibilities (Fig. 63.1): (1) noninferiority is demonstrated, (2) it is uncertain, or (3) it is excluded, if the 95% confidence interval of a study is respectively (1) entirely on the right side of the margin of noninferiority, (2) crosses the margin, (3) is entirely left from the margin. The margin of noninferiority is of a rather subjective nature, and, usually, defined by expert investigators as the margin of undisputed clinical relevance (Mercola 2011; Snapinn 2000). From Fig. 63.1 it can be easily perceived that investigators benefit from wide margins, increasing the chance of a positive study, and that, with *very* wide margins, it becomes virtually impossible to reject noninferiority. Scientists (Mercola 2011; Snapinn 2000), statisticians (Hung and Wang 2004; Pocock 2003; Allen and Seaman 2007), and regulatory agencies (Anonymous 2011a,b) have expressed their worries about this practice. Recently, the EMEA (European Medicines Agency) has declared that noninferiority trials will not be accepted as proof of efficacy in Alzheimer's and Parkinson's trials, while the FDA (Food & Drug Administration) formally rejected the use of noninferiority trials in the development of antimicrobial drugs for chronic bronchitis (Anonymous 2011b).

T.J. Cleophas and A.H. Zwinderman, *Statistics Applied to Clinical Studies*,
DOI 10.1007/978-94-007-2863-9_63, © Springer Science+Business Media B.V. 2012

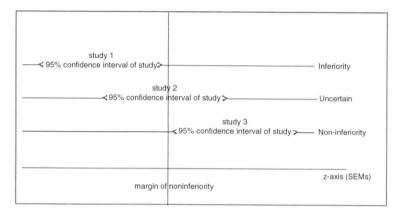

Fig. 63.1 Traditional results of noninferiority trials

In the past 4 years recommendations have been given regarding margins based on counted criteria rather than experts' view (Anonymous 2011a). Also the requirement of including various null-hypothesis tests and tests against historical placebo data have been proposed (Kaul and Diamond 2006; Piaggio et al. 2006). The current chapter reviews proposals, and shows, using data examples, how they can be readily included in the study protocol and data-analysis.

2 A Novel Approach

2.1 Basing the Margins of Noninferiority on Counted Criteria

The reason for performing a noninferiority trial is, that comparison versus placebo is less ethical, if alternative efficacious products are known. The EMEA guidelines for noninferiority margins recommends that margins of noninferiority be constructed with the help of the summaries of the information known about the relative efficacy of these known products (Anonymous 2011a). As an alternative approach the EMEA recommends to survey practitioners on the range of differences that they consider to be important, and choose the margin based on a summary statistic of their responses (Anonymous 2011b). Some flexibility is useful and can be included. For example, in the situation where a test product is anticipated to have a safety advantage over the reference product, a larger margin could be justified, as some loss of efficacy might be accepted in exchange for the safety benefit. Other circumstances which may warrant such consideration include a more convenient route of administration, more convenient posology, advantages on secondary endpoints etc.

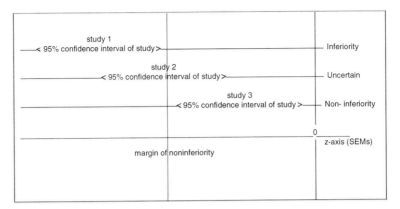

Fig. 63.2 In study 3 the presence of both noninferiority and a significant difference from zero is observed

2.2   Testing the Presence of Both Noninferiority and a Significant Difference from Zero

The result of a clinical trial is often expressed as its t-value or, with qualitative data, its z-value.

t = (mean result)/SEM,
z = (proportion of responders)/SEM,
SEM = standard error of the mean result or of the proportion of responders.

The unit of t- values is not mmol/l, or mg, etc, but rather SEM-units. SEM-units are often called standardized results of studies, and can be obtained by dividing the mean result by its standard error.

For example, a mean result of 2.4 mmol/l with an SEM of 1.2 mmol/l would produce a t-value of 2.4/1.2=2.0 SEM-units.

A t - value > 2.0 or < −2.0 SEM - units indicates a result distant from zero at $p < 0.05$
A t - value > 2.6 or < −2.6 SEM - units indicates a result distant from zero at $p < 0.01$
A t - value > 3.1or < −3.1 SEM - units indicates a result distant from zero at $p < 0.002$.

A t- or z-value >2.0 or <−2.0 SEM-units also indicates that the 95% confidence interval of the trial does not cross zero on the x-axis (in statistics often called z-axis), because this 95% confidence interval is >2±2 SEM-units or <−2±2 SEM-units (Fig. 63.2).

This means that in the given example noninferiority based on the defined margin is demonstrated, but at the same time the new treatment is significantly worse than the standard treatment at $p<0.05$. The meaning of noninferiority in the given situation has become very limited. The CONSORT Group (Consolidated Standards of

Reporting Trials) (Kaul and Diamond 2006) advised that, although this peculiar situation may not occur often, it is a real risk with wide margins of noninferiority.

2.3 Testing the New Treatment Versus Historical Placebo Data

Kaul and Diamond (Kim 1997) recently proposed that placebo-controlled data of the standard treatment be added to any noninferiority trial, because a standard treatment without documented proof of superiority against placebo is not an adequate control treatment in a noninferiority study. Here we describe a novel method that includes historical placebo data in the analysis, and provides a good estimate of the new treatment compared to placebo.

If a controlled trial of a standard treatment versus placebo produces a t- or z-value of 3.0 SEM-units, and an equally large trial with a new treatment versus a standard treatment produces a t- or z-value of say 0.5 SEM-units, then $3 + 0.5 = 3.5$ SEM-units gives a good estimate of the comparison of the new treatment versus placebo. Or in summary:

$$\text{Standard} - \text{placebo} = 3 \text{ SEM - units} \quad (1)$$
$$\text{New} - \text{standard} \quad = 0.5 \text{ SEM - units} \quad (2)$$
$$(1) + (2) \quad \quad \quad = 3.5 \text{ SEM - units}$$

Table 63.1 gives an overview of possible results of comparisons of the new treatment versus placebo using the above method. If the t-value of placebo versus standard treatment is very large, then even poorly performing new compounds may be significantly better than placebo. If the t-value of placebo versus standard treatment is small, then the new compound will not easily perform better than placebo. If a noninferiority study is unable to demonstrate that, according to the above procedure, the new treatment is better than placebo, then the meaning of the noninferiority is very limited. The margin of noninferiority has probably been chosen too wide. We have to add here that the characteristics of the historical data should approximately match those of the new data, and that this information should be included in the report.

2.4 Including Prior Sample Size Calculations and p-Values

Usually, the results of noninferiority trials are reported as positive, uncertain, or negative (Fig. 63.1). Instead, just like with traditional trials methods for calculating p-values and prior sample sizes can be added to the protocol (Kim 1997). They are helpful to prevent lack of power, and to demonstrate the precision of the result. The following procedures can be followed. If in a noninferiority cholesterol study the expected difference between the new and standard treatment is, for example,

Table 63.1 If the t-value of standard treatment versus placebo is very large, then even poorly performing new compounds may perform significantly better than placebo. If the t-value of standard treatment versus placebo is small, then the new compound will less easily outperform placebo

Mean diff		P				P
New vs stand (SEM-units)	Stand vs placebo	New vs placebo	New vs stand	Stand vs placebo	New vs placebo	
−2	+4	2	S	−2	+2	0	NS
−1	+4	3	S	−1	+2	1	NS
0	+4	4	S	0	+2	2	S
+1	+4	5	S	+1	+2	3	S
+2	+4	6	S	+2	+2	4	S

NS not statistically significant, *S* statistically significant, *stand* standard treatment, *new* new treatment, *vs* versus, *diff* difference, *P* p-value

1.0 mmol/l with a standard deviation of 12 mmol/l, then we can determine the required sample size according to the underneath equation.

$$n = (Z\alpha + Z\beta)^2 * (SD/(D - mean))^2$$

$(Z\alpha + Z\beta)^2$ = power index = 7.8 with α = type I error = 5%, and β = type II error = 80%,

D = margin of noninferiority,
* = sign of multiplication.

With a defined D-value of −4 mmol/l,

$$n = 7.8 * (12/(-4-1))^2 = 45 \text{ patients per group.}$$

The above study would provide a $t - value = (D - mean)/SEM$
$$= (D - mean)/(SD/\sqrt{n})$$
$$= (-4-1)/(12/\sqrt{45})$$
$$= -2.8 \text{ SEM - units,}$$

corresponding with a p-value of 0.005. Noninferiority is demonstrated with a p-value of 0.005.

3 Examples

In the underneath examples we assess noninferiority using three steps.

1. The 95% confidence interval is tested against the set margin.
2. The null-hypothesis of no difference between new and standard is tested.
3. The null-hypothesis of no difference between new and a placebo is tested.

3.1   Example 1

Two inhalers "New" and "Standard" used for the relief of asthma attacks were compared in a non-inferiority study using morning peak expiratory flow rate (l/min) as the primary measurement. The margin of noninferiority was set at −15 l/min. The results of the trial were as follows:

Mean morning peak expiratory flow on treatment:

New = 420 ml/min (150 patients)
Standard = 416 ml/min (150 patients)
Mean difference between new and standard = 4 ml/min.
Estimated standard error of the mean of the difference, SEM = 5 ml/min.

1. The distance of the mean difference from the margin = −15−4 = −19 ml/min = −19/5 SEM-units = −3.8 SEM-units. A t-value of −3.8 SEMs-units corresponds to a p-value of 0.0001. Non-inferiority is demonstrated with a p-level as low as 0.0001.
2. A mean result of 4 ml/min = 4/5 = 0.8 SEM-units. The 95% confidence interval of this mean result 0.8 ± 2 SEM-units is between −1.2 and +2.8 SEM-units, and does not cross the 0 value on the z -axis, and, so, the mean difference between standard and new is not significantly different from zero.
3. A similarly sized placebo-controlled trial of the standard treatment versus placebo produces a t-value of 3.0 SEM-units. The comparison of the new treatment versus placebo equals 3.0 + 0.8 = 3.8 SEM-units. The new treatment is, thus, significantly better than placebo at t = 3.8 SEM-units, corresponding with a p-value of 0.0001.

Both the lack of a significant difference between standard and new, and the significant difference between new and placebo support the presence of noninferiority of the new treatment versus the standard treatment.

3.2   Example 2

A sleeping pill parallel study compares in 236 patients the numbers of sleeping hours of two compounds. Based on prior studies a margin of noninferiority of −6.4 h was defined. The mean difference between the new and standard treatment was −3.3 h, with an estimated standard error of 1.5 h.

1. The distance of the mean difference from the boundary = −6.4 + 3.3 h = −3.1 h = −3.1/1.5 SEM-units = −2.05 SEM-units. A t-value of −2.05 SEMs-units corresponds to a p-value of 0.04. Non-inferiority is demonstrated with a p = 0.04.
2. A mean difference of −3.3 h = −3.3/1.5 = −2.2 SEM-units. The 95% confidence interval of this mean result −2.2 ± 2 SEM-units is between −4.2 and −0.2 SEM-units,

and does not cross the 0 value on the z-axis, and, so, the mean difference between standard and new is significantly different from zero. The new treatment, although noninferior according to the set margin, performs at the same time significantly worse than standard treatment.

3. A similarly sized placebo-controlled trial of the standard treatment versus placebo produces a t-value of 4.5 SEM-units. The comparison of the new treatment versus placebo equals $-2.2+4.5$ SEM-units$=2.3$ SEM-units. The new treatment is, thus, significantly better than placebo at $t=2.3$ SEM-units, corresponding with a p - value of 0.021.

The presence of noninferiority is supported by the significant superiority of the new compound against placebo. However, the significantly worse performance against the standard treatment undermines these findings. We have to admit that the margin of noninferiority in this example was taken very wide: -6.4 h equals -4.26 SEM-units, and was based on arbitrary criteria rather than summary statistics of published data.

3.3   Example 3

In a hypertension of two groups of 100 patients each a new antihypertensive drug is compared to a standard treatment. A margin of noninferiority of -24 mmHg is set a priori. The mean difference between the new and standard treatment$=-4.5$ mmHg, with an estimated standard error of 9 mmHg.

1. The distance of the mean difference from the boundary$=-24+4.5$ mmHg $=-19.5$ mmHg$=19.5/9=2.2$ SEM-units. A t-value of 2.2 corresponds with a p-value of 0.028. Non-inferiority is demonstrated at p$=0.028$.
2. A mean difference of -4.5 mmHg$=-4.5/9=-0.5$ SEM-units. The 95% confidence interval of this mean result -0.5 ± 2 SEM-units is between -2.5 and 1.5 SEM-units, and does cross the 0 value on the z-axis, and so the mean difference between standard and new is not significantly different from zero. The new treatment is noninferior according to the set margin, and at the same time not significantly worse than the standard treatment supporting its noninferiority.
3. A similarly sized placebo-controlled trial of the standard treatment versus placebo produces a t-value of 2.3 SEM-units. The comparison of the new treatment versus placebo equals $-0.5+2.3=1.8$ SEM-units. The new treatment is, thus, not significantly better than placebo.

The presence of noninferiority is supported the lack of a significant difference between new and standard. However, these findings are undermined by the lacking superiority of the new compound against placebo.

3.4   Example 4

In a cholesterol study of two groups of 80 patients each a new compound is compared to a standard treatment. A margin of −1.4 mmol/l is set a priori. The mean difference between the new and standard treatment = −0.63 mmol/l, with an estimated standard error of 0.30 mmol/l.

1. The distance of the mean difference from the boundary = −1.4+0.63 mmol/l = −0.77 mmol/l = −0.77/0.3 = 2.57 SEM-units. A t-value of 2.57 corresponds with a p-value of 0.01. Non-inferiority is demonstrated at p = 0.01.
2. A mean difference of −.63 mmol/l = −0.63/0.30 = −2.1 SEM-units. The 95% confidence interval of this mean result −2.1 ± 2 SEM-units is between −4.1 and −0.1 SEM-units, and does not cross the 0 value on the z-axis, and so the mean difference between standard and new is significantly different from zero. The new treatment is noninferior according to the set margin, but at the same time significant worse than the standard treatment which does not support its noninferiority.
3. A similarly sized placebo-controlled trial of the standard treatment versus placebo produces a t-value of 2.4 SEM-units. The comparison of the new treatment versus placebo equals −0.63 + 2.4 = 1.77 SEM-units. The new treatment is, thus, not significantly better than placebo.

The presence of noninferiority is undermined both by the significant difference between new and standard and by the lack of efficacy of the new treatment against placebo. Also in this example the margin of noninferiority was taken very wide: −1.4 mmol/l = −4.7 SEM-units. It was again based on arbitrary criteria rather than summary statistics of published data.

4   Discussion

We propose that current arbitrary margins of noninferiority, based on clinical arguments, be replaced with methods of assessment based on statistical reasoning. It not only provides more precise results as demonstrated in the examples, but also helps to prevent expert investigators from being seduced into producing too wide margins. The following procedures are recommended: (1) basing the margin of noninferiority on counted rather than arbitrary criteria, (2) null-hypothesis tests of no difference between the new and standard treatment, and (3) null-hypothesis tests of no difference between the new treatment and a placebo. A summary of the procedures proposed and an example designed and analyzed according to the novel procedures are given in the Tables 63.2 and 63.3 respectively.

Some additional special points of noninferiority studies should be mentioned. A comparative trial is valid when it is blinded, randomized, explicit, accurate statistically and ethically. The same is true for a noninferiority trial. However, a

Table 63.2 Summary of the proposed novel approach to noninferiority testing, including the construct of the noninferiority margin

A. Basing margins of noninferiority on counted rather than arbitrary criteria
1. Construct the margin of noninferiority with the help of the summary of the published data of these products (alternatively construct it with the help of the summary statistic of the responses to a survey on the range of differences considered to be important by practitioners)
2. Determine a priori the sample size with the help of the equation

$$n = (Z\alpha + Z\beta)^2 * (SD / (D - mean))^2,$$

where $(Z\alpha + Z\beta)^2$ = powerindex, D = margin of noninferiority, * = sign of multiplication
3. Calculate a p-value for the level of noninferiority according to the equation

$$t - value = (D - mean) / SEM,$$

where SEM = standard error of the mean
B. Test the null-hypothesis of no difference between the new and standard treatment
C. Test the null-hypothesis tests of no difference between the new treatment and a placebo. The placebo result must be obtained from adequate historical data

Noninferiority studies should be reported together with the p-values as calculated above (A3). Unequivocal noninferiority is demonstrated only if the p-value is <0.05 (A3), and if the p-value for the difference between new and standard is >0.05 (B), and the p-value for the difference between new and a placebo is <0.05 (C)

---

problem arises with the intention to treat analysis. Intention to treat patients are analyzed according to their randomized treatment irrespective of whether they actually received the treatment. The argument is that it mirrors what will happen when a treatment is used in practice. In a comparative parallel group study the inclusion of protocol violators in the analysis tend to make the results of the two treatments more similar. In a noninferiority study this effect may bias the study towards a positive result, being the demonstration of noninferiority. A possibility is to carry out both intention-to-treat-analysis and completed-protocol-analysis. If no difference is demonstrated, we conclude that the study's data are robust (otherwise called sensitive, otherwise called precise), and that the protocol-analysis did not introduce major sloppiness into the data. Sometimes, efficacy and safety endpoints are analyzed differently: the former according to the protocol analysis simply because important endpoint variables are missing in the population that leaves the study early, and intention to treat analysis for the latter, because safety variables frequently include items such as side effects, drop-offs, morbidity and mortality during trial. Either endpoint can of course be assessed in a noninferiority trial, but we must consider that an intention to treat analysis may bias the noninferiority principle towards overestimation of the chance of noninferiority.

Another special point to be considered is that crossover studies of different compounds may have a negative correlation between the treatments (Cleophas 2000), and this causes loss of sensitivity of demonstrating noninferiority. Fortunately, most crossover studies have a positive correlation, and, so, the crossover design is generally quite sensitive to assess equivalence.

Table 63.3 Example of a non-inferiority study designed and analyzed according to the novel approach proposed

Two parallel-groups of patients with rheumatoid arthritis are treated with either a standard or a new nonsteroidal anti-inflammatory drug (NSAID). The reduction of gamma globuline levels (g/l) after treatment was used as the primary estimate of treatment success

A. Determination of the margin of noninferiority, the required sample, and the p-value of the study result

    1. The left boundaries of the 95% confidence intervals of previously published studies of the Standard NSAID versus various alternative NSAIDS were never lower than −8 g/l. And, so, the margin was set at −8 g/l

    2. Based on a pilot-study with the novel compound the expected mean difference was 0 g/l with an expected standard deviation of 32 g/l. This would mean a required sample size of

$$n = \text{power index} * \left(SD / \left(\text{margin} - \text{mean} \right) \right)^2$$

$$n = 7.8 * \left(32 / \left(-8 - 0 \right) \right)^2 = 125 \text{ patients per group. } (* = \text{sign of multiplication}).$$

       A power index of 7.8 takes care that noninferiority is demonstrated with a power of about 80% in this study

    3. The mean difference between the new and standard NSAID was calculated to be 3.0 g/l With an SEM of 4.6 g/l. This meant that the t-value of the study equalled

$$t = \left(\text{margin} - \text{mean} \right) / SEM = \left(-8 - 3 \right) / 4.6 = -2.39 \text{ SEM} - \text{units.}$$

       This t-value corresponds with a p-value of 0.017. Non-inferiority is demonstrated at p=0.017

B. Testing the significance of difference between the new and the standard treatment

    The mean difference between the new and standard treatment equalled 3.0 g/l with a SEM of 4.6 g/l. The 95% confidence of this result is 3.0±2*4.6, and is between −6.2 and 12.2 g/l (*=sign of multiplication). This interval does cross the zero value on the z-axis, which means no significant difference from zero (p>0.05)

C. Testing the significance of difference between the new treatment and placebo

    A similarly sized published trial of the standard treatment versus placebo produced a t-value of 2.83, and, thus a p-value of 0.0047. The t-value of the current equals 3.0/4.6=0.65 SEM-units. The add-up sum 2.83+0.65=3.48 is a good estimate of the comparison of the new treatment versus placebo. A t-value of 3.48 corresponds with a p-value of 0.0005. The would mean that the new treatment is significantly better than placebo at p=0.0005

We conclude that (1) noninferiority is demonstrated at p=0.017, that (2) a significant difference between the new and standard treatment is rejected at p>0.05, and that (3) the new treatment is significantly better than placebo at p=0.0005. Non-inferiority has, thus, been unequivocally demonstrated in this study

Non-inferiority testing according to the procedure proposed in this paper can also be included in traditional efficacy analyses of treatment comparisons. It may help solving important future clinical issues like the one in the next example. The treatment of hypertension is believed to follow a J-shape curve, where overtreatment produces increased rather than reduced mortality/morbidity. A different theory would tell you that the more intensive the therapy the better the result. This latter theory was tested in the HOT trial (Hansson et al. 1998), but could not be confirmed: high dosage antihypertensive therapy was not significantly better than medium-dosage therapy. Probably it was not worse either, however, unfortunately, this was not tested in the report. The study would definitely have been powerful to test this question, and, moreover, it would have solved a major so far unsolved discussion.

An additional advantage of routinely testing noninferiority according to the above procedure, is, that it helps preventing well-designed studies from going down in history as just "negative" studies that did not prove anything and are more likely not to be published, leading to unnecessary and costly repetition of research. If such "negative" studies are capable of rejecting the chance of inferiority, they may be reconsidered as a study that is not completely negative and may be rightly given better priority for being published.

We conclude that expert investigators traditionally set arbitrary margin of noninferiority based on clinical arguments, and benefit from wide margins. As an alternative and more meaningful approach to noninferiority testing we propose to use

1. margins of noninferiority based on counted rather than arbitrary criteria,
2. null-hypothesis tests of no difference between the new and standard treatment,
3. null-hypothesis tests of no difference between the new treatment and a placebo.

5   Conclusions

Noninferiority trials have been criticized for their wide margins of noninferiority, making it virtually impossible to reject noninferiority. Recommendations have been given to replace the practice of arbitrarily set margins. This chapter reviews various alternative methods of assessment based on statistical reasoning.

Four examples are given.

1. In a 300 patient parallel group study of two inhalers for asthma noninferiority was demonstrated at $p = 0.0001$. This result was supported by both the lack of a significant difference between the standard and new inhaler, and the presence of a significant difference between the new inhaler and a placebo at $p = 0.0001$.
2. In a 236 patient parallel-group sleeping pill study noninferiority was demonstrated at $p = 0.04$. The presence of noninferiority was supported by a significant superiority of the new compound against a placebo at $p = 0.021$. However, the significantly worse performance against the standard treatment undermined these findings.
3. In a 200 patient hypertension study of two treatment groups noninferiority was demonstrated at $p = 0.028$. The presence of noninferiority was supported by the lack of a significant difference between the new and the standard treatment. However, these findings were undermined by the lacking superiority of the new compound against a placebo.
4. In a 160 patients parallel-group cholesterol study noninferiority was demonstrated at $p = 0.01$.

The presence of noninferiority was undermined both by the significant difference between the new and the standard treatment, and by the lack of efficacy of the new treatment against a placebo.

We conclude that expert investigators traditionally set arbitrary margin of noninferiority based on clinical arguments, and that they benefit from wide margins. As an alternative and more meaningful approach to noninferiority testing we propose to use

1. margins based on counted rather than arbitrary criteria,
2. null-hypothesis tests between the new and standard treatment,
3. null-hypothesis tests between the new treatment and a placebo.

References

Allen IE, Seaman CA (2007) Superiority, equivalence, and non-inferiority. Qual Prog 40(2):52–54. http://www.asq.org. Accessed 15 Dec 2011

Anonymous (2011a) European Medicines Agency guideline on the choice of the non-inferiority margin. www.emea.eu.int. Accessed 15 Dec 2011

Anonymous (2011b) Scrip clinical research, new FDA and EMEA draft guidelines. www.scripnews. com. Accessed 15 Dec 2011

Cleophas TJ (2000) Crossover trials should not be used to test one treatment against another treatment with a different chemical class/mode of action. J Clin Pharmacol 40:1503–1508

Hansson L, Zanchetti A, Carruthers SG et al (1998) Effects of intensive blood-pressure lowering and low-dose treatment in patients with hypertension: principal results of the Hypertension Optimal Treatment (HOT) randomised trial. Lancet 351:1755–1762

Hung HMJ, Wang SJ (2004) Multiple testing of noninferiority hypotheses in active controlled trials. J Biopharm Stat 14:327–335

Kaul S, Diamond GA (2006) Good enough: a primer on the analysis and interpretation of noninferiority trials. Ann Intern Med 145:62–69

Kim JS (1997) Determining sample size for testing equivalence and noninferiority. Medical Device Link. www.devicelink.com. Accessed 15 Dec 2011

Mercola J. Lying with statistics. http://randomjohn.wordpress.com. Accessed 15 Dec 2011

Piaggio G, Elbourne DR, Altman DG, Pocock SJ, Evans SJ (2006) Reporting of noninferiority and equivalence randomized trials, an extension of the CONSORT Statement. JAMA 295:1152–1160

Pocock SJ (2003) The pros and cons of noninferiority trials. Fundam Clin Pharmacol 17:483–490

Snapinn SM (2000) Noninferiority trials. Curr Control Trials 1:19–21

Chapter 64
Time Series

1 Introduction

Time series often appear as a sequence of unpaired or paired data observed through time. Examples include the incidence of nosocomial infection in a hospital, course of analgesia during surgery, seasonal variations in hospital admissions, waveform of electroencephalogram potentials, analysis of ambulatory blood pressures, the course of any disease through time. In fact, time series are encountered in virtually every field of medicine. The analysis of time series traditionally focuses on the identification of patterns, and the prediction of future observations. Unlike Kaplan-Meier methodology which assesses the time to a single event in a group of patients, time series deals with multiple repeated observations and/or events either paired or unpaired.

Four specific questions are most often assessed.

1. Is there a trend in the magnitude or frequency of events through time.
2. Are there cyclic patterns in the long term data?
3. Is an event correlated with other events in time?
4. Is there a point in time at which a pattern changes?

The first question has already been addressed in Chap. 27: for binary data a chi-square trend test, for continuous data linear regression is available. Both tests will be more sensitive than standard chi-square or t-tests if a trend is in the data, because they only have one degree of freedom.

The current chapter addresses cyclic patterns in longitudinal data that can be analyzed using auto correlation. Second, it addresses whether two variables that are related at the start of the observation remain related through time. Third, whether change points can be identified, which is a particularly important issue with time series.

In this chapter we will also briefly address modern computationally intensive methods like ARMA (autoregressive moving averages) and wavelet analysis, and, finally, we will underscore that smoothing is helpful with wild patterns in the data, and how it can be done.

T.J. Cleophas and A.H. Zwinderman, *Statistics Applied to Clinical Studies*,
DOI 10.1007/978-94-007-2863-9_64, © Springer Science+Business Media B.V. 2012

2   Autocorrelation

A correlation coefficient r is a measure of the correlation between two correlated
data sets. This has been explained, for example, in Chap. 14. It varies between −1
and +1, and it equals the cross product of the deviations of observations from their
means. If the correlated data sets are not taken at a point of time but instead taken
sequentially through time, then the correlation between them is termed *serial correlation*. A serial correlation in which the second of the matching set is a repeat of
the first is called an *autocorrelation*. If the second is a different variable, then the
serial correlation is a *cross correlation*. The method of autocorrelation tells us
whether a single variable such as disease severity is seasonal.

Observations through time may be correlated with themselves. A set of observations through time is taken as the first set, and the same set is taken as the second,
except in a lagged form (Fig. 64.1).

Original series	First-order pairs	Second-order pairs
1	1 4	1 6
4	4 6	4 3
6	6 3	6 5
3	3 5	3 2
5	5 2	5 7
2	2 7	
7		

If the autocorrelation coefficient retreats from 1.00 as the lag increases and then
returns to nearly 1.00, then we know that we have a periodically recurring disease.
If that lag is 12 months, then the disease will be seasonal. A plot of autocorrelation
depending on lag is termed a correlogram. Periodicities in a time series can be seen
easily in a correlogram as the time values at which the autocorrelation coefficient
approached 1.00.

3   Cross Correlation

The method of cross correlation tells us whether two variables are related through
time. For example, the correlation of infant malaria between malaria-free and
infected mothers are followed for 2 years. The study should tell us how close the
two variables (malaria-free and infected mothers) are through time. The correlation
is based on the difference between them, not on their behavior through time. Thus,
if they both rise or fall together, the correlation is high even though the pattern may
not be simple. Serial correlations can also be calculated with one of the sets lagged
behind the other. The severity of a disease having a 2 week incubation period can be
correlated with the symptoms observed during exposure to the infection. By varying

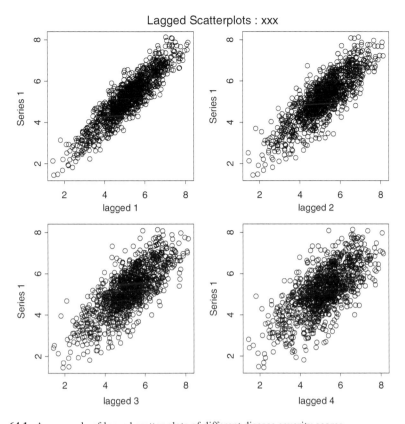

Fig. 64.1   An example of lagged scatter plots of different disease severity scores

the lag we may even be able to find the incubation period. Also, by knowing the incubation period, finding lagged cross correlations may be helpful to identify severity of exposure.

Another example of cross correlation with lag is given. A group of people who recently traveled in a tropical country contract a new type of viral disease. The dates of visits and symptom onset are correlated with various lags. The lag that provides the largest cross correlation coefficient estimates the average incubation time. These examples are given by Riffenburgh (1999).

4   Change Points

A very important issue with time series is the establishment of change points. A change point indicates that a difference in the pattern of the time series has occurred. Various methods for assessment are available but most of them are very complex.

One simple method is called "moving the F-value", and it works very well. It will be briefly discussed.

Variances of samples moving along the timeline are calculated, and then divided by its baseline variance. In this way changing F-values are created. A critical F-value is defined, and once the time series passes this critical F-value, we will conclude that a serious change point has been reached.

Observation	Correlation	Moving F-value	Moving F
323	0.9104	...	...
324	0.9111	...	...
...	...	...	...
331	0 1.9172	...	1.605
332	0.9183	...	1.749
333	0.9196	0.001398	1.912
334	0.9210	0.001601	2.190
335	0.9225	0.001826	2.498
336	0.9242	...	...
....	...	...	...
343	0.9412	...	...
344	0.9443	...	...

In the above example the critical F-value was 2.20. The statistic crosses the line at observation no 335, which is taken as the point of change from a rather horizontal pattern of observations to a more sloped one.

5   Discussion

Some time series contain wild patterns of values, and very often a potential pattern of sequences is obscured by the wide variability of the data. A potential pattern can, then, be better discerned if the variability about the data is reduced, otherwise called smoothed. Smoothing is not needed with very small samples, because here no patterns can be detected anyway. However with large samples smoothing is useful and smoothed data can, subsequently, be further tested with the methods as reviewed above. Many methods for smoothing exist, including convolution filters using moved averages, recursive filters using autoregression, exponential smoothing as used in SPSS (2011), kernel regression (Chap. 24), and splines (Chap. 24) etc. However, simpler methods of smoothing are useful and an example is given. The underneath figures show a wild pattern of data from a time series. Simply, taking the median of every subsequent seven values gives an idea of a slightly increasing trend. If instead the mean values of every subsequent 50 values are given, an even better pattern of the rising pattern of the data is suggested. Performing a regression analysis of the second order with the mean values as independent variable provided a very good fit of these data with a p-value as small as 0.001 (Fig. 64.2).

As with much of statistics more sophisticated methods accounting effects of potential biases are, generally, available. One example is the ARMA (autoregressive

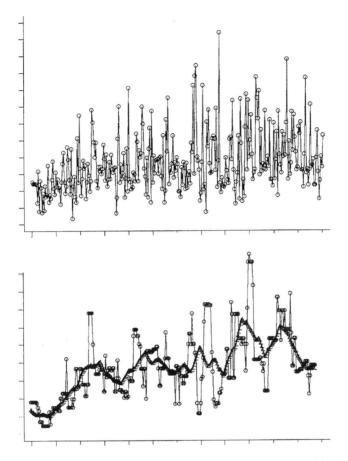

Fig. 64.2 *Upper graph* gives a wild pattern of data from a time series. Simply, taking the medians (*thin line lower graph*) of every subsequent seven values gives an idea of a slightly increasing trend. If instead the mean values of every subsequent 50 values are given (*fat line lower graph*), an even better pattern of the rising pattern of the data is suggested (From Riffenburgh (1999), with permission from the editor)

moving average) method, a combination of the MA (moving averages) and AR (autoregressive) models, providing better fit for some data sets, but at the same time at risk of power loss if for one reason or another the data do not fit well. Also the wavelet theory for describing time series is a relevant though computationally intensive method. It assesses brief oscillations like seismographic and heart monitor displays, but also audio and image signals. The software program S-plus (2011) provides the module Discrete Wavelet Transform which can be and has been used for purpose like blood pressure, heart rate and ECG analyses, DNA analyses, protein analyses, climatology, general signal processing, image processing etc. Terminology includes mother wavelets (i.e. the wavelet functions) and the father wavelets (i.e. the scaling functions) (Fig. 64.3).

Fig. 64.3 Example of a wavelet function consisting of the sum of father and mother wavelets instead of a sum of sines and cosines like with Fourier analysis

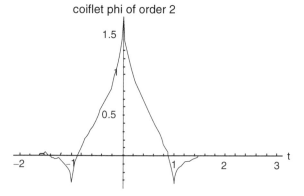

6   Conclusions

Background: Time series often appear as a sequence of unpaired or paired data observed through time, and are encountered in virtually every field of medicine.

Objectives: To address cyclic patterns in longitudinal data that can be analyzed using auto correlation. Second, to address how two variables that are related at the start of the observation can be assessed through time. To address how change points in time series can be identified.

Results:

1. If the correlated data sets are not taken at a point of time but instead taken sequentially through time, then the correlation between them is termed *serial correlation*. A serial correlation in which the second of the matching set is a repeat of the first is called an *autocorrelation*.
2. If the second is a different variable, then the serial correlation is a *cross correlation*.
3. "Moving the F-value" establishes change points in time series.
4. With time series data smoothing is useful and smoothed data can, subsequently, be further used for testing the data.
5. The ARMA (autoregressive moving average) method is a sophisticated method for better fit of some types of time series.
6. The wavelet theory enables to assess quantitatively time series consisting of oscillation patterns.

Conclusions: The analysis of time series focuses on the identification of data patterns and the prediction of future observations, and is an increasingly important subject in the field of clinical data analysis.

References

Riffenburgh RH (1999) Statistics in medicine. Academic, San Diego
SPSS. www.spss.com. Accessed 15 Dec 2011
S-plus. www.s-plus.com. Accessed 15 Dec 2011

Chapter 65
Odds Ratios and Multiple Regression Models, Why and How to Use Them

1 Introduction

In observational studies odds ratios (ORs) and multiple regressions models are commonly used for respectively the surrogate measurements of relative risks and the assessments of independent risk factors. In clinical trials both of them can be used for different purposes. Odds ratios unlike chi-square tests provide a direct insight in the strength of the relationship: odds ratios describe the probability that patients with a certain treatment will have the event compared to those without. Multiple regression models can reduce the data spread due to certain patient characteristics like differences in baseline values, and thus, improve the precision of the treatment comparison. Despite these advantages these methods are not routinely used for the evaluation of clinical trials. The current chapter was written (1) to emphasize the great potential of odds ratios and multiple regression models in clinical trials, (2) to illustrate the ease of use, and (3) to familiarize the non-mathematical readership of this book with these important methods for clinical trials.

2 Understanding Odds Ratios (ORs)

As stated recently by Guyatt and Rennie, while clinicians have an intuitive understanding of risks and even risk ratios, and gamblers of odds, no one, with the possible exception of a few statisticians, intuitively understands ORs (Guyatt and Rennie 2001). The clinical perception of ORs may be difficult. Yet, they have obtained an important place in observational research, particularly, unmatched case-control studies. Because, in such studies, patients are selected on the basis of their disease, and controls are just a small sample from the target population, it is impossible to calculate either the absolute or the relative risk of a disease. Instead,

T.J. Cleophas and A.H. Zwinderman, *Statistics Applied to Clinical Studies*,
DOI 10.1007/978-94-007-2863-9_65, © Springer Science+Business Media B.V. 2012

$$\text{the OR} = \frac{\text{the odds of a disease in a group exposed to a risk factor}}{\text{the odds of the same disease in a group unexposed to the risk factor}}$$

can be used as a surrogate measure for the relative risk of disease. ORs can, however, also be used for different purposes. In clinical trials, particularly, those using events as endpoints like cardiovascular trials, ORs can be used as an alternative to the traditional χ^2 – test for assessing patients with versus without an event. Apart from the p-values, χ^2 – tests do not provide an insight in the strength of the relationship. Instead, ORs measure the magnitude of association, and, in addition, describe the probability that people with a certain treatment will have the event compared to people without the treatment. Despite this advantage ORs are not routinely used for the evaluation of clinical trials.

2.1   Odds Ratios (ORs) as an Alternative Method to χ^2-Tests for the Analysis of Binary Data

The odds is the probability that an event happens divided by the chance that it does not so.

Event	Yes	No (numbers of patients)
Treatment-1	p	q
Treatment-2	r	s

With treatment-1 the probability or risk of an event can be described by p/(p+q), with treatment-2 by r/(r+s), the ratio of p/(p+q) and r/(r+s)=risk ratio (RR).

The odds of an event from treatment-1 is different. It equals p/q, and the ratio of two odds, p/q and r/s is called the odds ratio (OR). In case-control studies ORs are used as a surrogate measure for RRs, because p/(p+q) in such studies is, simply, nonsense. Let us assume:

	Event-group	No-event-group	Target population (numbers of patients)
Risk factor (treatment)	32 (p)	4(q)	4,000
No risk factor (no treatment)	24 (r) +	52 (s) +	52,000
	56	56	

The risk factor could be a treatment. The no-event-group group is just a random sample from the target population, but the ratio r/s is that of target population. Suppose 4=4,000 and 52=52,000, then the magnitude of

$$\frac{p/(p+q)}{r/(r+s)} \text{ is suddenly close to } \frac{p/q}{r/s} \; .$$

This means that the OR in this situation is a good approximation of the RR of the target population. In clinical trials things are different. Both ORs and RRs can be meaningfully used. An OR or RR of 1.0 indicates no difference between treatment-1 and -2. The more distant from 1.0, the larger the difference between the two treatments where the OR is always more distant than the RR. An advantage of the RR is that it truly reflects the magnitude of the increased risk, e.g., a risk of ½ in group-1 and ¼ in group-2 produces a RR of ½/¼ = 2, a twice increased risk. The OR of these data produces the result $1/(1/3) = 3$, a three times increased odds ratio, which is clinically somewhat more difficult to understand. However an increased OR can still be interpreted as an increased probability of events in patients with the treatment compared to those without the treatment. For clinical trials advantages of the ORs compared to the RRs include:

1. ORs can be used as an alternative to the widely used χ^2 – tests for analyzing 2×2 contingency tables, while RRs can not because they use different cells (Bland and Altman 2000).
2. Statistical software uses rarely RRs, and mainly ORs. (BUGS y WinBUGS 2011; S plus 2011; Stata 2011; StatsDirect 2011; StatXact 2011; True Epistat 2011; SAS 2011; SPSS Statistical Software 2011)
3. Computations using RRs are less sensitive than those using ORs. This is due to ceiling problems, risks run from 0 to 1, odds from 0 to infinity (Zwinderman et al. 1998).
4. Unlike RRs, ORs are the basis of modern methods like meta-analyses of clinical trials (Zwinderman 2006), propensity scores for assessment of confounding (Cleophas and Zwinderman 2007), logistic regression for subgroup analysis (Rubin 1997), Cox regression for proportional hazard ratios (Cleophas 2005) etc.

2.2   How to Analyze Odds Ratios (ORs)

If we take many samples from a target population, the mean results of those samples usually follow a normal frequency distribution, meaning that the value in the middle will be observed most frequently and the more distant from the middle the less frequently a value will be observed. For example, we will have only 5% chance to find a result more than 2 standard errors (SEs) (or more precisely 1.96 SEs) distant from the middle. The same is true with proportional data. Many statistical tests make use of the normal distribution to make predictions. Figure 65.1 shows, e.g., how the normal distribution theorem is used to reject the null-hypothesis of no difference from zero.

A problem with ORs is that they are not normally distributed. And so, the above approach to making predictions cannot be applied. Figure 65.2 upper graph shows how skewed the frequency distribution of ORs, actually, can be. Suppose the OR of a representative sample is 0.25. Then it can be demonstrated that the chance of finding a lower or higher OR the next time are far from equal (Fig. 65.2 upper graph). Chances can be expressed in the form of 95% confidence intervals which are for the

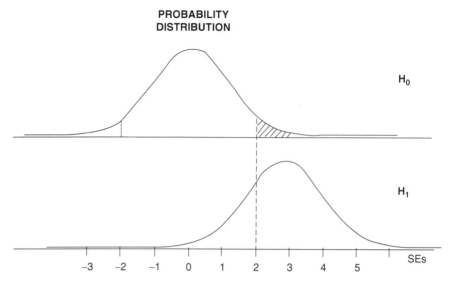

Fig. 65.1 H_1 = graph based on the data of a sample with standard errors distant from zero (SEs) as unit on the x-axis. H_0 = same graph with a mean value of 0. We make a giant leap from the sample to the entire population, and we can do so because the sample is assumed to be representative for the entire population. H_1 = also the summary of the means of many samples similar to our sample. H_0 = also the summary of the means of many samples similar to our sample, but with an overall effect of 0. Our mean not 0 but 2.9. Still it could be an outlier of many samples with an overall effect of 0. If H_0 is true, then our sample is an outlier. We can't prove, but calculate the chance/probability of this possibility. A mean result of 2.9 SEs is far distant from 0: suppose it belongs to H_0. Only 5% of H_0 trials >2.0 SEs distant 0. The chance that it belongs to H_0 is thus <5%. We conclude that we have <5% chance to find this result, and, therefore, reject this small chance

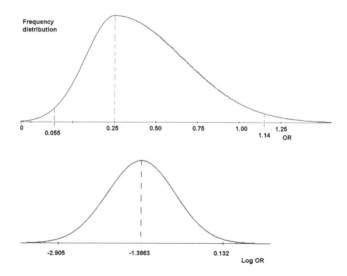

Fig. 65.2 *Upper graph*: frequency distribution of an OR of 0.25 with 95% confidence interval; *lower graph* logarithmic transformation of the *upper graph*

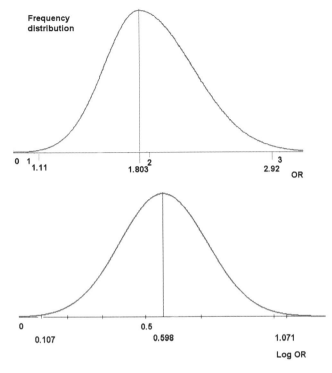

Fig. 65.3 *Upper graph*: frequency distribution of an OR of 1.803 with 95% confidence interval; *lower graph* logarithmic transformation of the *upper graph*

given example between 0.055 and 1.14. With an OR of 1.803 the 95% confidence interval is between 1.11 and 2.92 (Fig. 65.3 upper graph) The frequency distributions are not symmetrical around the observed sample OR. This asymmetry is, especially, noticeable when the sample OR is low (Fig. 65.2 upper graph). Statisticians were very happy to observe that something wonderful happened when on the x-axis of the frequency distribution curve the OR was replaced with the logarithm of the OR (log OR). A close to normal distribution was observed (Figs. 65.2 and 65.3 lower graphs). This means that the log OR can be used for testing ORs. We should add that throughout the text the term log indicates the natural logarithm (logarithm with base e).

As explained in Fig. 65.1, if the log OR is more than 2 SEs distant from a log OR of 0, the null-hypothesis of no difference from 0 is rejected. Our result is, then, significantly different from 0 at p <0.05.

Event	Yes	No (numbers of patients)
Treatment-1	p	q
Treatment-2	r	s

If OR $(=p/q/r/s)=1$, then no difference exists between treatment-1 and -2.
If OR $=1$, then log OR $=0$.

With normal distributions, if a mean result is >2 SEs distant from 0, it will be significantly different from 0 at $p<0.05$. Also, if log OR is >2 SEs distant from 0, it will be significantly different from 0 at $p<0.05$.

Examples

Study 1	`< --.-- >`	log OR >2SEs distant from $0 \rightarrow p<0.05$
Study 1	`< --.-- >`	log OR >2SEs distant from $0 \rightarrow p<0.05$
Study 1	`< --.-- >`	log OR >2SEs distant from $0 \rightarrow p<0.05$

Log OR $=0$ (OR $=1.0$)

In order to proceed we need to know the standard errors of the log odds ratios. For the calculation of a standard error of the log odds ratios a mathematical trick called the quadratic approximation (Anonymous 2011) has to be used. Most functions f(x) can be represented by a power series near some point a:

$$f(x) = c_0 + c_1(x-a) + c_2(x-a)^2 + c_3 \ldots \ldots$$

where $c_0, c_1, c_3 \ldots$ are constants.

If we put $x=a$ in the equation, then all terms after the first are 0, and $f(a)=c_0$.
If we differentiate the equation, then we have

$$f'(x) = c_1 + 2c_2(x-a) + 3c_3(x-a)^2 \ldots$$

If we put again $x=a$, then $f'(a)=c_1$
If we take the second differentiation, we have

$$f''(x) = 2c_2 + 6c_3(x-a) + 12c_4 \ldots$$

$$f''(a) = 2c_2 \text{ or } c_2 = f''(a)/2.$$

As the right end terms of the equation soon will be very small, we can stop right here and neglect these terms. This means that f(x) can be described as

$$f(x) = f(a) + f'(a)(x-a) + \frac{f''}{2}(a)(x-a)^2$$

Even $f(a) + f'(a)(x-a)$ is a good approximation of $f(x)$.

This quadratic approximation formula can be conveniently used to develop a formula for the standard errors of odds ratios as follows:

$$\log(x) = \log(a) + (x-a)\log'(a)$$

$\log'(a)$ denotes the first derivative of $\log(a)$, the slope of the graph of $\log(a)$ against a which equals $1/a$.

Adding or subtracting a constant to a variable leaves its standard error unchanged and multiplying by a constant has the effect of multiplying the standard error by that constant. Applying these rules under the assumption that the variable x is close to (a) we can further deduce:

$$se \log (x) = \frac{se\ x}{x}$$

If the variable is an odds, we can calculate the standard error of the log odds according to

$$se \log (odds) = \frac{se\ odds}{odds}$$

	Number responders	Non-responders
Treatment-0	p	q
Treatment-1	r	s

If in an experiment of $(p+q)$ patients there are p responders to a treatment, the odds of responding is p/q. The standard error of the odds is given by the formula se

$$odds = \sqrt{\left[p(p+q)/q^3 \right]}.$$

We can now readily calculate the standard error of the log (odds).

$$Se \log (odds) = \frac{se\ odds}{odds} = \frac{\sqrt{\left[p(p+q)/q^3 \right]}}{p/q} = \sqrt{(1/p+1/q)}.$$

More relevant to us than the standard error of an odds is the standard error of an OR.

The odds of responding in treatment-group-0 is p/q, in treatment-group-1 it is r/s. The standard error of the log (OR) is given by the formula $\sqrt{(1/p+1/q+1/r+1/s)}$.

2.3   Real Data Examples of Simple OR Analyses

The first example given is from the data in Fig. 65.2 left side.

Event	Yes	No (numbers of patients)
Treatment-1	5 (p)	10 (q)
Treatment-2	10 (r)	5 (s)

$$OR = p/q/r/s = 0.25,$$

$$\log OR = -1.3863,$$

$$\text{SEM log OR} = \sqrt{(1/p+1/q+1/r+1/s)} = 0.7746,$$
$$\text{log OR} \pm 2 \text{ SEMs} = -1.3863 \pm 1.5182,$$
$$= \text{between} - 2.905 \text{ and } 0.132.$$

Now turn the log numbers into real numbers by the antilog button of the pocket calculator.

$$= \text{between } 0.055 \text{ en } 1.14.$$

This result "crosses" 1.0, and, so, it is not significantly different from 1.0. The second example given is from Fig. 65.3 right side.

Event	Yes	No (numbers of patients)
Treatment-1	77	62
Treatment-2	103	46

$$\text{OR} = 103 / 46 / 77 / 62 = 2.239 / 1.242 = 1.803,$$
$$\text{log OR} = 0.589,$$
$$\text{SEM log OR} = \sqrt{(1/103+1/46+1/77+1/62)} = 0.245,$$
$$\text{log OR} \pm 2 \text{ SEMs} = 0.589 \pm 2(0.245),$$
$$= 0.589 \pm 0.482,$$
$$= \text{between } 0.107 \text{ and } 1.071.$$

Turn the log numbers into real numbers by the antilog button of the pocket calculator.

$$= \text{between } 1.11 \text{ and } 2.92,$$
$$\text{significantly different from } 1.0.$$

The p-value of this difference can be calculated using the t-test.
$t = \text{log OR/SEM} = 0.589/0.245 = 2.4082$, which according to the t-table means a p-value <0.02.

2.4   Real Data Examples of Advanced OR Analyses

Odds ratios are also the basis of many modern methods like various logistic regression models used to adjust for subgroup analyses. A simple example of a logistic model is given.

	Responders	Non-responders
New treatment (group-1)	17 (p)	4 (q)
Control treatment (group-2)	19 (r)	28 (s)

The odds of responding are p/q and r/s,

$$\text{odds ratio}(OR) = (p/q)/(r/s)$$

$$= \frac{\text{odds of responding group} - 1}{\text{odds of responding group} - 2}$$

As there is a linear relationship between treatment modality and log odds of responding, we use a loglinear regression model called binary logistic regression instead of a linear regression model.

The linear regression model $y = a + bx$
is transformed into: $\log \text{odds} = a + bx$.

Log odds is the dependent variable, and x is the independent variable (treatment modality: 1 if the patient is given the new treatment, 0 if control).

Instead of $\log \text{odds} = a + bx$
we can describe the equation as $\text{odds} = e^{a+bx}$,
if new treatment, then x $= 1$, and $\text{odds} = e^{a+b}$,
if control treatment, then x $= 0$, and $\text{odds} = e^{a}$
the ratio of two treatments $\text{odds ratio} = e^{a+b}/e^{a} = e^{b}$.

Software calculates the best b for given data,

if $b = 0$, then $e^{b} = OR = 1$,
if b significantly > 0, then the OR significantly > 1, and there is a significant difference between the new treatment and control.

The results are

	Coefficients	SEM	t	p
a	−1.95	0.53	.....	.....
b	1.83	0.63	2.9	0.004

We can conclude that b = significantly different from 0, and that there is, thus, a significant difference between new treatment and control, the odds of cure is $e^{1.83} = 6.2339$ times greater in the treatment group than it is in the control group.

The logistic model can adjust for subgroups as demonstrated underneath:

	Responders	Non-responders	Responders	Non-responders
	>50 years		<50 years	
Group-1 (new treatment)	4	12	13	2
Group-2 (control treatment)	9	16	10	12

Software calculates best fit b- and a-values for data:

	Coefficients	SEM	t	p
a > 50	−2.37	0.65		
a < 50	−1.54	0.59		
b > 50	1.83	0.67	2.7..	0.007
b < 50	1.83	0.67	2.7..	0.007

We can conclude here that the b-values are identical and both significantly different from 0. There is, thus, a significant difference between the new and control treatment also after age-class adjustment. In both subgroups the new treatment is better than control, which strengthens the earlier conclusions from these data.

3   Multiple Regression Models to Reduce the Spread in the Data

Small precision results in lack of power to reject null hypotheses and wide confidence intervals for parameter estimates. Certain patient characteristics in randomized controlled trials may cause spread in the data even if the characteristics are equally distributed among the treatment groups and do not interact with the treatment modalities. As an example, sulfonurea-compounds are efficacious for the treatment of diabetes type II. In a parallel-group clinical trial 36 patients with diabetes type II were treated with a potent (glibencamide) and a non-potent sulfonurea-compound (tolbutamide). Efficacy of treatment was assessed by fasting glucose. In the glibencamide group fasting glucose after treatment was 7.50 with standard deviation 2.01 mmol/l, in the tolbutamide group 8.50 with standard error 1.76 mmol/l. The difference in efficacy equals 8.50–7.50 = 1.00 mmol/l glucose with a pooled standard error of 0.94 mmol/l. According to the unpaired t-test this difference was not significant ($p > 0.05$). These data can also be assessed by a linear regression model with on the x-axis the treatment modality (0 = glibencamide; 1 = tolbutamide), and on the y-axis treatment efficacy (fasting glucose), (Fig. 65.4, left graph). The regression coefficient (direction coefficient) of the regression line equals $b = 1.00$ mmol/l with standard error 0.94 mmol/l, $p > 0.05$: exactly the same result as that obtained by an unpaired t-test. However, the regression model enables to add a second variable: the presence of beta-cell failure defined as a fasting glucose >8.0 mmol/l. After adjustment for this second variable the treatment efficacy b was unchanged (1.00 mmol/l), but standard errors fell from 0.94 to 0.53 mmol/l, with a significance of difference between the two treatment modalities at $p < 0.05$ (Fig. 65.4, right graph). This initial lack of precision was not caused by confounding, because in either subgroup the number of patients receiving glibencamide was similar to that receiving tolbutamide. Also interaction could not explain the lack of precision, because the difference in treatment efficacy in the two subgroups was similar. By appropriate data modeling some of the variability is removed from the data, and a more precise data comparison is produced. So far,

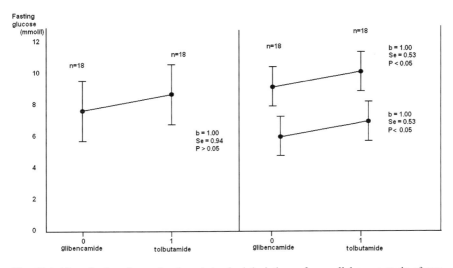

Fig. 65.4 Mean fasting glucose levels and standard deviations of a parallel-group study of two treatments for diabetes type II. *Left graph*: linear regression of overall data. *Right graph*: the same analysis after adjustment for the presence of beta cell failure or not (fasting glucose >8 mmol/l)

data modeling has not been emphasized in the analysis of prospective randomized clinical trials, and special statistical techniques need to be applied including the transformation of parallel-group data into regression data and the addition of covariates to the models (Cleophas 2003, 2005). We should emphasize that low precision in a clinical trial may be caused by a biased study due to the presence of confounding or interacting variables. Adjusting such variables will, of course, improve precision. In the present chapter we demonstrate that some covariates even if they are no confounding or interacting variables, may contribute to increasing precision of the data analysis.

3.1 A Linear Regression Model for Increasing Precision

The underneath data present a parallel-group trial comparing efficacy of a new laxative versus control laxative.

Patient no	Treatment modality (new = 0, control = 1)	Response = stool frequency after treatment (4 week stools)	Baseline stool frequency (4 week stools)
1	0	24	8
2	0	30	13
3	0	25	15
4	1	35	10
5	1	39	9
6	0	30	10

(continued)

(continued)

Patient no	Treatment modality (new = 0, control = 1)	Response = stool frequency after treatment (4 week stools)	Baseline stool frequency (4 week stools)
7	0	27	8
8	0	14	5
9	1	39	13
10	1	42	15
11	1	41	11
12	1	38	11
13	1	39	12
14	1	37	10
15	1	47	18
16	0	30	13
17	1	36	12
18	0	12	4
19	0	26	10
20	1	20	8
21	0	43	16
22	0	31	15
23	1	40	14
24	0	31	7
25	1	36	12
26	0	21	6
27	0	44	19
28	1	11	5
29	0	27	8
30	0	24	9
31	1	40	15
32	1	32	7
33	0	10	6
34	1	37	14
35	0	19	7

SPSS statistical software is used for analysis (SPSS Statistical Software 2011). First, enter the data or a data-file, e.g., from Excel (Excel by Windows 2011). Then command: statistics; regression; linear.

The underneath results are presented.

The mean difference in response between new treatment and control = 9.824 stools per 4 weeks (se = standard error = 2.965). The t-test produces a t-value of 9.824/2.965 = 3.313, and the t-table gives a p-value of <0.01. A linear regression according to

$y = a + bx$

with y = response and x = treatment modalities (0 = new treatment, 1 = control), a = intercept, and b = regression coefficient, produces a similar result

$b = 9.824$
$se_b = 2.965$
$t = 3.313$
p-value = 0.020
95% confidence interval 4.013–15.635.

Improved precision of this data analysis is a possibility if we extend the regression model by including a second explanatory-variable = baseline stool frequency according to

$y = a + b_1 x_1 + b_2 x_2$
with x_1 = treatment modalities (0 = new treatment, 1 = control),
x_2 = baseline stool frequencies, and b-values are partial regression coefficients.

This produces the following results

$b_1 = 6.852$
$se_{b1} = 1.792$
$t = 3.823$
p-value = 0.001
95% confidence intervals 3.340–10.364.

Now, the 95% confidence interval for the treatment effect is substantially narrower than the previously presented confidence interval. So, by adjusting for the baseline stool frequencies an improved precision is obtained as demonstrated by a smaller confidence interval, a larger t-value, and a smaller p-value. We should of course answer the questions: is baseline stool a (1) confounding or (2) interacting variable. For answering question (1) we perform a simple linear regression analysis of the variables x_1 versus x_2 which shows that the two variables are independent of one another ($p > 0.05$). X_2 is, thus, not a confounding variable. For answering question (2) a multiple linear regression is used with x_1, x_2, and x_3 as interacting variable given by $x_1 \cdot x_2$ (x_1 times x_2). This analysis shows that x_3 is not a significant determinant of treatment response ($p > 0.05$). There is, thus, no interaction between the two independent variables in the model. This means that increased precision to predict treatment response is obtained by including the baseline stool into the model, and that this model is otherwise unbiased by confounding or interaction (more examples are given in Chap. 18).

3.2   A Logistic Regression Model for Increasing Precision

Consider the underneath two by two contingency table.

	Numbers responders	Numbers non-responders
Treatment 1	30 a	45 b
Treatment 2	45 c	30 d

The odds-ratio-of-responding equals a/b/c/d=30/45/45/30=0.444. The natural logarithmic (ln) transformation of this odds ratio equals −0.8110. The approximate standard error of this logarithmic transformation is given by

$$\sqrt{(1/a+1/b+1/c+1/d)}=\sqrt{(1/30+1/45+/1/30+1/45)}=0.333.$$

A t-test of these data produces a t-value of 0.8110/0.333=2.435. According to the t-table this odds-ratio is significantly different from an odds ratio of 1.0 with a p-value of 0.015.
Logistic regression according to the model

ln odds-of-responding=a+bx
with x=treatment modality (0 or 1),
a=intercept, and b=regression coefficient,

produces the same result.
SPSS statistical software is again used to calculate the best b-values for the data given.

First enter the data or an Excel data file.
The command: statistics; regression; binary logistic.
The underneath results are presented.

b=0.8110
se$_b$=0.333
odds ratio of responding to treatment 1/treatment 2=2.250 with 95% confidence interval 1.613–3.139,
p-value = 0.015.

	Over 50 years		Under 50 years	
	Responders	Non-responders	Responders	Non-responders
Treatment 1	18	20	12	25
Treatment 2	31	8	14	22

Improved precision of the statistical analysis is a possibility if we control for age groups using the underneath multiple logistic regression model

ln odds-of-responding=a+b$_1$ x$_1$ +b$_2$ x$_2$
with x$_1$ =treatment modalities (0=treatment 1, 1=treatment 2)
x$_2$ =age classes (0=< 50 years, 1 =>50 years)
b-values are regression coefficients.

The following results are obtained:

b$_1$ =0.867
se$_{b1}$ =0.350
odds ratio of responding to treatment 1/treatment 2=2.380 with 95% confidence interval 1.677–3.377,
p-value = 0.012.

After adjustment for age class improved precision to test the efficacy of treatment has been obtained as demonstrated by a smaller p-value. Is this increased precision due to unmasked confounding or interaction? For answering these questions we perform a simple binary logistic regression of the variables x_1 versus x_2 which shows that the two variables are independent of one another ($p > 0.05$). X_2 is not a confounding variable. A multiple binary logistic regression is used with x_1, x_2 and x_3 as interacting variable given by $x_1 \cdot x_2$ (x_1 times x_2). This analysis shows that x_3 is not a significant determinant of treatment response ($p > 0.05$). There is, thus, no interaction between the two independent variables in the model. This means increased precision to predict treatment response has been obtained by including the age-category as covariate into the model, and that, like the previous example, it is unbiased by confounding or interaction.

4   Discussion

Advantages of the ORs compared to the RRs include (1) that, unlike RRs, they can be used as an alternative to the widely used χ^2 – tests for analyzing binary data in clinical trials, (2) that software for ORs is widely available, (3) that unlike RRs, ORs do not suffer from ceiling problems, and (4) that they are the basis of many modern methods like logistic regression, and Cox regression. An advantage of ORs compared to the traditional χ^2 – tests is that ORs provide, in addition to p-values, a direct insight in the strength of the relationship: odds ratios describe the probability that people with a certain treatment will have the event compared to people without the treatment.

For the analysis of ORs the logarithms of the ORs should be used. Data results are obtained by turning the logarithmic numbers into real numbers by using their antilogarithms.

A limitation of the ORs is that, although they adequately present the relative benefits of a treatment compared to control, they do not tell us anything about the absolute benefits. For that purpose information about baseline risks or likelihoods are required. For example, with an odds ratio of cure of treated versus baseline of 5, and a baseline likelihood of cure of 10 out of 1,000 patients, the number of cured will increase to approximately 50 out of 1,000, with a baseline of 100 out of 1,000 patients, it will do so to approximately 500 out of 1,000.

ORs, despite a fairly complex mathematical background, are easy to use, even for non-mathematicians, and they are the basis of many modern methods for analyzing clinical data including multivariable methods.

Multiple regression analysis of confounding variables, although routinely used in retrospective observational studies, is not emphasized in prospective studies like randomized clinical trials (RCTs). The randomization process ensures that differences in potential confounders are the result of chance. If differences are statistically significant, multiple regression analysis can be used for adjustment. Multiple regression can, also, be used in prospective studies for a different purpose. Certain patient characteristics in RCTs may cause substantial spread in the data even if they are equally distributed. Including such data in the efficacy analysis may increase precision and power in the data analysis. When the dependent variable is a change score, as in the first example, the baseline level is the first candidate to be considered, because it is almost certainly associated with the change score. When the dependent variable is an odds ratio, like in the second example, gender or age-category are adequate candidates.

We should emphasize that it has to be decided prior to the trial and stated explicitly in the trial protocol whether a regression model will be applied, because post hoc decisions regarding regression modeling like any other post hoc change in the raises the risk of statistical bias due to multiple testing. Naturally, there is less opportunity for modeling in a small trial than in a large trial. There is no general rule about which sample sizes are required for sensible regression modeling, but one rule-of-thumb is that at least ten times as many patients are required as the number of variables in the model. This would mean that a data set of at least 30 is required if we wish to include a single covariate in the model for the purpose of improving precision. With every additional covariate in the model an extra regression weight must be estimated, which rapidly leads to a decreased rather than improved precision.

Regression analysis can be adequately used for improving precision of efficacy analysis. Application of these models is very easy since many computer programs are available. For a successful application the fit of the regression models should, however, always be checked for example by scatter plots, or in case of doubt by goodness of fits tests, and the covariate selection should be sparse.

We do hope that this chapter will stimulate clinical investigators to use odds ratios and multiple regression models more often.

5   Conclusions

Odds ratios (ORs) unlike χ^2 – tests provide a direct insight in the strength of the relationship between treatment modalities and treatment effects. Multiple regression models can reduce the data spread due to certain patient characteristics, and thus, improve the precision of the treatment comparison. Despite these advantages the use of these methods in clinical trials is relatively uncommon.

This chapter (1) emphasizes the great potential of odds ratios and multiple regression models as a basis of modern methods, (2) illustrates their ease of use, and (3) familiarizes the non-mathematical scientific community with these important methods.

Advantages of the ORs are multiple:

1. They describe the probability that people with a certain treatment will have an event compared to people without the treatment, and are, therefore, a welcome alternative to the widely used χ^2 – tests for analyzing binary data in clinical trials.
2. Statistical software of ORs is widely available.

3. Computations using risk ratios (RRs) are less sensitive than those using ORs.
4. ORs are the basis for modern methods like meta-analyses, propensity scores, logistic regression, Cox regression etc.

For analysis logarithms of the ORs have to be used, results are obtained by calculating antilogarithms. A limitation of the ORs is that they present relative benefits but not absolute benefits. ORs, despite a fairly complex mathematical background, are easy to use, even for non-mathematicians.

Both linear and logistic regression models can be adequately applied for the purpose of improving precision of parameter estimates like treatment effects. We caution that, although application of these models is very easy with computer programs widely available, the fit of the regression models should always be carefully checked, and the covariate selection should be carefully considered and sparse.

We do hope that this chapter will stimulate clinical investigators to use odds ratios and multiple regression models more often.

References

Anonymous. Explanation of the quadratic approximation. www.math.tamu.edu/~kfu/Quadratic Approximation.pdf. Accessed 15 Dec 2011

Bland JM, Altman DG (2000) The odds ratio. BMJ 320:1468

BUGS y WinBUGS. http://www.mrc-bsu.cam.ac.uk/bugs, http://cran.r-project.org. Accessed 15 Dec 2011

Cleophas TJ (2003) The sense and non-sense of regression modeling for increasing precision of clinical trials. Clin Pharmacol Ther 74:295–297

Cleophas TJ (2005) Problems with regression modeling for the analysis of clinical trials. Int J Clin Pharmacol Ther 43:23–29

Cleophas TJ, Zwinderman AH (2007) Statistical primer for cardiovascular research, meta-analysis. Circulation 115:2870–2875

Excel by Windows. http://www.excel.com. Accessed 15 Dec 2011

Guyatt G, Rennie D (2001) Users guide to the medical literature-a manual for evidence based clinical practice by the Evidence-Based Medicine Working Group. AMA Press, Chicago, pp 356–357

Rubin DB (1997) Estimating causal effects from large data sets using propensity scores. Ann Intern Med 127:757–763

S-plus. http://www.mathsoft.com/splus. Accessed 15 Dec 2011

SAS. http://www.prw.le.ac.uk/epidemiol/personal/ajs22/meta/macros.sas. Accessed 15 Dec 2011

SPSS Statistical Software. http://www.spss.com. Accessed 15 Dec 2011

Stata. http://www.stata.com. Accessed 15 Dec 2011

StatsDirect. http://www.camcode.com. Accessed 15 Dec 2011

StatXact. http://www.cytel.com/products/statxact/statact1.html. Accessed 15 Dec 2011

True Epistat. http://ic.net/~biomware/biohp2te.htm. Accessed 15 Dec 2011

Zwinderman AH (2006) Subgroup analysis using multiple regression, confounding, interactions, synergism. In: Cleophas TJM, Zwinderman AH, Cleophas TF (eds) Statistics applied to clinical trials. Springer, Dordrecht, pp 125–140

Zwinderman AH, Niemeijer MG, Kleinjans HA, Cleophas TJ (1998) Application of item response modelling for quality of life assessments: effect of two nitrate treatment regimens in stable angina pectoris. In: Kuhlmann J, Mrozikiewicz A (eds) What should a clinical pharmacologist know to start a clinical trial. Zuckschwerdt Verlag, New York, pp 40–48

Chapter 66
Statistics Is No "Bloodless" Algebra

1 Introduction

Because biological processes are full of variations, statistics can not give you certainties, but only chances. What kind of chances? Basically, the chances that prior hypotheses are true or untrue. The human brain excels in making hypotheses. We make hypotheses all the time, but they may be untrue. For example, when you were a kid, you thought that only girls could become doctors, because your family doctor was a girl. Later on this hypothesis appeared to be untrue. In clinical medicine we currently emphasize that hypotheses may be equally untrue and must be assessed prospectively with hard data. That's where statistics comes in, and that is where at the same time many a clinician starts to become nervous, loses his/her self-confidence, and is more than willing to leave his/her data to the statistical consultant who subsequently runs the data through a whole series of statistical tests of SAS (SAS Statistical Software 2011) or SPSS (SPSS Statistical Software 2011) or comparable statistical computer software to see if there are any significances. The current chapter was written to emphasize that the above scenario of analyzing clinical trial data is bad practice and frequently kills the data, and that biostatistics can do more for you than provide you with a host of irrelevant p-values.

2 Statistics Is Fun Because It Proves Your Hypothesis Was Right

Statistics is fun, particularly, for the clinical investigator. It is not mathematics, but a discipline at the interface of biology and mathematics. This means that maths is used to answer the biological questions. The scenario as described above does not answer reasonable biological questions. It is called data dredging and is the source of a lot of

T.J. Cleophas and A.H. Zwinderman, *Statistics Applied to Clinical Studies*,
DOI 10.1007/978-94-007-2863-9_66, © Springer Science+Business Media B.V. 2012

misinterpretations in clinical medicine. A statistical analysis should be confined to testing of the prior hypotheses. The problem with multiple statistical tests can be explained by gambling 20 times with a chance of success of 5%. You can be sure that after the game you will get $(1-0.05)^{20} = (0.95)^{20} = 0.36 = 36\%$ chance to win a prize. This result is, however, not based on any significant effect but rather on the play of chance. Now, don't let it happen to your trial. Also, a statistical result that does not confirm your prior belief, don't trust it. Make sure that the simplest univariate tests are used for your prospective trial data, because they are adequate and provide the best power. Fancy multivariate procedures are not in place to answer your prior hypotheses. Statistics is fun, because it generally confirms or largely confirms your prior hypotheses, which is appropriate because they were based on sound clinical arguments. If they don't, this is peculiar and should make you anxious to find out why so: imperfections within the design or execution of the trial? (Cleophas 1999) It is fun to prove your hypothesis was right, or to find out what you did overlook. Another fun thing with statistics, although completely different and by far not so important, is the method of secondary analyses: it does not prove anything, but it is kind of sports and gives you new and sound ideas for further research.

3   Statistical Principles Can Help to Improve the Quality of the Trial

Over the past decades, the randomized controlled trial has entered an era of continuous improvement and has gradually become accepted as the most effective way of determining the relative efficacy and toxicity of a new therapy, because it controls for placebo and time effects. However, even sensitive and properly designed and executed trials do not always confirm hypotheses to be tested, and conclusions are not always confirmed by subsequent trials. Although the former may be due to wrong hypotheses, the latter is likely to be due to the presence of certain imperfections within the design and execution, and analysis of the trial itself. Such principles could include (Cleophas and Zwinderman 2000): (1) giving every effort to avoid asymmetries in the treatment groups (Chap. 1, stratification issues), (2) emphasis on statistical power rather than just null-hypothesis testing (Chap. 5), (3) assessing asymmetries of outcome variables in order to determine the most important determinants of clinical benefit (Chap. 17), (4) accounting routinely for Type III errors of mistakenly believing that an inferior treatment is superior (Chap. 5), (5) routinely weighing the odds of benefits against the odds of risks of new treatments.

4   Statistics Can Provide Worthwhile Extras to Your Research

The classical two-parallel-groups design for clinical drug trials is a rather dull activity and is, essentially, unable to answer many current scientific questions. Also, it is laborious, and in the clinical setting sometimes ethically or financially impossible.

Examples of what the classical clinical trial design cannot manage: (1) assess multimodal therapies, (2) account historical data, (3) safeguard ethics and efficacy during the course of long-term trials, (4) study drugs, before well-established toxicity information is available, (5) account the possibility of therapeutic equivalence between test and reference treatment, (6) study multiple treatments in one trial, (7) adjust change scores for baseline levels. Alternative designs for such purposes: (1) factorial designs (Chap. 1) (Farewell and Dángio 1981), (2) historical controls designs (Chap. 1) (Sacks et al. 1982), (3) group-sequential interim analysis designs (Chap. 6) (Pocock 1988), (4) sequential designs for continuous monitoring (Chap. 6) (Whitehead 1998), (5) therapeutic equivalence designs (Chap. 4), (6) multiple crossover-periods/multiple parallel-groups designs (Lauter 1996), (7) increased precision designs through multivariable adjustment (Chap. 18). There is, of course, the increased risks of type I/II errors, and the possible loss of some of the validity criteria with the novel designs. However, provided that such possibilities are adequately accounted for in the design stage of the trial, the novel designs are acceptedly valid, and offer relevant scientific, ethical, and financial extras.

5 Statistics Is Not Like Algebra Bloodless

Statistics is not like algebra bloodless, and requires a lot of biological thinking and just a little bit of mathematics. For example, mathematically we need representative sample sizes to make meaningful inferences about the whole population. Yet, from a biological point of view, this is less true: the first datum encountered in a clinical situation of complete ignorance provides the greatest amount of information from any one datum an investigator will encounter. For example, consider a new disease for which there is no knowledge whatsoever about the order of magnitude of time of exposure, time of incubation, time of appearance of subsequent symptoms. The first patient for whom we know such data provides a great deal of information.

Another example of biological rather than mathematical thinking involves the issue of making the test parameters alpha and beta flexible. They are mostly set at respectively 5% and 20%. A 20% beta is, however, larger than is appropriate in many cases. For example, when the false positive is worse for the patient than the false negative, as in case of testing a drug for non-life threatening illness with the drug having severe side effects, the 5% and 20% choices for alpha and beta are reasonable. However, in testing treatment for cancer, the rate of false negatives is worse for the patient, and so, the ratio beta/alpha should be reduced.

A third example of biological thinking is the inclusion of a "safety factor" when estimating prior to a trial the sample size required. Usually the required sample size is calculated from a pilot study or from results quoted in the literature. However, these data are not the actual data from our study, and not using the real data may introduce an error. Also, the data as used for sample size calculation are subject to randomness error. Due to such errors the alpha and beta errors upon which our sample size is based may be larger than we thought. Because of these possibilities we should add a "safety factor" to the sample size as calculated, and make our sample size somewhat larger than the calculated one, e.g., 10% larger. This is more important, the more uneasy we are about the ultimate result of the study being in agreement with the estimate used for sample size calculation.

6   Statistics Can Turn Art into Science

Traditionally, the science of medicine is considered to be based on experimental evidence, while the art of science is supposed to be based on trust, sympathy, the threatened patient, and other things that no one would believe that could ever be estimated by statistical methods. It is true that factors, of psychosocial and personal nature, are difficult to measure, but it is not impossible to do so. At first, quality of life assessments were based on the amount of primary symptoms, e.g., pain scores etc. Increasingly it is recognized that it should be based on factors like feeling of well-being, social performance. Along this line of development, the art of medicine is more and more turned into science, e.g., with modern quality of life assessments addressing general feeling of well-being, physical activity domains etc. Statistical analyses can be readily performed on validated quality of life indices or any other measurements of effectiveness as developed (Chap. 38). It follows that this development is going to accomplish something that was only shortly believed to be impossible: turning the art of medicine into the science of medicine.

7   Statistics for Support Rather Than Illumination?

In 1948 the first randomized controlled trial was published (Medical Research Council 1948). Until then, observations had been largely uncontrolled. Initially, trials frequently did not confirm hypotheses to be tested. This phenomenon was attributed to little sensitivity due to small samples, as well as inappropriate hypotheses based on biased prior trials. Additional flaws were being recognized and, subsequently better accounted for: carryover effects due to insufficient washout from previous treatments, time effects due to external factors and the natural history of conditions being studied, bias due to asymmetry between treatment groups, lack of sensitivity due to a negative correlation between treatment responses etc. Currently, due to the complexity of trials, clinicians increasingly leave the thinking to statisticians, a practice which is essentially wrong and produces flawed research, because bio-research requires a lot of biological thinking and no more than a bit of statistics. Moreover, a statistician can do much more for you than provide you with a host of irrelevant p-values, but he/she can only do so, if you intuitively know what statistics can and what it cannot answer. Like Professor M. Hills, the famous statistician of London, used to say, clinicians often use statistics as a drunk uses a lantern standard, for support rather than illumination. Illumination can be obtained by exploring your clinical intuition against a mathematical background.

8 Statistics Can Help the Clinician to Better Understand Limitations and Benefits of Current Research

Medical literature is currently snowed under with mortality trials, showing invariably a highly significant 10–30% relative increase in survival. Mortality is considered an important endpoint, and this may be so. Yet, a relative increase in survival of 10–30% generally means in absolute terms an increase of no more than 1–2%. Mortality is an insensitive variable of the effects of preventive medicine that is begun when subjects are middle-aged. At such ages the background noise associated with senescence becomes high. The endpoints better be reduction in morbidity so far. In addition, many clinicians know that patients would prefer assessment of quality of life and reduced morbidity rather than 1–2% increased survival in return for long term drug treatment with considerable side effects. Relative risk reductions are frequently overinterpreted by clinicians in terms of absolute risk reductions. And so are underpowered p-values: a p-value of 0.05 after all means the chance of a type II error of 50%.

On the other hand, statistics can do a lot more for clinicians than calculating p-values and relative risk reductions. Multivariable analyses can be used not only for exploring new ideas, but also for increasing precision of point estimates in a trial. Benefit/risk analyses of trial data are helpful to provide relevant arguments for clinical decision making, and they are particularly so when their ratios are assessed quantitatively. Statistics can provide us with wonderful meta-analyses of independent trials to find out whether scientific findings are consistent and can be generalized across populations.

9 Limitations of Statistics

Of course, we should avoid giving a non-stop laudatio of statistics only. It is time that we added a few remarks on its limitations and possible disadvantages in order to express a more balanced opinion. Statistics is at the interface of mathematics and biology. Therefore, it gives no certainties, only chances. What chances? For example, chances that hypotheses are true or untrue. We generally reject the null-hypothesis of no effect at $p < 0.05$. However, $p = 0.05$ means 5% chance of a type I error of finding a difference where there is none, and 50% chance of a type II error of finding no difference where there is one. It pictures pretty well how limited statistical inferences can be. In addition to the risks of type I and type II errors, there is the issue of little clinical relevance in spite of statistically significant findings. A subanalysis of the SOLVD study (Yusuf et al. 1992) found no symptoms of angina pectoris in 85.3% of the patients on enalapril and in 82.5% of the patients on placebo (difference statistically significant at $p < 0.001$). In situations like this, one has to wonder about the clinical relevance of the small difference. This is even more so when one considers that an active compound generally causes more side-effects than does a placebo. Finally, we have to consider the point of bias. Arguments have been raised that controlled clinical trials although they adjust for placebo effects and time effects, are still quite vulnerable to other biases, e.g., psychological biases and selection biases. In clinical trials, as opposed to regular patient care, patients are generally highly compliant; their high compliance is an important reason for participating in the trials in the first place. They have a positive attitude towards the trial and anticipate personal benefit from it, a mechanism which is known as the Hawthorne effect (Campbell et al. 1995). Alternatively, patients selected for a trial often refuse to comply with randomization which may render unrepresentative samples (Cleophas 1997). Statistics has great difficulty in handling such effects and is, essentially, unable to make sense of unrepresentative samples. Not being familiar with statistics raises a two-way risk: you're not only missing the benefit of it but also fail to adequately recognize the limitations of it.

10   Conclusions

1. Statistics is fun for the clinical investigator because it generally confirms or l largely confirms his/her prior hypotheses.
2. Accounting some simple statistical principles can help the clinical investigator reduce imperfections in the design and execution of clinical trials.
3. For the clinical investigator getting a good command of non-classical study designs can provide worthwhile extras to his/her research.
4. Statistics is not like algebra, because it requires a lot of biological thinking and just a little bit of mathematics.
5. Statistical analyses can be readily performed on such modern quality of life assessments like general feeling of well-being, physical activity domains, psychosocial performance etc.
6. Along this line the art of medicine is more and more being turned into scientific evidence.
7. Statistics can do a lot for the clinical investigator if he/she intuitively knows what statistics can and what it cannot answer.
8. Statistics can help clinical investigators to interpret more adequately limitations as well as benefits of current clinical research.
9. Statistics has, of course, limitations of its own. It can not give certainties, only chances.
10. Statistical significance does not automatically indicate clinical relevance. Statistical methods can not test every possible source of bias in a trial.

Not being familiar with statistics raises a two-way risk: you're not only missing the benefit of it but also fail to adequately recognize its limitations. We hope that this book will be an incentive for readers to improve their statistical skills in order to better understand the statistical data as published in the literature and to be able to take better care of their own experimental data.

References

Campbell JP, Maxey VA, Watson WA (1995) Hawthorne effect: implications for prehospital research. Ann Emerg Med 26:590–594

Cleophas TJ (1997) The use of a placebo-control group in clinical trials. Br J Clin Pharmacol 43:219–221

Cleophas TJ (1999) Methods for improving drug trials. Clin Chem Lab Med 37:1035–1041

Cleophas TJ, Zwinderman AH (2000) Limits of randomized trials, proposed alternative designs. Clin Chem Lab Med 38:1217–1223

Farewell VT, Dángio GJ (1981) Report of the National Wilms' Tumor Study Group. Biometrics 37:169–176

Lauter J (1996) Exact t and F-tests for analyzing studies with multiple endpoints. Biometrics 52:964–970

Medical Research Council (1948) Streptomycin treatment of pulmonary tuberculosis. Br Med J 2:769–782

Pocock SJ (1988) Clinical trials. A practical approach. Wiley, New York

Sacks H, Chalmers TC, Smith H (1982) Randomized versus historical controls for clinical trials. Am J Med 72:233–240

SAS Statistical Software, New York, NY, USA, www.SAS.com. Accessed 15 Dec 2011

SPSS Statistical Software, Chicago, IL, USA, www.SPSS.com. Accessed 15 Dec 2011

Whitehead J (1998) Planning and evaluating sequential trials (PEST, version 3). University of Reading. Reading. www.reading.ac.uk/mps/pest/pest.html. Accessed 15 Dec 2011

Yusuf S, Pepine CJ, Garces C (1992) Effect of enalapril on myocardial infarction and angina pectoris in patients with low ejection fraction. Lancet 340:1173–1178

Chapter 67
Bias Due to Conflicts of Interests, Some Guidelines

1 Introduction

The controlled clinical trial, the gold standard for drug development, is in jeopardy. The pharmaceutical industry rapidly expands it's commend over clinical trials. Scientific rigor requires independence and objectivity. Safeguarding such criteria is hard with industrial sponsors, benefiting from favorable results, virtually completely in control. The recent Good Clinical Practice Criteria adopted by the European Community (Anonymous 1997) were not helpful, and even confirmed the right of the pharmaceutical industry to keep everything under control. Except for the requirement that the trial protocol should be approved by an external protocol review board, little further external monitoring of the trial is required in Europe today. The present chapter was written to review flawed procedures jeopardizing the credibility of current clinical trials, and to look for possible solutions to the dilemma between sponsored industry and scientific independence.

2 The Randomized Controlled Clinical Trial as the Gold Standard

Controlled clinical trials began in the UK with James Lind, on H.M.S. Salisbury, a royal Frigate, by the end of the 18th century. However, in 1948 the first randomized controlled trial was actually published by the English Medical Research Council in the British Medical Journal (Medical Research Council 1948). Until then, published observations had been uncontrolled. Initially, trials frequently did not confirm hypotheses to be tested. This phenomenon was attributed to little sensitivity due to small samples, as well as inappropriate hypotheses based on biased prior trials. Additional flaws were being recognized and, subsequently were better accounted

T.J. Cleophas and A.H. Zwinderman, *Statistics Applied to Clinical Studies*,
DOI 10.1007/978-94-007-2863-9_67, © Springer Science+Business Media B.V. 2012

for: carryover effects due to insufficient washout from previous treatments, time effects due to external factors and the natural history of the condition under study, bias due to asymmetry between treatment groups, lack of sensitivity due to a nega-tive correlation between treatment responses etc. Such flaws mainly of a technical nature have been largely implemented and lead to trials after 1970 being of signifi-cantly better quality than before. And so, the randomized clinical trial has gradually become accepted as the most effective way of determining the relative efficacy and toxicity of new drug therapies. High quality criteria for clinical trials include clearly defined hypotheses, explicit description of methods, uniform data analysis, but, most of all, a valid design. A valid design means that the trial should be made independent, objective, balanced, blinded, controlled, with objective measurements. Any research but, certainly, industrially-sponsored drug research where sponsors benefit from favorable results, benefits from valid designs.

3 Need for Circumspection Recognized

The past decade focused, in addition to technical aspects, on the need for circum-spection in planning and conducting clinical trials (Cleophas et al. 2002). As a consequence, prior to approval, clinical trial protocols started to be routinely scrutinized by different circumstantial organs, including ethic committees, institutional and federal review boards, national and international scientific organizations, and monitoring committees charged with conducting interim analyses. And so things seems to be developing just fine until something else emerged, the rapidly expand-ing commend of the pharmaceutical industry over clinical trials. Scientific rigor requires independence and objectivity of clinical research, and safeguarding such principles is hard with sponsors virtually completely in control.

4 The Expanding Commend of the Pharmaceutical Industry Over Clinical Trials

Today megatrials are being performed costing billions of dollars paid by the indus-try. Clinical research has become fragmented among many sites, and the control of clinical data often lies exclusively in the trial sponsor's hands (Montaner et al. 2001). A serious issue to consider here is adherence to scientific criteria like objec-tivity, and validity criteria like blindness during the analysis phase. In the USA, the FDA audits ongoing registered trials for scientific validity. However, even on-site-audits can hardly be considered capable of controlling each stage of the trial. Not any audits are provided by the FDA's European counterparts. Instead, in 1991, the European Community endorsed the Good Clinical Practice (GCP) criteria devel-oped (Anonymous 1997) as a collaborative effort of governments, industries, and the profession. For each of the contributing parties benefits are different. Governments are interested in uniform guidelines and uniform legislation. For the profession the main incentives are scientific progress, and the adherence to scientific and validity criteria. In contrast, for the pharmaceutical industry a major incentive is its commercial interest. And so, the criteria are, obviously, a compromise. Scientific criteria like clearly defined prior hypotheses, explicit description of methods, uniform data analyses are broadly stated in the guidelines given (Anonymous 1997). However, scientific criteria like instruments to control independence and objectivity of research are not included. Validity criteria like control groups and blinding are recognized, but requirements like specialized monitoring teams consistent of a group of external independent investigators guiding such criteria, and charged with interim analysis and stopping rules are not mentioned. And so, the implementation of the Good Clinical Practice Criteria is not helpful for the purpose of safeguarding scientific independence. Instead, they confirmed the right of the pharmaceutical industry to keep everything under control.

5   Flawed Procedures Jeopardizing Current Clinical Trials

Flawed procedures jeopardizing current clinical trials are listed in Table 67.1. Industries, at least in Europe, are allowed to choose their own independent protocol review board prior to approval. Frequently, a pharmaceutical company chooses one-and-the-same-board for all of its (multicenter) studies. The independent protocol review board may approve protocols, even if the research is beyond its scope of expertise, for example, specialized protocols like oncology-protocols without an oncologist among its members. Once the protocol is approved, little further external review is required in Europe today. Due to recent European Community Regulations, health facilities hosting multicenter trials are requested to refrain from scientific or ethic assessment. Their local committees may assess local logistic aspects of the trial but no more than that. And so, the once so important role of local committees

Table 67.1 Flawed procedures jeopardizing current clinical trials

1.	Pharmaceutical industries, at least in Europe, are allowed to choose their own independent review board prior to approval
2.	The independent protocol review board approves protocol even if the research is beyond the scope of its expertise
3.	Health facilities hosting multicenter research are requested to refrain from ethic or scientific assessment after approval by the independent review board
4.	Trial monitors are often employees of pharmaceutical industry
5.	Data control is predominantly in the hands of the sponsor
6.	Interim analyses are rarely performed by independent groups
7.	The scientific committee of a trial consists largely of guests (names of prominent physicians attached to the study) and graphters (for the purpose of giving the work more impact)
8.	The analysis and report is produced by *ghosts* (clinical associates at the pharmaceutical companies) and is after a brief review co-signed by the *guests* and *graphters*

to improve the objectivity of sponsored research is minimized. Another problem with the objectivity of industrially-sponsored clinical trials is the fact that the trial monitors are often employees of the pharmaceutical industry. Furthermore, data control is predominantly in the hands of the sponsor. Interim analyses are rarely performed by independent groups. The scientific committee of the trial consists largely of prominent but otherwise uninvolved physicians attached to the study, the so-called *guests*. Analysis and report of the trial is generally produced by clinical associates at the pharmaceutical companies, the *ghosts*, and, after a brief review, co-signed by prominent physicians attached to the study the so-called *graphters*.

6 The Good News

The Helsinki guidelines rewritten in the year 2000 have been criticized (Diamant 2002) for its incompleteness regarding several ethical issues, e.g., those involving developing countries. However, these independently written guidelines also included important improvements. For the first time the issue of conflict of interests has been assessed in at least five paragraphs. Good news is also the American FDA's initiative to start auditing sponsored trials on site. In May 1998 editors of 70 major journals have endorsed the Consolidated Standards of Reporting Trials Statement (CONSORT) in an attempt to standardize the way trials are conducted, analyzed and reported. The same year, the Cochrane Collaborators together with the British journals The Lancet and The British Medical Journal have launched the "Unpublished Paper Amnesty Movement", in an attempt to reduce publication bias. There is also good news from the basis. For example, in 30 hospitals in the Netherlands local ethic committees, endorsed by the Netherlands Association of Hospitals, have declared that they will not give up scrutinizing sponsored research despite approval by the independent protocol review board.

In our educational hospital house officers are particularly critical of the results of industrially-sponsored research even if it is in the Lancet or the New England Journal of Medicine, and they are more reluctant to accept results not fitting in their prior concept of pathophysiology, if the results are from industrially-sponsored research. Examples include: ACE-inhibitors for normotensive subjects at risk for cardiovascular disease (HOPE Study (Slcight et al. 2001)), antihypertensive drugs for secondary secondary prevention of stroke in elderly subjects (PROGRESS Study (PROGRESS Collaborative Group 2001)), beta-blockers for heart failure (many sponsored studies, but none of them demonstrating an unequivocal improvement of cardiac performance (Meyer and Cleophas 2001)), cholesterol-lowering treatment for patients at risk of cardiovascular disease but normal LDL-cholesterol levels (Heart Protection Study), hypoglycemic drugs for prediabetics (NAVIGATOR Study). As a matter of fact, all of the above studies are based on not so sensitive univariable analyses. When we recently performed a multivariable analysis of a secondary prevention study with statins, we could demonstrate that patients with normal LDL-cholesterol levels did not benefit (Cleophas and Zwinderman 2003).

7 Further Solutions to the Dilemma Between Sponsored Research and the Independence of Science

After more than 50 years of continuous improvement, the controlled clinical trial has become the most effective way of determining the relative efficacy and toxicity of new drug therapies. This gold standard is, however, in jeopardy due to the expanding commend of the pharmaceutical industry. Mega-trials are not only paid for by the industry but also designed, carried-out, and analyzed by the industry. Because objectivity is at stake when industrial money mixes with the profession (Relman et al. 2001) it has been recently suggested to separate scientific research and the pharmaceutical industry. However, separation may not be necessary, and might be counterproductive to the progress of medicine. After all, pharmaceutical industry has deserved substantial credits for developing important medicines, while other bodies including governments have not been able to develop medicines in the past 40 years, with the exception of one or two vaccines. Also, separation would mean that economic incentives are lost not only on the part of the industry but also on the part of the profession while both are currently doing well in the progress of medicine. Money *was* and *is* a major motive to stimulate scientific progress. Without economic incentives from industry there may soon be few clinical trials. Circumspection from independent observers during each stage of the trial has been recognized as an alternative for increasing objectivity of research and preventing bias (Cleophas et al. 2002). In addition, tight control of study data, analysis, and interpretation by the commercial sponsor is undesirable. It not only raises the risk of biased interpretation, but also limits the opportunities for the scientific community to use the data for secondary analyses needed for future research (Montaner et al. 2001). If the pharmaceutical industry allows the profession to more actively participate in different stages of the trial, scientific research will be better served, and reasonable biological questions will be better answered. First on the agenda will have to be the criteria for adequate circumspection (Table 67.2). Because the profession will be more convinced of its objective character, this allowance will not be counterproductive to the sales. Scientific research will be exciting again, confirming prior hypotheses, and giving new and sound ideas for further research.

Table 67.2 Criteria for adequate circumspection

1.	Disclosure of conflict of interests and the nature of it from each party involved
2.	Independent ethical and scientific assessment of the protocol
3.	Independent monitoring of the conduct of the trial
4.	Independent monitoring of data management
5.	Independent monitoring of statistical analysis including the cleaning-up of the data
6.	The requirement to publish even if data do not fit in the commercial interest of the sponsor
7.	Requirement that interim analyses be performed by an independent group

8   Conclusions

The controlled clinical trial, the gold standard for clinical research, is in jeopardy. The pharmaceutical industry rapidly expands its commend over clinical trials. Scientific rigor requires independence and objectivity. Safeguarding such criteria is hard with industrial sponsors, benefiting from favorable results, virtually completely in control. The objective of this chapter was to review flawed procedures jeopardizing the credibility of trials, and to look for possible solutions to the dilemma between sponsored industry and scientific independence.

Flawed procedures jeopardizing current clinical trials could be listed as follows. Industries, at least in Europe, are allowed to choose their own independent protocol review board prior to approval. The independent protocol review board approves protocols even if the research is beyond the scope of its expertise. Health facilities hosting multicenter trials are requested to refrain from scientific or ethic assessment of the trial. Trial monitors are often employees of industry. Data control is predominantly in the hands of the sponsor. Interim analyses are rarely performed by independent groups. The scientific committee of the trial consists largely of prominent but otherwise uninvolved physicians attached to the study. Analysis and report of the trial is generally provided by clinical associates at the pharmaceutical companies and, after a brief review, co-signed by prominent physicians attached to the study.

Possible solutions to the dilemma between sponsored industry and scientific independence could include the following. Circumspection from independent observers during each stage of the trial is desirable. In contrast, tight control of study data, analysis, and interpretation by the commercial sponsor is not desirable. If, instead, pharmaceutical industry allows the profession to more actively participate in different stages of the trial, scientific research will be better served, reasonable biological questions will be better answered, and, because the profession will be more convinced of the objective character of the research, it will not be counterproductive to the sales.

References

Anonymous (1997) International guidelines for good clinical practice. NEFARMA (Netherlands Association of Pharmaceutical Industries), Utrecht

Cleophas TJ, Zwinderman AH (2003) Efficacy of HMG-CoA reductase inhibitors dependent on baseline cholesterol levels, secondary analysis of the Regression Growth Evaluation Statin Study (REGRESS). Br J Clin Pharmacol 56:465–466

Cleophas TJ, Zwinderman AH, Cleophas TF (2002) Statistics applied to clinical trials, self-assessment book. Kluwer, Boston

Diamant JC (2002) The revised declaration of Helsinki – is justice served. Int J Clin Pharmacol Ther 40:76–83

Medical Research Council (1948) Streptomycin treatment of pulmonary tuberculosis. Br Med J 2:769–782

Meyer FP, Cleophas TJ (2001) Meta-analysis of beta-blockers in heart failure. Int J Clin Pharmacol Ther 39:561–563 and 39:383–388

Montaner JS, O'Shaughnessy MV, Schechter MT (2001) Industry-sponsored clinical research: a double-edged sword. Lancet 358:1893–1895

PROGRESS Collaborative Group (2001) Randomised trial of a perindopril-based blood-pressure lowering regimen among 6105 individuals with previous stroke or transient ischaemic attack. Lancet 358:1033–1041

Relman AJ, Cleophas TJ, Cleophas GI (2001) The pharmaceutical industry and continuing medical education. JAMA 286:302–304

Sleight P, Yusuf S, Pogue J, Tsuyuki R, Diaz R, Probsfield J (2001) Blood pressure reduction and cardiovascular risk in HOPE Study. Lancet 358:2130–2131

Appendix

T-Table

v	Q = 0.4	0.25	0.1	0.05	0.025	0.01	0.005	0.001
	2Q = 0.8	0.5	0.2	0.1	0.05	0.02	0.01	0.002
1	0.325	1. 000	3.078	6.314	12.706	31.821	63.657	318.31
2	.289	0.816	1.886	2.920	4.303	6.965	9.925	22.326
3	.277	.765	1.638	2.353	3.182	4.547	5.841	10.213
4	.171	.741	1.533	2.132	2.776	3.747	4.604	7.173
5	0.267	0.727	1.476	2.015	2.571	3.365	4.032	5.893
6	.265	.718	1.440	1.943	2.447	3.143	3.707	5.208
7	.263	.711	1.415	1.895	2.365	2.998	3.499	4.785
8	.262	.706	1.397	1.860	2.306	2.896	3.355	4.501
9	.261	.703	1.383	1.833	2.262	2.821	3.250	4.297
10	0.261	0.700	1.372	1.812	2.228	2.764	3.169	4.144
11	.269	.697	1.363	1.796	2.201	2.718	3.106	4.025
12	.269	.695	1.356	1.782	2.179	2.681	3.055	3.930
13	.259	.694	1.350	1.771	2.160	2.650	3.012	3.852
14	.258	.692	1.345	1.761	2.145	2.624	2.977	3.787
15	0.258	0.691	1.341	1.753	2.131	2.602	2.947	3.733
16	.258	.690	1.337	1.746	2.120	2.583	2.921	3.686
17	.257	.689	1.333	1.740	2.110	2.567	2.898	3.646
18	.257	.688	1.330	1.734	2.101	2.552	2.878	3.610
19	.257	.688	1.328	1.729	2.093	2.539	2.861	3.579
20	0.257	0.687	1.325	1.725	2.086	2.528	2.845	3.552
21	.257	.686	1.323	1.721	2.080	2.518	2.831	3.527
22	.256	.686	1.321	1.717	2.074	2.508	2.819	3.505
23	.256	.685	1.319	1.714	2.069	2.600	2.807	3.485
24	.256	.685	1.318	1.711	2.064	2.492	2.797	3.467
25	0.256	0.684	1,316	1.708	2.060	2.485	2.787	3.450
26	.256	.654	1,315	1.706	2.056	2.479	2.779	3.435
27	.256	.684	1,314	1.701	2.052	2.473	2.771	3.421
28	.256	.683	1,313	1.701	2.048	2.467	2.763	3.408
29	.256	.683	1.311	1.699	2.045	2.462	2.756	3.396

(continued)

T.J. Cleophas and A.H. Zwinderman, *Statistics Applied to Clinical Studies*,
DOI 10.1007/978-94-007-2863-9, © Springer Science+Business Media B.V. 2012

T-Table   (continued)

v	Q=0.4	0.25	0.1	0.05	0.025	0.01	0.005	0.001
	2Q=0.8	0.5	0.2	0.1	0.05	0.02	0.01	0.002
30	0.256	0.683	1.310	1.697	2.042	2.457	2.750	3.385
40	.255	.681	1.303	1.684	2.021	2.423	2.704	3.307
60	.254	.679	1.296	1.671	2.000	2.390	2.660	3.232
120	.254	.677	1.289	1.658	1.950	2.358	2.617	3.160
∞	.253	.674	1.282	1.645	1.960	2.326	2.576	3.090

v = degrees of freedom for t-variable, Q = area under the curve right from the corresponding t-value, 2Q tests both right and left end of the total area under the curve
Unpaired non-parametric test: Mann-Whitney test

Chi-square distribution

df	Two-tailed P-value			
	0.10	0.05	0.01	0.001
1	2.706	3.841	6.635	10.827
2	4.605	5.991	9.210	13.815
3	6.251	7.815	11.345	16.266
4	7.779	9.488	13.277	18.466
5	9.236	11.070	15.086	20.515
6	10.645	12.592	16.812	22.457
7	12.017	14.067	18.475	24.321
8	13.362	15.507	20.090	26.124
9	14.684	16.919	21.666	27.877
10	15.987	18.307	23.209	29.588
11	17.275	19.675	24.725	31.264
12	18.549	21.026	26.217	32.909
13	19.812	22.362	27.688	34.527
14	21.064	23.685	29.141	36.124
15	22.307	24.996	30.578	37.698
16	23.542	26.296	32.000	39.252
17	24.769	27.587	33.409	40.791
18	25.989	28.869	34.805	42.312
19	27.204	30.144	36.191	43.819
20	28.412	31.410	37.566	45.314
21	29.615	32.671	38.932	46.796
22	30.813	33.924	40.289	48.268
23	32.007	35.172	41.638	49.728
24	33.196	36.415	42.980	51.179
25	34.382	37.652	44.314	52.619
26	35.563	38.885	45.642	54.051
27	36.741	40.113	46.963	55.475
28	37.916	41.337	48.278	56.892
29	39.087	42.557	49.588	58.301
30	40.256	43.773	50.892	59.702
40	51.805	55.758	63.691	73.403
50	63.167	67.505	76.154	86.660
60	74.397	79.082	88.379	99.608
70	85.527	90.531	100.43	112.32
80	96.578	101.88	112.33	124.84
90	107.57	113.15	124.12	137.21
100	118.50	124.34	135.81	149.45

F-distribution

df of denominator	2-tailed P-value	1-tailed P-value	Degrees of freedom (df) of the numerator												
			1	2	3	4	5	6	7	8	9	10	15	25	500
1	0.05	0.025	647.8	799.5	864.2	899.6	921.8	937.1	948.2	956.6	963.	968.6	984.9	998.1	1017.0
1	0.10	0.05	161.4	199.5	215.7	224.6	230.2	234.0	236.8	238.9	240.5	241.9	245.9	249.3	254.1
2	0.05	0.025	38.51	39.00	39.17	39.25	39.30	39.33	39.36	39.37	39.39	39.40	39.43	39.46	39.50
2	0.10	0.05	18.51	19.00	19.16	19.25	19.30	19.33	19.35	19.37	19.38	19.40	19.43	19.46	19.49
3	0.05	0.025	17.44	16.04	15.44	15.10	14.88	14.73	14.62	14.54	14.47	14.42	14.25	14.12	13.91
3	0.10	0.05	10.13	9.55	9.28	9.12	9.01	8.94	8.89	8.85	8.81	8.79	8.70	8.63	8.53
4	0.05	0.025	12.22	10.65	9.98	9.60	9.36	9.20	9.07	8.98	8.90	8.84	8.66	8.50	8.27
4	0.10	0.05	7.71	6.94	6.59	6.39	6.26	6.16	6.09	6.04	6.00	5.96	5.86	5.77	5.64
5	0.05	0.025	10.01	8.43	7.76	7.39	7.15	6.98	6.85	6.76	6.68	6.62	6.43	6.27	6.03
5	0.10	0.05	6.61	5.79	5.41	5.19	5.05	4.95	4.88	4.82	4.77	4.74	4.62	4.52	4.37
6	0.05	0.025	8.81	7.26	6.60	6.23	5.99	5.82	5.70	5.60	5.52	5.46	5.27	5.11	4.86
6	0.10	0.05	5.99	5.14	4.76	4.53	4.39	4.28	4.21	4.15	4.10	4.06	3.94	3.83	3.68
7	0.05	0.025	8.07	6.54	5.89	5.52	5.29	5.12	4.99	4.90	4.82	4.76	4.57	4.40	4.16
7	0.10	0.05	5.59	4.74	4.35	4.12	3.97	3.87	3.79	3.73	3.68	3.64	3.51	3.40	3.24
8	0.05	0.025	7.57	6.06	5.42	5.05	4.82	4.65	4.53	4.43	4.36	4.30	4.10	3.94	3.68
8	0.10	0.05	5.32	4.46	4.07	3.84	3.69	3.58	3.50	3.44	3.39	3.35	3.22	3.11	2.94
9	0.05	0.025	7.21	5.71	5.08	4.72	4.48	4.32	4.20	4.10	4.03	3.96	3.77	3.60	3.35
9	0.10	0.05	5.12	4.26	3.86	3.63	3.48	3.37	3.29	3.23	3.18	3.14	3.01	2.89	2.72
10	0.05	0.025	6.94	5.46	4.83	4.47	4.24	4.07	3.95	3.85	3.78	3.72	3.52	3.35	3.09
10	0.10	0.05	4.96	4.10	3.71	3.48	3.33	3.22	3.14	3.07	3.02	2.98	2.85	2.73	2.55
15	0.05	0.025	6.20	4.77	4.15	3.80	3.58	3.41	3.29	3.20	3.12	3.06	2.86	2.69	2.41
15	0.10	0.05	4.54	3.68	3.29	3.06	2.90	2.79	2.71	2.64	2.59	2.54	2.40	2.28	2.08
20	0.05	0.025	5.87	4.46	3.86	3.51	3.29	3.13	3.01	2.91	2.84	2.77	2.57	2.40	2.10
20	0.10	0.05	4.35	3.49	3.10	2.87	2.71	2.60	2.51	2.45	2.39	2.35	2.20	2.07	1.86
30	0.05	0.025	5.57	4.18	3.59	3.25	3.03	2.87	2.75	2.65	2.57	2.51	2.31	2.12	1.81

(continued)

F-distribution (continued)

df of denominator	2-tailed P-value	1-tailed P-value	Degrees of freedom (df) of the numerator												
			1	2	3	4	5	6	7	8	9	10	15	25	500
30	0.10	0.05	4.17	3.32	2.92	2.69	2.53	2.42	2.33	2.27	2.21	2.16	2.01	1.88	1.64
50	**0.05**	**0.025**	**5.34**	**3.97**	**3.39**	**3.05**	**2.83**	**2.67**	**2.55**	**2.46**	**2.38**	**2.32**	**2.11**	**1.92**	**1.57**
50	0.10	0.05	4.03	3.18	2.79	2.56	2.40	2.29	2.20	2.13	2.07	2.03	1.87	1.73	1.46
100	**0.05**	**0.025**	**5.18**	**3.83**	**3.25**	**2.92**	**2.70**	**2.54**	**2.42**	**2.32**	**2.24**	**2.18**	**1.97**	**1.77**	**1.38**
100	0.10	0.05	3.94	3.09	2.70	2.46	2.31	2.19	2.10	2.03	1.97	1.93	1.77	1.62	1.31
1000	**0.05**	**0.025**	**5.04**	**3.70**	**3.13**	**2.80**	**2.58**	**2.42**	**2.30**	**2.20**	**2.13**	**2.06**	**1.85**	**1.64**	**1.16**
1000	0.10	0.05	3.85	3.00	2.61	2.38	2.22	2.11	2.02	1.95	1.89	1.84	1.68	1.52	1.13

Paired non-parametric test: Wilcoxon signed rank test, the table uses smaller of the two rank numbers

N pairs	P<0.05	P<0.01
7	2	0
8	2	0
9	6	2
10	8	3
11	11	5
12	14	7
13	17	10
14	21	13
15	25	16
16	30	19

P<0.01 levels

$n_2\downarrow$ / $n_1\rightarrow$	2	3	4	5	6	7	8	9	10	11	12	13	14	15
4			10											
5		6	11	17										
6		7	12	18	26									
7		7	13	20	27	36								
8	3	8	14	21	29	38	49							
9	3	8	15	22	31	40	51	63						
10	3	9	15	23	32	42	53	65	78					
11	4	9	16	24	34	44	55	68	81	96				
12	4	10	17	26	35	46	58	71	85	99	115			
13	4	10	18	27	37	48	60	73	88	103	119	137		
14	4	11	19	28	38	50	63	76	91	106	123	141	160	
15	4	11	20	29	40	52	65	79	94	110	127	145	164	185
16	4	12	21	31	42	54	67	82	97	114	131	150	169	
17	5	12	21	32	43	56	70	84	100	117	135	154		
18	5	13	22	33	45	58	72	87	103	121	139			
19	5	13	23	34	46	60	74	90	107	124				
20	5	14	24	35	48	62	77	93	110					
21	6	14	25	37	50	64	79	95						
22	6	15	26	38	51	66	82							
23	6	15	27	39	53	68								
24	6	16	28	40	55									
25	6	16	28	42										
26	7	17	29											
27	7	17												
28	7													

Table uses difference of added up rank numbers between group 1 and group 2

Unpaired non-parametric test: Mann-Whitney test

P<0.05 levels

$n_1 \rightarrow$	2	3	4	5	6	7	8	9	10	11	12	13	14	15
$n_2 \downarrow$														
5				15										
6		10		16	23									
7		10		17	24	32								
8			11	17	25	34	43							
9		6	11	18	26	35	45	56						
10		6	12	19	27	37	47	58	71					
11		6	12	20	28	38	49	61	74	87				
12		7	13	21	30	40	51	63	76	90	106			
13		7	14	22	31	41	53	65	79	93	109	125		
14		7	14	22	32	43	54	67	81	96	112	129	147	
15		8	15	23	33	44	56	70	84	99	115	133	151	171
16		8	15	24	34	46	58	72	86	102	119	137	155	
17		8	16	25	36	47	60	74	89	105	122	140		
18		8	16	26	37	49	62	76	92	108	125			
19	3	9	17	27	38	50	64	78	94	111				
20	3	9	18	28	39	52	66	81	97					
21	3	9	18	29	40	53	68	83						
22	3	10	19	29	42	55	70							
23	3	10	19	30	43	57								
24	3	10	20	31	44									
25	3	11	20	32										
26	3	11	21											
27	4	11												
28	4													

Table uses difference of added up rank numbers between group 1 and group 2

Index

A

Accuracy of diagnostic tests, 509–518,
  545–552, 555–568
Accuracy ROC curves, 516
Advanced analysis of variance (ANOVA),
  607–617
  repeated measurements experiments,
    587–592, 615
  type II ANOVA, random
    effects models, 615
  type III ANOVA, mixed effects models, 615
Adjusted mutual information, 604
AIC (Akaike information criterion), 286
Alpha, type I error, 80, 713
Alternative hypothesis, hypothesis-1, 120
Altman-Bland method or plot, 550
Analysis of covariance (ANCOVA), 402, 591
Analysis of variance (ANOVA), 8, 24, 38, 466
  balanced / unbalanced, 27
  one-way / two-way, 27
  with / without replication, 27
Artificial intelligence, 627–635
  activity and inactivity phases, 628
  artificial neural networks, 627
  back propagation, 627
  best fit outcome, 628
  bootstrapping, 628
  commands on SPSS, 630
  distribution free method, 627
  hidden layers, 629
  iteration, 628
  layers of artificial neurons, 627
  layers of neurons, 627
  multilayer perceptron, 630
  negative weights in matrices, 629
  non linear data, 627
  propagation of signals, 628
  signal-transfers, 628
  SPSS add-on module, 634
  three-layer perceptron model, 628
  transduction of imputed information, 627
  weighted signal transfers from one layer
    to another, 628
Average, 34

B

Bartlett's test, 494
Bavry's program, 409
Bayes' rule, 524
Bayes' theorem, 450
Benefit-risk analyses, 717
Beta, type II error, 77, 679
Between-group variance, 7
Bhattacharya modeling, 301–311
  Bhattacharya Gaussian curves, 303
  delta log values, 302
  first derivative of Gaussian curve, 303
  Food and agricultural organization, 301
  kernel histograms, 301
  quasi-gaussianizing, 301
  subset analysis, 310
  unmasking Gaussian curves, 301
Bias 1, 470
Binary data, 8, 52–53, 317
Binary partitioning, 579–584
  binary digits, 583
  CART (classification
    and regression trees), 579
  classification and regression trees, 579
  cut-off decision trees, 579
  entropy method, 582
  magnitude of impurity, 582
  weighted impurity cut-off, 583

Binomial distribution, 8, 42
Bioavailability, 588
Bioequivalence, 70–71, 489, 492
Bland-Altman plot or method, 566
Bonferroni inequality, 2, 144
Bonferroni t-test, 31
Bootstrap, 332
Box-Cox algorithm, 184

C
Carryover effect, 405, 415
Categorical data, 243–252
    categorical variables, 243
    cohort study, 248
    dummy variables, 251
    multinomial logistic regression, 251
    ordered logistic regression, 251
    process of recoding, 251
Censored data, 54
Central tendency, 489
Chi-square curves left end, 123, 141–142
Chi-square curves right end, 123
Chi-square distribution, 460
Chi-square goodness of fit test, 460
Chi-square Mc Nemar's test, 51
Chi-square test for multiple tables, 46, 490
Cigetivectors, 525
Cluster analysis, 604
Complex functions, 525
Confidence intervals (95%), 6, 41,
        455–467
    of chi-square distributions, 466
    of F distributions, 466
Conflicts of interests, 721–726
CONSORT (Consolidated standards of
        reporting trials), 377, 387
Contingency table, 8
Continuous data, 8
Controlled clinical trials, 721–722
Correlation coefficient (r), 162–168
Correlation matrix, 173
Correlation ratio, 502
Covariate (concomitant variable), 182
Cox regression, Cox proportional hazard
        model, 209–212
Cronbach's alpha, 424, 426
Crossover studies with binary responses,
        407–413
    assessment of carryover and treatment
        effect, 408
    examples, 410–412
    results, 409–410
    statistical model for testing treatment and
        carryover effects, 409

Crossover studies with continuous variables,
        397–405
    hypothesis testing, 399–400
    mathematical model, 398
    statistical power of testing, 400–403
C-statistic vs. logistic regression, 516,
        535–543
    concordance-(c-) statistic, 535–543
    logistic regression for assessing qualitative
        tests, 543
    smooth ROC curves, 540
Cumulative tail probability, 410
Curvilinear regression, 187–196
    Fourier modeling, 195
    methods, statistical models, 188–190
    polynomial modeling, 195
    results, 190–194

D
Data cleaning, 119
    deleting the errors, 119
    maintaining the outliers, 119
Data dispersion, 149–158
    data without measure of dispersion, 150
    overdispersion, 155
Data dredging, 713
Data mining, 451, 604
Data stream clustering, 604
Delta-method, 524, 525
Dependent variable, 174, 178, 205
Dersimonian and Laird model for
        heterogeneity, 373
Diagnostic meta-analyses, 527–533
Diagnostic tests. *See* Qualitative diagnostic
        tests; Quantitative diagnostic tests
Direction coefficient, 209
Discriminant ability, 516
Disease Activity Scale (DAS) of Fuchs, 115
Dose concentration relationships, 495
Dose response relationships, 495
Dunnett method, 107
Duplicate standard deviations, 188, 508
Durbin-Watson test, 184

E
Efficacy data, 15–38
    null-hypothesis testing
        of complex data, 27
    null-hypothesis testing of 3 or more paired
        samples, 21–22
    null hypothesis testing of three or more
        unpaired samples, 21–22
    overview, 15–16

paired data with a negative correlation, 28–33
the principle of testing statistical significance, 16–18
rank testing, 33–35
rank testing for 3 or more samples, 36–38
three methods to test statistically a paired sample, 22–25
unpaired t-test, 19–21
Equiprobable intervals, 470
Equivalence testing, 69–75
    equivalence testing, a new gold standard?, 72–73
    overview of possibilities with equivalence testing, 70–71
    validity of equivalence trials, 73
Ethical issues, 721–726
E-value, 128
Evidence-based medicine, 499
Excel files, 164
Exploratory analyses, 173–174, 363
Exponential regression models, 351
Extreme exclusion criteria, 477

F
False positive / negatives, 535
False positive trials, 103–107
    adjusted p-values, 105–106
    Bonferroni tests, 103–106
    composite endpoint procedures, 106
    least significant difference test, 105
    pragmatic solutions, 107
F-distribution, 464–467
Fisher-exact test, 61
Fixed effect model for heterogeneity, 374, 384
Flipping a coin, 152
Food and Drug Administration (FDA), 722
Fourier analysis, 187
Frailty, 363
Friedman test, 36–37
F test, 348. *See also* Analysis of variance (ANOVA)
Funnel plot, 371
Fuzzy logic, 639–649
    dose-response effects, 640–644
    fuzzy memberships, 641
    fuzzy methodologies, 648
    fuzzy modeling, 648
    fuzzy plots, 640
    fuzzy statistics, 647
    fuzzy truths, 639
    linguistic membership names, 641
    linguistic rules, 640

time-response effects, 644–647
triangular fuzzy sets, 640
universal space, 640

G
Gaussian curve, 4
Genetic data, 445–452
    data mining, 447–448
    genetics, 447–448
    genomics, 448–452
    proteonomics, 447–448
    terminology, 446–447
Ghost, guest and graphter writers, 721–726
Good clinical practice criteria, 721–726
Goodness of fit, 195, 471–472
Grizzle model for assessment of crossover, 405

H
Haplotype, 446
Harvard Graphics, 190
Hawthorne effect, 718
Hazard ratio, 210–212
Helsinki Declaration, 721–726
Heterogeneity, 372–376, 384–385
Heteroscedasticity, 165
Hierarchical cluster analysis, 447–448
Hierarchical liner model, 604
High quality criteria for studies, 376
Histogram, 4
Hochberg´s procedure, 106
Homogeneity, 369–377, 381
Homoscedasticity, 176, 179
Honestly significant difference (HSD), 106
Hosmer-Lemeshow test, 184
Hotelling's T-square, 116
Hung's model, 135
Hypothesis, data, stratification, 1–14
    different types of data: continuous data, 3–8
    different types of data: correlation coefficient, 10–12
    different types of data: proportions, percentages and contingency table, 8–10
    factorial designs, 13–14
    general considerations, 1–2
    randomized *versus* historical controls, 13
    stratification issues, 12–13
    two main hypotheses in drug trials: efficacy and safety, 2–3
Hypothesis-driven data analysis, 452

I

ICC. *See* Intraclass correlation
Incidence analysis and scientific method,
    659–663
  chi-square test, 660
  CIA (Critical incident analysis), 659
  CIT (Critical incident technique), 659
  95 % confidence intervals, 661
  log likelihood ratio test, 661
  PRISMA (Prevention and recovery system
    for monitoring and analysis), 659
  TRIPOD (method based
    on tripod theory), 659
  z-test, 660
Independent review board, 723
Independent variable, 175, 179, 208
Indicator variable, 178
Inferiority testing, 91–93
Intention to treat analysis, 73
Interaction, 337–351
  analysis of variance, 341–342
  definitions, 337
  incorrect methods for testing, 339–340
  regression modeling, 343–345
  t-tests, 339
Interaction effects, 337–351
Interaction terms, 337–351
Interim analyses, 95–101
  continuous sequential statistical
    techniques, 99–101
  group-sequential design of interim
    analysis, 99
  interim analysis, 96–99
  monitoring, 95–96
Intraclass correlation coefficient,
    503, 568
Intraclass correlations, 503, 568.
    See also Cronbach's alpha
I^2 statistic, 385
Item response modeling, 433–442
  BILOG-MG software, 434
  ceiling effects, 433
  clinical and laboratory testing,
    438–439
  computer assisted adaptive testing, 433
  Egret software, 434
  expected ability a posteriori (EAP), 437
  latent trait analysis (LTA)-2, 435
  LTA software, 434
  MULTILOG software, 434
  OPLM software, 434
  quality of life assessment, 435–438
  Rasch models, 433
  RSP software, 434

K

Kaplan Meier curves, 55–56,
    210–211
Kappa, 502–503, 567
Katz´s method, 9
Kendall Tau test, 365–378, 551
Kernel regression, 690
Kolmogorov-Smirnov test, 471–472
Kruskall-Wallis test, 37–38

L

Laplace transformations, 213–215
Latent class analysis, 604
Least significance difference (LSD) procedure,
    105, 109–116
Levene's test, 494
Left and χ^2 table, 123, 134
Likelihood ratio, 61–68, 183, 446
Linear regression principles, 161–185,
    199–203
  another real data example of multiple
    linear regression, 173–174
  more on paired observations,
    162–164
  multiple linear regression, 166–168
  multiple variables analyses, 176
  multivariate analyses, 176
  univariate analyses, 176
  using statistical software for simple linear
    regression, 164–166
Logarithmic transformation, log-transformed
    ratios, 12, 59–60
Logistic regression, 199–218, 227–231
  pseudo-R2 measures, 207
  R2-like measures, 207
Log likelihood ratio tests, 61–68
  normal approximations, 62–64
  numerical problems, 61–62
  quadratic approximation, 64–66
Log rank test, 56

M

Mann-Whitney test, 15, 34, 35, 37
Mantel-Haenszl summary, chi-square test,
    55–56
Markov models, 212–213
Markov predictors, 153–154
McNemar's odds ratio, 59
McNemar's test, 51–53
Mean, 3
Measure of concordance, 516
Median absolute deviation (MAD), 490

Medline database, 368
Mendelian experiment, 133
Meta-analysis, 365–388
    clearly defined hypotheses, 367–368
    discussion, where are we now?, 377–378
    examples, 366–367
    new developments, 386–388
    pitfalls, 383–386
    scientific framework, 381–383
    strict inclusion criteria, 368
    thorough search of trials, 368
    uniform data analysis, 369–377
Meta-analysis of diagnostic tests, 527–533
Meta-analysis of regression data, 391–396
Meta-regression, 391–396
    heterogeneous meta-analyses, 391–394
    multiple linear meta-regression, 394
Microarrays, 449, 451
Microarrays, normalized ratios of, 450
Minimization, 12–13
Missing data, 253–265
    closest neighbour observed, 253, 254
    hot deck imputation, 257
    imputation of missing data, 254
    LOCF (last observation
        carried forward), 259
    means imputated, 261
    module Missing Value Analysis
        SPSS, 258
    multiple imputations, 261–265
    regression-substitution, 254–255
Mixed effects models, 607–615
Mixed linear models for repeated measures,
    593–604
    build nested terms, 596, 601
    mixed models, 593, 599–604
Mixture model, 450
Monte Carlo methods
    analyzing continuous data, 621–622
    analyzing proportional data, 622–623
    principles, 620
Multicenter research, 723
Multicollinearity, 173, 176
Multidimensional scaling, 604
Multiple linear regression, 173–174, 176
Multiple r, multiple r-square, 169–171
Multiple statistical inferences, 109–116
    multiple comparisons, 109–113
    multiple variables, 113–116
Multiple variables analysis, 175–176
Multistage regression, 233–241
    decomposition of correlation, 239
    linear regression modeling, 234
    multistage least squares method, 237–238

multistep regression, 240
    path analysis, 234–236, 238–239
    path statistic, 241
    problematic variable, 237–239
    2SLS (two stage least squares), 237
    standardized regression coefficient, 236
    two-path statistic, 236
Multivariate analysis, 176, 289–298
    inflated type I error, 289
    MANOVA (multiple analysis of variance),
        289–298
    multiple outcome variables, 289
    multivariate logistic regression, 298
    multivariate probit regression, 296–297
    path analysis, 290–291
    probit regression modeling, 289
    STATA Software, 296, 297
Multivariate analysis of variance (MANOVA),
    176, 289–298

N
Nearest neighbor search, 604
Negative correlation, 28
Newman Keuls. *See* Student-Newman-Keuls
    method
Non-inferiority testing, 91–93
Non linear relationships, splines, 277–287
    ACE (alternating conditional expectations)
        package, 280–281
    Akaike information criterion (AIC), 286
    AVAS (additive and variance stabilization
        for regression) package, 280–281
    box Cox transformation, 280–281
    cubic regression, 283–285
    curvilinear data, 281–282
    generalized additive models, 283
    generalized linear methods, 279
    guesstimates, 277
    iterations, 277
    kernel frequency distributions, 285
    lambda calculus, 283
    LOESS (locally weighted scatter plot
        smoothing, 285
    logit transformation, 278–281
    low order polynomial regression, 283
    mathematical spline methods, 277
    mechanical spline method, 277
    Michaelis-Menten relationship, 279
    probit transformation, 278–281
    smooth shapes, 277
    spline modeling, 282–285
    subsequent knots, 283
    trial and error method, 280–281

Non-mem (nonlinear mixed effects regression models), 214
Non-normal data, 479–481
Non-parametric tests, 33–35
Normal distribution, 5, 456–458
Normalized ratio, 450
Normal test, 59
Null-hypotheses, 5
Numbers needed to treat (NNTs), 150–151

O

Observational data, 60
Odds, 8
Odds of responding, 207
Odds ratio (OR), 8, 55–59, 366, 367
One-way ANOVA, 27
Optimism corrected c-statistic, 516
Ordinal data, 113, 373
Overall accuracy, 509, 517
Overdispersion, 155–157

P

Paired Wilcoxon test, 34–35
Parabolas, 525
Partial regression coefficients, 169
Peak trough relationships, 495
Pearson's correlation coefficient, 172
Peer-review system, 377
Phase I-IV trials, 1
Pocock criterium for stopping a trial, 97–99
Point estimates or estimators, 370
Poisson distribution, 8, 41
Poisson regression, 267–274
    events per time unit, 267
    generalized linear models, 271, 273
Polynomial analysis, 187–196
Pooled standard error, 20
Pooling data, 365–378
Posterior odds, 446–448
Post-hoc analysis in clinical trials, 227–231
    examples, 228–230
    logistic regression analysis, 227, 229
    logistic regression equation, 230–231
    multiple variables methods, 227
Power computations, 80–86
    for continuous data, 80
    for equivalence testing, 81
    for proportions, 80–81
    using the t-table, 81–86
Power curves, 401

Power indexes, 87–91
Precision, 555, 558
Primary variables, 182
Prior odds, 446–448
Probability, 8
Probability density, 5, 7
Probability distribution, 4, 77
Product-limit, 54
Propensity score matching, 329–336
    calculation of propensity scores, 329–330
    Caliper matching, 332
    kernel matching, 332
    Mahalanobis metric matching, 332
    nearest neighbor watching, 332
    observational data, 329
    propensity scores, 329
    propensity scores for adjusting, 331–332
    propensity scores for matching, 332–333
    stratification matching, 332
    subclassification, 329
Proportion, 8
Proportion of variance, 501–502
Pseudo-R2 measures, 207, 550
Publication bias, 371–372, 377–378
Pubmed, 233
P-values, 111–130
    < 0.0001, 124–126
    > 0.95, 123–124
    common misunderstandings, 122
    interpretation, 120–121
    tables for high p-values, 141–144

Q

Quadratic approximation, 525
Qualitative diagnostic tests, 509–518
    bivariate model, 296–297
    Cohen's kappas, 502–503, 557, 567
    confidence intervals, 519–525
    c-statistic, 516, 535–543
    delta method, 524–525
    diagnostic odds ratios, 528–531
    kappas, 502–503, 557, 567
    meta-analyses, 527–533
    optimism corrected c-statistic, 516, 535–343
    overall accuracy, 509–511
    perfect and imperfect tests, 511–513
    ROC curves, 515–516, 531
    sensitivity, 509, 527

specificity, 509, 527
S statistic, 529
standard errors, 519–525
STARD statement, 558
summary ROC curves, 531–532, 557, 564–565
threshold for positive tests, 513–516
uncertainty, 519–525
validation, 509–518
Quality-of-life (QOL) assessment in clinical trials, 423–431
defining QOL in a subjective or objective way, 425
lack of sensitivity of QOL-assessments, 426–427
odds ratio analysis of effects of patient characteristics on QOL data provides increased precision, 427–429
patients' opinion is an important independent-contributor to QOL, 425–426
some terminology, 423–425
Quantitative diagnostic tests, 545–552
Altman-Bland plots, 550–552
Barnett's tests, 567
confidence intervals, 547–548
Deming regression, 550–552
duplicate standard deviations, 500, 561, 567
intraclass correlation vs. duplicate test, 505, 567
intraclass correlation vs. gold test, 567
Kendall rank correlation, 551
least squares, 549
linear regression correct method, 555, 561
linear regression incorrect method, 555, 559–562
paired t-tests, 550–551
Passing Bablok regression, 551, 552
repeatability coefficients, 503, 508, 561–562, 567
squared correlation coefficients, 548–550

R
Randbetween, 484
Random effect model for heterogeneity, 373–374
Randomization, 469
Randomization assumption, 469
Randomness, 469–485
non-normal data, 479–481

testing, 469–478
testing normality, 481
what in case of non-normality, 482–483
Randomness error. *See* Systematic error
Randomness of survival data test, 472–473
Random sampling, 119, 469
Rasch item response models, 207
Receiver operating characteristic (ROC) curves, 515, 517, 527–528, 560–561, 580–582
Regression analysis, 161–176
Regression coefficient (b), 162, 163
Regression line, 11, 12, 187
Regression plane, 168, 171–172
Regression sum of squares, 25
Relationship among statistical distributions, 455–467
chi-square can be used for multiple samples of data, 462–465
examples of data where variance is more important than mean, 462
normal distribution, 456–458
null-hypothesis testing with the chi-square distribution, 459–461
null-hypothesis testing with the normal or the t-distribution, 458–459
relationship between the normal distribution and chi-square distribution, 459–461
variances, 456
Relative risks, 370–371
Reliability (= reproducibility), 151–152
Repeated measurements ANOVA, 26–27
Representative samples, 5
Reproducibility assessments, 499–508
incorrect methods, 503–504
qualitative data, 502–503
quantitative data, 151, 500–502
Required sample size, 86–93
for continuous data, 88–89
for equivalence testing, 90–91
for proportional data, 89–90
Residual variation, 26, 178, 184
Risk, 8
Ritchie joint pain score, 115
R2-like statistic, 207, 550
Robustness (sensitivity) of data, 386
ROC curves. *See* Receiver operating characteristic (ROC) curves
R-square, 164, 170

S

Safety data, 41–60
    chi-square to analyze more than two
        unpaired proportions, 48–51
    four methods to analyze two unpaired
        proportions, 42–48
    McNemar's test for paired proportions, 51
    survival analysis, 54–56
Safety factor, 715, 716
SAS Statistical Software, 111, 713
Scatter plot, 180
Scientific method in everyday practice,
    654–655
Scientific rigor, 721–726
SD (standard deviation) of a proportion, 9
Second derivatives, 525
Second order polynomes, 525
Secondary variables, 114
SEM (standard error) of a proportion, 9
Sensitivity (robustness) of data, 556–558
Shapiro Wilks' test, 484
Skewed data, 10, 11
Spearman rank correlation test, 176
Specificity, 509–518
Spread in the data, 509
SPSS Statistical Software, 111, 164, 713
Standard deviation, 4
Standard error of the mean, 5
STARD (Standards of Reporting of Diagnostic
    Accuracy), 149, 157
STARD statement, 528–531, 558
Statistical analysis of genetic data, 445–452
    genetics, genomics, proteonomics data
        mining, 447–448
    genomics, 448–452
    some terminology, 446–447
Statistical power and sample size
        requirements, 77–93
    calculation of required sample size,
        rationale, 86–87
    calculations of required sample sizes,
        methods, 87–91
    emphasis on statistical power rather than
        null-hypothesis testing, 78–80
    power computations, 80–81
    testing not only superiority but also
        inferiority of a new treatment
        (type III error), 91–93
    what is statistical power, 77–78
Statistical principles can help to improve the
    quality of the trial, 714
Statistics can help the clinician to better
    limitations of statistics, 714
    understand limitations and benefits of
        current research, 717

Statistics can provide worthwhile extras to
    your research, 714–715
Statistics can turn art into science, 716
Statistics for support
    rather than illumination?, 716
Statistics is fun because it proves your
    hypothesis was right, 713–714
Statistics is no "bloodless" algebra,
    713–718
Statistics is not like algebra bloodless, 715
Stepwise multiple regression analysis, 172
Stopping rules, 99
Studentized statistic, 112
Student-Newman-Keuls method,
    106, 107, 111
Student t-test, 18–21
Structural data analysis, 604
Subgroup analysis using multiple linear
        regression: confounding, interaction,
        and synergism, 177–185
    confounding, 181–182
    estimation, and hypothesis testing, 183
    example, 178
    goodness-of-fit, 183–185
    increased precision of efficacy,
        180–181
    interaction and synergism, 182–183
    model, 178–180
    selection procedures, 185
Sum of products, 165, 403
Sum of squares, 7
Superiority testing, 665–672
    clinical superiority, 667–669
    graphs for assessments, 667
    studies not meeting endpoints, 666
Supervised data analysis, 451
Surrogate endpoints, 569–578
    confidence intervals, 572–574
    prespecified boundary of validity, 570
    regression modeling, 574–576
    require sample size, 571–572
    surrogate markers, 572–574
    validation, 574–576
Surrogate risk ratios, 8
Synergism, 182–183
Systematic error, 345

T

Tables, 729–734
    chi-squared distribution, 730
    F-distribution, 731–732
    Mann-Whitney test, 733–734
    t-table, 729–730
    Wilcoxon rank sum test, 733

T-distribution, 7
Test statistic, 16
Therapeutic index, 364
Time-dependent factor analysis,
    353–364
  changing lifestyles, 353
  Cox regression without time-dependent
    predictors, 354–356
  Cox regression with segmented time-
    dependent predictors, 359–362
  Cox regression with time-dependent
    predictors, 356–359
  Multiple Cox regression with segmented
    time-dependent predictors, 362–363
  predictors changing across time, 353
Time effect, 400
Time series, 687–692
  AR (autoregressive) models, 691
  autocorrelation, 688
  autoregressive moving
    averages (ARMA), 687
  change points in time, 689–690
  convolution filters, 690
  correlations with other events in time, 688
  correlogram, 688
  critical F-value, 690
  cross correlation, 688–689
  cyclic patterns, 687
  Discrete Wavelet Transformation, 691
  exponential filters, 690
  father wavelet, 691
  kernel regression, 690
  MA (moving averages) models, 691
  mother wavelet, 691
  moving the F-value, 690
  recursive filters, 690
  serial correlation, 692
  simpler methods of smoothing, 690
  splines, 690
  trend analysis, 687
  wavelet analysis, 687
  wavelet theory, 691
  wild patterns in the data, 687
Treatment by period
  interaction, 337–351, 397
Trend testing, 313–318
  chi-square test for trends, 314–315
  linear regression for trends, 315–316
Trial monitors, 721–726
Triangular test, 100
True positives / negatives, 512

Tukey's honestly significant difference (HSD)
    method, 106, 107, 111
Type I error, 77, 96, 98
Type II error, 77, 79
Type III error, 91–93

U
Univariate analysis, 176
Unpaired ANOVA, 22
Unpaired data, 6, 11
Unpaired t-test, 19–21
Unpublished paper amnesty movement,
    366, 377
Unrandomness, 470
Unsupervised data analysis, 451

V
Validation diagnostic tests, 509–518, 545–552,
    555–568
Validity, 1, 509
Validity criteria, 721–726
Variability analysis, 487–496
  index for variability, 489–490
  one sample, 490–492
  three or more samples,
    493–494
  two samples, 492–493
Variables, 2
  dependent/independent, 2, 162–163, 178,
    204–205
  exposure/outcome, 2
  indicator/outcome, 2, 178
Variance, 3, 183–184

W
Wald statistic, 183
Whitehead's arguments, 100, 101
White's test, 165
Wilcoxon rank sum test, 34–36
Wilcoxon signed rank test, 34–36
Within-group variance, 7

Z
Z-axis, 77
Z-distribution, 9
Z-test for binomial or binary data, 43,
    460–461

Printed by Publishers' Graphics LLC
MO20120524